Medical and Health Genomics: Latest Findings

Medical and Health Genomics: Latest Findings

Edited by Victor Fargo

hayle
medical

New York

Hayle Medical,
750 Third Avenue, 9th Floor,
New York, NY 10017, USA

Visit us on the World Wide Web at:
www.haylemedical.com

ISBN: 978-1-63241-651-3

Cataloging-in-Publication Data

Medical and health genomics: latest findings / edited by Victor Fargo.
p. cm.
Includes bibliographical references and index.
ISBN 978-1-63241-651-3
1. Genomics. 2. Medical genetics. 3. Health--Genetic aspects. 4. Human genetics.
5. Genetic disorders. I. Fargo, Victor.
RB155 .M43 2019
616.042--dc23

Contents

Preface

Every book is initially just a concept; it takes months of research and hard work to give it the final shape in which the readers receive it. In its early stages, this book also went through rigorous reviewing. The notable contributions made by experts from across the globe were first molded into patterned chapters and then arranged in a sensibly sequential manner to bring out the best results.

Genomics is an interdisciplinary field of science, which is concerned with the structure, function, mapping, evolution and editing of genomes. It has numerous applications in the field of medicine. Genomic data of large populations when combined with modern informatics for disease research, can provide comprehensive insights into the genetic bases of disease and drug response. Medical genomics is increasingly becoming relevant in the understanding of common diseases. A patient with a suspected genetic disease undergoes a diagnostic evaluation that is tailored to account for the signs and symptoms presented, in order to establish a differential diagnosis. This is done for inborn errors of metabolism, chromosomal disorders and single gene disorders. Genetic syndromes arise due to alterations of chromosomes or genes. This book provides comprehensive insights into the field of medical and health genomics. It consists of contributions made by international experts. In this book, using case studies and examples, constant effort has been made to make the understanding of the difficult concepts of medical genomics as easy and informative as possible, for the readers.

It has been my immense pleasure to be a part of this project and to contribute my years of learning in such a meaningful form. I would like to take this opportunity to thank all the people who have been associated with the completion of this book at any step.

Editor

Integrative analyses of genes and microRNA expressions in human trisomy 21 placentas

Ji Hyae Lim[1,2], You Jung Han[3], Hyun Jin Kim[1], Moon Young Kim[3], So Yeon Park[1], Youl-Hee Cho[2*] and Hyun Mee Ryu[1,3*] (iD)

Abstract

Background: The most frequent chromosomal aneuploidy is trisomy 21 (T21) that is caused by an extra copy of chromosome 21. The imbalance of whole genome including genes and microRNAs contributes to the various phenotypes of T21. However, the integrative association between genes and microRNAs in the T21 placenta has yet to be determined.

Methods: We analyzed the expressions of genes and microRNAs in the whole genomes of chorionic villi cells from normal and T21 human fetal placentas based on our prior studies. The functional significances and interactions of the genes and microRNAs were predicted using bioinformatics tools.

Results: Among 110 genes and 34 microRNAs showing significantly differential expression between the T21 and normal placentas, the expression levels of 17 genes were negatively correlated with those of eight microRNAs in the T21 group. Of these 17 genes, 10 with decreased expression were targeted by five up-regulated microRNAs, whereas seven genes with increased expression were targeted by three down-regulated microRNAs. These genes were significantly associated with hydrogen peroxide-mediated programmed cell death, cell chemotaxis, and protein self-association. They were also associated with T21 and its accompanying abnormalities. The constructed interactive signaling network showed that seven genes (three increased and four decreased expressions) were essential components of a dynamic signaling complex ($P = 7.77e\text{-}16$).

Conclusions: In this study, we have described the interplay of genes and microRNAs in the T21 placentas and their modulation in biological pathways related to T21 pathogenesis. These results may therefore contribute to further research about the interaction of genes and microRNAs in disease pathogenesis.

Keywords: Gene expression, MicroRNA, Placenta, Trisomy 21, Whole genome

Background

Trisomy 21 (T21) is the most frequent chromosome aneuploidy affecting 1 in 700 live births [1]. Individuals with T21 have an increased risk of various congenital abnormalities, including eye, cardiac, gastrointestinal, renal and urinary tract defects [2]. These defects are generally considered to originate from gene dosage imbalance between the trisomic genes on chromosome 21 and the

disomic genes on other chromosomes. Therefore, studies of T21 have focused mainly on expression levels of the chromosome 21-derived genome in various tissues from subjects with the condition [3–5]. However, the severity and incidence of those phenotypic abnormalities are variable within the T21 population, possibly due to the genetic and epigenetic backgrounds of each individual.

MicroRNAs (miRNAs) are small (18~ 25-nucleotide-long) non-coding endogenous RNAs. They regulate expression of genes at the post-transcriptional level by regulating mRNA stability and translation [6–9]. More than 1000 miRNAs are expected to participate in regulating over 60% of all the genes [10, 11]. Hence, miRNAs

* Correspondence: yhcho@hanyang.ac.kr; hmryu@yahoo.com
[2]Department of Medical Genetics, College of Medicine, Hanyang University, 222, Wangsimni-ro, Seongdong-gu, Seoul 04763, South Korea
[1]Laboratory of Medical Genetics, Medical Research Institute, Cheil General Hospital and Women's Healthcare Center, Seoul, South Korea
Full list of author information is available at the end of the article

seem to be involved in almost all cellular processes, such as cell apoptosis, differentiation, development, and proliferation [12, 13]. Moreover, changes in their expression levels are reported in various human diseases such as cancer, cardiovascular disease, mental retardation, fetal growth restriction, Alzheimer's disease, and T21 [14–19]. For this reason, great attentions are currently devoted to miRNA research.

In our previous studies, we profiled expression levels of genome-wide miRNAs and genes in placental samples from normal and T21 fetuses using microarray analyses [20, 21]. Our results demonstrated that 34 miRNAs (16 up-regulated and 18 down-regulated) and 110 genes (77 up-regulated and 33 down-regulated) were significantly differentially expressed in the T21 placenta compared with that in normal placentas. Moreover, these miRNAs targeted 76 genes on chromosome 21, suggesting a relationship between genetic and epigenetic changes in the placentas of fetuses with T21. However, the association between genes and miRNA expressions in the whole genome has not yet been determined in the T21 placenta, and the functional significances of these genetic and epigenetic interactions are also unclear. Therefore, an integrative investigation of human genes and miRNAs in the whole genome might be important in understanding the complex genetic-epigenetic mechanisms involved in the pathogenesis of T21 associated abnormalities.

The miRNAs and genes differentially expressed between the placentas of normal and T21 fetuses were found in our previous data [20, 21], and in this study we could identify genes showing a negative correlation with miRNAs, and explored the biological function and molecular pathways of the identified genes using various bioinformatics tools.

Methods

Study subjects

The placenta cells were collected by the chorionic villi sampling (CVS) from first-trimester pregnant women. The written informed consents were obtained from participants in compliance with the Declaration of Helsinki. The institutional review board approval was received from the Ethics Committee at Cheil General Hospital (#CGH-IRB-2011-85). The fetal karyotype was analyzed by standard protocols using the Giemsa banding procedure. All trisomy samples used in this study were completely T21, and all normal samples were completely euploid.

Expression profiling of genome-wide whole genes and miRNAs

Expression of genes and miRNAs in the whole genomes was analyzed based on our previous studies [20, 21]. In brief, total RNA was extracted from normal and T21 fetal placentas. An RNA quantity, quality, and integrity

number were measured by an Agilent 2100 Bioanalyzer (Agilent Technologies, CA, USA) and a NanoVue Plus spectrophotometer (GE Healthcare, London, UK). Expression profiles of whole genes were determined using the Affymetrix GeneChip Human Genome U133 Plus 2. 0 Array (Affymetrix Inc., Santa Clara, CA, USA) [21]. The miRNAs expressions were profiled using Human miRNA Microarray kit, 8 × 60 K (based on miRBase release 16.0, Agilent Technologies) [20]. Differences in expressions of genes and miRNAs between the T21 and normal groups were considered significant at a P-value of < 0.05. The Benjamini–Hochberg procedure was used to set the false discovery rate (FDR) at 0.05 [22].

Functional annotation of the candidate genes

All target genes of the 34 miRNAs differentially expressed in T21 were compared with 110 genes differentially expressed in T21 using the VENNY tool (http://bioinfogp.cnb.csic.es/tools/venny_old/index.html). The genes showing a negative correlation with miRNAs in terms of expression were selected as candidates for functional annotation. The web-based gene set analysis toolkit (http://www.webgestalt.org/webgestalt_2013) was used for gene ontology (GO) analysis, Kyoto encyclopedia of genes and genomes (KEGG) pathway analysis, and disease-associated analysis. The Search Tool for the Retrieval of Interacting Genes database (STRING; http://version10.string-db.org/) is a database to retrieve and display protein-protein interactions, including both physical and functional interactions. STRING was used to analyze an interaction of candidate genes.

Statistical analyses

The clinical characteristics were analyzed by the Mann-Whitney U-test and χ^2-test. In all tests, a value of $P < 0.05$ was considered statistically significant (SPSS Inc., Chicago, IL, USA).

Results

Study subjects were constructed with 10 women with euploid fetuses and seven women with T21 fetuses. The CVS from five euploid and three T21 placentas were used for expression profiling of genome-wide whole genes [20], and those from the other five euploid and four T21 placentas were used for miRNA expression analysis [21]. Table 1 shows the clinical characteristics of the subjects. At the time of CVS, there were no significant differences between the two groups with regard to maternal and fetal characteristics ($P > 0.05$ for all).

Based on our previous studies, we had analyzed the expression levels of over 47,000 genes and 1349 miRNAs in the whole human genome. Thirty-four miRNAs were differentially expressed (16 up-regulated and 18 down-regulated) in the T21 placentas relative to that in the

Table 1 Clinical characteristics of the study population

Characteristics	mRNA profiling			microRNA profiling			Total subjects		
	Trisomy 21 ($n=3$)	Normal ($n=5$)	P value	Trisomy 21 ($n=4$)	Normal ($n=5$)	P value	Trisomy 21 ($n=7$)	Normal ($n=10$)	P value
Maternal Age (years)	34.6 ± 3.8	37.4 ± 3.9	0.853	30.3 ± 2.2	34.2 ± 3.1	0.628	32.1 ± 3.6	35.8 ± 3.7	0.062
Gestational age (weeks)	12.0 ± 0.0	12.2 ± 0.4	0.092	12.2 ± 0.4	12.4 ± 0.7	0.071	12.1 ± 0.4	12.3 ± 0.6	0.454
Body mass index (kg/m^2)	22.3 ± 3.7	24.4 ± 6.2	0.545	21.8 ± 3.3	21.5 ± 1.2.2	0.874	22.0 ± 3.2	22.9 ± 4.7	0.659
Gravidity	2.7 ± 1.2	2.8 ± 0.8	0.446	1.8 ± 1.0	3.0 ± 1.6	0.210	2.1 ± 1.1	2.9 ± 1.2	0.201
Nuchal translucency (mm)	3.7 ± 1.4	4.9 ± 1.9	0.402	4.2 ± 0.8	3.3 ± 1.5	0.377	4.0 ± 1.0	4.1 ± 1.8	0.862
Nullipara	2	1	0.146	2	1	0.524	4	2	0.162
Gender-ratio (female:male)	1:2	1:4	1.000	1:3	1:4	1.000	2:5	2:8	1.000

normal placentas. The number of predicted target genes of the up-regulated and down-regulated miRNAs was 7421 and 6058, respectively (Fig. 1). The 110 genes showing significant differential expression between the T21 and normal placentas were identified, of which 77 genes were up-regulated and 33 genes were down-regulated in the T21 group. The 110 genes and 34 miR-NAs were selected for the analysis of genetic-epigenetic association in the T21 placenta. In the analysis of the miRNA-gene associations, 17 genes showed a negative correlation with eight miRNAs in terms of expression (Fig. 1 and Table 2). These 17 genes were selected as candidate genes for the functional annotation.

In the *in-silico* analysis using the 17 candidate genes, GO annotation and disease association analyses were performed by a statistical hypergeometric test (Table 3). In the "biological process" category of GO annotation, the candidate genes, *HGF* and *MAP3K5*, were significantly associated with hydrogen peroxide-mediated programmed cell death (adj*P* = 0.0008). The *F2RL1*, *HGF*, and *JAM3* genes were associated with cell chemotaxis (adj*P* = 0. 0435). Protein self-association (adj*P* = 0.0172) in the molecular function category of GO annotation was significantly associated with genes, *AGA* and *DYRK1A*. However, none of the candidate genes were associated with the "cellular component" category of GO annotation. The disease associations of the candidate genes are shown in Table 4. The most statistically significant association with candidate genes, *AGA*, *DYRK1A*, *SETD4*, and *TTC3*, was found in mental retardation (adj*P* = 0.0014). Besides this, the candidate genes were also significantly associated with T21, neurobehavioral manifestations, chromosome disorders, osteoarthritis, and fibrosis (adj*P* < 0.05 for all).

An interaction of the candidate genes was predicted by STRING tool (Fig. 2). The list of the identified candidate genes was used to reveal their functional interactions. Each node represents a protein, and each edge represents an interaction. Thicker lines represent stronger associations. On the basis of 17 genes showing a negative correlation with miRNAs, the part of the dynamic signaling complex in

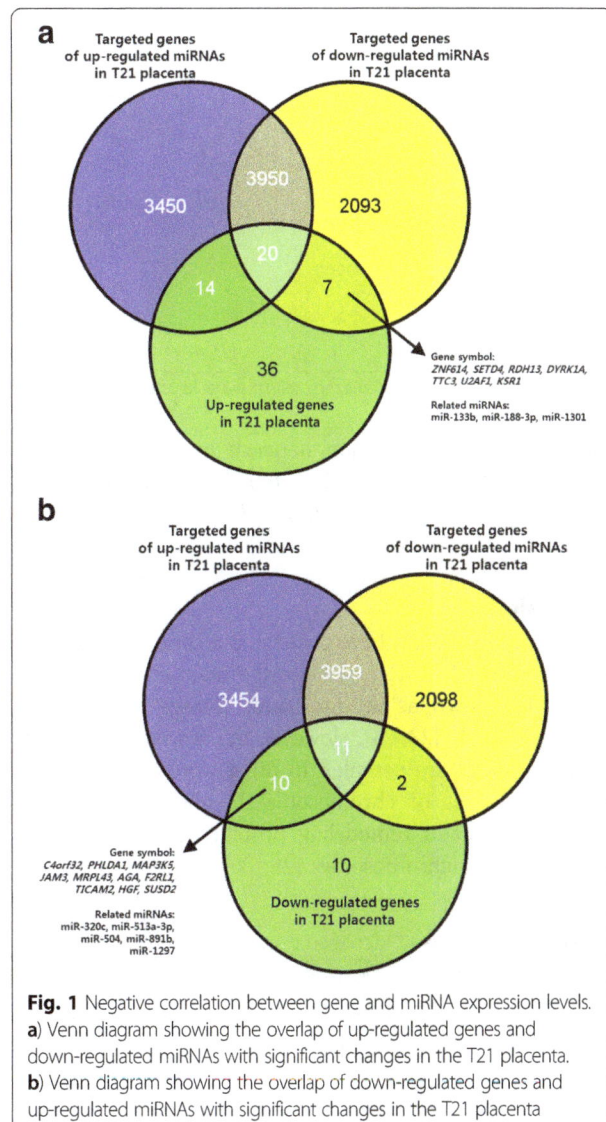

Fig. 1 Negative correlation between gene and miRNA expression levels. **a)** Venn diagram showing the overlap of up-regulated genes and down-regulated miRNAs with significant changes in the T21 placenta. **b)** Venn diagram showing the overlap of down-regulated genes and up-regulated miRNAs with significant changes in the T21 placenta

Table 2 Expression changes of microRNA and genes showing negative correlation in the T21 placenta

Expression pattern of mRNAs in the T21 placenta	Gene Symbol	Fold intensity	P value	FDR	Chr	microRNAs showing negative correlation				
						mir	Fold intensity	P value	FDR	Chr
Up-regulation	DYRK1A	1.530	0.013	0.008	21	mir-188-3p	4.301	0.004	0.007	X
	KSR1	1.805	0.013	0.006	17	mir-1301	6.571	0.016	0.046	2
	RDH13	1.634	0.016	0.018	19	mir-188-3p	4.301	0.004	0.007	X
	SETD4	1.696	0.007	0.009	21	mir-1301	6.571	0.016	0.046	2
	TTC3	1.678	0.037	0.045	21	mir-133b	5.470	0.001	0.001	6
	U2AF1	1.856	0.007	0.025	21	mir-133b	5.470	0.001	0.001	6
	ZNF614	1.615	0.043	0.040	19	mir-188-3p	4.301	0.004	0.007	X
Down-regulation	AGA	1.520	0.005	0.002	4	mir-513a-3p	4.192	0.013	0.040	X
	C4orf32	1.798	0.017	0.015	4	mir-504,	3.848	0.006	0.012	X
						mir-513a-3p	4.192	0.013	0.040	X
						mir-891b	4.407	0.014	0.041	X
	F2RL1	1.846	0.006	0.004	5	mir-513a-3p	4.192	0.013	0.040	X
						mir-1297	8.045	0.012	0.036	13
	HGF	2.404	0.020	0.014	7	mir-1297	8.045	0.012	0.036	13
	JAM3	1.885	0.032	0.013	11	mir-320c	2.558	0.002	0.002	18
	MAP3K5	1.617	0.033	0.029	6	mir-513a-3p	4.192	0.013	0.040	X
						mir-891b	4.407	0.014	0.041	X
	MRPL43	2.611	0.020	0.016	10	mir-504	3.848	0.006	0.012	X
	PHLDA1	1.905	0.027	0.010	12	mir-513a-3p	4.192	0.013	0.040	X
						mir-891b	4.407	0.014	0.041	X
						mir-1297	8.045	0.012	0.036	13
	SUSD2	2.324	0.024	0.008	22	mir-1297	8.045	0.012	0.036	13
	TICAM2	1.604	0.043	0.033	5	mir-891b	4.407	0.014	0.041	X

rawP: p value from hypergeometric test, adjP: p value adjusted by the multiple test adjustment

the constructed interaction network included three up-regulated (*U2AF1*, *DYRK1A*, and *KSR1*) and four down-regulated genes (*MRPL43*, *F2RL1*, *TICAM2*, and *MAP3K5*) (Fig. 2C).

Discussion

To date, most studies have confirmed a gene dose effect of chromosome 21 in T21, because the main etiology of T21 has been known as an imbalance dosage of genes on chromosome 21 [23, 24]. However, the downstream consequences of T21 are complex. In other words, gene expression imbalances of chromosome 21 affect transcription factors, chromatin remodeling proteins, or related molecules on other chromosomes [25, 26]. These suggest that

genomic dosage changes of chromosome 21 in T21 could be relatively subtle or massively disruptive to various genes on other chromosomes. Therefore, as well as primary gene dosage effects in pathogenesis T21, secondary (downstream) effects of disomic genes on other chromosomes are also likely to have a major role in T21. In gene expression process of the human genome, the miRNAs affect as key regulators. They induce mRNA degradation of target genes by perfect binding to target mRNAs or inhibit their translation by imperfect complementary binding to the 3′ untranslated region [27, 28]. Moreover, these miRNAs are involved in the occurrence and development of various diseases [14–19]. Therefore, understanding the whole genomic changes that contribute to the various phenotypes of T21 is

Table 3 GO analysis of identified genes

	Pathway	GeneSymbol	rawP	adjP
BP	Hydrogen peroxide-mediated programmed cell death	HGF, MAP3K5	0.000002	0.0008
	Cell chemotaxis	F2RL1, HGF, JAM3	0.0003	0.0435
MF	Protein self-association	AGA, DYRK1A	0.0004	0.0172

BP Biological process, *MF* Molecular function, *GO* gene ontology, *rawP* p value from hypergeometric test, *adjP* p value adjusted by the multiple test adjustment

Table 4 Disease association of identified genes

Disease	GeneSymbol	rawP	adjP
Mental Retardation	AGA, DYRK1A, SETD4, TTC3	0.0001	0.0014
Down Syndrome	DYRK1A, SETD4, TTC3	0.0004	0.0028
Trisomy	DYRK1A, TTC3	0.0016	0.0056
Neurobehavioral Manifestations	DYRK1A, SETD4, TTC3	0.0016	0.0056
Chromosome Disorders	DYRK1A, SETD4, TTC3	0.0021	0.0059
Osteoarthritis	F2RL1, JAM3	0.0036	0.0084
Fibrosis	F2RL1, HGF	0.0098	0.0196

rawP: *p* value from hypergeometric test, adjP: *p* value adjusted by the multiple test adjustment

becoming a major goal in T21 research. A comprehensive investigation of genes and miRNAs in the whole genome may improve our understanding of the genetic-epigenetic interactions of T21.

In this study, we investigated the genes and miRNAs with abnormal expression in placentas from T21 fetuses compared with that in euploid fetuses and found 17 genes that

were negatively regulated by miRNAs in the T21 placentas. Among them, seven genes had increased and 10 had decreased expression. Of the seven genes with increased expression, four genes were on chromosome 21 and were target genes of three down-regulated miRNAs in the T21 placenta. The 10 genes with decreased expression in the T21 placenta were located on the various chromosomes

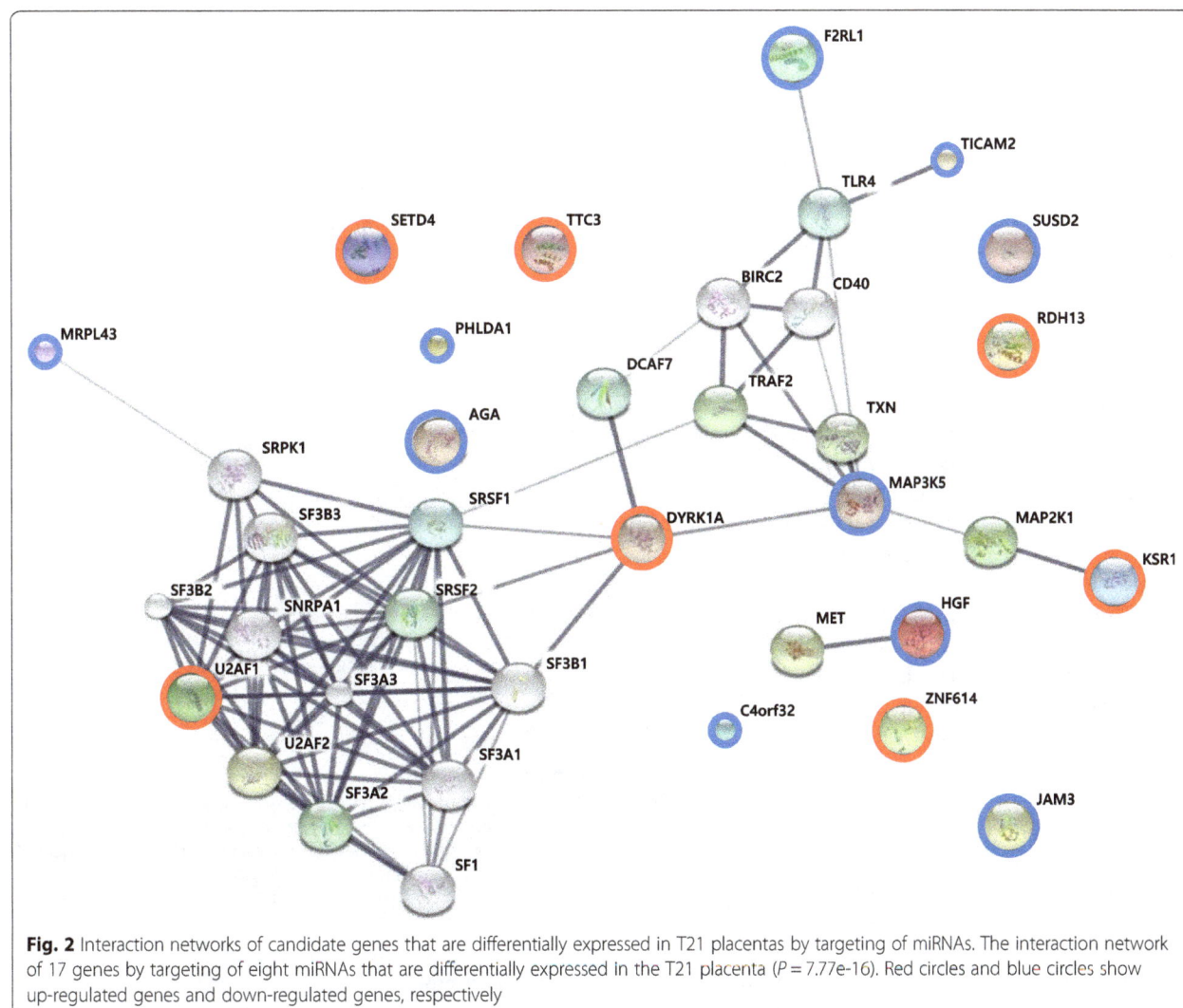

Fig. 2 Interaction networks of candidate genes that are differentially expressed in T21 placentas by targeting of miRNAs. The interaction network of 17 genes by targeting of eight miRNAs that are differentially expressed in the T21 placenta (*P* = 7.77e-16). Red circles and blue circles show up-regulated genes and down-regulated genes, respectively

and were target genes of five up-regulated miRNAs. Half of the eight miRNAs of interest are on the X-chromosome. Most of the tested samples were from males (Table 1). In male spermatogenesis, epigenetic changes play a crucial role in meiotic sex chromosome inactivation (MSCI) and escape. Escape from MSCI characterizes a set of miRNA genes such as mir-221, mir-374, mir-470 and mir-741 [29]. Up to 86% of the X-linked miRNAs escape MSCI during male spermatogenesis [30]. This is likely to have little impact in association between gene and miRNA expression of tested male samples.

Additionally, by in silico pathway-based exploratory analysis, we found an interaction network of three up-regulated genes (*U2AF1*, *DYRK1A*, and *KSR1*) and four down-regulated genes (*MRPL43*, *F2RL1*, *TICAM2*, and *MAP3K5*) in the T21 placenta. Our network showed the possibility of the processes involving *DYRK1A* and *MAP3K5*, being in the genetic-epigenetic mechanisms related to T21 pathophysiology. The DYRK1A protein is a member of the dual-specificity tyrosine-regulated kinases (DYRKs), and has the ability to phosphorylate serine/threonine and tyrosine residues. Its gene is located in the Down syndrome critical region of chromosome 21. DYRK1A overexpression alters both the phosphorylation of tau and alternative splicing factor, and causes an imbalance of 3R- and 4R-tau in the T21 brain [31]. In neurons, the hyperphosphorylation and accumulation of tau into neurofibrillary tangles (NFTs) was found to characterize some neurodegenerative disorders, known as taupathies, Alzheimer's disease being among them [32]. Tau has an important impact on the organization of the cytoskeleton in neurons and, in particular, in the regulation of axonal transport. Therefore, it is considered a strong candidate gene for the neuronal degeneration associated with Down syndrome [33]. Interestingly, researchers have identified molecules that can modulate splicing, selectively targeting DYRK1A and cyclin-dependent kinase-like 1 [34, 35], thus opening up new avenues for T21 therapy. Mitogen-activated protein kinase kinase kinase 5 (MAP3K5) acts as an essential molecule of the MAPK signal transduction. It plays an important role in the cascades of cellular responses evoked by changes in the environment, and mediates the signals that determine cell fate, such as differentiation and survival. In particular, by activating MAPKs, MAP3K5, mediates signaling pathways involved in both the differentiation and survival of neuronal cells. MAP3K5-null mice show impairment of long-term recognition memory, in addition to hyperactivity in a novel environment, and superior motor coordination [36]. Therefore, MAP3K5 seems a good candidate for explaining the mechanisms underpinning intellectual disability and epilepsy [37]. Our results showed that miRNAs negatively regulated the expression of their target genes

DYRK1A and *MAP3K5* in T21, likely through their transcriptional regulatory mechanisms of translational repression or mRNA degradation. Thus, our finding suggests that expression changes of miRNAs that target DYRK1A and MAP3K5 could lead to the changed levels of these two genes in T21, thereby playing a key part in the role of *DYRK1A* and *MAP3K5* in T21 pathogenesis.

In this study, different CVS samples were used for gene expression profiling and for miRNA expression analysis. The amount of material from CVS available for analysis was limited. Because fetal placenta samples at the first-trimester pregnancy were very difficult to obtain, a small amount of chorionic villus were obtained per case. Therefore, as this study was limited by its small sample size, a larger-scale study is needed to clarify the findings.

Conclusions

To our best knowledge, this is the first study to survey whole genes and miRNAs in placentas of T21 fetuses. This study shows that 17 genes and eight miRNAs were differentially expressed between euploid and T21 fetuses and they were negatively regulated in T21. Furthermore, our results propose that many biological pathways that have been implicated in T21 and its complications are possibly regulated by these genes. Therefore, the present work provides a variety of information that may give to a better understanding of genetic-epigenetic modulations in T21.

Abbreviations

CVS: Chorionic villus sampling; miRNA: microRNA; T21: Trisomy 21

Acknowledgments

The authors thank all staffs to participate in this study; Jin Woo Kim, Da Eun Lee, Bom Yi Lee, Ju Yeon Park, Do Jin Kim, Shin Young Kim, Yeon Woo Lee, Ah Rum Oh, Shin Young Lee, So Min Seo, Kyoung Mee Han, and Hwa Jin Choi.

Funding

The publication of this article was funded by grants (HI16C0628) from the Korea Health Technology R&D Project through the Korea Health Industry Development Institute (KHIDI), funded by the Ministry of Health & Welfare, Republic of Korea.

Authors' contributions

Conception and design: JHL, YHC, and HMR. Experimental part, analysis and interpretation of data: JHL, HJK, and SYP. Preparation of the manuscript: JHL, YJH, HJK, and MYK. Sample collection and maintaining patient database: YJH, MYK, and HMR. Principal investigator of the project: YHC and HMR. All authors read and approved the final manuscript.

Competing interests

The authors declare that they have no competing interests.

Author details
[1]Laboratory of Medical Genetics, Medical Research Institute, Cheil General Hospital and Women's Healthcare Center, Seoul, South Korea. [2]Department of Medical Genetics, College of Medicine, Hanyang University, 222, Wangsimni-ro, Seongdong-gu, Seoul 04763, South Korea. [3]Department of Obstetrics and Gynecology, Cheil General Hospital and Women's Healthcare Center, Dankook University College of Medicine, 1-19, Mookjung-dong, Chung-gu, Seoul 100-380, South Korea.

References
1. Mégarbané A, Ravel A, Mircher C, Sturtz F, Grattau Y, Rethoré MO, Delabar JM, Mobley WC. The 50th anniversary of the discovery of trisomy 21: the past, present, and future of research and treatment of trisomy 21. Genet Med. 2009;11:611–6.
2. Korenberg JR, Kawashima H, Pulst SM, Ikeuchi T, Ogasawara N, Yamamoto K, Schonberg SA, West R, Allen L, Magenis E, et al. Molecular definition of a region of chromosome 21 that causes features of the Down syndrome phenotype. Am J Hum Genet. 1990;47:236–46.
3. Li CM, Guo M, Salas M, Schupf N, Silverman W, Zigman WB, Husain S, Warburton D, Thaker H, Tycko B. Cell type-specific over-expression of chromosome 21 genes in fibroblasts and fetal hearts with trisomy 21. BMC Med Genet. 2006;7:24.
4. Giannone S, Strippoli P, Vitale L, Casadei R, Canaider S, Lenzi L, D'Addabbo P, Frabetti F, Facchin F, Farina A, Carinci P, Zannotti M. Gene expression profile analysis in human T lymphocytes from patients with Down syndrome. Ann Hum Genet. 2004;68:546–54.
5. Mao R, Wang X, Spitznagel EL Jr, Frelin LP, Ting JC, Ding H, Kim JW, Ruczinski I, Downey TJ, Pevsner J. Primary and secondary transcriptional effects in the developing human Down syndrome brain and heart. Genome Biol. 2005;6:R107.
6. Bushati N, Cohen SM. microRNA functions. Annu Rev Cell Dev Biol. 2007;23:175–205.
7. Kloosterman WP, Plasterk RH. The diverse functions of microRNAs in animal development and disease. Dev Cell. 2006;11:441–50.
8. MicroRNAs BDP. Genomics, biogenesis, mechanism, and function. Cell. 2004;116:281–97.
9. Valencia-Sanchez MA, Liu J, Hannon GJ, Parker R. Control of translation and mRNA degradation by miRNAs and siRNAs. Genes Dev. 2006;20:515–24.
10. Friedman RC, Farh KK, Burge CB, Bartel DP. Most mammalian mRNAs are conserved targets of microRNAs. Genome Res. 2009, 19:92–105.
11. Kozomara A, Griffiths-Jones S. miRBase: annotating high confidence microRNAs using deep sequencing data. Nucleic Acids Res. 2014;42(Database issue):D68–73.
12. Pillai RS, Bhattacharyya SN, Filipowicz W. Repression of protein synthesis by miRNAs: how many mechanisms? Trends Cell Biol. 2007;17:118–26.
13. Krützfeldt J, Stoffel M. MicroRNAs: a new class of regulatory genes affecting metabolism. Cell Metab. 2006;4:9–12.
14. Adams BD, Kasinski AL, Slack FJ. Aberrant regulation and function of microRNAs in cancer. Curr Biol. 2014;24:R762–76.
15. Condorelli G, Latronico MV, Cavarretta E. microRNAs in cardiovascular diseases: current knowledge and the road ahead. J Am Coll Cardiol. 2014;63:2177–87.
16. Szulwach KE, Jin P, Alisch RS. Noncoding RNAs in mental retardation. Clin Genet. 2009;75:209–19.
17. Huang L, Shen Z, Xu Q, Huang X, Chen Q, Li D. Increased levels of microRNA-424 are associated with the pathogenesis of fetal growth restriction. Placenta. 2013;34(7):624.
18. Provost P. MicroRNAs as a molecular basis for mental retardation, Alzheimer's and prion diseases. Brain Res. 2010;1338:58–66.
19. Siew WH, Tan KL, Babaei MA, Cheah PS, Ling KH. MicroRNAs and intellectual disability (ID) in Down syndrome, X-linked ID, and fragile X syndrome. Front Cell Neurosci. 2013;7:41.
20. Lim JH, Kim DJ, Lee DE, Han JY, Chung JH, Ahn HK, Lee SW, Lim DH, Lee YS, Park SY, Ryu HM. Genome-wide microRNA expression profiling in placentas of fetuses with Down syndrome. Placenta. 2015;36:322–8.
21. Lim JH, Han YJ, Kim HJ, Kwak DW, Park SY, Chun SH, Ryu HM. Genome-wide gene expression analysis in the placenta from fetus with trisomy 21. BMC Genomics. 2017;18:720.
22. Benjamini Y, Hochberg Y. Controlling the false discovery rate: a practical and powerful approach to multiple testing. J R Statist Soc B. 1995;57:289–300.
23. Korenberg JR, Chen XN, Schipper R, Sun Z, Gonsky R, Gerwehr S, Carpenter N, Daumer C, Dignan P, Disteche C, et al. Down syndrome phenotypes: the consequences of chromosomal imbalance. Proc Natl Acad Sci US A. 1994;91:4997–5001.
24. Pritchard MA, Kola I. The "gene dosage effect" hypothesis versus the "amplified developmental instability" hypothesis in Down syndrome. J Neural Transm Suppl. 1999;57:293–303.
25. FitzPatrick DR. Transcriptional consequences of autosomal trisomy: primary gene dosage with complex downstream effects. Trends Genet. 2005;21:249–53.
26. Lockstone HE, Harris LW, Swatton JE, Wayland MT, Holland AJ, Bahn S. Gene expression profiling in the adult Down syndrome brain. Genomics. 2007;90:647–60.
27. Filipowicz W, Bhattacharyya SN, Sonenberg N. Mechanisms of posttranscriptional regulation by microRNAs: are the answers in sight? Nat Rev Genet. 2008;9:102–14.
28. Du T, Zamore PD. microPrimer: the biogenesis and function of microRNA. Development. 2005;132:4645–52.
29. Berletch JB, Yang F, Disteche CM. Escape from X inactivation in mice and humans. Genome Biol. 2010;11:213.
30. Song R, Ro S, Michaels JD, Park C, McCarrey JR, Yan W. Many X-linked microRNAs escape meiotic sex chromosome inactivation. Nat Genet. 2009;41:488–93.
31. Bardoni B, Abekhoukh S, Zongaro S, Melko M. Intellectual disabilities, neuronal posttranscriptional RNA metabolism, and RNA-binding proteins: three actors for a complex scenario. Prog Brain Res. 2012;197:29–51.
32. Ittner LM, Götz J. Amyloid-β and tau–a toxic pas de deux in Alzheimer's disease. Nat Rev Neurosci. 2011;12:65–72.
33. Wegiel J, Kaczmarski W, Barua M, Kuchna I, Nowicki K, Wang KC, Wegiel J, Yang SM, Frackowiak J, Mazur-Kolecka B, Silverman WP, Reisberg B, Monteiro I, de Leon M, Wisniewski T, Dalton A, Lai F, Hwang YW, Adayev T, Liu F, Iqbal K, Iqbal IG, Gong CX. Link between DYRK1A overexpression and several-fold enhancement of neurofibrillary degeneration with 3-repeat tau protein Down syndrome. J Neuropathol Exp Neurol. 2011;70:36–50.
34. Giraud F, Alves G, Debiton E, Nauton L, Théry V, Durieu E, Ferandin Y, Lozach O, Meijer L, Anizon F, Pereira E, Moreau P. Synthesis, protein kinase inhibitory potencies, and in vitro antiproliferative activities of meridianin derivatives. J Med Chem. 2011;54:4474–89.
35. Rosenthal AS, Tanega C, Shen M, Mott BT, Bougie JM, Nguyen DT, Misteli T, Auld DS, Maloney DJ, Thomas CJ. An inhibitor of the Cdc2-like kinase 4 (Clk4). In: Probe reports from the NIH molecular libraries program [internet]. Bethesda (MD): National Center for biotechnology information (US); 2010–. 2010 mar 29 [updated 2011 Mar 3].
36. Kumakura K, Nomura H, Toyoda T, Hashikawa K, Noguchi T, Takeda K, Ichijo H, Tsunoda M, Funatsu T, Ikegami D, Narita M, Suzuki T, Matsuki N. Hyperactivity in novelenvironment with increased dopamine and impaired noveltypreference in apoptosis signal-regulating kinase 1 (ASK1)-deficient mice. Neurosci Res. 2010;66:313–20.
37. Nguyen LS, Jolly L, Shoubridge C, Chan WK, Huang L, Laumonnier F, Raynaud M, Hackett A, Field M, Rodriguez J, Srivastava AK, Lee Y, Long R, Addington AM, Rapoport JL, Suren S, Hahn CN, Gamble J, Wilkinson MF, Corbett MA, Gecz J. Transcriptome profiling of UPF3B/NMD-deficient lymphoblastoid cells from patients with various forms of intellectual disability. Mol Psychiatry. 2012;17:1103–15.

2

Rare variants in the splicing regulatory elements of EXOC3L4 are associated with brain glucose metabolism in Alzheimer's disease

Jason E. Miller[1,5], Manu K. Shivakumar[1], Younghee Lee[2], Seonggyun Han[2], Emrin Horgousluoglu[3], Shannon L. Risacher[3], Andrew J. Saykin[3], Kwangsik Nho[3*], Dokyoon Kim[1,4*] and for the Alzheimer's Disease Neuroimaging Initiative

Abstract

Background: Alzheimer's disease (AD) is one of the most common neurodegenerative diseases that causes problems related to brain function. To some extent it is understood on a molecular level how AD arises, however there are a lack of biomarkers that can be used for early diagnosis. Two popular methods to identify AD-related biomarkers use genetics and neuroimaging. Genes and neuroimaging phenotypes have provided some insights as to the potential for AD biomarkers. While the field of imaging-genomics has identified genetic features associated with structural and functional neuroimaging phenotypes, it remains unclear how variants that affect splicing could be important for understanding the genetic etiology of AD.

Methods: In this study, rare variants (minor allele frequency < 0.01) in splicing regulatory element (SRE) loci from whole genome sequencing (WGS) in the Alzheimer's Disease Neuroimaging Initiative (ADNI) cohort, were used to identify genes that are associated with global brain cortical glucose metabolism in AD measured by FDG PET-scans. Gene-based associated analyses of rare variants were performed using the program BioBin and the optimal Sequence Kernel Association Test (SKAT-O).

Results: The gene, EXOC3L4, was identified as significantly associated with global cortical glucose metabolism (FDR (false discovery rate) corrected $p < 0.05$) using SRE coding variants only. Three loci that may affect splicing within EXOC3L4 contribute to the association.

Conclusion: Based on sequence homology, EXOC3L4 is likely a part of the exocyst complex. Our results suggest the possibility that variants which affect proper splicing of EXOC3L4 via SREs may impact vesicle transport, giving rise to AD related phenotypes. Overall, by utilizing WGS and functional neuroimaging we have identified a gene significantly associated with an AD related endophenotype, potentially through a mechanism that involves splicing.

Keywords: Alternative splicing, Imaging genomics, Alzheimer's disease, Whole genome sequencing, Rare variants

* Correspondence: knho@iupui.edu; dkim@geisinger.edu
[3]Department of Radiology and Imaging Sciences, Indiana University School of Medicine, Indianapolis, IN, USA
[1]Biomedical and Translational Informatics Institute, Geisinger Health System, Danville, PA, USA
Full list of author information is available at the end of the article

Background

Late-onset Alzheimer's disease (LOAD) is a progressive common neurodegenerative disorder that causes problems with memory, thinking, and behavior and pathologically characterized by the presence of amyloid deposition and neurofibrillary tangles in the brain [1, 2]. 5.5 million Americans are estimated to have AD in 2017 and the number of Americans with AD is rapidly increasing because of the growing number of older adults [1]. Currently, there is no available cure for AD. As a result, without earlier diagnosis and early disease-modifying intervention, the total number of individuals with AD is predicted to quadruple by 2050, causing a great economic and social burden [1]. Furthermore, a biomarker for early diagnosis could benefit clinical trials for AD by precisely classifying prognosis, stage, and determining a clinical endpoint [3]. Thus, AD related research is increasingly important, especially as it relates to early diagnosis.

Genetic variation may play an essential role in AD pathogenesis [4]. Recently, a large-scale genome-wide association study (GWAS) identified and validated more than 22 susceptibility genes for LOAD [5]. After the success of GWAS for common SNPs, large-scale whole exome and genome sequencing studies have successfully identified several rare risk variants for LOAD [6–9]. Recently, the genetics of AD has been investigated in the context of imaging data. By combining information from genetic architecture, functional neuroimaging, and multi-omics data, genetic variation associated with AD-related imaging biomarkers

have been identified and thus the potential influence of genetic variation on brain structure and function related to AD pathophysiology [10, 11]. Furthermore, imaging endophenotypes can substantially increase statistical detection power of genetic association analysis through the use of quantitative traits as phenotypes [12].

Rare and low-frequency variants play an important role in the heritability of disease. However, the spurious nature of rare variants makes them difficult to run an association test. With so few occurrences of the variant at a given loci most tests will be underpowered [13]. In order to overcome this problem, variants can be grouped together by prior biological knowledge, such as genes, conserved loci, and pathways [14–16]. This strategy will accumulate effects of rare variants within a knowledge-driven region and reduce the number of statistical tests, thereby increasing the power to detect an association. Additionally, focusing on specific types of variants, such as those that lead to non-synonymous changes can also reduce the multiple testing burden and provide a potential explanation for the gene associated with the phenotype [17]. An attractive category of variant for studying AD are those that impact splicing.

Alternative splicing (AS) is an important gene regulatory mechanism underlying neurological function and development [18]. While motifs along splice junctions have been well studies, the effect of genetic variants in splicing regulatory elements (SREs) is less understood in the context of AD. There are multiple types of SREs that

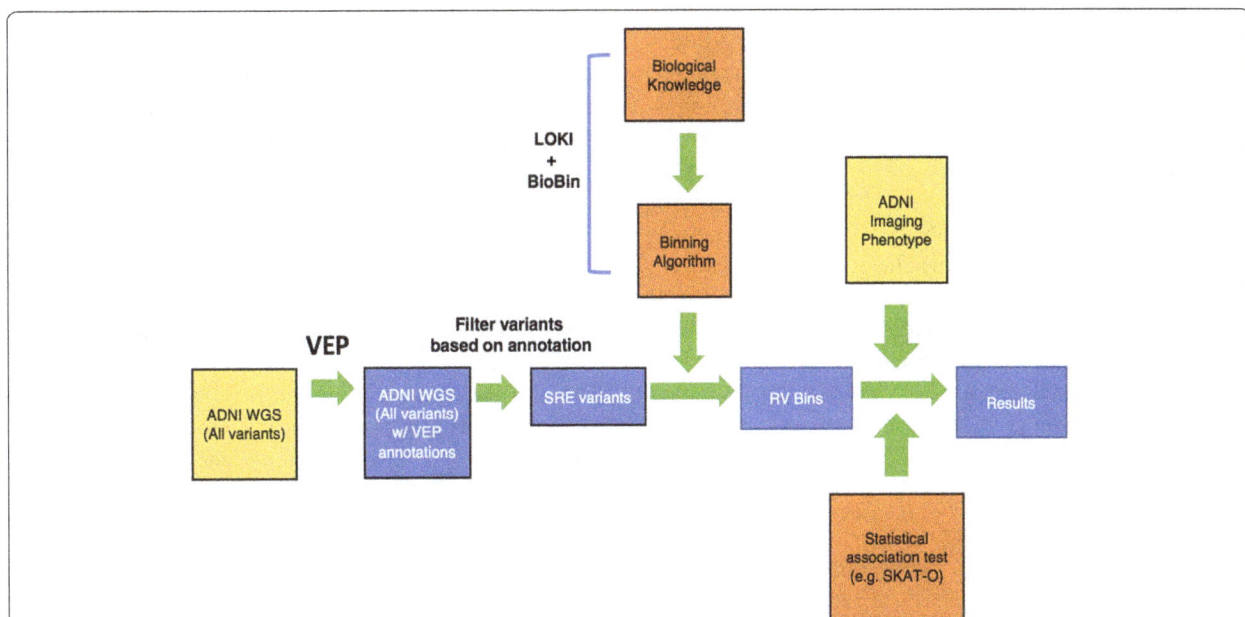

Fig. 1 Workflow describing rare SRE variant association test using imaging phenotype data. Diagram of how rare variants (RV) from whole-genome sequencing (WGS) data were tested for an association with ADNI imaging data. WGS variants were annotated with VEP then filtered for those that reside in SRE loci (i.e., ESE, ESS, and ISE). Variants were then binned into genes using annotations from LOKI. SKAT-O was then used to test genes for an association with the ADNI imaging endophenotype

Table 1 Summary statistics of variables used as covariates in association study

Demographics and Covariates	Values (N = 695)
Sex (M/F)	391/304
Age in years (Mean/Std)	72.95 (+/− 7.05)

can impact splicing in different ways including intronic splicing enhancers (ISE), intronic splicing silencers (ISS), exonic splicing enhancers (ESE), and exonic splicing silencers (ESS) [19]. However, the significance of SRE in relation to AD related phenotypes remains unknown. In this study, an imaging genomics approach was taken to investigate AD by identifying rare variants within SREs associated with a neuroimaging phenotype using ADNI data. The Alzheimer's Disease Neuroimaging Initiative (ADNI) has provided publically available whole-genome sequencing (WGS) data, along with imaging phenotypes. BioBin, an open-source program that was developed to group or bin the variants using information from multiple databases, was employed to bin rare variants from ADNI WGS data [14]. Gene-based analyses were performed using the optimal Sequence Kernel Association Test (SKAT-O), which maximizes power by adaptively using the data to optimally combine the burden test and dispersion test.

Methods
Study sample
All whole-genome sequencing (WGS) and imaging data came from the Alzheimer's Disease Neuroimaging Initiative (ADNI) cohort. The cohort used here was made up of participants with cognitive normal (CN), early mild cognitive impairment (EMCI), late MCI (LMCI), and AD. The demographic data, along with sequencing and imaging data were downloaded from the ADNI data repository (http://www.loni.usc.edu/ADNI/). All participants provided written informed consent and study protocols were approved by participating sites' Institutional Review Board. WGS was performed using blood-derived genomic DNA samples from ADNI participants. Sequencing was performed using 100 bp paired-end reads on the Illumina HiSeq2000 platform (www.illumina.com). As previously described using Broad GATK and BWA-mem, reads were

mapped and aligned to the human genome (build 37), then variants were called [8, 20].

Neuroimaging analysis
Pre-processed [18F] FDG PET scans were downloaded from the LONI (http://loni.usc.edu). As previously described in detail, these FDG scans (Co-registered, Averaged, Standardized Image and Voxel Size, Uniform Resolution) were already averaged, aligned to a standard space, re-sampled to a standard image and voxel size (2 × 2 × 2 mm), smoothed to a uniform resolution, and intensity normalized [21]. The pre-processed images were aligned to each individual's MRI scan at the same visit and normalized to MNI space using SPM8 as previously described [22]. The intensity of the resulting scans was re-scaled to a pons reference region and then the final [18F] FDG standardized uptake value ratio (SUVR) images were created. A global cortical glucose metabolism measured from [18F] FDG-PET scans was used as an AD-related quantitative endophenotype with age at baseline and sex as covariates.

Variant annotation
The VCF file containing 695 non-Hispanic Caucasian participants with imaging phenotype, covariates and genomic data was annotated using the variant effect predictor (VEP) package [23]. The variant_effect_predictor.pl script was applied to the VCF file using cache, refseq, and pick flags. Variants were then selected if they were also annotated with an SRE element. Sequences and organization of SREs in humans were identified using previously developed method [19, 24] which required the use of dbSNP version 137 and hg19 reference genome [25, 26]. In brief, this method predicts hexamer motifs associated with the following types of SREs associated with exon skipping events: intronic splicing enhancer (ISE), exonic splicing enhancer (ESE), and exonic splicing silencer (ESS). The program *twoBitToFa* was used to find the genome sequences surrounding the SNPs of interest with hg19 reference [27]. 11-mer sequences were interrogated surrounding the SNPs (5 bp on each side) using the hexamer motifs. While ESE and ESS were coding SNPs, the ISE were defined as intronic SNPs. Using the published methods [19], an SRE was counted if there was a match between a hexamer motif and any part of the

Table 2 Top 5 genes associated with imaging phenotype using ISE variants only

Gene	Unique Loci	Variants across cohort	SKAT-O p-value	FDR corrected p-value
TNFAIP2	7	10	2.47E-05	0.123
STK35	56	148	3.09E-05	0.123
PWRN1	34	101	4.15E-05	0.123
EXOC3L4	8	21	6.11E-05	0.123
TMEM182	23	67	6.22E-05	0.123

Table 3 EXOC3L4 gene is associated with imaging phenotype using ESE/ESS variants only

Gene	Unique Loci	Variants across cohort	SKAT-O p-value	FDR corrected p-value
EXOC3L4	4	16	7.48E-06	0.038

11-mer, and associated with exon skipping. ISE SNPs were included based on the exons bordering the intron in which the SNP was located.

Variant binning, association test, and analysis

BioBin was used to group rare variants by genic region (minor allele frequency (MAF) < 0.01). BioBin uses gene annotations from LOKI (the library of knowledge integration), which contains a number of widely used publically available databases such as NCBI Entrez, UCSC Genome Browser, Kyoto Encyclopedia of Genes and Genomes (KEGG), Reactome, Genome Ontology (GO) and others. Association tests were performed using SKAT-O [28], adjusting for age and sex. The minimum bin size included in the association test was five variants across samples. The bins were tested for an association with global brain cortical glucose metabolism measured by FDG PET scans (often referred to as the "imaging phenotype"). For both annotation and BioBin, the GRCh37 assembly was specified. Finally, the false discovery rate for BioBin output p-values was then calculated in R using the p.adjust function, using the "FDR" method. Variant effect analysis using PROVEAN and SIFT was performed online at http://provean.jcvi.org [29–31]. The UCSC genome browser was used to visualize the ECO3L4 gene along with splicing isoforms and protein domains [25].

Results

First, variants from the ADNI WGS study were selected that were located in the SRE coding and/or ISE loci (Fig. 1). Next BioBin was employed to bin variants with minor allele frequency (MAF) less than 0.01 into their respective genes. SKAT-O was used to test if these rare variants in each gene were associated with the phenotype derived from FDG PET scans from ADNI. These associations were adjusted for covariates such as age and sex to reduce the effect of confounding variables (Table 1). The p-values were adjusted for multiple testing, and genes with a false discovery rate (FDR) less than 0.05 were considered significant, while those with FDR < 0.1 were suggestive of statistical significance. Using ISE variants, there were no genes that had a significant association with the imaging phenotype (Table 2). However, using SRE coding variants (i.e., ESE and ESS), EXOC3L4 was identified as having a genome-wide significant (FDR < 5%) association with the imaging phenotype (Table 3 and Fig. 2). PROVEAN and SIFT predictions for variants in EXOC3L4 were considered neutral and tolerated, respectively, which suggests SRE annotations offer novel insight into the consequence of rare variants. Also, the sequence homology between EXOC3L4 and exocyst complex components suggests SRE sites are within the Sec6 domain, indicating these splicing elements could have a functional impact on the protein (uniprot.org). Alternatively, when combining both sets of variants there were several genes which were only

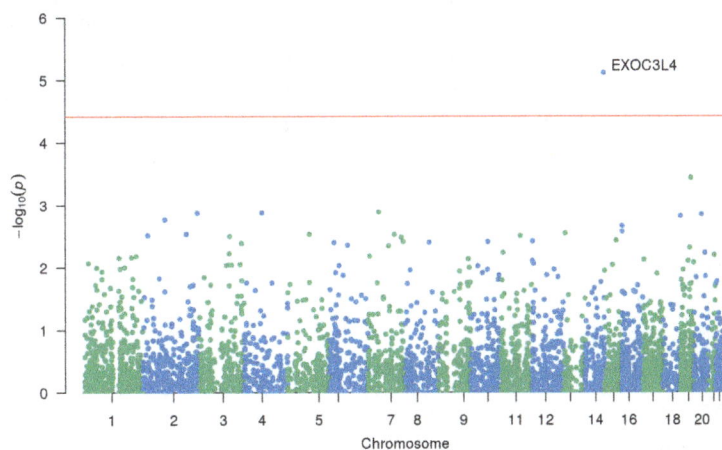

Fig. 2 Manhattan plot of p-values from association between genes and the imaging phenotype using SRE coding variants. Manhattan plot which shows the results from the association test between the imaging phenotype and each gene tested using SKAT-O. Only variants that fell into SRE coding loci were used. The blue and red lines represent 0.05 p-value and 0.05 FDR cutoffs, respectively

Table 4 Top 5 genes associated with imaging phenotype using ESE/ESS and ISE variants

Gene	Unique Loci	Variants across cohort	SKAT-O p-value	FDR corrected p-value
TNFAIP2	8	14	1.20E-05	0.094
EXOC3L4	10	35	1.99E-05	0.094
STK35	56	148	3.09E-05	0.094
STEAP4	7	13	3.23E-05	0.094
PWRN1	34	101	4.15E-05	0.097

suggestive of having a significant (FDR < 10%) association with the imaging phenotype (Table 4). In summary, SRE coding annotations provided increased power to detect *EXOC3L4* as having an association with the imaging phenotype.

To investigate the association with *EXOC3L4* further, each of the four loci in *EXOC3L4* with rare variants were interrogated to define their contribution to the association. This analysis was performed by removing each SNP individually then rerunning the association test to retrieve a *p*-value for only *EXOC3L4* (Table 5). After removing SNPs rs10142287, rs9324055, or rs148718670, *EXOC3L4* had a *p*-value that was less significant compared to the original *p*-value of *EXOC3L4* with 4 variants. These effects are unlikely to be caused purely by the number of variants at each locus removed, as only one or three variants were removed, suggesting there is something specific about the loci which leads to the association with the phenotype. As shown in the UCSC genome browser (Fig. 3), there is evidence that alternative splicing of *EXOC3L4* can lead to the existence of a transcript that skips the second exon which harbors two SNPs within ESE sites, rs10142287 and rs9324055. The skipped exon is part of a region encoding the Sec6 domain (Fig. 3). These results help explain why variability in SRE sites of *EXOC3L4* could impact the phenotype through a mechanism involving AS. On the other hand, removing the rs117708804 SNP resulted in an increase in significance as illustrated by the lower *p*-value, suggesting that *EXOC3L4* can absorb variation at this locus, and that variants here may be spurious or not important for the context of this association.

Discussion

Although very little is known about *EXOC3L4* or its orthologues, BLAST search results using its amino acid sequence suggests it is likely to be an exocyst complex component (uniprot.org). This information lends itself to a number of possible models for how *EXOC3L4* may be involved in AD. In mammals, the exocyst complex is an eight-subunit complex that is ubiquitously expressed [32]. The exocyst proteins are important for vesicle trafficking along with SNARE proteins [33, 34]. It has been suggested that SNARE proteins are important for glucose uptake in the context of proper neuronal function [35]. And the imaging phenotype from this study, FDG PET-scans, quantifies global brain cortical glucose metabolism in AD. Additionally, vesicle transport is used for lysosomal transport, such as seen in autophagy [36]. AD is defined by the accumulation of proteins like amyloid plaques, which can be removed via the autophagy-lysosome pathway [37]. There is evidence that defects in this autophagy process can lead to AD [38]. Thus, our results suggest a model where variants in *EXOC3L4* that are located in SRE coding loci may alter the function of the protein through exon skipping, which may inhibit proper vesicle transport. Moreover, these variants may lead to AD related phenotypes.

Evidence suggests the exocyst plays important roles in embryogenesis, neuronal cell polarity, and cell motility [32]. *EXOC3L4* shares high sequence similarity with M-seq (also known as *TNFaip2*), a protein that shares structural similarity to *Sec6* (uniprot.org). It has been suggested that *TNFaip2* has a role in filopedia development in neurons [32]. Thus, if *EXOC3L4* does not carry out its function through interactions with the exocyst

Table 5 Characterization of EXOC3L4 rare variant loci

rsID	Consequence	p-value[a]	SRE type	Variants across cohort
rs117708804	missense	4.32E-07	ESE, ESS	11
EXOC3L4		7.48E-06[b]		16
rs10142287	synonymous	1.58E-04	ESE	1
rs9324055	missense	1.59E-04	ESE	1
rs148718670	missense	1.68E-04	ESE	3

[a]SKAT-O p-value results after removing the variant from EXOC3L4
[b]SKAT-O p-value result using all variants from EXOC3L4

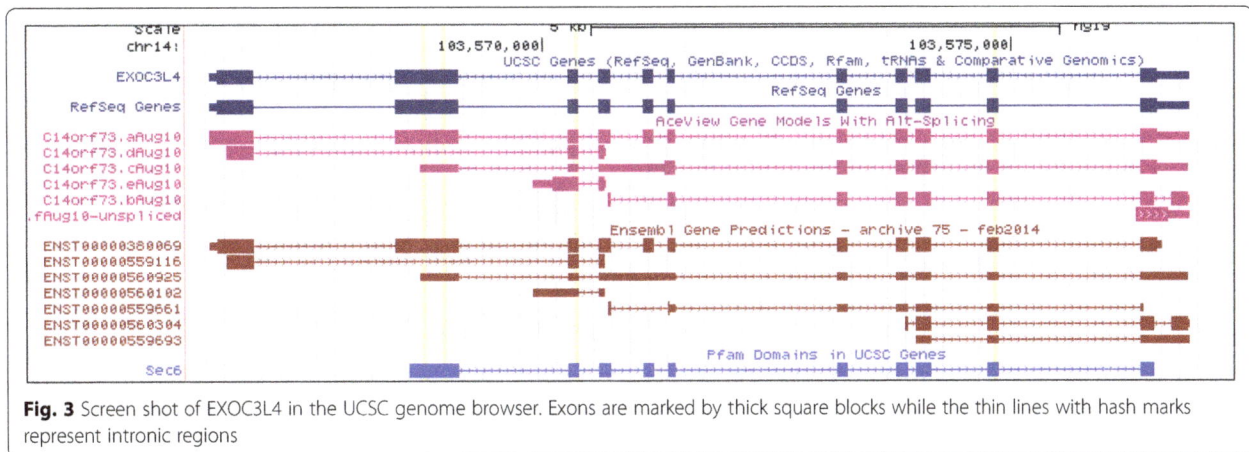

Fig. 3 Screen shot of EXOC3L4 in the UCSC genome browser. Exons are marked by thick square blocks while the thin lines with hash marks represent intronic regions

complex, there is evidence that exocyst-like proteins are important for neuronal cell function through an alternative mechanism.

One limitation of this study is the samples size. *TNFAIP2* was only suggestive of statistical significance, however it is another protein that is functionally relevant to SNARE proteins and thus vesicle transport (uniprot.org). Since only few samples contained the rare variants, it will be important for this study to be replicated in another independent cohort. Additionally, since these are associations it will be important to perform follow-up experiments to identify a causal link between *EXOC3L4* and AD. None the less, these results suggest more genes that contain rare variants in SRE loci, and are important for proper exocytosis and autophagy, are likely to be identified in studies with increased sample size. In summary, annotating variants as SRE provides novel insight as to how rare variants may be useful when finding an association between an imaging phenotype and genetic variants in the context of AD.

Conclusions

In this study, we set out to find associations between a neuroimaging phenotype and rare SRE variants from WGS in AD. While it is common to perform a gene-wise association test, we hypothesized that the power of this study could be increased by focusing on functionally relevant loci such as those that impact splicing. Furthermore, associations with annotated regions can lead to easier interpretation afterward. Thus, rare variants that fell into SRE loci from WGS from the ADNI cohort were collapsed into genes using BioBin. These rare variants were used in an association test for an imaging phenotype and *EXOC3L4* was identified as having a statistically significant association. And while intronic elements did not detect a statistically significant association, exonic splicing elements did. In summary, utilizing prior biological

knowledge in the form of splicing elements serves as an important means to identify genotype-phenotype relationships with respect to imaging data and AD.

Abbreviations
FDG: Fluorodeoxyglucose; LOAD: Late-onset Alzheimer's Disease; WGS: Whole-genome sequencing

Acknowledgments
Data used in preparation of this article were obtained from the Alzheimer's Disease Neuroimaging Initiative (ADNI) database (adni.loni.usc.edu). As such, the investigators within the ADNI contributed to the design and implementation of ADNI and/or provided data but did not participate in analysis or writing of this report. A complete listing of ADNI investigators can be found at: http://adni.loni.usc.edu/wp-content/uploads/how_to_apply/ADNI_Acknowledgement_List.pdf

Funding
Data collection and sharing for this project was funded by the Alzheimer's Disease Neuroimaging Initiative (ADNI) (National Institutes of Health Grant U01 AG024904) and DOD ADNI (Department of Defense award number W81XWH-12-2-0012). ADNI is funded by the National Institute on Aging, the National Institute of Biomedical Imaging and Bioengineering, and through generous contributions from the following: Alzheimer's Association; Alzheimer's Drug Discovery Foundation; BioClinica, Inc.; Biogen Idec Inc.; Bristol-Myers Squibb Company; Eisai Inc.; Elan Pharmaceuticals, Inc.; Eli Lilly and Company; F. Hoffmann-La Roche Ltd. and its affiliated company Genentech, Inc.; GE Healthcare; Innogenetics, N.V.; IXICO Ltd.; Janssen Alzheimer Immunotherapy Research & Development, LLC.; Johnson & Johnson Pharmaceutical Research & Development LLC.; Medpace, Inc.; Merck & Co., Inc.; Meso Scale Diagnostics, LLC.; NeuroRx Research; Novartis Pharmaceuticals Corporation; Pfizer Inc.; Piramal Imaging; Servier; Synarc Inc.; and Takeda Pharmaceutical Company. The Canadian Institutes of Health Research is providing funds to support ADNI clinical sites in Canada. Private sector contributions are facilitated by the Foundation for the National Institutes of Health (www.fnih.org). The grantee organization is the Northern California Institute for Research and Education, and the study is coordinated by the Alzheimer's Disease Cooperative Study at the University of California, San Diego. ADNI data are disseminated by the Laboratory for Neuro Imaging at the University of Southern California. Samples from the National Cell Repository for AD (NCRAD), which receives government support under a cooperative agreement grant (U24 AG21886) awarded by the National Institute on Aging (AIG), were used in this study. Funding for the WGS was provided by the Alzheimer's Association and the Brin Wojcicki Foundation. This project is funded, in part, under a grant with the Pennsylvania Department of Health (#SAP 4100070267) and NLM R01 LM012535 and NIA R03 AG054936. The Department specifically disclaims responsibility for any analyses, interpretations or conclusions. The cost of publication was funded by Dokyoon Kim's startup fund at Geisinger.

Authors' contributions

All authors contributed substantively to this work. JEM, YL, KN, and DK were involved in study conception and design. JEM, MKS, YL, KN, EH, DK, SH, and AJS were involved in data organization, whole genome sequencing analysis and statistical analyses. AJS was involved in coordination and data collection and processing for ADNI. JEM, MKS, KN and DK drafted the report and prepared all figures and tables. All authors were involved in reviewing and editing of the manuscript and approved it.

Competing interests

The authors declare they have no competing interests.

Author details

[1]Biomedical and Translational Informatics Institute, Geisinger Health System, Danville, PA, USA. [2]Department of Biomedical Informatics, University of Utah School of Medicine, Salt Lake City, UT 84106, USA. [3]Department of Radiology and Imaging Sciences, Indiana University School of Medicine, Indianapolis, IN, USA. [4]Huck Institute of the Life Sciences, Pennsylvania State University, University Park, PA, USA. [5]Present Address: Department of Genetics, Institute for Biomedical Informatics, Perelman School of Medicine, University of Pennsylvania, Philadelphia, PA, USA.

References

1. Alzheimer's A. 2015 Alzheimer's disease facts and figures. Alzheimers Dement. 2015;11(3):332–84.
2. Bloom GS. Amyloid-beta and tau: the trigger and bullet in Alzheimer disease pathogenesis. JAMA Neurol. 2014;71(4):505–8.
3. Beach TG. A review of biomarkers for neurodegenerative disease: will they swing us across the valley? Neurol Ther. 2017;6(Suppl 1):5–13.
4. Tanzi RE. The genetics of Alzheimer disease. Cold Spring Harb Perspect Med. 2012;2(10)
5. Lambert JC, Ibrahim-Verbaas CA, Harold D, Naj AC, Sims R, Bellenguez C, DeStafano AL, Bis JC, Beecham GW, Grenier-Boley B, et al. Meta-analysis of 74,046 individuals identifies 11 new susceptibility loci for Alzheimer's disease. Nat Genet. 2013;45(12):1452–8.
6. Cruchaga C, Karch CM, Jin SC, Benitez BA, Cai Y, Guerreiro R, Harari O, Norton J, Budde J, Bertelsen S, et al. Rare coding variants in the phospholipase D3 gene confer risk for Alzheimer's disease. Nature. 2014;505(7484):550–4.
7. Guerreiro R, Wojtas A, Bras J, Carrasquillo M, Rogaeva E, Majounie E, Cruchaga C, Sassi C, Kauwe JS, Younkin S, et al. TREM2 variants in Alzheimer's disease. N Engl J Med. 2013;368(2):117–27.
8. Nho K, Horgusluoglu E, Kim S, Risacher SL, Kim D, Foroud T, Aisen PS, Petersen RC, Jack CR Jr, Shaw LM, et al. Integration of bioinformatics and imaging informatics for identifying rare PSEN1 variants in Alzheimer's disease. BMC Med Genomics. 2016;9(Suppl 1):30.
9. Steinberg S, Stefansson H, Jonsson T, Johannsdottir H, Ingason A, Helgason H, Sulem P, Magnusson OT, Gudjonsson SA, Unnsteinsdottir U, et al. Loss-of-function variants in ABCA7 confer risk of Alzheimer's disease. Nat Genet. 2015;47(5):445–7.
10. Nho K, Kim S, Horgusluoglu E, Risacher SL, Shen L, Kim D, Lee S, Foroud T, Shaw LM, Trojanowski JQ, et al. Association analysis of rare variants near the APOE region with CSF and neuroimaging biomarkers of Alzheimer's disease. BMC Med Genet. 2017;10(Suppl 1):29.
11. Saykin AJ, Shen L, Yao X, Kim S, Nho K, Risacher SL, Ramanan VK, Foroud TM, Faber KM, Sarwar N, et al. Genetic studies of quantitative MCI and AD phenotypes in ADNI: progress, opportunities, and plans. Alzheimers Dement. 2015;11(7):792–814.
12. Shen L, Thompson PM, Potkin SG, Bertram L, Farrer LA, Foroud TM, Green RC, Hu X, Huentelman MJ, Kim S, et al. Genetic analysis of quantitative phenotypes in AD and MCI: imaging, cognition and biomarkers. Brain Imaging Behav. 2014;8(2):183–207.
13. Lee S, Abecasis GR, Boehnke M, Lin X. Rare-variant association analysis: study designs and statistical tests. Am J Hum Genet. 2014;95(1):5–23.
14. Moore CB, Wallace JR, Frase AT, Pendergrass SA, Ritchie MD. BioBin: a bioinformatics tool for automating the binning of rare variants using publicly available biological knowledge. BMC Med Genomics. 2013;6(Suppl 2):S6.
15. Moore CB, Wallace JR, Frase AT, Pendergrass SA, Ritchie MD. Using BioBin to explore rare variant population stratification. Pac Symp Biocomput. 2013:332–43.
16. Basile AO, Wallace JR, Peissig P, McCarty CA, Brilliant M, Ritchie MD. Knowledge driven binning and Phewas analysis in Marshfield personalized medicine research project using Biobin. Pac Symp Biocomput. 2016;21:249–60.
17. Kim D, Basile AO, Bang L, Horgusluoglu E, Lee S, Ritchie MD, Saykin AJ, Nho K. Knowledge-driven binning approach for rare variant association analysis: application to neuroimaging biomarkers in Alzheimer's disease. BMC Med Inform Decis Mak. 2017;17(Suppl 1):61.
18. Vuong CK, Black DL, Zheng S. The neurogenetics of alternative splicing. Nat Rev Neurosci. 2016;17(5):265–81.
19. Lee Y, Gamazon ER, Rebman E, Lee Y, Lee S, Dolan ME, Cox NJ, Lussier YA. Variants affecting exon skipping contribute to complex traits. PLoS Genet. 2012;8(10):e1002998.
20. Nho K, West JD, Li H, Henschel R, Bharthur A, Tavares MC, Saykin AJ. Comparison of multi-sample variant calling methods for whole genome sequencing. IEEE Int Conf Systems Biol. 2014;2014:59–62.
21. Jagust WJ, Bandy D, Chen K, Foster NL, Landau SM, Mathis CA, Price JC, Reiman EM, Skovronsky D, Koeppe RA, et al. The Alzheimer's disease neuroimaging initiative positron emission tomography core. Alzheimers Dement. 2010;6(3):221–9.
22. Risacher SL, Kim S, Nho K, Foroud T, Shen L, Petersen RC, Jack CR Jr, Beckett LA, Aisen PS, Koeppe RA, et al. APOE effect on Alzheimer's disease biomarkers in older adults with significant memory concern. Alzheimers Dement. 2015;11(12):1417–29.
23. McLaren W, Pritchard B, Rios D, Chen Y, Flicek P, Cunningham F. Deriving the consequences of genomic variants with the Ensembl API and SNP effect predictor. Bioinformatics. 2010;26(16):2069–70.
24. Gamazon ER, Konkashbaev A, Derks EM, Cox NJ, Lee Y. Evidence of selection on splicing-associated loci in human populations and relevance to disease loci mapping. Sci Rep. 2017;7(1):5980.
25. Fujita PA, Rhead B, Zweig AS, Hinrichs AS, Karolchik D, Cline MS, Goldman M, Barber GP, Clawson H, Coelho A, et al. The UCSC genome browser database: update. Nucleic Acids Res. 2011;39(Database issue):D876–82.
26. Yeo G, Hoon S, Venkatesh B, Burge CB. Variation in sequence and organization of splicing regulatory elements in vertebrate genes. Proc Natl Acad Sci U S A. 2004;101(44):15700–5.
27. Kent WJ. BLAT--the BLAST-like alignment tool. Genome Res. 2002;12(4):656–64.
28. Lee S, Emond MJ, Bamshad MJ, Barnes KC, Rieder MJ, Nickerson DA, Team NGESP-ELP, Christiani DC, Wurfel MM, Lin X. Optimal unified approach for rare-variant association testing with application to small-sample case-control whole-exome sequencing studies. Am J Hum Genet. 2012;91(2):224–37.
29. Choi Y, Sims GE, Murphy S, Miller JR, Chan AP. Predicting the functional effect of amino acid substitutions and indels. PLoS One. 2012;7(10):e46688.
30. Choi Y. A fast computation of pairwise sequence alignment scores between a protein and a set of single-locus variants of another protein. In: Proceedings of the ACM conference on bioinformatics, computational biology and biomedicine. Orlando, Florida: ACM; 2012. p. 414–7.
31. Ng PC, Henikoff S. Predicting deleterious amino acid substitutions. Genome Res. 2001;11(5):863–74.
32. Martin-Urdiroz M, Deeks MJ, Horton CG, Dawe HR, Jourdain I. The exocyst complex in health and disease. Front Cell Dev Biol. 2016;4:24.
33. Wu B, Guo W. The exocyst at a glance. J Cell Sci. 2015;128(16):2957–64.
34. He B, Guo W. The exocyst complex in polarized exocytosis. Curr Opin Cell Biol. 2009;21(4):537–42.
35. Park SJ, Jung YJ, Kim YA, Lee-Kang JH, Lee KE. Glucose/oxygen deprivation and reperfusion upregulate SNAREs and complexin in organotypic hippocampal slice cultures. Neuropathology. 2008;28(6):612–20.
36. Moreau K, Renna M, Rubinsztein DC. Connections between SNAREs and autophagy. Trends Biochem Sci. 2013;38(2):57–63.
37. Zare-Shahabadi A, Masliah E, Johnson GV, Rezaei N. Autophagy in Alzheimer's disease. Rev Neurosci. 2015;26(4):385–95.
38. Nixon RA. The role of autophagy in neurodegenerative disease. Nat Med. 2013;19(8):983–97.

3

Comprehensive genomic diagnosis of non-syndromic and syndromic hereditary hearing loss in Spanish patients

Rubén Cabanillas[1*†], Marta Diñeiro[1†], Guadalupe A. Cifuentes[1], David Castillo[2], Patricia C. Pruneda[2], Rebeca Álvarez[1], Noelia Sánchez-Durán[1], Raquel Capín[1], Ana Plasencia[3], Mónica Viejo-Díaz[3], Noelia García-González[3], Inés Hernando[3], José L. Llorente[3], Alfredo Repáraz-Andrade[4], Cristina Torreira-Banzas[4], Jordi Rosell[5], Nancy Govea[5], Justo Ramón Gómez-Martínez[3], Faustino Núñez-Batalla[3], José A. Garrote[6], Ángel Mazón-Gutiérrez[7], María Costales[3,7], María Isidoro-García[8], Belén García-Berrocal[8], Gonzalo R. Ordóñez[2] and Juan Cadiñanos[1*] ⓘ

Abstract

Background: Sensorineural hearing loss (SNHL) is the most common sensory impairment. Comprehensive next-generation sequencing (NGS) has become the standard for the etiological diagnosis of early-onset SNHL. However, accurate selection of target genomic regions (gene panel/exome/genome), analytical performance and variant interpretation remain relevant difficulties for its clinical implementation.

Methods: We developed a novel NGS panel with 199 genes associated with non-syndromic and/or syndromic SNHL. We evaluated the analytical sensitivity and specificity of the panel on 1624 known single nucleotide variants (SNVs) and indels on a mixture of genomic DNA from 10 previously characterized lymphoblastoid cell lines, and analyzed 50 Spanish patients with presumed hereditary SNHL not caused by *GJB2/GJB6*, *OTOF* nor *MT-RNR1* mutations.

Results: The analytical sensitivity of the test to detect SNVs and indels on the DNA mixture from the cell lines was > 99.5%, with a specificity > 99.9%. The diagnostic yield on the SNHL patients was 42% (21/50): 47.6% (10/21) with autosomal recessive inheritance pattern (*BSND*, *CDH23*, *MYO15A*, *STRC* [n = 2], *USH2A* [n = 3], *RDX*, *SLC26A4*); 38.1% (8/21) autosomal dominant (*ACTG1* [n = 3; 2 de novo], *CHD7*, *GATA3* [de novo], *MITF*, *P2RX2*, *SOX10*), and 14.3% (3/21) X-linked (*COL4A5* [de novo], *POU3F4*, *PRPS1*). 46.9% of causative variants (15/32) were not in the databases. 28.6% of genetically diagnosed cases (6/21) had previously undetected syndromes (Barakat, Usher type 2A [n = 3] and Waardenburg [n = 2]). 19% of genetic diagnoses (4/21) were attributable to large deletions/duplications (*STRC* deletion [n = 2]; partial *CDH23* duplication; *RDX* exon 2 deletion).

Conclusions: In the era of precision medicine, obtaining an etiologic diagnosis of SNHL is imperative. Here, we contribute to show that, with the right methodology, NGS can be transferred to the clinical practice, boosting the yield of SNHL genetic diagnosis to 50–60% (including *GJB2/GJB6* alterations), improving diagnostic/prognostic accuracy, refining genetic and reproductive counseling and revealing clinically relevant undiagnosed syndromes.

Keywords: Hereditary, Hearing loss, Precision, Diagnostics, NGS, Gene panel

* Correspondence: rcabanillas@imoma.es; jcb@imoma.es
†Rubén Cabanillas and Marta Diñeiro contributed equally to this work.
[1]Instituto de Medicina Oncológica y Molecular de Asturias (IMOMA) S. A,
Avda. Richard Grandío s/n, 33193 Oviedo, Spain
Full list of author information is available at the end of the article

Background

Congenital profound deafness affects ~ 1 in 1000 live births and an additional 1 in 1000 children will suffer from hearing loss (HL) before becoming adult [1]. Up to 60% of congenital/early-onset sensorineural HL (SNHL) is caused by genetic factors and often appears in the absence of a family history for deafness. Although alterations in the *GJB2* and *GJB6* genes *(DNFB1* locus) account for a large proportion of cases in different populations (10–40%) [2, 3], many cases remain undiagnosed after *GJB2/GJB6* testing. This is not surprising given the extreme genetic and phenotypic heterogeneity of HL, with more than 400 syndromes that include HL as a feature and more than 100 genes associated with nonsyndromic SNHL [1]. With next-generation sequencing (NGS) technology, it has become feasible and affordable to routinely sequence a large number of genes per patient [4]. Therefore, genetic diagnosis of SNHL has evolved from single-mutation Sanger sequencing to comprehensive multi-gene testing, and NGS has become the new standard of care [5].

Accordingly, once a case of newborn SNHL is confirmed, testing for congenital cytomegalovirus infection and NGS are recommended [6]. Obtaining a SNHL genetic diagnosis has a number of advantages for patients and parents [7]: it provides information about genetic heritability; it helps diagnosing or excluding syndromic causes of HL to better define medical and educational needs; it can also provide information about the evolution of the HL and/ or of its associated syndromic features, improving prognostic accuracy; and it can prevent other unnecessary and costly testing [5]. Furthermore, a genetic diagnosis can contribute to prevent triggers such as aminoglycosides in mitochondrial mutation carriers [8], or even to improve treatment selection, including future mutation-driven clinical trials [9, 10].

In order to implement targeted NGS into the clinical practice, there is an urgent need to solve a number of issues such as the selection of the most efficient gene panel, the achievement of high analytical specificity and sensitivity, and the establishment of pipelines able to unambiguously define the clinical impact of genetic variants [11]. Therefore, the aims of this study are: (1) to present the development and validation of a NGS-based approach for the genetic diagnosis of patients with hereditary syndromic and non-syndromic SNHL; (2) to pinpoint and resolve the main problems associated with the introduction of targeted NGS into routine deafness diagnostics; (3) to evaluate the panel's performance and diagnostic yield; and (4) to initiate a comprehensive catalogue of the Spanish genome-wide SNHL variation spectrum.

Methods

Purpose of test

The aim of the performed test (OTOgenics™) was to detect the molecular basis of individual clinical diagnoses of sensorineural or mixed hearing loss after non-genetic causes had been explored and not identified.

Design of panel content: Rationale for inclusion of specific genes

Genes associated with prelingual, postlingual and adult-onset sensorineural or mixed HL, either symmetric or asymmetric, irrespective of the pattern of inheritance, and including both syndromic and non-syndromic forms, were considered. To generate a preliminary gene list, the professional version of the Human Gene Mutation Database (HGMD) was queried to identify genes associated to HL, using as search keywords a list of phenotypes potentially related to hearing defects (Additional file 1). The resulting gene list was manually curated by analysis of the literature and information available in the databases (HGMD, OMIM, PubMed, GeneReviews, and the Hereditary Hearing Loss Homepage; last accessed 19/09/2017) to identify those fulfilling the following criteria: I) the gene had been associated to sensorineural and/or mixed HL phenotypes (as opposed to exclusively conductive HL), II) there existed published evidence supporting the gene-phenotype association in at least two independent families and III) at least one of the existing publications demonstrated convincing cosegregation of phenotype with gene variants. Based on the curation results, a tiered classification system was devised as previously proposed by Abou Tayoun et al. [11]. Genes with strong/moderate association with HL (fulfilling criteria I, II and III described above, and corresponding mainly to Evidence level 3 according to Abou Tayoun et al. [11]) formed tier 1, while genes with weak/preliminary association (fulfilling criterion I, but not criteria II and/or III, and corresponding mainly to Evidence level 2 according to Abou Tayoun et al. [11]) were grouped in tier 2. The panel evolved with revision of newly published literature, yielding versions v1, v2 and v3 (Additional file 2, Additional file 3 and Table 1, respectively). v1–2 were used during the research and development phase of the study, whereas v3 was considered the first clinical-grade version of the panel. 32 cases were analyzed with v1, 13 with v2 and 5 with v3 (Additional file 4).

Sample types

4 ml of peripheral blood in conventional EDTA-tubes or ≥ 200 ng of germline genomic DNA (quantitated by a fluorimetric method) were required per patient.

Sample preparation and evaluation of genomic DNA integrity

Germline genomic DNA was isolated as previously described [12] and calculation of its DNA integrity number (DIN) was performed using the Genomic DNA ScreenTape Assay on a TapeStation 4200 system (Agilent Technologies,

Table 1 Tier 1 and tier 2 genes included in the OTOgenics™ panel (v3)

Tier 1 (154 genes): genes with strong/moderate association with SNHL[#]

ABHD12 NM_001042472.2	BSND NM_057176.2	CLRN1 NM_174878.2	DIABLO NM_019887.5	FTO NM_001080432.2	HSD17B4 NM_000414.3	MARVELD2 NM_001038603.2	MYO3A NM_017433.4	P2RX2 NM_174873.2	PTPN11 NM_002834.3	SLC52A3 NM_033409.3	TMIE NM_147196.2
ACTB NM_001101.3	CABP2 NM_016366.2	COCH NM_004086.2	DIAPH1 NM_005219.4	GATA3 NM_001002295.1	ILDR1 NM_001199799.1	MASP1 NM_139125.3	MYO6 NM_004999.3	PAX3 NM_181457.3	PTPRQ NM_001145026.1	SLITRK6 NM_032229.2	TMPRSS3 NM_024022.2
ACTG1 NM_001614.3	CACNA1D NM_000720.3	COL2A1 NM_001844.4	DNMT1 NM_001130823.1	GIPC3 NM_133261.2	KARS NM_001130089.1	MIR96 NR_029512.1	MYO7A NM_000260.3	PCDH15 NM_033056.3	RAF1 NM_002880.3	SMPX NM_014332.2	TPRN NM_001128228.2
ADGRV1 NM_032119.3	CCDC50 NM_178335.2	COL4A3 NM_000091.4	ECHS1 NM_004092.3	GJB2 NM_004004.5	KCNE1 NM_000219.5	MITF NM_000248.3	MYO15A NM_016239.3	PDZD7 NM_001195263.1	RDX NM_002906.3	SNAI2 NM_003068.4	TRIOBP NM_001039141.2
AIFM1 NM_004208.3	CDH23 NM_022124.5	COL4A4 NM_000092.4	EDN3 NM_207034.2	GJB3 NM_024009.2	KCNJ10 NM_002241.4	MSRB3 NM_198080.3	NARS2 NM_024678.5	PEX1 NM_000466.2	RMND1 NM_017909.3	SOX10 NM_006941.3	TSPEAR NM_144991.2
ALMS1 NM_015120.4	CEACAM16 NM_001039213.3	COL4A5 NM_000495.4	EDNRB NM_000115.3	GJB6 NM_006783.4	KCNQ1 NM_000218.2	MT-CO1 NC_012920.1	NDP NM_000266.3	PEX2 NM_000318.2	SERAC1 NM_032861.3	SPATA5 NM_145207.2	USH1C NM_005709.3
ANKH NM_054027.4	CHD7 NM_017780.3	COL9A1 NM_001851.4	EPS8L2 NM_022772.3	GPSM2 NM_013296.4	KCNQ4 NM_004700.3	MT-RNR1 NC_012920.1	NLRP3 NM_004895.4	PEX3 NM_003630.2	SERPINB6 NM_004568.5	STRC NM_153700.2	USH1G NM_173477.4
AP1S1 NM_001283.3	CIB2 NM_006383.3	COL11A1 NM_001854.3	ESPN NM_031475.2	GRHL2 NM_024915.3	LARS2 NM_015340.3	MT-TH NC_012920.1	OPA1 NM_015560.2	PEX5 NM_001131025.1	SIX1 NM_005982.3	SYNE4 NM_001039876.1	USH2A NM_206933.2
ATP1A3 NM_152296.4	CISD2 NM_001008388.4	COL11A2 NM_080680.2	ESRRB NM_004452.3	GRXCR1 NM_001080476.2	LHFPL5 NM_182548.3	MT-TK NC_012920.1	OSBPL2 NM_144498.2	PEX6 NM_000287.3	SLC17A8 NM_139319.2	TBC1D24 NM_001199107.1	WFS1 NM_006005.3
ATP6V1B1 NM_001692.3	CLCNKA NM_004070.3	DCAF17 NM_025000.3	EYA1 NM_000503.5	HARS2 NM_012208.3	LHX3 NM_014564.3	MT-TL1 NC_012920.1	OTOA NM_144672.3	PEX26 NM_017929.5	SLC19A2 NM_006996.2	TECTA NM_005422.2	WHRN NM_015404.3
BCAP31 NM_001139441.1	CLCNKB NM_000085.4	DDX11 NM_030653.3	EYA4 NM_004100.4	HGF NM_000601.4	LOXHD1 NM_144612.6	MT-TS1 NC_012920.1	OTOF NM_194248.2	POU3F4 NM_000307.4	SLC26A4 NM_000441.1	TIMM8A NM_004085.3	XYLT2 NM_022167.3
BCS1L NM_004328.4	CLDN14 NM_144492.2	DFNA5 NM_004403.2	FGF3 NM_005247.2	HOXA1 NM_005522.4	LRP2 NM_004525.2	MYH9 NM_002473.5	OTOG NM_001277269.1	POU4F3 NM_002700.2	SLC33A1 NM_004733.3	TJP2 NM_004817.3	
BRAF NM_004333.4	CLPP NM_006012.2	DFNB59 NM_001042517.1	FGFR3 NM_000142.4	HOXB1 NM_002144.3	LRTOMT NM_001145308.4	MYH14 NM_024729.3	OTOGL NM_173591.3	PRPS1 NM_002764.3	SLC52A2 NM_024531.4	TMC1 NM_138691.2	

Tier 2 (45 genes): genes with weak/preliminary association with SNHL[#]

ADCY1 NM_021116.2	COL4A6 NM_001847.3	CRYM NM_001888.4	ELMOD3 NM_032213.4	FGFR1 NM_023110.2	GTF2IRD1 NM_016328.2	KITLG NM_000899.4	NDUFA13 NM_015965.6	SIX5 NM_175875.4	TK2 NM_004614.4	TP63 NM_003722.4
ATP2B2 NM_001683.3	COL9A2 NM_001852.3	DCDC2 NM_016356.4	EPS8 NM_004447.5	FGFR2 NM_000141.4	HMX2 NM_005519.1	MAF NM_005360.4	NFIX NM_001271043.2	SLC4A11 NM_032034.3	TMEM132E NM_001304438.1	
ATP6V1B2 NM_001693.3	COL9A3 NM_001853.3	DIAPH3 NM_001042517.1	FAM65B NM_014722.3	FOXI1 NM_012188.4	HMX3 NM_001105574.1	MARS2 NM_138395.3	PNPT1 NM_033109.4	SLC9A1 NM_003047.4	TMPRSS5 NM_030770.3	
BDP1 NM_018429.2	COQ6 NM_182476.2	DSPP NM_014208.3	FBLN1 NM_006486.2	GRXCR2 NM_001080516.1	HOMER2 NM_004839.3	MCM2 NM_004526.3	SEMA3E NM_012431.2	SLC26A5 NM_198999.2	TNC NM_002160.3	

[#]Sensorineural hearing loss

Santa Clara, CA, USA), following the manufacturer's instructions.

Library preparation, target enrichment and sequencing

Library preparation was performed on genomic DNA physically sheared by ultrasonication on a Covaris S2 instrument (Covaris, MA, USA). For library construction and gene target enrichment by hybrid capture, the SureSelectXT protocol was followed, as previously described [12]. This approach has a series of advantages over other library construction and target enrichment methods. Thus, libraries from randomly fragmented DNA show higher complexities than PCR-based ones, enabling the identification and removal of PCR duplicates (important for the accurate identification of low frequency variants present in mosaic patients) [13]. Additionally, capture probes, although laborious to use, are more tolerant to mismatches than PCR primers, circumventing issues of allelic dropout (underrepresentation or absence of an existing allele in the library) caused by polymorphisms in the hybridization sequence that can be observed in amplification-based assays [13]. Finally, capturing and sequencing at least all coding exons of every targeted gene, and not just hotspots, facilitates creating background references for CNV calling. Sequencing was performed on a NextSeq500 sequencer (Illumina, CA, USA), following the manufacturers specifications. The optimized NGS diagnostic pipeline (OTOgenics™) targets the coding exons and intron-exon junctions of 199 genes (v3) (Table 1).

Bioinformatics for variant identification and annotation

NGS results were processed using the bioinformatics software HD Genome One (DREAMgenics, Oviedo, Spain), certified with IVD/CE-marking. The pipeline has been adapted from the one previously described as part of the ONCOgenics NGS platform [12], the performance of which has been externally evaluated through participation in the Oncogene Panel Testing schemes organized by the European Molecular Genetics Quality Network (EMQN), obtaining satisfactory results (maximum genotyping score) for three consecutive years (2015, 2016 and 2017). The analysis workflow was at follows:

FASTQ read generation, alignment and duplicate removal

FASTQ reads were generated from base call files (BCL) produced by the Illumina NextSeq500 sequencing platform using the bcl2fastq2 v2.19 Conversion Software (https://support.illumina.com/sequencing/sequencing_software/bcl2fastq-conversion-software.html). Raw FASTQ files were evaluated using quality control checks from FastQC (http://www.bioinformatics.babraham.ac.uk/projects/fastqc/) and Trimmomatic was employed to remove low quality bases, adapters and other technical sequences. Each FASTQ file was aligned to the human reference genome (GRCh37/

hg19 before 2017; GRCh38/hg38 afterwards) using BWA-mem [14] generating sorted BAM files with SAMtools [15]. Reads from the same libraries were then merged and optical and PCR duplicates were removed using Picard (http://broadinstitute.github.io/picard/).

SNV/Indel identification

SNVs and indels were identified using a variation of Sidrón algorithm, previously described [16], with the following parameters: total read depth ≥ 6, mutated allele count ≥3, variant frequency ≥ 0.1, base quality ≥20, mapping quality ≥30. Stricter criteria (total read depth ≥ 10, mutated allele count ≥4) were applied before the selection of reportable variants. Manual inspection was then carried out to discard false positives and avoid missing true variants not meeting those criteria (i.e long indels with underestimated frequencies).

CNV identification

The detection of CNVs was performed with an adapted version of the exome2cnv algorithm, incorporating a combination of read depth and allelic imbalance computations for copy number assessment. The algorithm employs a background of pooled samples processed using the same capturing protocol and sequencing technology [12, 17]. For increased sensitivity in the detection of large homozygous deletions, genomic regions with no sequencing coverage in an individual sample, but showing proper coverages in the remaining samples, were identified.

Variant annotation

Variants were annotated using several databases containing functional (Ensembl, CCDS, RefSeq, Pfam), populational (dbSNP, 1000 Genomes, ESP6500, ExAC) and disease-related (Clinvar, HGMD professional) information, as well as 12 scores from algorithms for prediction of the impact caused by nonsynonymous variants on the structure and function of the protein (SIFT [18], Poly-Phen2 [19], PROVEAN [20], Mutation Assessor [21], Mutation Taster [22], LRT [23], MetaLR, MetaSVM [24], FATHMM, FATHMM-MKL [25] and M-CAP [26]), and 1 score (GERP++) for evolutionary conservation of the affected nucleotide [27].

Analytical sensitivity and specificity

The analytical sensitivity and specificity of our panel to detect SNVs/indels was calculated using the v3 probe set to evaluate 1624 total variants (1503 SNVs + 121 indels) with allelic frequency ≥ 0.1, following a procedure similar to that previously described [12]. Briefly, 10 immortal lymphoblastoid cell lines, corresponding to 10 individuals whose genomes/exomes had been sequenced by the 1000 Genomes and HapMap projects, were obtained from the Coriell Institute: NA20298 (ASW), NA12872 (CEU), NA18570 (CHB), HG00320 (FIN), HG00110 (GBR), A18960 (JPT), NA19020

Comprehensive genomic diagnosis of nonsyndromic and syndromic hereditary hearing loss in Spanish...

19

(LWK), NA19794 (MXL), HG00740 (PUR) and NA18486 (YRI). Cell lines were cultured according to the protocols provided by Coriell, their DNAs isolated and mixed in equimolecular amounts. An NGS library was prepared, captured using the custom probe and sequenced in 20% of a NextSeq500 MidOutput run (2×75 sequencing cycles). Variants were called as described in the previous section and the results compared to those expected according to the genomic information available for these cell lines.

Interfering highly homologous regions

Regions with < 100% callability at DP20 (i.e. with less than 100% of the target bases covered by ≥20 reads) in > 50% of v3 cases were considered as potential conflictive regions (Additional file 5). Those showing high homology to at least another region of the GRCh38 human reference genome are listed in Additional file 6. Realignment of the NGS results with reference sequences containing only the panel genes affected by these conflictive regions was performed, as previously described for the *PMS2* gene [12], followed by validation, using gene-specific analyses (i.e. Long-Range PCR followed by Sanger sequencing) of putative pathogenic/likely pathogenic SNV and indel variants [28].

Variant filtering, interpretation, classification and diagnostic yield

Database resources to evaluate gene variants included HGMD professional, OMIM, PubMed, dbSNP, 1000 Genomes Project, ESP, ExAC, and ClinVar. A minor allele frequency (MAF) cut-off of 5% was applied to variants considered as pathogenic (DM) by HGMD or as pathogenic/likely pathogenic by ClinVar, as well as to those variants predicted to create a null allele (nonsense, frameshift causing premature STOP codons, canonical splicing-site disruption, ATG-loss and complete exon deletions/duplications). A MAF cut-off of 1%, as suggested by Shearer et al. [29], was applied to all other variants predicted to affect the sequence/expression of the protein (for protein-coding genes) or of the RNA (for non-coding genes).

Clinical classification of all variants from v1 and v2 cases was performed as described [12]. For v3 cases, only variants that could potentially explain the SNHL phenotype of the probands, based on zygosity of the variant, presence of additional variants on the same gene and mode of inheritance of the audiologic phenotypes associated to the gene, were further considered. After that, variants were clinically classified according to the American College of Medical Genetics and Genomics (ACMG) guidelines as pathogenic (class 5), likely pathogenic (class 4), uncertain significance (class 3), likely benign (class 2) and benign (class 1) [30]. Class 3–5 variants were thoroughly curated searching the literature and databases for clinically relevant data. Class 3–5 variants were reported for tier 1 genes. To reduce the interpretation burden of tier 2 genes, only class 4–5 variants affecting genes whose associated putative phenotype matched the patient's phenotype were evaluated and reported.

Diagnostic yield (generally described as the likelihood that a test or procedure will provide the information needed to establish a diagnosis) was defined as the percentage of tested patients with pathogenic/likely pathogenic variants capable of explaining their HL phenotype.

Variant validation

Pathogenic/likely pathogenic variants considered responsible for SNHL were validated by approaches alternative to NGS. SNVs/indels were validated by PCR + Sanger sequencing. For validation and breakpoint identification of the partial *CDH23* duplication (exons 11–15) and the *RDX* exon 2 deletion multiple PCR reactions were performed. *STRC* CNVs were validated with a qPCR assay able to distinguish *STRC* from the *pSTRC* pseudogene [28] as well as by MLPA (MRC-Holland, Amsterdam, The Netherlands; cat.# P64-DIS). Primers used in validation PCRs are described in Additional file 7). Segregation was determined in 8/8 (100%) relatives with available biospecimens.

Reportable range

Reportable variants had to be supported by ≥4 independent reads, with a total read depth ≥ 10, belonging to genes from Tier 1 (consistently associated) and showing allelic frequencies in the sample ≥ 0.1. Variants considered responsible or likely responsible for the phenotype of the patient additionally needed to have been validated by a method alternative to NGS to be considered reportable. Occasionally, a variant from a Tier 2 gene fulfilling all other criteria could be reportable, as long as the phenotype of the patient was compatible with the phenotype considered in the existing publications supporting the gene-phenotype association of the Tier 2 gene.

Reference range

Only variants consistent with the mode of inheritance of the auditory phenotypes associated with the gene they affect (for instance, biallelic variants on a gene with a recessive phenotype) were evaluated according to ACMG/AMP guidelines and their resulting clinical classification was reported [30]. For those classified as pathogenic, likely pathogenic or VUS, additional information supporting their clinical classification was provided. Those classified as benign or likely benign were considered to lay within the reference range of results and, thus, no further details about them were provided. The remaining variants (not consistent with the mode of inheritance of the auditory phenotypes associated with the genes they affect) were included in the reports for informative purposes but were not considered responsible for the patient's phenotype.

Sample tracking

A series of 6 SNPs on Tier 1 genes, with population MAFs between 0.463 and 0.483, were selected for sample tracking: rs10864198 on *USH2A* (MAF = 0.4531; ExAC); rs7598901 on *ALMS1* (MAF = 0.4736, 1000 Genomes); rs2228557 on *COL4A4* (MAF = 0.4657; ExAC), rs7624750 on *OPA1* (MAF = 0.4683; ExAC), rs734312 on *WFS1* (MAF = 0.4633; ExAC), and rs2438349 on *ADGRV1* (MAF = 0.4830; ExAC). The genotypes identified by the NGS pipeline were compared to those obtained from the corresponding TaqMan qPCR genotyping assays (cat #: C_31803731_10, C_29307975_10, C_11523965_10, C_2715859_10, C_2401729_1 and C_16236492_10, respectively; Applied Biosystems, CA, USA) run on a 7900HT Fast Real-Time PCR System (Applied Biosystems, CA, USA). All samples showed coincident genotypes for all SNPs on both platforms.

Patient population

Between September 2014 and March 2017, 50 consecutive patients (21 male, 29 female) with syndromic/non-syndromic SNHL were selected after excluding non-genetic causes and causative variants in the *DFNB1 (GJB2/GJB6)*, *OTOF* and *MT-RNR1* loci, considered the most frequent causes of hereditary deafness in Spain [7, 31]. Consent was obtained from patients or their parents. The study was approved by the Comité de Ética de Investigación del Principado de Asturias (research project #75/14). The ages at SNHL onset ranged between 0 to 47 years (median: 12 years). 20 cases (40%) were congenital. To identify syndromic SNHL, a clinical geneticist evaluated the patients. 2/50 patients were diagnosed (pre-test) of Alport and CHARGE syndromes. Other 3 patients presented with potentially syndromic complications, without fulfilling criteria for known syndromes.

Results

Panel validation

Performance of targeted NGS

Mean coverage of tier 1 genes was 445× for v1, 515× for v2 and 1121× for v3, and 98.87, 99.56 and 99.95% of their target bases were covered by 20 or more reads, respectively (these calculations exclude the *STRC* and *OTOA* genes due to their high homology to other genomic regions). The minimum, average and maximum coverage (average read depth of all target bases of the gene) and callabilities (% of the target bases of the gene with minimum read depths of 10, 20, 50 and 100 reads per each target base of the gene) for every tier 1 and tier 2 gene on samples analysed with OTOgenics v3 is shown in Additional file 5. In v3 cases, regions from tier 1 genes with less than 100% coverage with a minimum of 20 reads (DP20) and specific positions within those regions affected by such limitation were included in each individual patient's report.

Analytical sensitivity and specificity

Prior to its use in the diagnostic setting, the clinical version of the panel (v3) was evaluated for sensitivity and specificity on a genotyped mixture of 10 lymphoblastoid cell lines. 1617/1624 variants with allele frequency ≥ 0.1 were detected (1497/1503 SNVs and 120/121 indels), yielding a sensitivity of 0.9957 (> 99.5%). Additionally, 1,034,047/1034817 true negative positions of the target region were called by the platform as not bearing SNVs or indels, representing a specificity of 0.9992 (> 99.9%).

Orthogonal validation of sequencing results

All variants considered responsible for the SNHL phenotypes of the probands (Table 2) were successfully validated by approaches alternative to NGS. These included 25 instances of SNVs or indels (validated by PCR and Sanger sequencing) and 4 CNVs: 1 heterozygous partial duplication of *CDH23* (exons 11–15), 1 homozygous deletion of *RDX* exon 2 (both validated by breakpoint-specific PCR) and 2 homozygous *STRC* whole gene deletions (validated by qPCR and MLPA). Apart from these, 4 samples had heterozygous *STRC* CNVs (3 deletions and 1 duplication) all of which were validated by qPCR and MLPA (Additional file 8). These results indicate that our CNV calling procedure is highly specific.

Performance at interfering highly homologous regions

Genomic regions with high sequence homology cause misalignment of sequencing data and represent a major challenge for short-read NGS technologies. Out of the 199 genes included in the v3 panel, *STRC*, *OTOA*, *ESPN* and *KCNE1* contain a total of 22 interfering highly homologous regions (as defined in the Methods section), most of which overlap with those previously identified by Mandelker et al. [32] (Additional file 6). To avoid missing clinically relevant variants present in those target regions, the panel NGS reads from all samples were realigned to reference sequences containing only the *STRC*, *OTOA*, *ESPN* and *KCNE1* loci, as previously described by us for the *PMS2* gene in a cancer panel [12]. This approach revealed that all samples might potentially carry a pathogenic variant in the *STRC* gene: c.4057C > T, p.Gln1353* (coincident with the reference sequence for exon 20 from the *pSTRC* pseudogene). To unequivocally discriminate the origin of this variant, LR-PCR specific for the *STRC* gene followed by Sanger sequencing was performed as described [28]. This approach discarded the potential genic origin of the variant in 28/50 samples; not enough DNA was available from 1 sample and no LR-PCR product was obtained from 21. Of note, the average genomic DNA Integrity Number (DIN) of the 28 samples with successful LR-PCR was significantly higher than that of the remaining 21 samples (8.71 vs 7.21; *p*-value = 1.8×10^{-4}; Student's T test), suggesting that DNA degradation precluded LR-PCR. Alternative approaches would be needed to discard or confirm the genic origin of the variant in those 21 samples.

Analysis of causative variants and diagnostic yield

Of 50 cases with severe-to-profound SNHL not caused by *GJB2/GJB6*, *OTOF* or *MT-RNR1* mutations, a genetic justification for their HL phenotype was found in 21 (42%) after identifying 31 pathogenic/likely pathogenic variants in 16 genes: *ACTG1*, *BSND*, *CDH23*, *CHD7*, *COL4A5*, *GATA3*, *MITF*, *MYO15A*, *P2RX2*, *POU3F4*, *PRPS1*, *RDX*, *SLC26A4*, *SOX10*, *STRC* and *USH2A* (Tables 2 and 3). Three more cases had recessive variants of uncertain significance in homozygosis (affecting the *LOXHD1* and *SLC26A4* genes) or in hemizygosis (affecting the *OTOA* gene: 1 SNV + heterozygous whole-gene *OTOA* deletion), which were suspicious of pathogenicity, but did not fulfill ACMG criteria and, thus, were not counted nor reported as positives (Table 4). Had they been counted, the diagnostic yield would have been 48% (24/50).

In our cohort, 47.6% (10/21) of the unambiguously molecularly diagnosed patients had autosomal recessive (AR) inheritance patterns, 38.1% (8/21) autosomal dominant (AD), and 14.3% (3/21) were X-linked (Table 2). The molecular basis of deafness was found in 44.4% (20/45) of the cases with symmetric SNHL, whereas only 1 of 5 cases with asymmetric SNHL was genetically diagnosed (Waardenburg syndrome caused by a *MITF* mutation) (Tables 2 and 3).

The most common SNHL causative genes in our prescreened population were *ACTG1* (3 patients), *USH2A* (3 patients) and *STRC* (2 patients). Interestingly, 2 of 3 pathogenic variants in *ACTG1* were de novo, as well as 1 *GATA3* and 1 *COL4A5* pathogenic variants.

CNV analysis identified causative variants in 4 of the 21 molecularly diagnosed patients (19%): 2 with a homozygous complete *STRC* deletion, 1 with a previously unreported partial *CDH23* duplication (exons 11–15) in compound heterozygosity with a second pathogenic variant (missense), and 1 with a homozygous *RDX* exon 2 deletion. One of the patients with a homozygous causative *STRC* deletion was also a carrier of a heterozygous substitution in *TECTA*, previously reported in the literature as a dominant pathogenic variant (c.3107G > A; p.Cys1036Tyr) [33]. However, reevaluation of this variant according to ACMG guidelines reclassified it as a variant of uncertain significance (it only fulfilled ACMG pathogenicity criteria PP1 and PP3).

In total, 451 variants, of which 406 were unique, in 121 distinct genes were identified in the full cohort of 50 patients: 394 variants in 97 genes were identified in tier 1. Tier 2 added 57 variants that contributed to the overall interpretation burden. No tier 2 variant was considered responsible for the SNHL phenotype (Fig. 1).

199/394 (50.5%) and 45/57 (78.9%) of the identified tier 1 and tier 2 variants, respectively, were absent from the

databases (HGMD professional and ClinVar). Fifteen of them (all from tier 1), were classified as pathogenic or likely pathogenic and responsible for the SNHL phenotype of the patient (Fig. 1). Globally, those 15 variants were considered responsible for the SNHL phenotype in 13 cases. As a result, 61.9% of the genetically diagnosed cases (13/21) were explained by variants not described in the databases (Fig. 2 and Table 2). Moreover, of 25 non-redundant variants classified as pathogenic (DM) by HGMD for hearing-related phenotypes, after looking for plausible published support in the literature, solid evidence could only be found for 13 of them (52%) (Additional file 9). Of the 12 variants considered DM by HGMD but, in our view, without enough supporting evidence, 3 (25%) were also considered as Pathogenic/Likely pathogenic by at least one ClinVar submitter (Additional file 9). To deal with these limitations, an average of 40 min of expert review was dedicated per variant. With an average of 9 variants per case, this represents 360 min (6 h) per case. These results highlight the importance of manual interpretation and curation for clinical classification of variants, even for those considered as (potentially) disease causing by reputable databases.

Increase of clinical sensitivity by analysis of syndromic genes on apparently non-syndromic SNHL

28.6% of the genetically diagnosed cases (6/21) had a previously unrecognized syndrome: Barakat (1 patient), Usher type 2A (3 patients) and Waardenburg (2 patients) (Table 2). These unexpected syndromic findings not only increased the diagnostic yield, but they provided diagnostics of utmost clinical relevance. Additionally, 6 patients carried pathogenic variants in genes associated with syndromic and non-syndromic conditions (Table 2): 1 had variants associated with Pendred syndrome and DFNB4, 1 with Bartter syndrome type IV and DFNB73, 1 with Usher syndrome 1D and DFNB12 and 3 with Baraitser-Winter type 2 and DFNA20/DFNA26. These patients will need close follow-up in case syndromic features develop.

Discussion

Hearing loss is one of the most genetically heterogeneous disorders known. 60% of cases are believed to be of genetic origin and 30% of them syndromic [34]. Due to its high diagnostic yield [35, 36], the newest ACMG guidelines include NGS testing in the standard SNHL diagnostic algorithm [1], whereas the use of non-genetic tests should be considered case-by-case, usually as a complement to genetic testing. However, except for the preeminent relevance of *GJB2* mutations, little is known about the frequency of SNHL variants in Europeans [9, 37].

Our results contribute to define the mutation spectra in the Spanish population, underlining the SNHL genetic heterogeneity, as the causative variants of 21 patients affected 16 different genes. The genes most commonly altered in

Table 2 Clinical and genetic characteristics of cases with causative mutations

Case ID	Pre-test phenotype	Pre-test suspected inheritance pattern	Time of deafness onset	Gene	Allele variants	Variant zygosity	ACMG[a] classification[30]	Fulfilled ACMG[a] pathogenicity criteria[30]	Present in HGMD and/or ClinVar[b]	Gene-associated phenotypes	Inheritance patterns of gene-associated phenotypes	Hidden syndrome
OTO.008	Bilateral non-syndromic sensorineural deafness	AR	Congenital	MYO15A	c.8050 T > C p.(Tyr2684His)	Heterozygous	Likely pathogenic	PM2, PM3, PP1, PP3	Yes	Non-syndromic sensorineural deafness (DFNB3)	AR	No
					c.8968-1G > T	Heterozygous	Pathogenic	PVS1, PM2, PP1	No			
OTO.001	Bilateral non-syndromic sensorineural deafness	AR	Congenital	STRC	Whole-gene deletion	Homozygous	Pathogenic	PVS1, PM2, PM3	Yes	Non-syndromic sensorineural deafness (DFNB16)	AR	No
OTO.033	Bilateral non-syndromic sensorineural deafness	AR	Childhood	STRC	Whole-gene deletion	Homozygous	Pathogenic	PVS1, PM2, PM3	Yes	Non-syndromic sensorineural deafness (DFNB16)	AR	No
OTO.050	Bilateral non-syndromic sensorineural deafness	AD / AR	Childhood	RDX	Exon 2 deletion	Homozygous	Likely pathogenic	PVS1, PM2	No	Non-syndromic sensorineural deafness (DFNB24)	AR	No
OTO.009	Bilateral non-syndromic sensorineural deafness	AR	Congenital	BSND	c.23G > A p.(Arg8Gln)	Homozygous	Likely pathogenic	PM1, PM2, PM5, PP3	No	Non-syndromic sensorineural deafness (DFNB73) / Bartter syndrome type IV	AR	Potential
OTO.006	Bilateral non-syndromic sensorineural deafness	AR	Childhood	SLC26A4	c.412G > T p.(Val138Phe)	Heterozygous	Pathogenic	PS3, PS(PM3), PP3	Yes	Non-syndromic sensorineural deafness (DFNB4) / Pendred syndrome	AR	Potential
					c.1370A > T p.(Asn457Ile)	Heterozygous	Likely pathogenic	PM1, PM2, PM3, PP3	Yes			
OTO.018	Bilateral non-syndromic sensorineural deafness	AR	Congenital	CDH23	c.4488G > C p.(Gln1496His)	Heterozygous	Pathogenic	PS3, PM2, PM3, PP1, PP3	Yes	Non-syndromic sensorineural deafness (DFNB12) / Usher syndrome type 1D	AR	Potential
					Duplication of exons 11–15	Heterozygous	Likely pathogenic	PM2, PM3, PM4	No			
OTO.004	Bilateral non-syndromic sensorineural deafness	AR	Childhood	USH2A	c.11864G > A p.(Trp3955*)	Homozygous	Pathogenic	PVS1, PS(PM3)	Yes	Usher syndrome type 2A	AR	Yes
OTO.005	Bilateral non-syndromic sensorineural deafness	AR	Congenital	USH2A	c.1724G > A p.(Cys575Tyr)	Homozygous	Likely pathogenic	PS(PM3), PM2, PP3	Yes	Usher syndrome type 2A	AR	Yes
OTO.014	Bilateral non-syndromic sensorineural deafness	AR	Congenital	USH2A	c.1724G > A p.(Cys575Tyr)	Heterozygous	Likely pathogenic	PS(PM3), PM2, PP3	Yes	Usher syndrome type 2A	AR	Yes
					c.1841-2A > G	Heterozygous	Pathogenic		Yes			

Table 2 Clinical and genetic characteristics of cases with causative mutations (Continued)

Case ID	Pre-test phenotype	Pre-test suspected inheritance pattern	Time of deafness onset	Gene	Allele variants	Variant zygosity	ACMG[a] classification[30]	Fulfilled ACMG[a] pathogenicity criteria[30]	Present in HGMD and/or ClinVar[b]	Gene-associated phenotypes	Inheritance patterns of gene-associated phenotypes	Hidden syndrome
								PVS1, PS(PM3), PS3, PM2				
OTO.003	Bilateral non-syndromic sensorineural deafness	AD	Childhood	P2RX2	c.178G > T p.(Val60Leu)	Heterozygous	Likely pathogenic	PS3, PM2, PP1	Yes	Non-syndromic sensorineural deafness (DFNA41)	AD	No
OTO.043	Bilateral non-syndromic sensorineural deafness	AD	Congenital	ACTG1	c.434C > G p.(Ser145Cys)	Heterozygous	Likely pathogenic	PM1, PM2, PP2, PP3	No	Non-syndromic sensorineural deafness (DFNA20/DFNA26) / Baraitser-Winter syndrome type 2	AD	Potential
OTO.023	Bilateral non-syndromic sensorineural deafness	AR	Childhood	ACTG1	c.548G > A p.(Arg183Gln)	Heterozygous	Likely pathogenic	PS2, PP(PM2), PP2, PP3	No	Non-syndromic sensorineural deafness (DFNA20/DFNA26) / Baraitser-Winter syndrome type 2	AD (de novo)	Potential
OTO.041	Bilateral non-syndromic sensorineural deafness	AR	Childhood	ACTG1	c.848 T > C p.(Met283Thr)	Heterozygous	Likely pathogenic	PS2, PM2, PP2	No	Non-syndromic sensorineural deafness (DFNA20/DFNA26) / Baraitser-Winter syndrome type 2	AD (de novo)	Potential
OTO.011	Unilateral non-syndromic sensorineural deafness	AD	Childhood	MITF	c.909G > A p.(Thr303Thr)	Heterozygous	Likely pathogenic	PS3, PM2, PP1	Yes	Waardenburg syndrome type 2A	AD	Yes
OTO.051	Bilateral non-syndromic sensorineural deafness	AR	Congenital	SOX10	c.135_154del p.(Ser45Argfs*15)	Heterozygous	Likely pathogenic	PVS1, PM2, PP3	No	Waardenburg syndrome type 2E	AD	Yes
OTO.019	Bilateral non-syndromic sensorineural deafness	AR	Congenital	GATA3	c.1018A > C p.(Asn340His)	Heterozygous	Likely pathogenic	PM1, PM2, PM6, PP2, PP3	No	Barakat syndrome	AD (de novo)	Yes
OTO.010	CHARGE syndrome	AD	Congenital	CHD7	c.235A > T p.(Lys79*)	Heterozygous	Pathogenic	PVS1, PM2, PP4	No	CHARGE syndrome	AD	No
OTO.015	Bilateral non-syndromic sensorineural deafness	AR	Childhood	POU3F4	c.692C > T p.(Thr231Ile)	Hemizygous (male)	Likely pathogenic	PM1, PM2, PP2, PP3	No	Non-syndromic sensorineural deafness (DFNX2/DFN3)	XR	No

Table 2 Clinical and genetic characteristics of cases with causative mutations (Continued)

Case ID	Pre-test phenotype	Pre-test suspected inheritance pattern	Time of deafness onset	Gene	Allele variants	Variant zygosity	ACMG[a] classification[30]	Fulfilled ACMG[a] pathogenicity criteria[30]	Present in HGMD and/or ClinVar[b]	Gene-associated phenotypes	Inheritance patterns of gene-associated phenotypes	Hidden syndrome
OTO.016	Bilateral non-syndromic sensorineural deafness	AD	Childhood	PRPS1	c.826C > T p.(Pro276Ser)	Hemizygous (male)	Likely pathogenic	PM1, PM2, PP2, PP3	No	Non-syndromic sensorineural deafness (DFNX1)	XD	No
OTO.007	Alport syndrome	AR	Childhood	COL4A5	c.3525_3529dup p.(Pro1117Leufs*124)	Hemizygous (male)	Pathogenic	PVS1, PM2, PM6	No	Alport syndrome	XD (de novo)	No

GenBank Accession and version numbers of the genes listed in the table: ACTG1 (NM_001614.3), BSND (NM_057176.2), CDH23 (NM_022124.5), CHD7 (NM_017780.3), COL4A5 (NM_000495.4), GATA3 (NM_001002295.1), MITF (NM_000248.3), MYO15A (NM_016239.3), P2RX2 (NM_174873.2), POU3F4 (NM_000307.4), PRPS1 (NM_002764.3), RDX (NM_002906.3), SLC26A4 (NM_000441.1), SOX10 (NM_006941.3), STRC (NM_153700.2), USH2A (NM_206933.2)

[a]American College of Medical Genetics and Genomics

[b]Yes: variants present in HGMD and/or Clinvar at the moment of clinical interpretation of the case; No: variants absent from both HGMD and ClinVar at the moment of clinical interpretation of the case

our pre-screened population were *ACTG1* (*n* = 3), *USH2A* (n = 3) and *STRC* (n = 3). Although variants in *USH2A* and *STRC* are often reported as common causes of SNHL [28, 37–40], the identification of *ACTG1* as the most frequent causative gene in our cohort is surprising.

ACTG1 variants are responsible for DFNA20/DFNA26 and type 2 Baraitser-Winter syndrome. None of our 3 cases has syndromic features to date, and all of them had early-onset profound SNHL, expanding the phenotypic spectrum of *ACTG1*, usually associated to post-lingual and progressive SNHL [41, 42], to prelocutive SNHL. Since none of the 3 causative variants had been described and 2 of them were de novo, a targeted hot-spot mutation assay or an AR oriented gene panel (the 2 de novo mutations took place in patients without familial background, simulating a recessive pattern) would have missed them. Therefore, the prevalence of *ACTG1* pathogenic variants could be higher, and its expression pattern more variable, than previously thought [43].

Our 38.1% rate of syndromic SNHL (8/21, including 2 syndromes diagnosed before and 6 after NGS genetic testing) is within expected rates. In contrast, our 38% incidence of AD and 14% of X-linked SNHL are higher than expected [44]. This might reflect the consequences of pre-screening, which excluded the most common AR (*GJB2/GJB6* and *OTOF*) and mitochondrial (*MT-RNR1*) mutations [2, 31, 45]. However, since in our patients 50% (4/8) of causative dominant variants were de novo (2 in *ACTG1*, 1 in *GATA3*; and 1 in *COL4A5*, Table 2) it might also be the consequence of using an unbiased NGS panel, able to identify unexpected de novo variants. Despite the limited size of our cohort, our de novo detection rate is strikingly similar to that reported recently in whole-exome sequencing (WES) studies for different clinical indications (37–68%) [35, 46].

A technical difficulty encountered for the implementation of a clinical-grade test was the presence of highly homologous pseudogene background for some of the target genes included in the panel (Additional file 6), especially *STRC* and *OTOA*. The measures proposed to deal with this problem (gene-restrictive realignment of sequencing results and validation of putative causative variants by gene-specific methods) should reduce misdiagnosis. Moreover, the *STRC* gene, one of the largest contributors to AR SNHL [28, 47, 48], is also a common site for large deletions [28], and CNVs can be refractory to general NGS approaches. As displayed in our population, where 19% of cases (4/21) were justified by CNVs, large genetic rearrangements are increasingly recognized as a common cause of genetic hearing loss, accounting for 13–19% of all causative variants [5, 48–50]. Therefore, CNV analysis should be a requirement for all patients undergoing genetic testing for SNHL. In this regard, our 100% validation rate of NGS-detected *STRC* CNVs by qPCR and MLPA is encouraging (Additional file 8).

Diagnostic rates of up to 60% are expected in patients with suspected AR congenital deafness. This percentage strongly declines for AD hearing loss, especially with the increase in the age of onset [5, 48]. In our series, as in most of published studies [5, 48, 51], prior to comprehensive genetic testing, patients were prescreened for common deafness mutations (in our cohort, *GJB2/GJB6*, *OTOF* and *MT-RNR1*, selected for their high prevalence in Spain [7, 31]). Mutations in the *GJB2* gene are among the most frequent causes for congenital hearing loss. The prevalence of its biallelic pathogenic mutations among non-syndromic SNHL cases ranges geographically from 0% to over 50% [3, 52–54]. Recent analyses show a worldwide and European prevalence of around 13%, increasing in < 5 year-old patients [2, 3]. In our laboratory, *GJB2/GJB6*, *OTOF* and *MT-RNR1* prescreening of 180 patients identified the cause of deafness in 34 (18.9%) (unpublished results). This figure, combined with the 42–48% diagnostic rate of our panel in pre-screened patients (48% considering as causative the highly suspicious variants of Table 4), allows us to estimate that combining prescreening with our panel will lead to a diagnosis in about 53–58% of patients.

Our 42–48% detection rate is slightly higher than the average reported with NGS-panels: 41% (10–83%) for a mix of pre-screened and not pre-screened patients [5, 9, 28, 48, 51]. Proper target region coverage and bioinformatics approaches shouldn't be underestimated for maximizing clinical sensitivity. Additionally, the inclusion of syndromic genes, revealing 'hidden syndromes', increased the diagnostic yield. The 6 a priori clinically unrecognized syndromes in our cohort diagnosed after genetic testing (Table 2), representing 28.6% of the genetically diagnosed cases, are a proof of concept of how NGS is changing medicine. In fact, undiagnosed syndromes in families with apparently non-syndromic SNHL are increasingly reported [55–58], expanding the phenotypes associated with SNHL-syndromes [35]. Moreover, 6 patients in our series had pathogenic variations in genes associated with both syndromic and non-syndromic HL: *CDH23* (Usher syndrome 1D and DFNB12), *ACTG1* (Baraitser-Winter syndrome type 2 and DFNA20/DFNA26), *BSND* (Bartter syndrome type IV and DNFB73) or *SLC26A4* (Pendred syndrome and DFNB4) (Table 2). Close follow-up of these patients is mandatory, since syndromic features may develop.

The clinical interpretation of genomic findings is a cornerstone of NGS diagnostic pipelines. Beyond deafness, a recent study indicated that as many as 30% of all disease-causing genetic variants cited in the literature may have been misinterpreted [59]. In our cohort, manual interpretation of variants required an average of 6 h/case, dedicated to in-depth review of the databases and scientific literature, under the perspective of the patient's phenotype and family history, which is imperative for accurate variant interpretation [11, 60].

Table 3 Clinical characteristics of cases without causative mutations

Case ID	Phenotype	Suspected inheritance pattern	Time of deafness onset
OTO.017	Bilateral non-syndromic sensorineural deafness	AR	Congenital
OTO.021	Bilateral sensorineural deafness. Nystagmus, strabismus, delay in psychomotor development and autism spectrum disorder	AR	Congenital
OTO.024	Bilateral non-syndromic sensorineural deafness	AR	Childhood
OTO.025	Bilateral non-syndromic sensorineural deafness	AR	Childhood
OTO.026	Unilateral non-syndromic sensorineural deafness	AR	Childhood
OTO.027	Bilateral non-syndromic sensorineural deafness	AR	Congenital
OTO.028	Bilateral non-syndromic sensorineural deafness	AR	Childhood
OTO.029	Unilateral non-syndromic sensorineural deafness	AR	Congenital
OTO.030	Unilateral sensorineural deafness. Connective tissue problems, digestive problems, urinary reflux and knee hypermobility	AR	Childhood
OTO.032	Unilateral non-syndromic sensorineural deafness	AR	Congenital
OTO.034	Bilateral non-syndromic sensorineural deafness	AR	Childhood
OTO.035	Bilateral non-syndromic sensorineural deafness	AR	Childhood
OTO.038	Bilateral non-syndromic sensorineural deafness	AR	Unknown
OTO.040	Bilateral non-syndromic sensorineural deafness	AR	Childhood
OTO.042	Bilateral non-syndromic sensorineural deafness	AR	Congenital
OTO.044	Bilateral non-syndromic sensorineural deafness	AR	Congenital
OTO.045	Bilateral non-syndromic sensorineural deafness	AR	Congenital
OTO.046	Bilateral non-syndromic sensorineural deafness	AR	Childhood
OTO.049	Bilateral non-syndromic sensorineural deafness	AR	Adulthood
OTO.052	Bilateral sensorineural deafness. Lobe of the auricular pavilion with grooves. Polysyndactyly in hands and feet. Hypospadias	AR	Congenital
OTO.053	Bilateral non-syndromic sensorineural deafness	AR	Childhood
OTO.036	Bilateral non-syndromic sensorineural deafness	AR/AD	Childhood
OTO.039	Bilateral non-syndromic sensorineural deafness	AR/AD	Adulthood
OTO.020	Bilateral non-syndromic sensorineural deafness	AD	Childhood
OTO.022	Bilateral non-syndromic sensorineural deafness	AD	Congenital
OTO.031	Bilateral non-syndromic sensorineural deafness	AD	Childhood
OTO.037	Bilateral non-syndromic sensorineural deafness	AD	Adulthood
OTO.047	Bilateral non-syndromic sensorineural deafness	AD	Childhood
OTO.048	Bilateral non-syndromic sensorineural deafness	AD	Childhood

To date, several studies using NGS for genetic diagnosis of deafness have been published, involving either gene panels or WES [5, 61]. When WES is ordered, sequenced regions not only include genes of interest ("targeted disease-specific panels" such as the one presented in this paper), but also all exons of all genes in the genome. Although WES avoids the need for specific gene panel enrichment, a literature-based selection of the genes involved in the pathology is anyway required for results intepretation. WES increases the requirements for sequencing resources, complicates the analysis and normally provides insufficient coverage of key target regions [29]. Moreover, WES carries

increased chance of secondary findings (variants identified in genes unrelated to the primary medical reason for testing [62]), which introduce noise into the genetic counseling procedure. A comparison of a disease-focused panel versus WES for inherited eye diseases found improved accuracy and performance of the disease-specific panel, a finding that can be translated to hearing loss panels [63]. For these reasons, disease-focused genetic tests have become the standard when evaluating hearing loss [64]. However, WES does have an advantage: the ability to identify alterations in genes not definitely associated with the disease yet. To minimize this disadvantage, a tiered approach was implemented: tier

Table 4 Clinical and genetic characteristics of cases with suspicious VUS#

Case ID	Pre-test phenotype	Pre-test suspected inheritance pattern	Time of deafness onset	Gene	Allele variants	Variant zygosity	ACMG¥ classification[30]	Fulfilled ACMG¥ pathogenicity criteria[30]	Gene-associated phenotype	Inheritance patterns of gene-associated phenotypes	Hidden syndrome
OTO.028	Bilateral non-syndromic sensorineural deafness	AR	Childhood	OTOA	Whole-gene deletion	Heterozygous	Pathogenic (likely pathogenic overriden to pathogenic)	PVS1, PM3	Non-syndromic sensorineural deafness (DFNB22)	AR	No
					c.1282G > T (p.Val428Phe)	Hemizygous	VUS#	PM2, PM3, PP2			
OTO.044	Bilateral non-syndromic sensorineural deafness	AR	Congenital	LOXHD1	c.3571A > G (p.Thr1191Ala)	Homozygous	VUS#	PM2, PP3	Non-syndromic sensorineural deafness (DFNB77)	AR	No
OTO.045	Bilateral non-syndromic sensorineural deafness	AR	Congenital	SLC26A4	c.695 T > G (p.Leu232Arg)	Homozygous	VUS#	PM1, PM2, PP3	Non-syndromic sensorineural deafness (DFNB4)/ Pendred syndrome	AR	Potential

#Variant/s of unknown significance

¥American College of Medical Genetics and Genomics

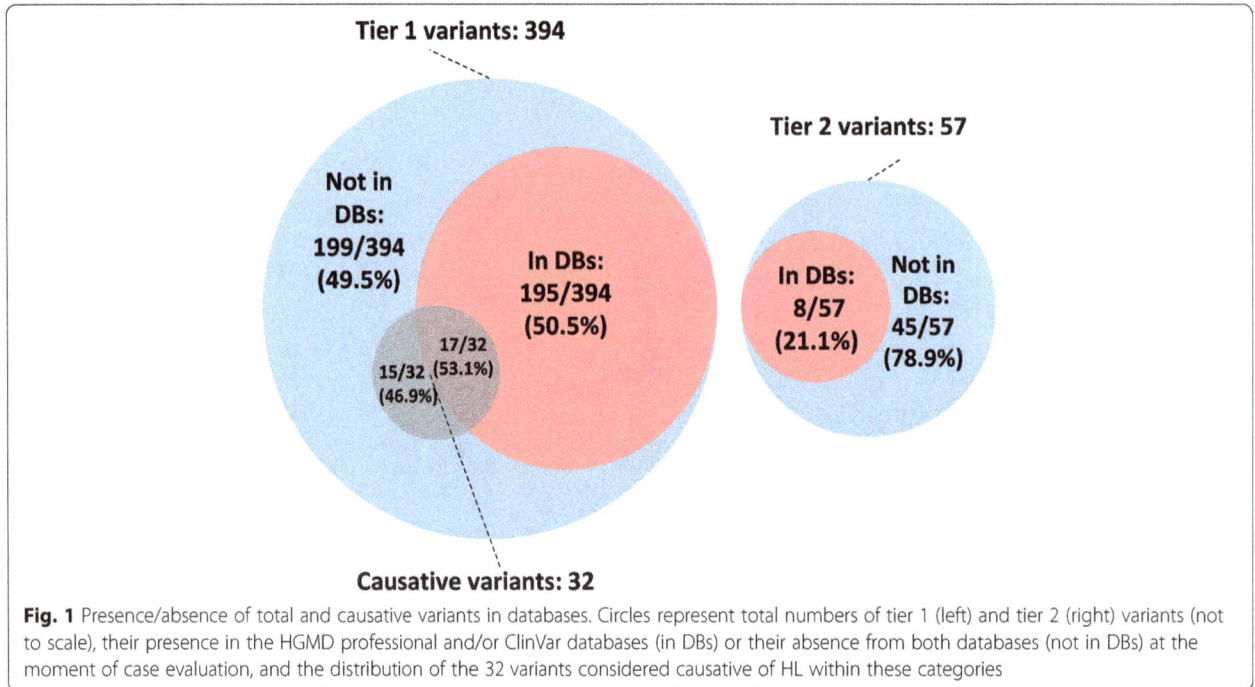

Fig. 1 Presence/absence of total and causative variants in databases. Circles represent total numbers of tier 1 (left) and tier 2 (right) variants (not to scale), their presence in the HGMD professional and/or ClinVar databases (in DBs) or their absence from both databases (not in DBs) at the moment of case evaluation, and the distribution of the 32 variants considered causative of HL within these categories

1 includes all genes consistently associated with SNHL, whereas tier 2 includes genes without sufficient clinical validity to be included in clinical testing. Non-systematic reporting of tier 2 genes reduces the uncertainty and simplifies the genetic counseling procedure. However,

meanwhile, it facilitates fast pipeline incorporation of clinically validated genes, as soon as confirmatory discoveries are published.

Conclusions

Our results underscore the importance of a comprehensive approach with careful gene selection to the genetic diagnosis of SNHL. Here, we contribute to show that, with the right methodology, NGS can be transferred to the clinical practice, boosting the yield of SNHL genetic diagnosis to 50–60% (including *GJB2/GJB6* alterations), improving diagnostic/prognostic accuracy, refining genetic and reproductive counseling and revealing clinically relevant undiagnosed syndromes. Lowering cost and increasing quality of WES and whole-genome sequencing (WGS) will probably prompt substitution of physical gene panels by non-targeted approaches. However, WES/WGS results are likely to be filtered through *in-silico* gene panels, based on a meticulously curated gene selection, such as the gene-set of the current panel. Thus, the methodology implemented on the present study is expected to be useful in the years to come. Since comprehensive genetic testing using NGS should be the standard of care for genetic evaluation of patients with SNHL, hereditary deafness should become a paradigm on the raising field of precision medicine. In this context, we expect that the use of the current platform, or others developed on the knowledge presented herein, will help to bring to the clinical arena the advantages of predictive and preventive SNHL genetic testing.

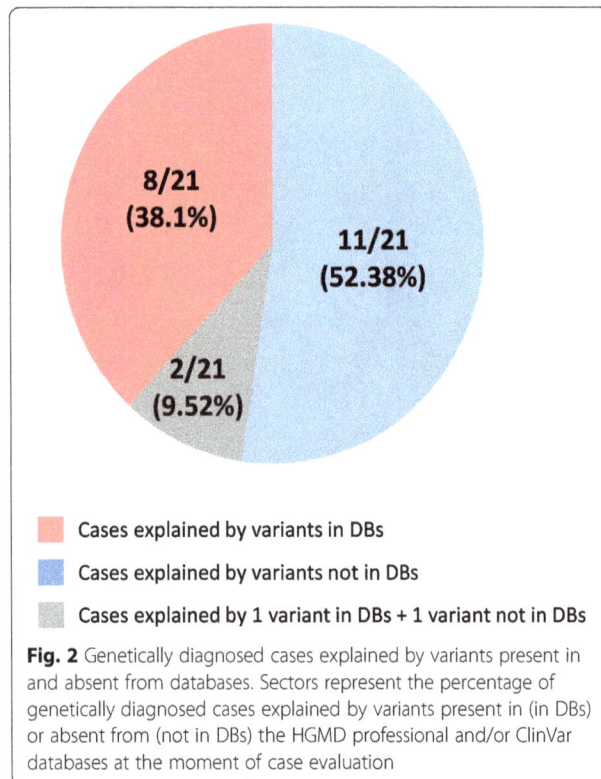

Fig. 2 Genetically diagnosed cases explained by variants present in and absent from databases. Sectors represent the percentage of genetically diagnosed cases explained by variants present in (in DBs) or absent from (not in DBs) the HGMD professional and/or ClinVar databases at the moment of case evaluation

Additional files

Additional file 1: List of phenotypes potentially related to hearing defects used as keywords for initial query on HGMD.

Additional file 2: Tier 1 and tier 2 genes included in v1 of the panel.

Additional file 3: Tier 1 and tier 2 genes included in v2 of the panel.

Additional file 4: Cases analyzed with each panel version.

Additional file 5: Coverages and callabilities for every tier 1 and tier 2 gene on v3 samples.

Additional file 6: Highly homologous conflictive regions.

Additional file 7: Primers used to validate causative (pathogenic and likely pathogenic) variants.

Additional file 8: Samples with STRC CNVs.

Additional file 9: Variants identified in our cohort classified as pathogenic (DM) by HGMD for hearing-related phenotypes.)

Abbreviations
ACMG: Americal college of medical genetics and genomics; AD: Autosomal dominant; AR: Autosomal recessive; CNVs: Copy number variations; DIN: DNA integrity number; HL: Hearing loss; NGS: Next-generation sequencing; SNHL: Sensorineural hearing loss; SNVs: Single nucleotide variants; WES: Whole-exome sequencing; WGS: Whole-genome sequencing

Acknowledgements
We are grateful to all participating patients and their families.

Funding
Work performed at IMOMA for this project was partially supported by a grant from Fundación María Cristina Masaveu Peterson. Work performed at DREAMgenics was partially supported by University of Oviedo Foundation grants (D.C., P.C.P.).

Authors' contributions
RuC participated in study design, interpretation of results and writing of the manuscript; MD performed most of the experimental work and contributed to interpretation of results; GAC contributed to experimental work and results interpretation; DC, PC and GRO, performed bioinformatic analyses; RA and NSD contributed to experimental work; RaC contributed to results interpretation; AP, MVD, NGG, IH, JLL. ARA, CTB, JR, NG, JRGM, FNB, JAG, AMG, MC, MIG and BGB provided patient samples and associated clinical data; JC participated in study design, interpretation of results and writing of the manuscript; all authors commented on the manuscript and approved the submitted version.

Competing interests
The following authors are currently employed by IMOMA or DREAMgenics, the companies involved in the development and exploitation of the OTOgenics™ platform: IMOMA: Ru.C. (Physician in Chief), M.D. (Clinical Molecular Geneticist), G.A.C. (Biotechnologist), N.S.D. (Lab. Technician), R.A. (Lab. Technician), Ra.C. (Molecular Biologist) and J.C. (Scientific Director); DREAMgenics: D.C. (Bioinformatitian), P.C.P. (Bioinformatitian) and G.R.O. (Bioinformatitian, C.S.O. and C.E.O.). G.R.O. is a shareholder of DREAMgenics. The other authors declare no conflict of interest.

Author details
[1]Instituto de Medicina Oncológica y Molecular de Asturias (IMOMA) S. A, Avda. Richard Grandío s/n, 33193 Oviedo, Spain. [2]Disease Research And Medicine (DREAMgenics) S. L., Oviedo, Spain. [3]Hospital Universitario Central de Asturias, Oviedo, Spain. [4]Hospital Álvaro Cunqueiro, Vigo, Spain. [5]Hospital Universitario Son Espases, Palma de Mallorca, Spain. [6]Hospital Universitario Río Hortega, Valladolid, Spain. [7]Hospital Universitario Marqués de Valdecilla, Santander, Spain. [8]Instituto de Investigación Biomédica de Salamanca, Salamanca, Spain.

References
1. Alford RL, Arnos KS, Fox M, Lin JW, Palmer CG, Pandya A, Rehm HL, Robin NH, Scott DA, Yoshinaga-Itano C, et al. American College of Medical Genetics and Genomics guideline for the clinical evaluation and etiologic diagnosis of hearing loss. Genet Med. 2014;16(4):347–55.
2. Burke WF, Warnecke A, Schoner-Heinisch A, Lesinski-Schiedat A, Maier H, Lenarz T. Prevalence and audiological profiles of GJB2 mutations in a large collective of hearing impaired patients. Hear Res. 2016;333:77–86.
3. Chan DK, Chang KW. GJB2-associated hearing loss: systematic review of worldwide prevalence, genotype, and auditory phenotype. Laryngoscope. 2014;124(2):E34–53.
4. Sabatini LM, Mathews C, Ptak D, Doshi S, Tynan K, Hegde MR, Burke TL, Bossler AD. Genomic sequencing procedure microcosting analysis and health economic cost-impact analysis: A Report of the Association for Molecular Pathology. J Mol Diagn. 2016;18(3):319–28.
5. Shearer AE, Smith RJ. Massively parallel sequencing for genetic diagnosis of hearing loss: the new standard of care. Otolaryngol Head Neck Surg. 2015; 153(2):175–82.
6. Nunez-Batalla F, Jaudenes-Casaubon C, Sequi-Canet JM, Vivanco-Allende A, Zubicaray-Ugarteche J, Cabanillas-Farpon R. Aetiological diagnosis of child deafness: CODEPEH recommendations. Acta Otorrinolaringol Esp. 2017;68(1):43–55.
7. Cabanillas Farpón R, Cadiñanos Bañales J. Hereditary hearing loss: genetic counselling. Acta Otorrinolaringol Esp. 2012;63(3):218–29.
8. Rahman S, Ecob R, Costello H, Sweeney MG, Duncan AJ, Pearce K, Strachan D, Forge A, Davis A, Bitner-Glindzicz M. Hearing in 44-45 year olds with m.1555A>G, a genetic mutation predisposing to aminoglycoside-induced deafness: a population based cohort study. BMJ Open. 2012;2:e000411.
9. Sommen M, Schrauwen I, Vandeweyer G, Boeckx N, Corneveaux JJ, van den Ende J, Boudewyns A, De Leenheer E, Janssens S, Claes K, et al. DNA diagnostics of hereditary hearing loss: a targeted resequencing approach combined with a mutation classification system. Hum Mutat. 2016;37(8):812–9.
10. Geleoc GS, Holt JR. Sound strategies for hearing restoration. Science. 2014; 344(6184):1241062.
11. Abou Tayoun AN, Al Turki SH, Oza AM, Bowser MJ, Hernandez AL, Funke BH, Rehm HL, Amr SS. Improving hearing loss gene testing: a systematic review of gene evidence toward more efficient next-generation sequencing-based diagnostic testing and interpretation. Genet Med. 2016;18(6):545–53.
12. Cabanillas R, Diñeiro M, Castillo D, Pruneda PC, Penas C, Cifuentes GA, de Vicente A, Durán NS, Álvarez R, Ordóñez GR, et al. A novel molecular diagnostics platform for somatic and germline precision oncology. Mol Genet Genomic Med. 2017;5(4):336–59.
13. Jennings LJ, Arcila ME, Corless C, Kamel-Reid S, Lubin IM, Pfeifer J, Temple-Smolkin RL, Voelkerding KV, Nikiforova MN. Guidelines for validation of next-generation sequencing-based oncology panels: A Joint Consensus Recommendation of the Association for Molecular Pathology and College of American Pathologists. J Mol Diagn. 2017;19(3):341–65.
14. Li H, Durbin R. Fast and accurate long-read alignment with burrows-wheeler transform. Bioinformatics. 2010;26(5):589–95.
15. Li H, Handsaker B, Wysoker A, Fennell T, Ruan J, Homer N, Marth G, Abecasis G, Durbin R, Genome project data processing S. The sequence alignment/map format and SAMtools. Bioinformatics. 2009;25(16):2078–9.
16. Puente XS, Pinyol M, Quesada V, Conde L, Ordonez GR, Villamor N, Escaramis G, Jares P, Bea S, Gonzalez-Diaz M, et al. Whole-genome sequencing identifies recurrent mutations in chronic lymphocytic leukaemia. Nature. 2011;475(7354):101–5.
17. Valdes-Mas R, Bea S, Puente DA, Lopez-Otin C, Puente XS. Estimation of copy number alterations from exome sequencing data. PLoS One. 2012;7(12):e51422.
18. Kumar P, Henikoff S, Ng PC. Predicting the effects of coding non-synonymous variants on protein function using the SIFT algorithm. Nat Protoc. 2009;4(7):1073–81.
19. Adzhubei IA, Schmidt S, Peshkin L, Ramensky VE, Gerasimova A, Bork P, Kondrashov AS, Sunyaev SR. A method and server for predicting damaging missense mutations. Nat Methods. 2010;7(4):248–9.
20. Choi Y, Sims GE, Murphy S, Miller JR, Chan AP. Predicting the functional effect of amino acid substitutions and indels. PLoS One. 2012;7(10):e46688.
21. Reva B, Antipin Y, Sander C. Predicting the functional impact of protein mutations: application to cancer genomics. Nucleic Acids Res. 2011;39(17):e118.
22. Schwarz JM, Cooper DN, Schuelke M, Seelow D. MutationTaster2: mutation prediction for the deep-sequencing age. Nat Methods. 2014;11(4):361–2.

23. Chun S, Fay JC. Identification of deleterious mutations within three human genomes. Genome Res. 2009;19(9):1553–61.

24. Dong C, Wei P, Jian X, Gibbs R, Boerwinkle E, Wang K, Liu X. Comparison and integration of deleteriousness prediction methods for nonsynonymous SNVs in whole exome sequencing studies. Hum Mol Genet. 2015;24(8):2125–37.

25. Shihab HA, Gough J, Mort M, Cooper DN, Day IN, Gaunt TR. Ranking non-synonymous single nucleotide polymorphisms based on disease concepts. Hum Genomics. 2014;8:11.

26. Jagadeesh KA, Wenger AM, Berger MJ, Guturu H, Stenson PD, Cooper DN, Bernstein JA, Bejerano G. M-CAP eliminates a majority of variants of uncertain significance in clinical exomes at high sensitivity. Nat Genet. 2016; 48(12):1581–6.

27. Davydov EV, Goode DL, Sirota M, Cooper GM, Sidow A, Batzoglou S. Identifying a high fraction of the human genome to be under selective constraint using GERP++. PLoS Comput Biol. 2010;6(12):e1001025.

28. Mandelker D, Amr SS, Pugh T, Gowrisankar S, Shakhbatyan R, Duffy E, Bowser M, Harrison B, Lafferty K, Mahanta L, et al. Comprehensive diagnostic testing for stereocilin: an approach for analyzing medically important genes with high homology. J Mol Diagn. 2014;16(6):639–47.

29. Shearer AE, Black-Ziegelbein EA, Hildebrand MS, Eppsteiner RW, Ravi H, Joshi S, Guiffre AC, Sloan CM, Happe S, Howard SD, et al. Advancing genetic testing for deafness with genomic technology. J Med Genet. 2013;50(9):627–34.

30. Richards S, Aziz N, Bale S, Bick D, Das S, Gastier-Foster J, Grody WW, Hegde M, Lyon E, Spector E, et al. Standards and guidelines for the interpretation of sequence variants: a joint consensus recommendation of the American College of Medical Genetics and Genomics and the Association for Molecular Pathology. Genet Med. 2015;17(5):405–24.

31. Gallo-Teran J, Morales-Angulo C, Rodriguez-Ballesteros M, Moreno-Pelayo MA, del Castillo I, Moreno F. Prevalence of the 35delG mutation in the GJB2 gene, del (GJB6-D13S1830) in the GJB6 gene, Q829X in the OTOF gene and A1555G in the mitochondrial 12S rRNA gene in subjects with non-syndromic sensorineural hearing impairment of congenital/childhood onset. Acta Otorrinolaringol Esp. 2005;56(10):463–8.

32. Mandelker D, Schmidt RJ, Ankala A, McDonald Gibson K, Bowser M, Sharma H, Duffy E, Hegde M, Santani A, Lebo M, et al. Navigating highly homologous genes in a molecular diagnostic setting: a resource for clinical next-generation sequencing. Genet Med. 2016;18(12):1282–9.

33. Hildebrand MS, Morin M, Meyer NC, Mayo F, Modamio-Hoybjor S, Mencia A, Olavarrieta L, Morales-Angulo C, Nishimura CJ, Workman H, et al. DFNA8/12 caused by TECTA mutations is the most identified subtype of nonsyndromic autosomal dominant hearing loss. Hum Mutat. 2011;32(7):825–34.

34. Toumpas CJ, Clark J, Harris A, Beswick R, Nourse CB. Congenital cytomegalovirus infection is a significant cause of moderate to profound sensorineural hearing loss in Queensland children. J Paediatr Child Health. 2015;51(5):541–4.

35. Retterer K, Juusola J, Cho MT, Vitazka P, Millan F, Gibellini F, Vertino-Bell A, Smaoui N, Neidich J, Monaghan KG, et al. Clinical application of whole-exome sequencing across clinical indications. Genet Med. 2016;18(7):696–704.

36. Millan F, Cho MT, Retterer K, Monaghan KG, Bai R, Vitazka P, Everman DB, Smith B, Angle B, Roberts V, et al. Whole exome sequencing reveals de novo pathogenic variants in KAT6A as a cause of a neurodevelopmental disorder. Am J Med Genet A. 2016;170(7):1791–8.

37. Hilgert N, Smith RJ, Van Camp G. Forty-six genes causing nonsyndromic hearing impairment: which ones should be analyzed in DNA diagnostics? Mutat Res. 2009;681(2–3):189–96.

38. Reardon W, Coffey R, Phelps PD, Luxon LM, Stephens D, Kendall-Taylor P, Britton KE, Grossman A, Trembath R. Pendred syndrome–100 years of underascertainment? QJM. 1997;90(7):443–7.

39. Bonnet C, Riahi Z, Chantot-Bastaraud S, Smagghe L, Letexier M, Marcaillou C, Lefevre GM, Hardelin JP, El-Amraoui A, Singh-Estivalet A, et al. An innovative strategy for the molecular diagnosis of usher syndrome identifies causal biallelic mutations in 93% of European patients. Eur J Hum Genet. 2016;24(12):1730–8.

40. Yoshimura H, Miyagawa M, Kumakawa K, Nishio SY, Usami S. Frequency of usher syndrome type 1 in deaf children by massively parallel DNA sequencing. J Hum Genet. 2016;61(5):419–22.

41. Kemerley A, Sloan C, Pfeifer W, Smith R, Drack A. A novel mutation in ACTG1 causing Baraitser-winter syndrome with extremely variable expressivity in three generations. Ophthalmic Genet. 2017;38(2):152 6.

42. Yuan Y, Gao X, Huang B, Lu J, Wang G, Lin X, Qu Y, Dai P. Phenotypic heterogeneity in a DFNA20/26 family segregating a novel ACTG1 mutation. BMC Genet. 2016;17:33.

43. Morin M, Bryan KE, Mayo-Merino F, Goodyear R, Mencia A, Modamio-Hoybjor S, del Castillo I, Cabalka JM, Richardson G, Moreno F, et al. In vivo and in vitro effects of two novel gamma-actin (ACTG1) mutations that cause DFNA20/26 hearing impairment. Hum Mol Genet. 2009;18(16):3075–89.

44. Sommen M, Wuyts W, Van Camp G. Molecular diagnostics for hereditary hearing loss in children. Expert Rev Mol Diagn. 2017;17(8):751–60.

45. Migliosi V, Modamio-Hoybjor S, Moreno-Pelayo MA, Rodriguez-Ballesteros M, Villamar M, Telleria D, Menendez I, Moreno F, Del Castillo I. Q829X, a novel mutation in the gene encoding otoferlin (OTOF), is frequently found in Spanish patients with prelingual non-syndromic hearing loss. J Med Genet. 2002;39(7):502–6.

46. Posey JE, Harel T, Liu P, Rosenfeld JA, James RA, Coban Akdemir ZH, Walkiewicz M, Bi W, Xiao R, Ding Y, et al. Resolution of disease phenotypes resulting from multilocus genomic variation. N Engl J Med. 2017;376(1):21–31.

47. Francey LJ, Conlin LK, Kadesch HE, Clark D, Berrodin D, Sun Y, Glessner J, Hakonarson H, Jalas C, Landau C, et al. Genome-wide SNP genotyping identifies the Stereocilin (STRC) gene as a major contributor to pediatric bilateral sensorineural hearing impairment. Am J Med Genet A. 2012;158A(2):298–308.

48. Zazo Seco C, Wesdorp M, Feenstra I, Pfundt R, Hehir-Kwa JY, Lelieveld SH, Castelein S, Gilissen C, de Wijs IJ, Admiraal RJ, et al. The diagnostic yield of whole-exome sequencing targeting a gene panel for hearing impairment in the Netherlands. Eur J Hum Genet. 2017;25(3):308–14.

49. Shearer AE, Kolbe DL, Azaiez H, Sloan CM, Frees KL, Weaver AE, Clark ET, Nishimura CJ, Black-Ziegelbein EA, Smith RJ. Copy number variants are a common cause of non-syndromic hearing loss. Genome Med. 2014;6(5):37.

50. Ji H, Lu J, Wang J, Li H, Lin X. Combined examination of sequence and copy number variations in human deafness genes improves diagnosis for cases of genetic deafness. BMC Ear Nose Throat Disord. 2014;14:9.

51. Likar T, Hasanhodzic M, Teran N, Maver A, Peterlin B, Writzl K. Diagnostic outcomes of exome sequencing in patients with syndromic or non-syndromic hearing loss. PLoS One. 2018;13(1):e0188578.

52. Gasparini P, Rabionet R, Barbujani G, Melchionda S, Petersen M, Brondum-Nielsen K, Metspalu A, Oitmaa E, Pisano M, Fortina P, et al. High carrier frequency of the 35delG deafness mutation in European populations. Genetic analysis consortium of GJB2 35delG. Eur J Hum Genet. 2000;8(1):19–23.

53. Estivill X, Fortina P, Surrey S, Rabionet R, Melchionda S, D'Agruma L, Mansfield E, Rappaport E, Govea N, Mila M, et al. Connexin-26 mutations in sporadic and inherited sensorineural deafness. Lancet. 1998; 351(9100):394–8.

54. Kenneson A, Van Naarden Braun K, Boyle C. GJB2 (connexin 26) variants and nonsyndromic sensorineural hearing loss: a HuGE review. Genet Med. 2002;4(4):258–74.

55. Wei X, Sun Y, Xie J, Shi Q, Qu N, Yang G, Cai J, Yang Y, Liang Y, Wang W, et al. Next-generation sequencing identifies a novel compound heterozygous mutation in MYO7A in a Chinese patient with usher syndrome 1B. Clin Chim Acta. 2012;413(23–24):1866–71.

56. Behar DM, Davidov B, Brownstein Z, Ben-Yosef T, Avraham KB, Shohat M. The many faces of sensorineural hearing loss: one founder and two novel mutations affecting one family of mixed Jewish ancestry. Genet Test Mol Biomarkers. 2014;18(2):123–6.

57. Lu Y, Zhou X, Jin Z, Cheng J, Shen W, Ji F, Liu L, Zhang X, Zhang M, Cao Y, et al. Resolving the genetic heterogeneity of prelingual hearing loss within one family: performance comparison and application of two targeted next generation sequencing approaches. J Hum Genet. 2014;59(11):599–607.

58. Qing J, Yan D, Zhou Y, Liu Q, Wu W, Xiao Z, Liu Y, Liu J, Du L, Xie D, et al. Whole-exome sequencing to decipher the genetic heterogeneity of hearing loss in a Chinese family with deaf by deaf mating. PLoS One. 2014;9(10):e109178.

59. Boycott KM, Vanstone MR, Bulman DE, MacKenzie AE. Rare-disease genetics in the era of next-generation sequencing: discovery to translation. Nat Rev Genet. 2013;14(10):681–91.

60. Maxwell KN, Hart SN, Vijai J, Schrader KA, Slavin TP, Thomas T, Wubbenhorst B, Ravichandran V, Moore RM, Hu C, et al. Evaluation of ACMG-guideline-based variant classification of Cancer susceptibility and non-Cancer-associated genes in families affected by breast Cancer. Am J Hum Genet. 2016;98(5):801–17.

61. Bademci G, Foster J 2nd, Mahdieh N, Bonyadi M, Duman D, Cengiz FB, Menendez I, Diaz-Horta O, Shirkavand A, Zeinali S, et al. Comprehensive analysis via exome sequencing uncovers genetic etiology in autosomal recessive nonsyndromic deafness in a large multiethnic cohort. Genet Med. 2016;18(4):364–71.

62. Kalia SS, Adelman K, Bale SJ, Chung WK, Eng C, Evans JP, Herman GE, Hufnagel SB, Klein TE, Korf BR, et al. Recommendations for reporting of secondary findings in clinical exome and genome sequencing, 2016 update (ACMG SF v2.0): a policy statement of the American College of Medical Genetics and Genomics. Genet Med. 2017;19(2):249–55.

63. Consugar MB, Navarro-Gomez D, Place EM, Bujakowska KM, Sousa ME, Fonseca-Kelly ZD, Taub DG, Janessian M, Wang DY, Au ED, et al. Panel-based genetic diagnostic testing for inherited eye diseases is highly accurate and reproducible, and more sensitive for variant detection, than exome sequencing. Genet Med. 2015;17(4):253–61.

64. Rehm HL. Disease-targeted sequencing: a cornerstone in the clinic. Nat Rev Genet. 2013;14(4):295–300.

4

Additional germline findings from a tumor profiling program

Neda Stjepanovic[1], Tracy L. Stockley[2,3], Philippe L. Bedard[1,2], Jeanna M. McCuaig[4], Melyssa Aronson[5], Spring Holter[5], Kara Semotiuk[5], Natasha B. Leighl[1], Raymond Jang[1], Monika K. Krzyzanowska[1], Amit M. Oza[1], Abha Gupta[1], Christine Elser[1], Lailah Ahmed[1,2], Lisa Wang[6], Suzanne Kamel-Reid[2,3], Lillian L. Siu[1,2] and Raymond H. Kim[1,2,5*] (iD)

Abstract

Background: Matched tumor-normal sequencing, applied in precision cancer medicine, can identify unidentified germline Medically Actionable Variants (gMAVS) in cancer predisposition genes. We report patient preferences for the return of additional germline results, and describe various gMAV scenarios delivered through a clinical genetics service.

Methods: Tumor profiling was offered to 1960 advanced cancer patients, of which 1556 underwent tumor-normal sequencing with multigene hotspot panels containing 20 cancer predisposition genes. All patients were provided with an IRB-approved consent for return of additional gMAVs.

Results: Of the whole cohort 94% of patients consented to be informed of additional germline results and 5% declined, with no statistically significant differences based on age, sex, race or prior genetic testing. Eight patients were found to have gMAVs in a cancer predisposition gene. Five had previously unidentified gMAVs: three in *TP53* (only one fulfilled Chompret's Revised criteria for Li-Fraumeni Syndrome), one in *SMARCB1* in the absence of schwannomatosis features and one a *TP53* variant at low allele frequency suggesting an acquired event in blood.

Conclusion: Interest in germline findings is high among patients who undergo tumor profiling. Disclosure of previously unidentified gMAVs present multiple challenges, thus supporting the involvement of a clinical genetics service in all tumor profiling programs.

Keywords: Germline mutation, Neoplasms/genetics, Neoplastic syndromes, Hereditary Cancer, Incidental findings, Secondary findings, Next generation sequencing

Background

Tumor profiling through next generation sequencing (NGS) has facilitated precision cancer therapies by identification of actionable tumor variants to guide cancer patient management [1]. Genetic analysis of tumor tissue can detect both acquired (somatic) aberrations found exclusively in the cancer cells, and inherited (germline, constitutional) variants. Often in molecular profiling of tumors, germline DNA from normal tissue is also tested to aid in filtering tumor-specific events by identification

and subtraction of germline variants [2]. However the analysis of germline DNA may identify pathogenic germline variants in cancer predisposition genes included in NGS molecular profiling panels [3]. The American Society of Clinical Oncology (ASCO) and the Clinical Sequencing Exploratory Research (CSER) Consortium Tumor Working Group, support the communication of medically relevant secondary or incidental germline findings from tumor profiling programs based on patient preferences [4, 5]. CSER defines secondary findings as "results that are unrelated to the diagnostic question, but are systematically sought and analyzed, while incidental findings are not sought out, but identified nonetheless" [6]. Recently, these findings have been collectively referred to as "additional findings" based on patients' preferences [7]. A number of NGS

* Correspondence: Raymond.Kim@utoronto.ca
[1]Division of Medical Oncology and Hematology, Princess Margaret Cancer Centre, 610 University Ave, Toronto, ON M5G 2M9, Canada
[2]Cancer Genomics Program, Princess Margaret Cancer Centre, 610 University Ave, Toronto, ON M5G 2M9, Canada
Full list of author information is available at the end of the article

tumor profiling programs have reported additional germline findings in actionable cancer predisposition genes with the frequency ranging between 4.3 and 17.5% of patients tested [8–11]. While studies designed to actively seek secondary gMAVs require considerable amount of analysis and resources, studies designed not to actively seek gMAV may also encounter additional findings incidentally. Although at a lower frequency, mechanisms to incorporate such additional findings into the clinical care of these patients should be considered. Tumor profiling programs may also provide a new avenue to identify individuals with a cancer predisposition syndrome with implications on their clinical management and families.

The Princess Margaret Cancer Centre completed accrual of two tumor profiling studies, the Integrated Molecular Profiling in Advanced Cancers Trial (IMPACT) and Community Oncology Molecular Profiling in Advanced Cancers Trial (COMPACT). Two targeted NGS panels of 48–50 genes were analyzed to inform precision cancer therapies in advanced cancer patients through paired tumor-germline sequencing [12]. Peripheral blood lymphocytes (PBL) were selected as representative of normal tissue to identify germline variants to aid in identification of tumor-specific variants. Although the variant analysis was not designed to detect all germline variants in cancer predisposition genes in the tested panels, the potential of detecting germline medically actionable variants (gMAVs) incidentally was recognized. Information about gMAVs was offered to the patients and disclosed only to those who provided consent. Here, we describe patient preferences in the return of additional gMAVs in cancer predisposition genes detected through tumor profiling, the types of variants detected and considerations in the interpretation and disclosure of the findings.

Methods

Patient cohort

The patient cohort consisted of advanced cancer patients who were candidates for clinical trials with targeted therapies and enrolled in the tumor profiling programs IMPACT or COMPACT (NCT01505400) (Fig. 1) [12]. Patients were age ≥ 18 years, with Eastern Cooperative Oncology Group (ECOG) performance status ≤1, had available formalin-fixed embedded archival tumor tissue and provided a blood sample to represent the germline DNA from PBL. At study registration all participants were asked to provide information regarding prior germline testing. Written informed consent for tumor profiling and germline co-analysis was obtained from all participants. An additional University Health Network Research Ethics Board-approved consent form for return of gMAVs was offered to the participants from June 2013 for IMPACT and January 2014 for COMPACT, until the closure of both trials in December 2015. Participants interested in

the return of gMAV results were asked to identify a delegate (preferably biologic relative), who could receive the results on their behalf if required. Demographic and clinical data were extracted from prospectively maintained databases and medical records.

Genetic analysis

DNA extraction and molecular analysis on PBLs or tumor FFPE tissue was performed as previously described [12]. NGS molecular test methods used included one of the following targeted amplicon cancer panels, designed to detect hotspot variants in regions of selected genes with known utility in somatic cancers: 1) TruSeq Amplicon Cancer Panel (TSACP; Illumina, San Diego, CA) sequenced on the MiSeq benchtop sequencer (Illumina), which included hotspot regions of 48 genes. (Additional file 1: Table S1) Sequence alignment and base calling used MiSeq Reporter (Illumina), followed by variant calling using NextGENe v.2.3.1 software (SoftGenetics, State College, PA) and data review using the Integrative Genomics Viewer (IGV, Broad Institute); or 2) Ion AmpliSeq Cancer Panel (ASCP; ThermoFisher Scientific, Waltham, MA) sequenced on the Ion Proton benchtop sequencer (ThermoFisher Scientific), which included hotspot regions of 50 genes (Additional file 1: Table S2) Sequence alignment and base calling was performed by Torrent Suite software (ThermoFisher Scientific) and analysis using NextGENe v.2.3.1 and IGV software.

Somatic variants identified met laboratory-defined thresholds of > 500× read coverage and allele frequency of > 10%. Recurrent mutations between 400-500X coverage or 5–10% allele fraction were reported if they were verified by an orthogonal molecular method. Three genes with read depth consistently falling below 500× on TSACP (*GNAS*, *HRAS*, *CDKN2A*) were not included in the data analysis.

Selected targeted hotspot regions (i.e. partial gene regions, not full gene/full exon sequences) of 20 genes which also have inherited cancer risk were included in the panels (Additional file 1: Table S1 and S2). For samples with insufficient DNA quality or quantity for either NGS panel, a custom multiplex genotyping assay was performed only on tumor tissue [12]. Tumor profiling with NGS methods was only performed when germline DNA was available. Germline and tumor samples from the same patient were tested using the same methods and analyses, and variants identified in tumor DNA were compared to variants identified in germline DNA to identify tumor-specific events. All NGS analyses used hg19, NCBI Build 37, as reference genome. All testing was performed in a laboratory accredited by the College of American Pathologists and certified to meet Clinical Laboratory Improvement Amendments.

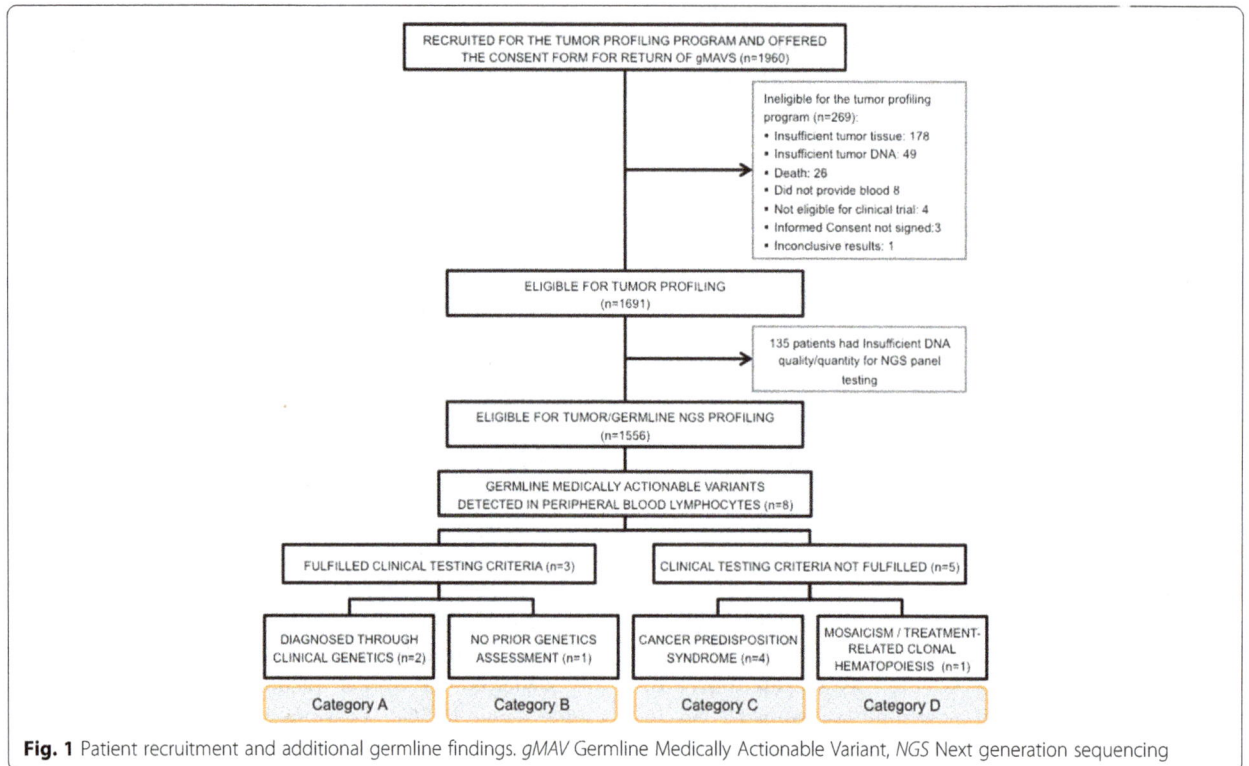

Fig. 1 Patient recruitment and additional germline findings. *gMAV* Germline Medically Actionable Variant, *NGS* Next generation sequencing

Determination of germline variants in cancer predisposition genes

Among the genes with targeted partial hotspot regions evaluated on the TSACP and ASCP NGS panels, 20 genes were related to cancer predisposition syndromes (Additional file 1: Tables S1–S3). Any germline variants detected in the select hotspot targeted regions of the cancer predisposition genes analyzed were investigated in online mutation databases (ClinVar, HGMD, IARC TP53, BIC), population variant databases (dbSNP, ExAC, 1000 Genomes) and relevant literature, and classified as pathogenic, likely pathogenic, uncertain significance, likely benign or benign using the variant assessment guidelines as specified by the American College of Medical Genetics [13]. The variant analysis approach was not specifically designed to systematically detect all germline variants as the focus of the data analysis was on primary detection of somatic acquired mutations. However, gMAVs were still identified incidentally. The gMAVs were defined as those germline variants which were pathogenic or likely pathogenic, were associated with a cancer predisposition syndrome and could have a clinical impact on the patient and/or prompt genetic testing in family members. gMAVs were considered as non-constitutional (mosaic or somatic event in PBL) when the allelic frequency of the variant in germline DNA was less than 25–30% based on validation data of the two NGS panels.

Return of germline medically actionable variants in cancer predisposition genes

A "Genomics Tumor Board" was developed which included medical oncologists, clinical molecular laboratory geneticists, genetic counsellors and a medical geneticist. All pathogenic or likely pathogenic variants from germline DNA analysis, as well as variants of conflicting interpretation for cancer predisposition syndromes were reviewed in conjunction with the personal and family history to determine clinical significance and potential management steps. Each case was discussed independently to determine whether germline results would be returned to patient or their delegate. If a cancer predisposition syndrome was previously identified through standard clinical routes, no further action was taken. For potentially newly uncovered gMAVs in cancer predisposition genes, patients who consented to return of additional findings or their delegate were contacted by the clinical genetics service, which comprised of a medical geneticist and genetic counsellor. Confirmation of the germline results on a new sample in an accredited clinical laboratory was required prior to being incorporated into the patient's medical record. Surveillance recommendations and familial cascade testing was conducted through standard clinical genetics routes (Additional file 2: Figure S1).

Statistical analysis

Descriptive statistics were used to summarize patient demographics (age, gender, race, tumor type, ECOG and prior germline testing). Comparisons between patients who consented for return of additional gMAVs and those who did not, were performed using t-test for age and Chi-Square test for gender, race, tumor type, ECOG and prior genetic testing. Differences with p-values of < 0.05 were considered statistically significant. All statistical analyses were conducted in SAS, version 9.4.

Results

Consenting rates and patients' preferences

A total of 1960 patients with a variety of malignancies were consented for IMPACT and COMPACT. The median age at enrollment to both studies was 58 years (range 18–89 years) and 67% of the population was female. Other relevant clinical characteristics are depicted in Fig. 2 and Additional file 1: Table S4. Of note, 18% (361/1960) patients did report already having clinical germline genetic testing which is consistent with the referral rates in our centre [14]. In the consent form 1844 (94%) agreed to the return of additional pathogenic germline results, 103 (5%) declined and 13 (1%) improperly filled the section regarding additional findings. There was no statistically significant difference by age, sex, race or prior genetic testing among the patients who consented for return of germline results and those who declined (Table 1).

Variants detected through germline DNA analysis

Samples from 1556 patients were tested with NGS panels, and eight patients were found to have gMAVs in cancer predisposition genes Fig. 1 and Table 2.

A variety of distinct scenarios were encountered in patients with gMAVs that were categorized as (Fig. 1):

A. Confirmation of a previously identified cancer predisposition syndrome
B. Identification of a cancer predisposition syndrome in a patient eligible for clinical genetic testing but not previously tested
C. Identification of a potential cancer predisposition syndrome in a patient ineligible for clinical genetic testing
D. A mosaic variant or somatic PBL variant likely not related to an inherited cancer predisposition

For category A patients (Table 2: patients 1 and 2) whose gMAVs were previously identified and disclosed by the clinical genetics service prior to the study, no further action was taken.

One category B patient (Table 2: patient 3) was identified. A woman, who fulfilled Chompret's Revised criteria for germline *TP53* genetic testing for Li-Fraumeni syndrome (LFS) [15] due to the history of multiple malignancies, however was not referred for a clinical genetics assessment and was found to have a pathogenic variant in *TP53* (c.473G > A; p.Arg158His) consistent with LFS. Unfortunately, the patient died of her malignancy prior to the availability of genetic results and the clinical confirmation could not be performed. Family members were referred for cascade testing on the *TP53* variant identified.

Category C included four patients (Table 2: patients 4–7) who did not meet genetic testing criteria for the identified gMAV at diagnosis of the disease. Patient 4 was a woman who did not meet Chompret's Revised criteria despite an extensive personal history of cancer. She was enrolled in the tumor profiling program due to a

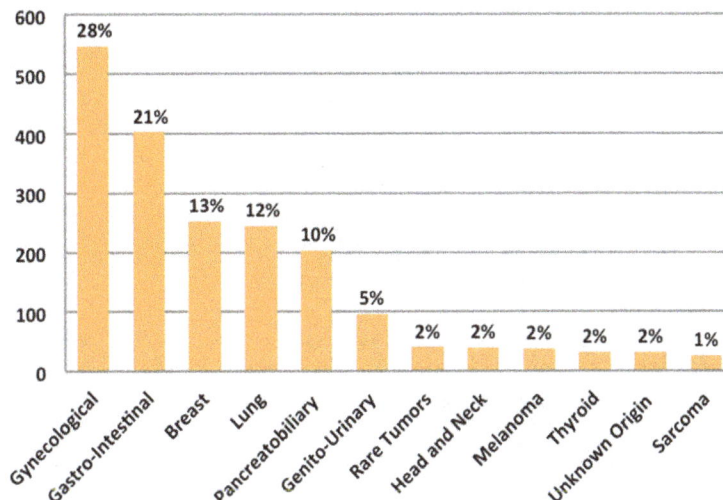

Fig. 2 Patients' characteristics – disease site

Table 1 Patients' characteristics and acceptance of the return of secondary germline Medically Actionable Variants

	Accepted n = 1844	Declined n = 103	p-value[†]
Age– years (mean)	57.6	57.6	> 0.95
Gender - n			p-value[‡]
Female	1235 (67%)	71 (69%)	> 0.68
Male	609 (33%)	32 (31%)	
Race - n			
White	1003 (54%)	56 (54%)	> 0.95
Asian	207 (11%)	16 (16%)	
Black	35 (2%)	1 (1%)	
Mixed	14 (1%)	0 (0%)	
Unknown	585 (32%)	30 (29%)	
Cancer site - n			
Gynecological	518 (28%)	25 (24%)	0.015
Gastrointestinal	382 (21%)	19 (18%)	
Breast	233 (13%)	18 (17%)	
Lung	227 (12%)	17 (17%)	
Pancreas	194 (11%)	8 (8%)	
Sarcoma	21 (1%)	5 (5%)	
Others	269 (15%)	11(11%)	
Prior genetic testing - n			
Yes	345 (19%)	15 (15%)	0.292
No	1499 (81%)	88 (85%)	
ECOG - n			
0	760 (41%)	37 (36%)	0.288
1	1084 (59%)	66 (64%)	

ECOG The Eastern Cooperative Oncology Group, *n* number. Values are expressed as mean (+/− standard deviation), except otherwise stated. [†] *T-d'Student test;* [‡] *Chi square test*

metastatic Her2+ breast cancer and germline DNA analysis revealed a pathogenic variant in *TP53* (c.817C > T; p.Arg273Cys). She presented a prolonged partial response on Her2 therapy and was enrolled in an LFS surveillance program [16] where she was found to have a lung adenocarcinoma. Patient 5, a man diagnosed with a gastroesophageal junction adenocarcinoma at age 29 years, and Patient 6, a man diagnosed with an ileocecal valve adenocarcinoma at age 36 years, were also found to harbor gMAVs in *TP53*. Interestingly, Patient 6 was found to have a c.467G > A (p.Arg156His) *TP53* germline variant, which in absence of other variants has been reported with conflicting interpretations in ClinVar [17], but when present in conjunction with an additional germline *TP53* variant has been associated with LFS [18]. The tumor analysis of Patient 6 did show another variant in *TP53* (c.742C > T; p.Arg248Trp). Given this potential association with LFS and the tumor results, the Genomic Tumor Board recommended return of this result and further *TP53* analysis to rule out LFS. Sanger sequencing and Multiplex Ligation–dependent Probe Amplification of *TP53* on another sample in a clinical molecular laboratory confirmed and classified the *TP53* c.467G > A variant as a variant of unknown significance, but no other germline variants in *TP53* were identified. Segregation analysis to further characterize the pathogenicity of this variant was not possible due to the unavailability of other family members with cancer history. Patient 7, a 75 year old man with esophageal cancer and no family history of note, was found to have a germline *SMARCB1* variant (c.143C > T; p.Pro48-Leu), which has been associated with schwannomatosis and multiple meningiomas [19]. The patient did not have any features of schwannomatosis, but was referred for

Table 2 Characteristics of patients with germline Medically Actionable Variants

Pt	Cat	Sex	Cancer (Age at diagnosis)	HCS	Variant in PBL (AF)
1	A	F	Desmoid tumor (32), Rectal cuff adenocarcinoma (43)	FAP	*APC* c.3927_3931del (p.Glu1309AspfsX4) (29%)
2	A	F	Embryonal Rhabdomyosarcoma (3), Thyroid (18), Peripheral Nerve Sheath Tumor (23), Renal leiomyosarcoma (29), Extraosseous sarcoma (31)	LFS	*TP53* c.743G > A (p.Arg248Gln) (48%)
3	B	F	Breast Cancer (39), Colorectal adenocarcinoma (39), Pleomorphic sarcoma (54), Lung Adenocarcinoma (55)	LFS	*TP53* c.473G > A (p.Arg158His) (57%)
4	C	F	Papillary Thyroid (28), Non-melanotic Skin Cancer (35), Breast Cancer (37), Lung Adenocarcinoma (39)	LFS	*TP53* c.817C > T (p.Arg273Cys) (53%)
5	C	M	Gastro-esophageal junction adenocarcinoma (29)	LFS	*TP53* c.818G > A (p.Arg273His) (52%)
6	C	M	Ileocecal valve adenocarcinoma (36)	LFS	*TP53* c.467G > A (p.Arg156His) (49%)
7	C	M	Esophageal adenocarcinoma (75)	Sch	*SMARCB1* c.143C > T (p.Pro48Leu) (72%)
8	D	F	Gallbladder Cancer (74)	N/A	*TP53* c.524G > A (p.Arg175His) (16%)

AF allele frequency, *Cat* category, *F* female, *FAP* familial adenomatous polyposis, *HCS* hereditary cancer syndrome, *LFS* Li-Fraumeni syndrome, *M* male, *Pt* patient, *Sch* schwannomatosis

neurologic assessment and familial testing did not identify the variant in the offspring.

Category D patient (Table 2: patient 8) was a 78 year old adopted woman with a diagnosis of cholangiocarcinoma at age 74, treated with gemcitabine/cisplatin in the metastatic setting prior to her enrollment in the tumor profiling program. PBL DNA analysis found a variant in *TP53* (c.524G > A; p.Arg175His), which has been associated with LFS [20] but was only present at a low allele frequency (16%). Negative cascade testing in the offspring and the absence of variants in *TP53* or other genes in the tumor, suggests that the finding may be due to mosaicism or more plausibly, a treatment related mutation limited to the blood [21, 22]. She declined a skin biopsy for mosaic studies because she was too unwell and shortly after passed away.

Discussion

Here, we describe the integration of a clinical genetics service in a tumor profiling program not specifically designed to actively seek nor comprehensively analyze germline medically actionable variants (gMAV). Despite this analytical approach of only analyzing gene hotspots, additional gMAVs were found incidentally and disclosed by a clinical genetics service. We also explore patients' preferences for the return of gMAVs in cancer predisposition genes. We are the first to describe the various scenarios and complexities in incorporating these additional findings into the clinical care of the study patients and families.

Patients expressed great interest in the return of gMAVs (94%), while minority declined (5%) or improperly filled in the consent form (1%). This is consistent with smaller studies such as Gray et al, who reported their experience in 69 lung, colorectal and breast cancer patients, and found that 87% of patients were willing to know about their inherited risk of cancer and 81% of patients agreed to the return of germline information regarding cancer risk and other medically actionable findings [23]. Yusuf et al, reported their experience in 100 breast cancer patients where 90% were willing to know about their cancer risk, while 87% of patients were also interested in other preventable/treatable diseases [24]. In another study from the same group, that included 1167 patients with multiple types of tumors, 99% of the cohort was in agreement to receive information about secondary germline findings [9]. More recently, a study of 413 breast, lung and colorectal cancer patients reported that 77% of patients were interested in germline variants of serious but preventable diseases, while only 56% were interested if the illness was unpreventable. In this study 49% of patients wanted to be informed about variants of unknown significance [25].

Patients' desire to be informed about additional germline findings remains high over time. Still, the demographic profile of the patients who decline or agree to the return of additional germline results has not been established. In our analysis, there were no statistically significant differences among the two groups in terms of sex, age, race, tumor type and ECOG status. Our cohort was heterogeneous, but with potential bias due to a high number of gynecological (28%) and breast cancer (13%) patients, which enriched the study with predominantly female population (67%).

Advanced cancer patients that are found to harbor previously unrecognized gMAVs in cancer predisposition genes can present multiple challenges for disclosure of the results even if they did consent for the return of additional findings. Alongside with molecular geneticists who determine the pathogenicity of a variant, a critical role is played by the clinical genetics team tasked to disclose germline results to the patient. For this purpose we depict four categories of results (Fig. 1) that highlight the complexity of genetic counseling [26]. Individuals who are eligible for genetic testing are often unrecognized and under-referred [27], and a tumor profiling program may identify a previously eligible patient (Category B) who did not have a genetics assessment. This underscores the importance of enquiring about personal and family cancer history in all cancer patients, especially in those undergoing a tumor molecular profiling that can reveal inherited variants.

On the other hand, current genetic testing criteria, such as Chompret's Revised criteria for *TP53* genetic testing (patients 4–6) do not capture all the cases and may miss individuals with less striking family histories or de novo cases (Category C). Other disorders such as schwannomatosis (Patient 7) may have low penetrance, making personal and family history unreliable for screening assessment. As exemplified in Patient 4, the identification of atypical hereditary cancer cases provides an opportunity for a patient to undergo appropriate surveillance and the detection of additional malignancies in at risk organs. The widespread use of NGS in tumor profiling programs may complement traditional routes of ascertaining patients and families with a cancer predisposition syndrome.

An emerging area of clinical uncertainty occurs when NGS testing identifies variants in PBL at allele frequency lower than expected for heterozygosity. These low allele frequencies are now detectable using NGS and may be due to a variety of causes such as post-zygotic mosaicism [28], age acquired clonal mosaicism [29, 30] or treatment-related clonal hematopoiesis [22, 28, 31]. This situation was observed in Category D and further follow-up studies are necessary to delineate the etiology of the NGS result, as post-zygotic mosaicism has implications on the family, while age acquired clonal mosaicism and treatment-related clonal hematopoiesis do not.

Our study revealed a total of eight patients with additional gMAVs in a cohort of 1556 advanced cancer patients who underwent NGS tumor profiling. This is likely an under-representation of the true prevalence of hereditary cancer syndromes in our cohort, as this study was not designed to systematically identify all germline genes and variants causing a hereditary cancer syndrome.

Despite these constraints a number of gMAVs were detected as additional findings. As numerous targeted panels perform tumor only sequencing, mostly for economic reasons, these gMAVs may be missed. Our study highlights the potential drawbacks of the tumor-only testing approach since patients were identified with constitutional variants that likely would have been considered somatic with tumor-only NGS panel testing. We also describe the benefit of integrating a tumor profiling program with a clinical genetics service to incorporate these findings into the clinical care of patients. This will ultimately identify more cancer predisposition families and, in turn, preventable cases of cancer.

Conclusions

Here, we describe the largest cohort reported so far to undergo a precision cancer medicine tumor profiling program, where germline DNA was used primarily to aid in filtering tumour variants. The normal DNA analysis resulted in a variety of returnable additional findings, disclosed through the incorporation of a clinical genetics service within the research study and into the clinical care of these families.

Abbreviations
ASCP: Ion AmpliSeq Cancer Panel; COMPACT: Community Oncology Molecular Profiling in Advanced Cancers Trial; ECOG: Eastern Cooperative Oncology Group; gMAV: germline medically actionable variant; IGV: Integrative Genomics Viewer; IMPACT: Integrated Molecular Profiling in Advanced Cancers Trial; LFS: Li-Fraumeni syndrome; NGS: Next generation sequencing; PBL: Peripheral blood lymphocytes; TSACP: TruSeq Amplicon Cancer Panel

Funding
The design of the study; collection, analysis, interpretation of data; and manuscript preparation was supported by the Princess Margaret Cancer Centre Cancer Genomics Program and the Princess Margaret Cancer Foundation, Division of Medical Oncology, University of Toronto, Cancer Care Ontario and Ontario Ministry of Health. The first author is supported in part by a translational research grant from the Spanish Society of Medical Oncology (SEOM).

Authors' contributions
NS, TS and RK analyzed and interpreted the patient data regarding the additional germline findings and were major contributors in writing the manuscript; PB, LS and SKR were involved in revising the manustript critically; JM, MA, SH, KS, NL, RJ, MK, AO, AG, CE and LA made substantial contributions to the acquisition of data; LW was responsible for the statistical analysis. All authors read and approved the final manuscript.

Competing interests
The authors declare that they have no competing interests.

Author details
[1]Division of Medical Oncology and Hematology, Princess Margaret Cancer Centre, 610 University Ave, Toronto, ON M5G 2M9, Canada. [2]Cancer Genomics Program, Princess Margaret Cancer Centre, 610 University Ave, Toronto, ON M5G 2M9, Canada. [3]Department of Clinical Laboratory Genetics & Department of Laboratory Medicine and Pathobiology, University of Toronto, 610 University Ave, Toronto, ON M5G 2M9, Canada. [4]Department of Molecular Genetics, University of Toronto, 610 University Ave, Toronto, ON M5G 2M9, Canada. [5]Zane Cohen Centre for Digestive Diseases, Mount Sinai Hospital, 60 Murray St, Toronto, ON M5T 3L9, Canada. [6]Department of Biostatistics, Princess Margaret Cancer Centre, 610 University Ave, Toronto, ON M5G 2M9, Canada.

References
1. Roychowdhury S, Iyer MK, Robinson DR, et al. Personalized oncology through integrative high-throughput sequencing: a pilot study. Science translational medicine. 2011;3(111):111ra121.
2. Jones S, Anagnostou V, Lytle K, et al. Personalized genomic analyses for cancer mutation discovery and interpretation. Science translational medicine. 2015;7(283):283ra253.
3. Catenacci DV, Amico AL, Nielsen SM, et al. Tumor genome analysis includes germline genome: are we ready for surprises? Int J Cancer. 2015;136(7): 1559–67.
4. Robson ME, Bradbury AR, Arun B, et al. American Society of Clinical Oncology policy statement update: genetic and genomic testing for Cancer susceptibility. J Clin Oncol. 2015;33(31):3660–7.
5. Raymond VM, Gray SW, Roychowdhury S, et al. Germline Findings in Tumor-Only Sequencing: Points to Consider for Clinicians and Laboratories. J Natl Cancer Inst. 2016;108(4):djv351.
6. Clinical Sequencing Exploratory Research Consortium Tumor Working G. Medically Actionable Secondary or Incidental Results. 2017; https://www.ashg.org/education/csertoolkit/medicallyactionable.html. Accessed 2 Jan 2018.
7. Tan N, Amendola LM, O'Daniel JM, et al. Is "incidental finding" the best term?: a study of patients' preferences. Genet Med. 2017;19(2):176–81.
8. Schrader KA, Cheng DT, Joseph V, et al. Germline variants in targeted tumor sequencing using matched normal DNA. JAMA oncology. 2016;2(1):104–11.
9. Meric-Bernstam F, Brusco L, Daniels M, et al. Incidental germline variants in 1000 advanced cancers on a prospective somatic genomic profiling protocol. Ann Oncol. 2016;27(5):795–800.
10. Seifert BA, O'Daniel JM, Amin K, et al. Germline analysis from tumor-germline sequencing dyads to identify clinically actionable secondary findings. Clin Cancer Res. 2016;22(16):4087–94.
11. Mandelker D, Zhang L, Kemel Y, et al. Mutation detection in patients with advanced Cancer by universal sequencing of Cancer-related genes in tumor and normal DNA vs guideline-based germline testing. JAMA. 2017;318(9): 825–35.
12. Stockley TL, Oza AM, Berman HK, et al. Molecular profiling of advanced solid tumors and patient outcomes with genotype-matched clinical trials: the Princess Margaret IMPACT/COMPACT trial. Genome med. 2016;8(1):109.
13. Richards S, Aziz N, Bale S, et al. Standards and guidelines for the interpretation of sequence variants: a joint consensus recommendation of the American College of Medical Genetics and Genomics and the Association for Molecular Pathology. Genet Med. 2015;17(5):405–24.
14. Demsky R, McCuaig J, Maganti M, Murphy KJ, Rosen B, Armel SR. Keeping it simple: genetics referrals for all invasive serous ovarian cancers. Gynecol Oncol. 2013;130(2):329–33.
15. Tinat J, Bougeard G, Baert-Desurmont S, et al. 2009 version of the Chompret criteria for li Fraumeni syndrome. J Clin Oncol. 2009;27(26):e108–9.
16. Villani A, Shore A, Wasserman JD, et al. Biochemical and imaging surveillance in germline TP53 mutation carriers with li-Fraumeni syndrome: 11 year follow-up of a prospective observational study. Lancet Oncol. 2016;17(9):1295–305.
17. de Martel C, Ferlay J, Franceschi S, et al. Global burden of cancers attributable to infections in 2008: a review and synthetic analysis. Lancet Oncol. 2012;13(6):607–15.
18. Quesnel S, Verselis S, Portwine C, et al. p53 compound heterozygosity in a severely affected child with li-Fraumeni syndrome. Oncogene. 1999;18(27): 3970–8.
19. Christiaans I, Kenter SB, Brink HC, et al. Germline SMARCB1 mutation and somatic NF2 mutations in familial multiple meningiomas. J Med Genet. 2011;48(2):93–7.

20. Bougeard G, Limacher JM, Martin C, et al. Detection of 11 germline inactivating TP53 mutations and absence of TP63 and HCHK2 mutations in 17 French families with Ii-Fraumeni or Ii-Fraumeni-like syndrome. J Med Genet. 2001;38(4):253–7.

21. Jacobs KB, Yeager M, Zhou W, et al. Detectable clonal mosaicism and its relationship to aging and cancer. Nat Genet. 2012;44(6):651–8.

22. Gillis NK, Ball M, Zhang Q, et al. Clonal haemopoiesis and therapy-related myeloid malignancies in elderly patients: a proof-of-concept, case-control study. Lancet Oncol. 2017;18(1):112–21.

23. Gray SW, Hicks-Courant K, Lathan CS, Garraway L, Park ER, Weeks JC. Attitudes of patients with Cancer about personalized medicine and somatic genetic testing. J Oncol Pract. 2012;8(6):329–35.

24. Yusuf RA, Rogith D, Hovick SR, et al. Attitudes toward molecular testing for personalized cancer therapy. Cancer. 2015;121(2):243–50.

25. Yushak ML, Han G, Bouberhan S, et al. Patient preferences regarding incidental genomic findings discovered during tumor profiling. Cancer. 2016;122(10):1588–97.

26. Goedde LN, Stupiansky NW, Lah M, Quaid KA, Cohen S. Cancer genetic Counselors' current practices and attitudes related to the use of tumor profiling. J Genet Couns. 2017;26(4):878–86.

27. Hampel H, Bennett RL, Buchanan A, et al. A practice guideline from the American College of Medical Genetics and Genomics and the National Society of genetic counselors: referral indications for cancer predisposition assessment. Genet Med. 2015;17(1):70–87.

28. Konnick EQ, Pritchard CC. Germline, hematopoietic, mosaic, and somatic variation: interplay between inherited and acquired genetic alterations in disease assessment. Genome med. 2016;8(1):100.

29. Jaiswal S, Fontanillas P, Flannick J, et al. Age-related clonal hematopoiesis associated with adverse outcomes. N Engl J Med. 2014;371(26):2488–98.

30. Xie M, Lu C, Wang J, et al. Age-related mutations associated with clonal hematopoietic expansion and malignancies. Nat Med. 2014;20(12):1472–8.

31. Wong TN, Ramsingh G, Young AL, et al. Role of TP53 mutations in the origin and evolution of therapy-related acute myeloid leukaemia. Nature. 2015;518(7540):552–5.

5

Min-redundancy and max-relevance multi-view feature selection for predicting ovarian cancer survival using multi-omics data

Yasser EL-Manzalawy[1,5,6], Tsung-Yu Hsieh[1,4,5], Manu Shivakumar[2], Dokyoon Kim[2,3*] and Vasant Honavar[1,3,4,5,6*]

Abstract

Background: Large-scale collaborative precision medicine initiatives (e.g., The Cancer Genome Atlas (TCGA)) are yielding rich multi-omics data. Integrative analyses of the resulting multi-omics data, such as somatic mutation, copy number alteration (CNA), DNA methylation, miRNA, gene expression, and protein expression, offer tantalizing possibilities for realizing the promise and potential of precision medicine in cancer prevention, diagnosis, and treatment by substantially improving our understanding of underlying mechanisms as well as the discovery of novel biomarkers for different types of cancers. However, such analyses present a number of challenges, including heterogeneity, and high-dimensionality of omics data.

Methods: We propose a novel framework for multi-omics data integration using multi-view feature selection. We introduce a novel multi-view feature selection algorithm, MRMR-mv, an adaptation of the well-known Min-Redundancy and Maximum-Relevance (MRMR) single-view feature selection algorithm to the multi-view setting.

Results: We report results of experiments using an ovarian cancer multi-omics dataset derived from the TCGA database on the task of predicting ovarian cancer survival. Our results suggest that multi-view models outperform both view-specific models (i.e., models trained and tested using a single type of omics data) and models based on two baseline data fusion methods.

Conclusions: Our results demonstrate the potential of multi-view feature selection in integrative analyses and predictive modeling from multi-omics data.

Keywords: Multi-omics data integration, Multi-view feature selection, Cancer survival prediction, Machine learning

* Correspondence: dkim@geisinger.edu; vhonavar@ist.psu.edu
[2]Biomedical and Translational Informatics Institute, Geisinger Health System, Danville, PA, USA
[1]Artificial Intelligence Research Laboratory, College of Information Sciences and Technology, Pennsylvania State University, University Park, PA 16802, USA
Full list of author information is available at the end of the article

Background

The advent of "big data" offers enormous potential for understanding and predicting health risks and intervention outcomes, as well as personalizing treatments, through integrative analysis of clinical, biomedical, behavioral, environmental, and even socio-demographic data. For example, recent efforts in cancer genomics under the Precision Health Initiative offer promising ways to diagnose, prevent, and treat many cancers [1]. Recent advances in high-throughput omics technologies offer cost-effective ways to acquire diverse types of genome-wide multi-omics data. For instance, Large-scale collaborative efforts such as the Cancer Genome Atlas (TCGA) and the International Cancer Genome Consortium (ICGC) are collecting multi-omics data for tumors along with clinical data for the patients. An important goal of these initiatives is to develop comprehensive catalogs of key genomic alterations associated for a large number of cancer types [2, 3].

Computational analyses of multi-omics data offer an unprecedented opportunity to deepen our understanding of complex underlying mechanisms of cancer that is essential for advancing precision oncology (See for example, [4–7]). Because different types of omics data have been shown to complement each other [8], there is a growing interest in effective methods for integrative analyses of multi-omics data [9–11]. The resulting methods have been successfully used to predict the molecular abnormalities that impact both clinical outcomes and therapeutic targets [5, 10, 12–16].

Effective approaches to integrative analyses and predictive modeling from multi-omics data have to address three major challenges [5]: i) the curse of dimensionality (i.e., the number of features p is very large compared to the number of samples n); ii) the differences in scales as well as sampling/collection bias and noise present in different omics data sets; iii) extracting and optimally combining, for the prediction task at hand, features that provide complementary information across different data sources. Unfortunately, baseline methods that simply concatenate the features extracted from the different data sources or analyze each data from each source separately and combine the predictions fail to satisfactorily address these challenges. Therefore, there is an urgent need for more sophisticated methods for integrative analysis and predictive modeling from multi-omics data [16].

The problem of learning predictive models from multi-omics data can be naturally formulated as a *multi-view learning* problem [17] where each omics data source provides a distinct view of the complex biological system. Multi-view learning offers a promising approach to developing predictive models by leveraging complementary information provided by the multiple data sources (views) to optimize the predictive performance of the resulting model [17]. The state-of-the-art learning algorithms attempt to learn a set of models, one from each view, and combine them so as to jointly optimize the predictive performance of the combined multi-view model. Some examples of multi-view learning algorithms include: multi-view support vector machines [18], multi-view Boosting [19], multi-view *k*-means [20], and clustering via canonical correlation analysis [21]. However, barring a few exceptions (e.g., multi-view feature selection methods [22], and multi-view representation learning [23]) the vast majority of existing multi-view learning algorithms are not equipped to effectively cope with the high-dimensionality of omics data [17]. Hence, predictive modeling from multi-omics data calls for effective methods for multi-view feature selection or dimensionality reduction.

Against this background, we present a general two-stage framework for multi-omics data integration. We introduce MRMR-mv, an adaptation of the well-known Min-Redundancy and Maximum-Relevance (MRMR) single-view feature selection algorithm to the multi-view setting. We provide, to the best of our knowledge, the first application of a multi-view feature selection method to predictive modeling from multi-omics data. We report the results of our experiments that compare the proposed approach with several baseline methods on the task of building a predictive model of cancer survival [13] using a TCGA multi-omics dataset composed of three omics data sources, copy number alteration (CNA), DNA methylation, and gene expression RNA-Seq. The results of our experiments show that: (i) the multi-view predictive models developed from multi-omics data outperform their single-view counterparts; and that (ii) the predictive models developed using MRMR-mv for multi-view feature selection outperform those developed using two baseline methods that combine multiple views into a single-view. These results demonstrate the potential of multi-view feature selection based approaches to multi-omics data integration.

Methods
Datasets

Normalized and preprocessed multi-omics ovarian cancer datasets (most recently updated on August 16, 2016), including genelevel copy number alteration (CNA), DNA methylation, and gene expression (GE) RNA-Seq data, were downloaded from UCSC Xena cancer genomic browser [24]. Table 1 summarizes the number of samples and features (e.g., genes) in each dataset. Clinical data about vital status and survival for the subjects were also downloaded from Xena server. Only the patients with CNA, methylation, RNA-Seq, and survival data were retained. Patients with survival time ≥3 years were labeled as long-term survivors while patients with survival time <3 years and vital status of 0 were labeled as short-term

Table 1 TCGA ovarian cancer omics data used in this study

Data source	Platform	Number of samples	Number of features	Number of features with high variance
CNA	Affymetrix SNP 6	579	24,777	7355
Methylation	Illumina Infinium HumanMethylation27k	616	27,579	6206
GE RNA-Seq	Illumina HiSeq	308	30,531	283

survivors. The resulting multi-view dataset consists of 215 samples, 127 of them are classified as long-term survivors. Each view was then pre-filtered and normalized as follows: i) features with missing values were excluded; ii) feature values in each sample were rescaled to lie in the interval [0,1]; iii) features with variance less than 0.02 were removed.

Notations

Table 2 summarizes convenient notations used in this work. For simplicity, we assumed a binary label for each sample. Note however, that Algorithms 1 and 2, described below, are also applicable to multi-class as well as numerically labeled data.

Minimum redundancy and maximum relevance feature selection

Unlike univariate feature selection methods [25] that return a subset of features without accounting for redundancy between the selected features, the minimum redundancy and maximum relevance (MRMR) feature selection algorithm [26] iteratively selects features that are *maximally relevant* for the prediction task and

minimally redundant with the set of already selected features. MRMR has been successfully used for feature selection in a number of applications including microarray gene expression data analysis [26, 27], prediction of protein sub-cellular localization [28], epileptic seizure [29], and protein-protein interaction [30].

While the exact solution to the problem of MRMR selection of $k = |S|$ features from a set of n candidates requires the evaluation of $O(n^k)$ candidate feature subsets, it is possible to obtain an approximate solution using a simple heuristic algorithm (see Algorithm 1) [26]. Algorithm 1 accepts as input: a labeled dataset D; a function $g:(x_i, x_j) \rightarrow R^+$ that quantifies the redundancy between any pair of features (e.g., the absolute value of Pearson's correlation coefficient); a function $f:(x_i, y) \rightarrow R^+$ that quantifies the relevance of a target feature for predicting the labels y (e.g., mutual information (MI) or F-statistic); and the number of features k to be selected using the MRMR criterion. In lines 1 and 2, the algorithm creates an empty set S and the feature with the maximum relevance for predicting y is added to S. In each of the subsequent $k - 1$ iterations (lines 3–5), the features that greedily approximate the MRMR criterion in Eq. 1 are successively

Table 2 Notations

Symbol	Definition and Description
$D = <X, y>$	Labeled dataset where $X \in R^{m \times n}$ is a matrix of m instances and n features, and $y \in \{0, 1\}^m$ is the binary class labels of the instances
x_i	i^{th} feature in X
$g(x_i, x_j)$	Function that returns the redundancy between two features x_i and x_j
$f(x_i, y)$	Function that returns the relevance between a feature x_i and class labels y
S	Indices of selected features
Ω	Indices of all features
Ω_S	Indices of candidate features $\Omega - S$
k	Number of features to be selected
v	Number of views in a multi-view dataset
$MVD = <(X^1, ..., X^v), y>$	Labeled multi-view dataset where $X^i \in R^{m \times n_i}$ is a matrix of m samples and n_i features and $y \in \{0, 1\}^m$ is the binary class labels of the instances in all views
$D^i = <X^i, y>$	i^{th} view in a multi-view dataset
x^i_j	j^{th} feature in X^i
S^i	Indices of selected features from i^{th} view
Ω^i	Indices of all features in i^{th} view
Ω_{S^i}	Indices of candidate features $\Omega^i - S^i$ in i^{th} view

added to S. Eq. 1 has two terms: the first term maximizes the relevance condition, whereas the second term minimizes the redundancy condition.

$$\text{argmax}_{j \in \Omega_S} \left(f(x_j, y) - \frac{1}{|S|^2} \sum_{l \in S} g(x_j, x_l) \right) \qquad (1)$$

Algorithm 1. MRMR

Require: $D = <X, y>, g, f, k$

1: $S \leftarrow \emptyset$

2: add $x_i = \text{argmax}_{j \in \Omega} f(x_j, y)$ to S

3: **for** $t = 1 : k - 1$ do

4:   add the feature that satisfies Eq. 1 to S

5: **end for**

6: **return** S

Multi-view minimum redundancy and maximum relevance feature selection

MRMR, or any single-view feature selection algorithm, can be trivially applied to multi-view data as follows: i) Apply MRMR separately to each view and then concatenate view-specific selected features. The major limitation of this approach is that it ignores the redundancy and complementarity of features across the views [31]; ii) Apply MRMR to a single-view dataset obtained by concatenating all the views. A key limitation of this approach is that it fails to explicitly account for the prediction task specific differences in the relative utility or relevance of the features extracted from the different views.

Here, we propose a novel multi-view feature selection algorithm, MRMR-mv, that adapts the MRMR algorithm to the multi-view setting. MRMR-mv (shown in Algorithm 2) accepts as input: a labeled multi-view dataset, MVD, with $v \geq 2$ views; a redundancy function g; a relevance function f; number of features to be selected k; and a probability distribution $P = \{p_1 \cdots p_v\}$ that models the relative importance of each view (or the prior probability that a view contributes a feature to the set of features selected by MRMR-mv). If each of the views is equally important, P should be a uniform distribution. MRMR-mv proceeds as follows. First, S^t is initialized for each view t to keep track of selected features from that view (lines 1–3). Second, the procedure *choice*, implemented in NumPy python library [32], is invoked to obtain k-1 views, sampled from with replacement, according to P, from the set of views. The list of sampled views is recorded in C (lines 4 and 5). Third, the maximally relevant feature across *all* of the views (say x^i_j, the jth feature in the ith view) is retrieved and the set (S^i) of the selected features for the corresponding view, i, is updated accordingly (line 6). Fourth, for each of the views in C, considered in turn and at each step t, the feature from the corresponding view that satisfies the

MRMR criterion with respect to the previously selected features from iterations (1 through t-1) is added to $S^{C[t]}$ (lines 7–10). Finally, the algorithm returns selected view-specific features $S^1, \cdots S^v$.

We note that MRMR-mv applies the MRMR criteria across all of the views, as opposed to the baseline methods that apply the criteria to each view separately or to the concatenation of all views. Thus MRMR-mv can select complementary features from within as well as across views. It can also assign different degrees of importance to the views to reflect any available information about their relative utility in the context of a given prediction task.

Algorithm 2. MRMR-mv

Require: $MVD = <(X^1, ..., X^v), y>, g, f, k, P = (p_i, ..., p_v)$

1: **for** $t = 1 : v$

2:   $S^t \leftarrow \emptyset$

3: **end for**

4: $V \leftarrow \{1, ..., v\}$

5: $C \leftarrow choice(V, k - 1, P)$

6: add $x^i_j = \text{argmax}_{i \in \{1,..,v\}} \text{argmax}_{j \in \Omega^i} f(x^i_j, y)$ to S^i

7: **for** $t = 1 : k - 1$ do

8:   $l \leftarrow C[t]$

9:   add $x^l_i = \text{argmax}_{j \in \Omega_{S^l}} (f(x^l_j, y) - \frac{1}{(t)^2} \sum_{q \in \{1,..,v\}} \sum_{h \in S^q} g(x^l_j, x^q_h))$ to S^l

10: **end for**

11: **return** $S = \{S^1, \cdots, S^v\}$

A two-stage feature selection framework for multi-omics data integration

Figure 1 shows our proposed two-stage framework for integrating multi-omics data for virtually any prediction task (e.g., predicting cancer survival or predicting clinical outcome). The input to our framework is a labeled multi-view dataset in the form $D^i = <X^i, y>$. Stage I includes view-specific filters that can be used to encapsulate any traditional single-view feature selection method (e.g., Lasso [33] or MRMR). Each filter has a gating signal that could be used to disable that filter in which case the disabled filter passes on no data to the 2nd stage. A special view-specific filter, called AllFilter, passes *all* of the input features without performing any feature selection. Stage II has a single filter that can encapsulate either a single-view or a multi-view feature selection method. If the 2nd stage filter encapsulates a single-view feature selection method, the feature selection method will be applied to the concatenation of the Stage II input. On the other hand, if the 2nd stage filter encapsulates a multi-view feature selection method (e.g., MRMR-mv), then the multi-view feature selection method will be applied to the multi-view input of Stage II. The framework supports two modes of operations: i) training mode, where each enabled filter will be

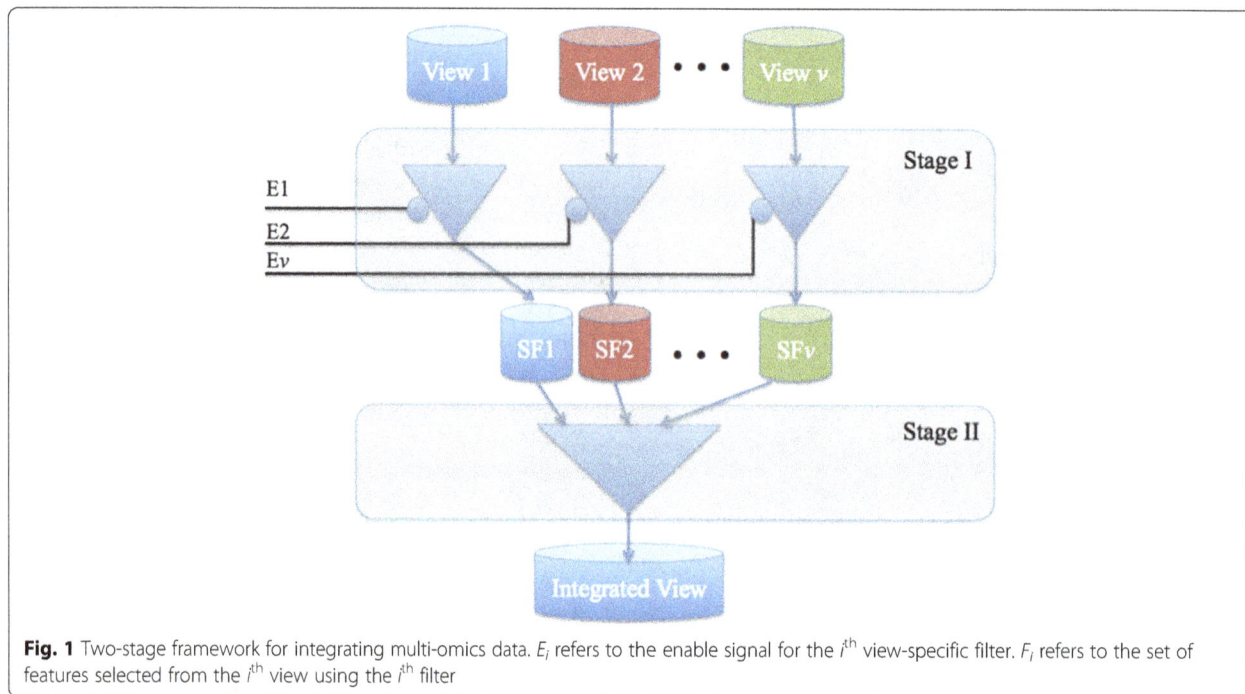

Fig. 1 Two-stage framework for integrating multi-omics data. E_i refers to the enable signal for the ith view-specific filter. F_i refers to the set of features selected from the ith view using the ith filter

trained using the input so as to produce the filtered version of the input; ii) test (or operation) mode, where test multi-view dataset is provided as input and the trained filters will output the selected features of the input data.

The framework can be easily customized so as to allow evaluation of different approaches of predictive modeling from multi-omics data. For example, to build a single-view model by applying the Lasso method to the ith view, we: set E_i to 1 and disable all other filters; pass Lasso feature selection method to the ith filter; use AllFilter as Stage II filter. Similarly, to apply MRMR to concatenated views, we: enable Stage I filters and use either AllFilter (to pass the input as is) or any single-view filter; and deploy MRMR as the Stage II filter.

Implementation

We implemented Algorithms 1 and 2 and the two-stage feature selection framework in Python using the scikit-learn machine learning library [34]. We will release the code as part of sklearn-fuse, a python library for data and model-based data fusion that is currently under development in our lab. In the mean time, the code for the methods described above will be made available to interested researchers upon request.

Experiments

We report results of experiments on the task of building a predictive model of cancer survival from an ovarian cancer multi-omics dataset derived from the TCGA database. The resulting data set is comprised of three views, namely, CNA, methylation, and gene expression RNA-Seq for each

patient along with the corresponding clinical outcomes (short-term versus long-term survival). Our first set of experiments consider single-view classifiers based on each of the 3 views to obtain view-specific models for comparison with the proposed multi-view models; The second set of experiments compare some of the representative instantiations of the two-stage multi-view feature selection framework in combination with some representative choices of (single-view) supervised algorithms for training the classifiers. In both cases, we experimented with three widely used machine learning algorithms for developing cancer survival predictors: i) Random Forest (RF) [35] with 500 trees; ii) eXtreme Gradient Boosting (XGB) [36] with 500 weak learners; ii) Logistic Regression (LR) [37] with L1 regularization. We used the implementations of these algorithms available in the Scikit-learn machine learning library [34].

For Stage I feature selection, we experimented with several feature selection methods implemented in Scikit-learn including: RF feature importance [35]; Lasso [33]; ElasticNet [38]; and Recursive Feature Elimination (RFE) [39]. However, due to space limitation, we describe only the results of the best performing method, Lasso with L1 regularization parameter set to 0.0001. In Stage II feature selection, we used MRMR as a baseline method and MRMR-mv for multi-view feature selection.

For both MRMR and MRMR-mv feature selection, we used the absolute value of Pearson's correlation coefficient as the redundancy function, g. For the relevance function, f, we experimented with three functions Chi2,

F-Statistic (F-Stat), and Mutual Information (MI). All functions are implemented in Scikit-learn.

We estimated the performance of the resulting classifiers on the task of predicting cancer survival using the 5-fold cross-validation (CV) procedure. Briefly, the dataset is randomly partitioned into five equal subsets. Four of the five subsets are collectively used to select the features and train the classifier and the remaining subset is held out for estimating the performance of the trained classifier. This procedure is repeated 5 times, by setting aside a different subset of the data for estimating model performance. The 5 results from all the folds are then averaged to report a single performance estimate. In our experiments we used the area under ROC curve (AUC) [40] to assess the predictive performance of classifiers. When the number of samples used to estimate the classifier performance is small, as is the case with the ovarian cancer data, the estimated performance can vary substantially across different random partitions of the data into 5 folds (see Section "Single-view models for predicting ovarian cancer survival" for details). To obtain a more robust estimate of performance, we ran the 5-fold cross-validation procedure 10 times (each using different partitioning of the data into 5 subsets) and reported the mean AUC estimated from the 10 5-fold CV experiments.

Results

Single-view models for predicting ovarian cancer survival

We evaluated RF, XGB, and LR classifiers trained using each of the individual views with the top k features selected using Lasso feature selection algorithm for choices of $k = 10, 20, 30, ..., 100$. Tables 3, 4 and 5 report the performance of the resulting classifiers averaged over 10 different 5-fold cross-validation experiments.

Table 3 Average AUC scores of RF, XGB, and LR models trained on CNA data, estimated using 10 runs of 5-fold cross validation

# Features	RF	XGB	LR
10	0.57	0.56	0.58
20	0.61	0.61	0.61
30	0.61	0.61	0.61
40	0.63	0.62	0.61
50	0.64	0.64	0.62
60	0.65	0.65	0.63
70	0.65	0.65	0.63
80	0.65	0.65	0.62
90	0.66	0.66	0.63
100	0.66	0.66	0.62
Max	0.66	0.66	0.63
Avg.	0.63	0.63	0.62

Table 4 Average AUC scores of RF, XGB, and LR models trained on methylation data, estimated using 10 runs of 5-fold cross validation

# Features	RF	XGB	LR
10	0.52	0.51	0.50
20	0.51	0.52	0.50
30	0.52	0.52	0.49
40	0.52	0.53	0.50
50	0.52	0.53	0.51
60	0.52	0.53	0.52
70	0.53	0.54	0.51
80	0.53	0.54	0.52
90	0.53	0.55	0.52
100	0.53	0.55	0.52
Max	0.53	0.55	0.52
Avg.	0.52	0.53	0.51

We observed that models built using only the methylation view performed marginally better than random guessing (i.e., the best observed average AUC in Table 5 is 0.55). In contrast, single-view models using CNA or RNA-Seq achieved higher average AUC scores of up to 0.66. These results are in agreement with those of previously reported studies (e.g., [13]). It should be noted that when the performance of single-view models is estimated using a single 5-fold cross-validation experiment (as opposed to average over 10 different cross-validation experiments), the best observed AUC scores were 0.70, 0.55, and 0.69 for models built from the CNA, methylation, and RNA-Seq views, respectively. The observed variability in performance among different 5-fold cross-validation experiments is expected because of the relatively small size of the ovarian cancer survival dataset. This finding underscores

Table 5 Average AUC scores of RF, XGB, and LR models trained on RNA-Seq data, estimated using 10 runs of 5-fold cross validation

# Features	RF	XGB	LR
10	0.58	0.57	0.59
20	0.60	0.58	0.61
30	0.61	0.60	0.63
40	0.62	0.61	0.64
50	0.62	0.61	0.65
60	0.63	0.60	0.66
70	0.63	0.60	0.64
80	0.64	0.60	0.65
90	0.63	0.61	0.65
100	0.64	0.61	0.65
Max	0.64	0.61	0.66
Avg.	0.62	0.60	0.64

the importance of using multiple CV experiments to obtain robust estimates and comparisons of classifier performance. Next, we show how integrating data sources (i.e., views) can further improve the predictive performance of the cancer survival predictors.

Integrative analyses of multi-omics data sources using multi-view feature selection

We used our two-stage feature selection framework (See Fig. 1) to construct multi-view (MV) models with the following settings. The input to the framework is two views, CNA and RNA-Seq. We chose not to use the methylation view because the performance of single-view models built using the methylation data performed marginally better than chance (see Section "Single-view models for predicting ovarian cancer survival"). For the Stage I filters, we used Lasso with L1 regularization parameter set to 0.0001 to select the top 100 features from CNA and RNA-Seq views, respectively.

For the Stage II filter, we used MRMR-mv with Pearson's correlation coefficient as the redundancy function and a uniform distribution for the selection probability parameter, P. Finally, we experimented with different multi-view models obtained using combinations of choices for the remaining MRMR-mv parameters, k and f. Specifically, we experimented with $k = 10, 20, ..., 100$ and the relevance function $f \in \{Chi2, F - Stat, MI, and\ CFM\}$, where CFM is the average of the other three relevance functions.

Figure 2 compares the performance of the different MV models described above. Interestingly, no single relevance function consistently outperforms other functions for different choices of the number of selected features, k, and machine learning algorithms. However, the best AUC of 0.7 is obtained using either $Chi2$ or MI relevance functions and RF classifier trained using the top 100 features. Hence, our final MV models will use $Chi2$ as the relevance function and the remaining MRMR-mv settings stated in the preceding paragraph.

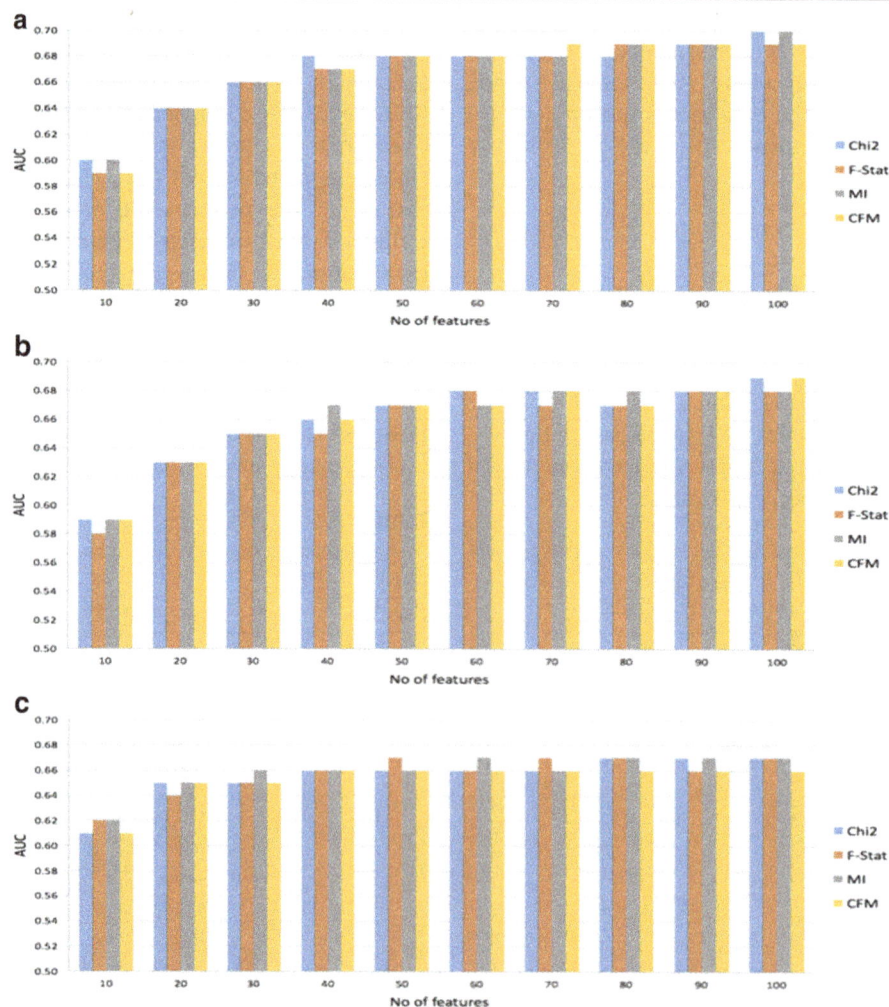

Fig. 2 Performance comparisons of multi-view models using four different relevance functions for MRMR-mv and three machine learning classifiers, **a**) RF, **b**). XGB, and **c**) LR

The selection probability parameter, P, in MRMR-mv algorithm controls the expected number of selected features from each view. Results shown in Fig. 2 have been produced using a uniform selection probability distribution. Although using a uniform distribution is reasonable since the best AUC score for the single-view models based on CNA or RNA-Seq is 0.66 (See Tables 3 and 5), it is interesting to examine the influence of P on the performance of our MV models. Let $P = (p_1, p_2)$ be the probability distribution where p_1 and p_2 denotes the sampling probability for CNA and RNA-Seq, respectively. In this experiment, we considered 11 different probability distributions obtained using $p_1 = \{0, 0.1, 0.2, ..., 1\}$. Then, for each choice of the number of selected features, k, we evaluated 11 MV models using RF algorithm and the same MRMR-mv settings described in the preceding subsection and the 11 different probability distributions for P. We used the percent relative range in the recorded AUC to assess the sensitivity of MV models to changes in P. Figure 3 shows the relationship between the number of selected MV features, k, and the sensitivity of MV models to changes in P. Interestingly, our results suggest that as the number of selected MV features increases, the resulting MV models become less sensitive to the selection probability distribution parameter P.

Multi-view vs. single-view models for predicting ovarian cancer survival

Figure 4 compares our final MV models with the following single-view models: i) SV_CNA, single-view models developed using CNA data source; ii) SV_RNA-Seq, single-view models developed using RNA-Seq data source; iii) SV_C, single-view models obtained by applying MRMR to the *concatenation* of the two views, CNA and RNA-Seq; iv) SV_S, single-view models obtained by applying MRMR *separately* to CNA and RNA-Seq views, respectively. In addition, Fig. 4 shows the results for a simple ensemble model that averages the predictions from SV_CNA and MV models. In general, MV and Ensemble models outperform SV models in most of the cases.

We noted some interesting observations from our experiments with each of the machine learning algorithms considered in our experiments. In the case of models developed using RF algorithm, MV and Ensemble models outperformed the four single-view models for all choices of the number of selected features, k. Ensemble models outperformed MV models for $k = 10, 20$, and 80. Baseline single-view models outperformed SV_CNA and SV_RNA-Seq for $k \leq 40$. The highest observed AUC was 0.7 and was obtained using the MV model and $k=100$. In the case of XGB based models, SV_S, MV, and Ensemble models outperformed the remaining single-view models. Ensemble models outperformed MV models for 8 out of 10 choices of k. Finally, for models developed using LR algorithm, SV_S, MV, and Ensemble models outperformed the other three single-view models. Regardless of which machine learning algorithm was used, SV_RNA-Seq and SV_C models had the lowest AUC in most of the cases reported in Fig. 4. Our results suggest that the best single-view model is more likely to perform better than models developed using concatenated views. Our results also suggest that either applying feature selection to each individual view or selecting features jointly using multi-view feature selection consistently outperform the best single-view model.

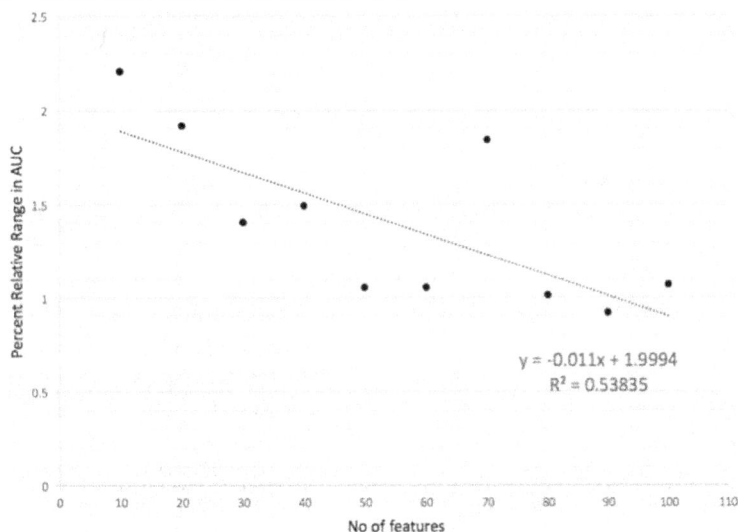

Fig. 3 Relationship between the number of selected MV features and sensitivity of MV models to changes in selection probability distribution P in terms of percent relative range in AUC

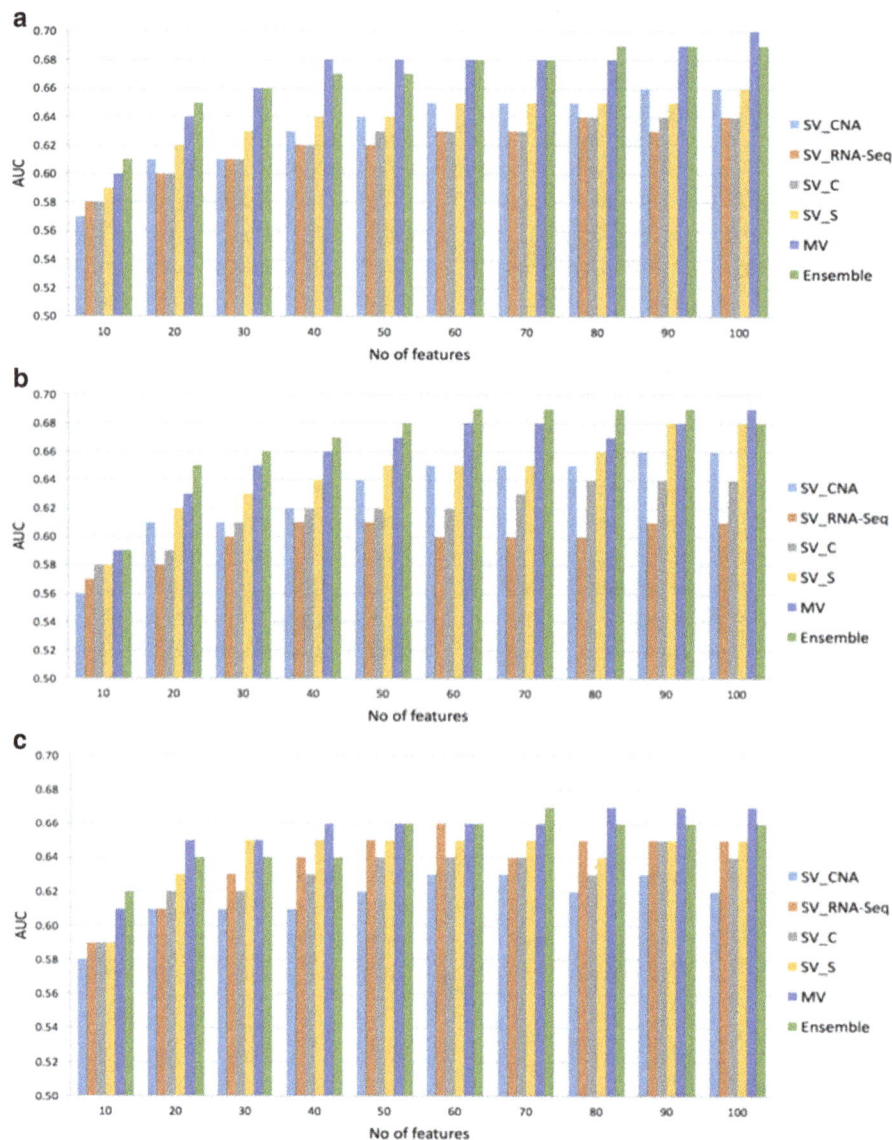

Fig. 4 Performance comparisons of final multi-view models with their single-view counterparts, for three different choices of machine learning algorithms: a) RF, b) XGB, and c) LR

Analysis of the top selected multi-view features

In order to get insights into the most discriminative features selected by our framework, we considered the top 100 features selected using MRMR-mv jointly from CNA and RNA-Seq views. To determine which features (genes) could serve as potential biomarkers for ovarian cancer survival, at each of the 50 iterations (resulting from running 5-fold procedure for 10 times), we scored each per-view input feature (input to our framework) by how many time it appears in the top 100 features. Table 6 summarizes the top 20 features from each view along with their normalized feature importance scores.

To examine the interplay between the top selected features from each view, we constructed an integrated network of interactions among the features using the cBio portal by integrating the biological interactions from public databases including NCI-Nature Pathway Interaction Database, Reactome, HPRD, Pathway Commons, and MSKCC Cancer Call Map [41]. Examination of the resulting network (Fig. 5) shows that *RPS19, PNOC, SFRP1* and *KCNJ16* are connected to other frequently altered genes, including *MYC or EIF3E* as oncogenes, from TCGA ovarian cancer dataset. In particular, ribosomal protein S19 (*RPS19*), which is known to be up-regulated in human ovarian and breast cancer cells and released from apoptotic tumor cells, was found to be associated with a novel immunosuppressive property [42]. Furthermore, *HTR3A* is targeted by several FDA approved cancer

Table 6 Top 20 features selected from CNA and RNA-Seq views

CNA	Score	RNA-Seq	Score
TBX18	0.44	OVGP1	0.56
TSHZ2	0.42	TOX3	0.54
RN7SL781P	0.42	SIX3	0.52
MAN1A2	0.42	HTR3A	0.50
KIF13B	0.40	FLG	0.48
DKFZP667F0711	0.36	SOSTDC1	0.48
CD70	0.36	EPYC	0.48
PRDM1	0.36	OBP2B	0.48
ZNF471	0.34	FBN3	0.46
RPS19	0.34	COL6A6	0.46
snoU13	0.34	NKAIN4	0.46
IRX1	0.32	LY6K	0.44
MIA	0.32	FABP6	0.44
LYPLA1	0.30	KIF1A	0.44
SHROOM3	0.30	KCNJ16	0.44
USP13	0.30	PNOC	0.42
SFRP1	0.28	TKTL1	0.42
CYP11A1	0.28	HLA-DRB6	0.42
ZMYM4	0.28	KRT14	0.42
APCDD1L	0.28	DPP10	0.40

drugs retrieved from PiHelper [43], an open source compilation of drug-target and antibody-target associations derived from several public data sources.

Finally, we performed a gene-set enrichment analysis to identify overrepresented GO terms in the two sets of top 20 features from CNA and RNA-Seq views. Specifically, we used the gene-batch tool in GOEAST (Gene Ontology Enrichment Analysis Software Toolkit) [44] with default parameters to import the gene symbols and to identify significantly overrepresented GO terms, for Biological Processes, Cellular Components and Molecular Function categories, in the CNA and RNA-Seq features sets. We found that the selected CNA gene set was enriched with 220 GO terms whereas the selected RNA-Seq gene set was enriched with 40 GO terms (See Additional files 1 and 2). Analysis of the GO terms enriched in the CNA gene set showed a significant overrepresentation of the molecular function GO terms related to hydrolase activity, oxidoreductase activity, and ion binding. Analysis of the GO terms enriched in the RNA-Seq gene set showed a significant over-representation of the molecular function GO terms related to transmembrane and substrate-specific transporter activity. We also used the Multi-GOEAST tool to compare the results of enrichment analysis of CNA and RNA-Seq gene sets. The graphical outputs of the Multi-GOEAST analysis results for top selected genes in CNA and RNA-Seq in Biological

Processes, Cellular Components and Molecular Function categories are provided in Additional files 3, 4 and 5. In these graphs, red and green boxes represent enriched GO terms only found in CNA and RNA-Seq, respectively. Yellow boxes represent commonly enriched GO terms in both sets of genes. The saturation degrees of all colors represent the significance of enrichment for corresponding GO terms. Interestingly, GO:0003777~microtubule motor activity term is only shared GO term between CNA and RNA-Seq enriched terms (see Additional file 5). We concluded that the CNA and RNA-Seq features selected by the proposed multi-view feature selection algorithm are non-redundant not only in terms of the genes selected from the CNA and RNA-Seq views but also in terms of their significantly overrepresented GO terms.

Discussion

We presented a two-stage feature selection framework for multi-omics data integration. The proposed framework can be customized in different ways to implement a variety of data integration methods. We described a novel instantiation of the proposed framework using multi-view feature selection. We introduced MRMR-mv, which extends MRMR, one of the state-of-the-art single-view feature selection methods, to the multi-view setting. We used the proposed two-stage framework to conduct a set of experiments to compare the performance of single-view and multi-view methods for predicting ovarian cancer survival from multi-omics data. The results of our experiments demonstrate the potential of the two-stage feature selection framework in general, and the MRMR-mv multi-view feature selection method in particular, in integrative analyses of and predictive modeling from multi-omics data.

Evaluation of single-view models for predicting ovarian cancer survival using methylation data alone showed very poor predictive performance where as those trained using CNA or RNA-Seq data showed substantially better predictive performance (with AUC between 0.64 and 0.66). Multi-view models that integrate mult-omics data using MRMR-mv, a multi-view feature selection method, were able to outperform single-view models. For example, multi-view models using the top 100 features selected by MRMR-mv from CNA and RNA-Seq data were able to achieve an AUC of 0.7. With the anticipated rapid increase in the size of multi-omics data, we can expect the predictive performance of such models to show corresponding improvements.

Further improvements can be expected from better techniques for coping with the ultra high-dimensionality and sparsity of multi-omics data. Of particular interest in this context are methods for pan-cancer analysis [45], multi-task learning [46], and incomplete multi-view learning [47], and multi-view representation learning [23].

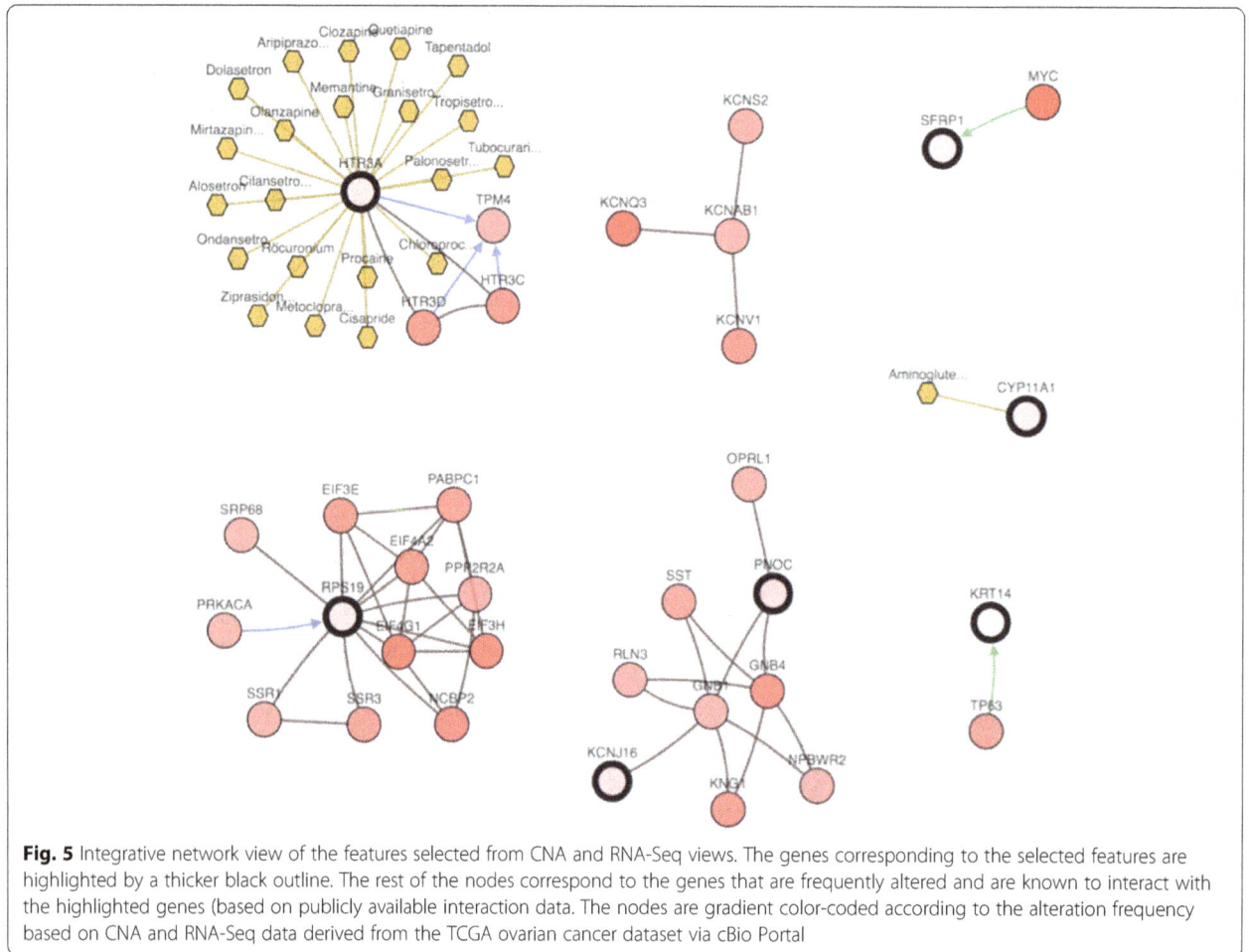

Fig. 5 Integrative network view of the features selected from CNA and RNA-Seq views. The genes corresponding to the selected features are highlighted by a thicker black outline. The rest of the nodes correspond to the genes that are frequently altered and are known to interact with the highlighted genes (based on publicly available interaction data. The nodes are gradient color-coded according to the alteration frequency based on CNA and RNA-Seq data derived from the TCGA ovarian cancer dataset via cBio Portal

MRMR-mv jointly selects (from multiple views) a compact yet most relevant subset of non-redundant features across multiple views for the prediction task at hand. Interestingly, the gene-set enrichment analysis of the top 20 genes selected by MRMR-mv from the CNA and RNA-Seq data shows that these genes are also non-redundant with respect to the GO terms that are significantly overrepresented in the CNA and RNA-Seq gene sets. If this observation is validated using other multi-omics datasets, MRMR-mv could be used to uncover, from multi-omics data, the underlying functional sub-networks that collectively orchestrate the biological processes that drive the onset and progression of diseases such as cancer. Ultimately, accurate and personalized prediction of clinical outcomes of different interventions and promising therapeutic targets for different cancer types will require advances in multi-view and multi-scale modeling that bring together information from different complementary data sources into cohesive explanatory, predictive, and causal models [48].

Conclusions

Developing multi-omics data-driven machine learning models for predicting clinical outcome, including cancer survival, is a promising cost-effective computational approach. However, the heterogeneity and extreme high-dimensionality of omics data present significant methodological challenges in applying the state-of-the art machine learning algorithms to training such models from multi-omics data. In this paper, we have described, to the best of our knowledge, the first attempt at applying multi-view feature selection to address these challenges. We have introduced a two-stage feature selection framework that can be easily customized to instantiate a variety of approaches to integrative analyses and predictive modeling from multi-omics data. We have proposed MRMR-mv, a novel maximum relevance and minimum redundancy based multi-view feature selection algorithm. We have applied the resulting framework and algorithm to build predictive models for ovarian cancer survival using multi-omics data derived from the Cancer Genome Atlas (TCGA).

We have demonstrated the potential of integrative analysis and predictive modeling of multi-view data in ovarian cancer survival prediction. Work in progress is aimed at further developing effective computational and statistical methods and tools for integrative analyses and modeling of multi-omics data, with particular emphasis on precision health applications.

Additional files

Additional file 1: GOEAST gene-batch output of enriched GO terms in the Biological Processes, Cellular Components and Molecular Function categories for CNA top selected genes.

Additional file 2: GOEAST gene-batch output of enriched GO terms in the Biological Processes, Cellular Components and Molecular Function categories for RNA-Seq top selected genes.

Additional file 3: Graphical output of Multi-GOEAST analysis results of Biological Processes GO terms in the top selected genes in CNA and RNA-Seq.

Additional file 4: Graphical output of Multi-GOEAST analysis results of Cellular Components GO terms in the top selected genes in CNA and RNA-Seq.

Additional file 5: Graphical output of Multi-GOEAST analysis results of Molecular Function GO terms in the top selected genes in CNA and RNA-Seq.

Abbreviations

AUC: Area under ROC curve; CNA: Copy number alteration; CV: Cross-validation; F-Stat: F-Statistic; GE: Gene expression; GOEAST: Gene Ontology Enrichment Analysis Software Toolkit; ICGC: International Cancer Genome Consortium; LR: Logistic Regression; MI: Mutual Information; MRMR: Min-Redundancy and Maximum-Relevance; MV: Multi-view; RF: Random Forest; RFE: Recursive Feature Elimination; TCGA: The Cancer Genome Atlas; XGB: eXtreme Gradient Boosting

Acknowledgments

We gratefully acknowledge the TCGA Consortium and all its members for the TCGA Project initiative, for providing sample, tissues, data processing and making data and results available. The results published here are in whole or part based upon data generated by The Cancer Genome Atlas pilot project established by the NCI and NHGRI. Information about TCGA and the investigators and institutions that constitute the TCGA research network can be found at http://cancergenome.nih.gov.

Funding

This project was supported in part by grants the National Institutes of Health (through grants NCATS UL1 TR000127, NCATS TR002014, NIGMS P50GM115318, NLM R01 NL012535 and NLM T32LM012415), the Pennsylvania Department of Health (SAP 4100070267), and the National Science Foundation (IIS 1636795). The project was also supported by the Edward Frymoyer Endowed Professorship in Information Sciences and Technology at Pennsylvania State University and the Sudha Murty Distinguished Visiting Chair in Neurocomputing and Data Science at the Indian Institute of Science [both held by Vasant Honavar] and the Pennsylvania State University Center for Big Data Analytics and Discovery Informatics (CBDADI) which is co-sponsored by the Institute for Cyberscience, the Huck Institutes of the Life Sciences, and the Social Science Research Institute at the university. The content, including specifically, analyses, interpretation, and conclusions, is solely the responsibility of the authors and does not necessarily represent the official views of the NIH, NSF, or the Pennsylvania Department of Health or other sponsors. The publication costs were covered by CBDADI.

Authors' contributions

YE, DK, and VH designed and conceived the research. YE developed and implemented the feature selection algorithm and the data integration framework. YE and TH ran the experiments. YE, TH, and MS performed the data analysis. YE drafted the manuscript. DK and VH edited the manuscript. All authors read and approved the final version of the manuscript.

Competing interests

The authors declare no conflict of interest.

Author details

[1]Artificial Intelligence Research Laboratory, College of Information Sciences and Technology, Pennsylvania State University, University Park, PA 16802, USA. [2]Biomedical and Translational Informatics Institute, Geisinger Health System, Danville, PA, USA. [3]The Huck Institutes of the Life Sciences, Pennsylvania State University, University Park, PA 16802, USA. [4]School of Electrical Engineering and Computer Science, Pennsylvania State University, University Park, PA 16802, USA. [5]The Center for Big Data Analytics and Discovery Informatics, Pennsylvania State University, University Park, PA 16802, USA. [6]The Clinical and Translational Sciences Institute, Pennsylvania State University, University Park, PA, USA.

References

1. Gagan J, Van Allen EM. Next-generation sequencing to guide cancer therapy. Genome Med. 2015;7(1):80.
2. Cancer Genome Atlas Research N. Comprehensive genomic characterization defines human glioblastoma genes and core pathways. Nature. 2008; 455(7216):1061–8.
3. Hudson TJ, Anderson W, Aretz A, Barker AD, Bell C, Bernabé RR, Bhan MK, et al. International network of cancer genome projects. Nature. 2010;464(7291):993–8.
4. Mo Q, Wang S, Seshan VE, Olshen AB, Schultz N, Sander C, Powers RS, Ladanyi M, Shen R. Pattern discovery and cancer gene identification in integrated cancer genomic data. Proc Natl Acad Sci. 2013;110(11):4245–50.
5. Wang B, Mezlini AM, Demir F, Fiume M, Tu Z, Brudno M, Haibe-Kains B, Goldenberg A. Similarity network fusion for aggregating data types on a genomic scale. Nat Methods. 2014;11(3):333–7.
6. Gligorijević V, Malod-Dognin N, Pržulj N. Integrative methods for analyzing big data in precision medicine. Proteomics. 2016;16(5):741–58.
7. Network CGAR. Integrated genomic and molecular characterization of cervical cancer. Nature. 2017;543(7645):378.
8. Kim D, Shin H, Sohn KA, Verma A, Ritchie MD, Kim JH. Incorporating inter-relationships between different levels of genomic data into cancer clinical outcome prediction. Methods. 2014;67(3):344–53.
9. Hanash S. Integrated global profiling of cancer. Nat Rev Cancer. 2004;4(8): 638–44.
10. Ritchie MD, Holzinger ER, Li R, Pendergrass SA, Kim D. Methods of integrating data to uncover genotype-phenotype interactions. Nat Rev Genet. 2015;16(2):85–97.
11. Lussier YA, Li H. Breakthroughs in genomics data integration for predicting clinical outcome. J Biomed Inform. 2012;45(6):1199–201.
12. Kim D, Joung JG, Sohn KA, Shin H, Park YR, Ritchie MD, Kim JH. Knowledge boosting: a graph-based integration approach with multi-omics data and genomic knowledge for cancer clinical outcome prediction. J Am Med Inform Assoc. 2015;22(1):109–20.
13. Kim D, Li R, Lucas A, Verma SS, Dudek SM, Ritchie MD. Using knowledge-driven genomic interactions for multi-omics data analysis: metadimensional models for predicting clinical outcomes in ovarian carcinoma. Journal of the American Medical Informatics Association. 2016; ocw165
14. Serra A, Fratello M, Fortino V, Raiconi G, Tagliaferri R, Greco D. MVDA: a multi-view genomic data integration methodology. BMC bioinformatics. 2015;16(1):261.

15. Kristensen VN, Lingjærde OC, Russnes HG, Vollan HKM, Frigessi A, Børresen-Dale A-L. Principles and methods of integrative genomic analyses in cancer. Nat Rev Cancer. 2014;14(5):299.

16. Huang S, Chaudhary K, Garmire LX. More is better: recent progress in multi-omics data integration methods. Front Genet. 2017;8:84.

17. Zhao J, Xie X, Xu X, Sun S. Multi-view learning overview: recent progress and new challenges. Information Fusion. 2017;38:43–54.

18. Huang C, Chung FL, Wang S. Multi-view L2-SVM and its multi-view core vector machine. Neural Netw. 2016;75:110–25.

19. Peng J, Aved AJ, Seetharaman G, Palaniappan K. Multiview boosting with information propagation for classification. IEEE Transactions on Neural Networks and Learning Systems. 2017;

20. Cai X, Nie F, Huang H: Multi-view k-means clustering on big data. In: Twenty-Third International Joint conference on artificial intelligence: 2013; 2013.

21. Chaudhuri K, Kakade SM, Livescu K, Sridharan K. Multi-view clustering via canonical correlation analysis. In: Proceedings of the 26th annual international conference on machine learning: 2009: ACM; 2009. p. 129–36.

22. Yang W, Gao Y, Shi Y, Cao L. MRM-lasso: a sparse multiview feature selection method via low-rank analysis. IEEE transactions on neural networks and learning systems. 2015;26(11):2801–15.

23. Wang W, Arora R, Livescu K, Bilmes J. On deep multi-view representation learning. In: International Conference on Machine Learning. 2015;2015:1083–92.

24. Goldman M, Craft B, Swatloski T, Cline M, Morozova O, Diekhans M, Haussler D, Zhu J. The UCSC cancer genomics browser: update 2015. Nucleic acids research. 2014; gku1073

25. Liu H, Motoda H: Feature selection for knowledge discovery and data mining, vol. 454: Springer Science & Business Media; 2012.

26. Ding C, Peng H. Minimum redundancy feature selection from microarray gene expression data. J Bioinforma Comput Biol. 2005;3(02):185–205.

27. El Akadi A, Amine A, El Ouardighi A, Aboutajdine D. A two-stage gene selection scheme utilizing MRMR filter and GA wrapper. Knowl Inf Syst. 2011;26(3):487–500.

28. Sakar O, Kursun O, Seker H, Gurgen F. Prediction of protein sub-nuclear location by clustering mRMR ensemble feature selection. In: Pattern Recognition (ICPR), 2010 20th International Conference on: 2010: IEEE; 2010. p. 2572–5.

29. Direito B, Duarte J, Teixeira C, Schelter B, Le Van Quyen M, Schulze-Bonhage A, Sales F, Dourado A. Feature selection in high dimensional EEG features spaces for epileptic seizure prediction. IFAC Proceedings Volumes. 2011; 44(1):6206–11.

30. Liu L, Cai Y, Lu W, Feng K, Peng C, Niu B. Prediction of protein–protein interactions based on PseAA composition and hybrid feature selection. Biochem Biophys Res Commun. 2009;380(2):318–22.

31. Zhang L, Zhang Q, Zhang L, Tao D, Huang X, Du B. Ensemble manifold regularized sparse low-rank approximation for multiview feature embedding. Pattern Recogn. 2015;48(10):3102–12.

32. Svd W, Colbert SC, Varoquaux G. The NumPy array: a structure for efficient numerical computation. Computing in Science & Engineering. 2011;13(2):22–30.

33. Tibshirani R. Regression shrinkage and selection via the lasso. J R Stat Soc Ser B Methodol. 1996:267–88.

34. Pedregosa F, Varoquaux G, Gramfort A, Michel V, Thirion B, Grisel O, Blondel M, Prettenhofer P, Weiss R, Dubourg V. Scikit-learn: machine learning in Python. J Mach Learn Res. 2011;12(Oct):2825–30.

35. Breiman L. Random forests. Mach Learn. 2001;45(1):5–32.

36. Chen T, Guestrin C. Xgboost: A scalable tree boosting system. In: Proceedings of the 22Nd ACM SIGKDD International Conference on Knowledge Discovery and Data Mining. ACM; 2016. p. 785–94.

37. Le Cessie S, Van Houwelingen JC. Ridge estimators in logistic regression. Appl Stat. 1992:191–201.

38. Zou H, Hastie T. Regularization and variable selection via the elastic net. Journal of the Royal Statistical Society: Series B (Statistical Methodology). 2005;67(2):301–20.

39. Guyon I, Weston J, Barnhill S, Vapnik V. Gene selection for cancer classification using support vector machines. Mach Learn. 2002;46(1):389–422.

40. Bradley AP. The use of the area under the ROC curve in the evaluation of machine learning algorithms. Pattern Recogn. 1997;30(7):1145–59.

41. Cerami E, Gao J, Dogrusoz U, Gross BE, Sumer SO, Aksoy BA, Jacobsen A, Byrne CJ, Heuer ML, Larsson E, et al. The cBio cancer genomics portal: an open platform for exploring multidimensional cancer genomics data. Cancer Discov. 2012;2(5):401–4.

42. Markiewski MM, Vadrevu SK, Sharma SK, Chintala NK, Ghouse S, Cho J-H, Fairlie DP, Paterson Y, Astrinidis A, Karbowniczek M. The ribosomal protein S19 suppresses antitumor immune responses via the complement C5a receptor 1. J Immunol. 2017;198(7):2989–99.

43. Aksoy BA, Gao J, Dresdner G, Wang W, Root A, Jing X, Cerami E, Sander C. PiHelper: an open source framework for drug-target and antibody-target data. Bioinformatics. 2013;29(16):2071–2.

44. Zheng Q, Wang X-J. GOEAST: a web-based software toolkit for Gene Ontology enrichment analysis. Nucleic acids research. 2008;36(suppl_2): W358–63.

45. Lengerich B, Aragam B, Xing EP. Personalized Regression Enables Sample-Specific Pan-Cancer Analysis. bioRxiv. 2018; 294496

46. Li Y, Wang J, Ye J, Reddy CK. A multi-task learning formulation for survival analysis. In: Proceedings of the 22nd ACM SIGKDD International Conference on Knowledge Discovery and Data Mining: 2016: ACM; 2016. p. 1715–24.

47. Xu C, Tao D, Xu C. Multi-view learning with incomplete views. IEEE Trans Image Process. 2015;24(12):5812–25.

48. Honavar VG, Hill MD, Yelick K: Accelerating science: a computing research agenda. arXiv preprint arXiv:160402006 2016.

6

Genome-wide association study identifies two loci influencing plasma neurofilament light levels

Jie-Qiong Li[1†], Xiang-Zhen Yuan[1†], Hai-Yan Li[2], Xi-Peng Cao[3], Jin-Tai Yu[1,3*], Lan Tan[1,3*], Wei-An Chen[4*] and Alzheimer's Disease Neuroimaging Initiative

Abstract

Background: Plasma neurofilament light (NFL) is a promising biomarker for Alzheimer disease (AD), which increases in the early stage of AD and is associated with the progression of AD. We performed a genome-wide association study (GWAS) of plasma NFL in Alzheimer's Disease Neuroimaging Initiative 1 (ADNI-1) cohort to identify novel variants associated with AD.

Methods: This study included 179 cognitively healthy controls (HC), 176 patients with mild cognitive impairment (MCI), and 172 patients with AD. All subjects were restricted to non-Hispanic Caucasian derived from the ADNI cohort and met all quality control (QC) criteria. Association of plasma NFL with the genetic variants was assessed using PLINK with an additive genetic model, i.e.dose-dependent effect of the minor alleles. The influence of a genetic variant associated with plasma NFL (rs7943454) on brain structure was further assessed using PLINK with a linear regression model.

Results: The minor allele (T) of rs7943454 in leucine zipper protein 2 gene (*LUZP2*) was associated with higher plasma NFL at suggestive levels ($P = 1.39 \times 10^{-6}$) in a dose-dependent fashion. In contrast, the minor allele (G) of rs640476 near *GABRB2* was associated with lower plasma NFL at suggestive levels ($P = 6.71 \times 10^{-6}$) in a dose-dependent effect in all diagnostic groups except the MCI group. Furthermore, the minor allele (T) of rs7943454 within *LUZP2* increased the onset risk of AD (odds ratio = 1.547, confidence interval 95% = 1.018–2.351) and was associated with atrophy of right middle temporal gyrus in the whole cohort in the longitudinal study ($P = 0.0234$).

Conclusion: GWAS found the associations of two single nucleotide polymorphisms (rs7943454 and rs640476) with plasma NFL at suggestive levels. Rs7943454 in *LUZP2* was associated with the onset risk of AD and atrophy of right middle temporal gyrusin the whole cohort. Using an endophenotype-based approach, we identified rs7943454 as a new AD risk locus.

Keywords: Genome-wide association study, Plasma NFL, Alzheimer disease, *LUZP2*, *GABRB2*, Genetic factors

* Correspondence: yu-jintai@163com; dr.tanlan@163.com; wzanan@126.com
Data used in preparation for this article were obtained from the Alzheimer's Disease Neuroimaging Initiative (ADNI) database (adni.loni.usc.edu). As such, the investigators within the ADNI contributed to the design and implementation of ADNI and/or provided data but did not participate in the analysis or writing of this report. A complete listing of ADNI investigators can be found at:http://adni.loni.usc.edu/wp-content/uploads/how_to_apply/ADNI_Acknowledgement_List.pdf.
†Equal contributors
[1]Department of Neurology, Qingdao Municipal Hospital, Qingdao University, No.5 Donghai Middle Road, Qingdao 266071, Shandong Province, China
[4]Department of Neurology, The First Affiliated Hospital of Wenzhou Medical University, Nanbaixiang Road, Wenzhou 325000, Zhejiang Province, China
Full list of author information is available at the end of the article

Background

Alzheimer disease (AD) is the main cause of dementia and one of the major challenges for health care across the world, which is characterized pathologically by extracellular accumulation of amyloid-β (Aβ), intracellular deposition of neurofibrillary tangles (NFT), neuronal loss and synaptic dysfunction [1]. Well-established cerebrospinal fluid (CSF) biomarkers including $Aβ_{42}$, total-tau (t-tau), phosphorylated tau (p-tau) have been used for the diagnosis of AD and monitoring its progression [2], but the their application is hampered by a high degree of invasiveness, complex operations and high costs. Biomarkers in peripheral blood are more appropriate screening tools for AD among old individuals to monitor AD progression. Interestingly, recent studies using ultrasensitive assay showed that plasma neurofilament light (NFL), the main component of neurofilaments (cytoskeletal protein of neurons), increased in patients with AD dementia and was associated with other established CSF and neuroimaging biomarkers of AD [3, 4]. Plasma NFL is a noninvasive biomarker for neuronal injury in AD compared with CSF biomarkers. Thus, it has the potential for monitoring AD progression [3].

AD is a clinically heterogeneous neurodegenerative disease with a strong genetic component. Genetic risk factors of AD impact the CSF or neuroimaging biomarkers through which they might modulate the process of AD [5]. Thus, biomarkers for AD may be used as endophenotypes to explore the genetic factors that impact their metabolism [6–8]. Based on the association between plasma NFL and AD, we performed a genome-wide association study (GWAS) using plasma NFL as an endophenotype of AD to explore genetic factors involved in plasma NFL metabolism. We hypothesized that these genetic factors may influence pathological change in AD.

Methods

Subjects

In this study, 172 AD patients, 176 subjects with mild cognitive impairment (MCI), and 179 healthy controls (HC) whose data met all quality control (QC) criteria were included from the Alzheimer's Disease Neuroimaging Initiative 1 (ADNI-1) cohort. The full cohort with plasma NFL and genotype data included 578 subjects. All the subjects were restricted to non-Hispanic Caucasian checked with their pedigree information checked to reduce potential bias of population stratification that might confound GWAS results. This step removed 40 subjects. After QC of the plasma NFL levels and removal of 11 outliers, there were 527 subjects with plasma NFL data left. The detailed demographic information and plasma NFL data have been shown in Table 1.

ADNI dataset

ADNI was launched in 2003 by the National Institute on Aging, the National Institute of Biomedical Imaging and Bioengineering, the Food and Drug Administration, private pharmaceutical companies and nonprofit organizations. ADNI was established to develop serial magnetic resonance imaging (MRI), positron emission tomography (PET), and a combination of biomarkers, neuropsychological and clinical assessment to improve early diagnosis and measure the progression of AD [9]. The ADNI database has three protocols (ADNI 1, ADNI 2 and ADNI Grand Opportunities (ADNI GO)) at present and recruited more than 1500 participants including normal older subjects, MCI and early AD in this research. More information is available on the website of ADNI (www. loni.ucla.edu/ADNI).

Plasma measurements and quality control

Plasma NFL was analyzed using the ultrasensitive Single Molecule array (Simoa) technique as previously described [10]. The assay used a combination of monoclonal antibodies and purified bovine NFL as a calibrator. Analytical sensitivity was < 1.0 pg/mL, and the NFL levels in all tested sample were above the detection limit. Further QC was performed to reduce the potential influence of extreme outliers on statistical results. Mean and standard deviations (SD) of baseline plasma NFL were calculated. Subjects who had a value which is 3-fold SD greater or smaller than the mean value ($< 42.8 - 3 \times 26.8$ pg/mL or $> 42.8 + 3 \times 26.8$ pg/mL) were removed from the analysis. This step removed 11 subjects.

Table 1 The demographic information of participants with plasma NFL data

Baseline diagnosis	AD	MCI	HC	Total
n	172	176	179	527
Age (years), mean ± SD (range)	76 ± 7 (56–91)	75 ± 8 (54–89)	76 ± 5 (62–90)	75 ± 7 (54–91)
Gender, male/female	90/82	117/59	103/76	310/217
APOE ε4 carrier (%)	66.9	52.8	26.8	48.6
Plasma NFL (pg/ml), mean ± SD[a]	48.7 ± 20.9	39.9 ± 17.7	32.8 ± 15.5	40.4 ± 19.3

Abbreviations: AD Alzheimer's disease, *APOE* Apolipoprotein E; *HC* healthy control, *MCI* mild cognitive impairment, *NFL* neurofilament light, *SD* standard deviation
[a]Plasma NFL levels were different across the 3 diagnostic groups ($P < 0.0001$). Tukey's multiple comparisons test showed that AD patients had higher plasma NFL levels compared with MCI group and healthy controls ($P < 0.001$). MCI group also had higher plasma NFL levels compared to healthy controls ($P = 0.0007$)

Genotyping and quality control

The ADNI 1 samples involved in this study were genotyped by Human 610-Quad BeadChip (Illumina, Inc., San Diego, CA). PLINK software (version 1.07) was used to explore the association of plasma NFL with the genetic variants using the following stringent criteria: minimum call rate for single nucleotide polymorphisms (SNPs) and individuals > 98%; minimum minor allele frequencies (MAF) > 0.20, Hardy-Weinberg equilibrium test $P > 0.001$. The restriction to SNPs with a minor allele frequency > 0.20 served to reduce the potential for false-positive results and enhance statistical power. An apolipoprotein E *(APOE)* genotyping kit was used to identify *APOE* alleles, which were defined by rs7412 and rs429358 [7].

Brain structure on MRI

The data of MRI brain structure were derived from UCSF FreeSurfer datasets, which were used to conduct association test of rs7943454in leucine zipper protein2 gene *(LUZP2)* with brain structure. The cerebral image segmentation and analysis were performed with the FreeSurfer version5.1 (http://surfer.nmr.mgh.harvard.edu/) based on the2010 Desikan-Killanyatlas [11]. The technical details of these procedures have been described in prior publications [12]. Brian regions have been reported to be closely associated with AD such as hippocampus, parahippocampus, middle temporal gyrus, posterior cingulate, precuneus and entorhinal cortex, which were selected as our regions of interest (ROI) to analyze their its associations with rs7943454.

Statistical analyses

Association studies of plasma NFL with the genetic variants were performed using PLINK (version 1.07) with the additive genetic model, i.e. dose-dependent effect of the minor allele. The analysis included a total of 30,1687 genotyped variants. To adjust for multiple testing, Bonferroni correction was applied and SNPs with corrected $p < 0.01$ (uncorrected $p < 3.31 \times 10-8$, i.e., 0.01/301687 markers) were considered genome-wide significant. And we secondarily examined SNPs with uncorrected p values less than $10–5$ to identify potential candidates. Age, gender and diagnosis were included as covariates. Bonferroni correction of the P values by the total number of acceptable quality SNPs was used for multiple test correction. Differences in continuous variables (plasma NFL levels, volume of regional brain) were examined using one-way analysis of variance (ANOVA), and Tukey's multiple comparisons test was used to perform the pairwise analysis after ANOVA. Genome-wide associations were visualized using a software program (R, version 3.4.0; The R Foundation). Regional associations were visualized with the Locus Zoom web tool (http://locuszoom.org/). Moreover, a multiple linear regression model was applied using PLINK to estimate coefficients for testing a possible correlation between brain structure and rs7943454. Age, gender, education, and APOE ε4status were used as covariates.

Results

Characteristics of included subjects

The information about these included subjects has been shown in Table 1. Briefly, 172 AD (82 women, 76 ± 7 years), 176 MCI (59 women, 75 ± 8 years) and 179 HC (76 women, 76 ± 5 years) subjects were recruited in this study. AD group had the highest frequency of ε4 allele within *APOE* gene (66.9%). AD patients (48.7 ± 20.9 pg/ml) had higher plasma NFL levels compared with MCI group (39.9 ± 17.7 pg/ml) and HC group (32.8 ± 15.5 pg/ml) ($P < 0.001$). MCI group also had higher plasma NFL levels compared to HC group ($P = 0.0007$). The sensitivity and specificity of plasma NFL used for the diagnosis of AD were 0.73 and 0.84 respectively. The area under the curve (AUC) of the model containing plasma NFL, age at baseline, gender, educational level and APOE ε4 genotype was 0.86 in predicting the onset of AD among HC controls group. By comparison, the AUROCs were 0.84 to 0.87 for CSF Aβ42, CSF t-tau, and CSF p-tau (Additional file 1: Figure S1).

SNPs associated with plasma NFL levels

There were 527 individuals with plasma NFL data as mentioned above. After adjusting for age, gender and diagnosis, two SNPs (rs7943454, rs640476) were identified associated with plasma NFL at suggestive levels of $P < 10^{-5}$ (Fig. 1a, Table 2). No SNPs with genome-wide significant association with plasma NFL levels was identified in this study.

The minor allele of rs7943454 (T) was associated with higher plasma NFL levels in a dose-dependent effect in all diagnostic groups (Fig. 2a). In contrast, the minor allele of rs640476 (G) showed association with lower plasma NFL levels in a dose-dependent effect in all diagnostic groups except the MCI group (Fig. 2b).

SNPs mapped closely to the two suggestive SNPs (rs7943454, rs640476) regions were also analyzed. These nearby SNPs showed association with plasma NFL levels at P levels lower than 0.01. However, these SNPs associated with plasma NFL also disappeared after controlling the genotype of the two suggestive SNPs (Fig. 1b and c, Fig. 1d and e). The results indicated that these nearby SNPs were driven by the two suggestive SNPs.

Rs7943454 and onset risk of AD

The International Genomics of Alzheimer's Disease Project (IGAP) is the largest genetic epidemiology investigation of AD risk to date. In 2013, the IGAP reported a grand-scale meta-analysis and identified 11 new susceptibility loci

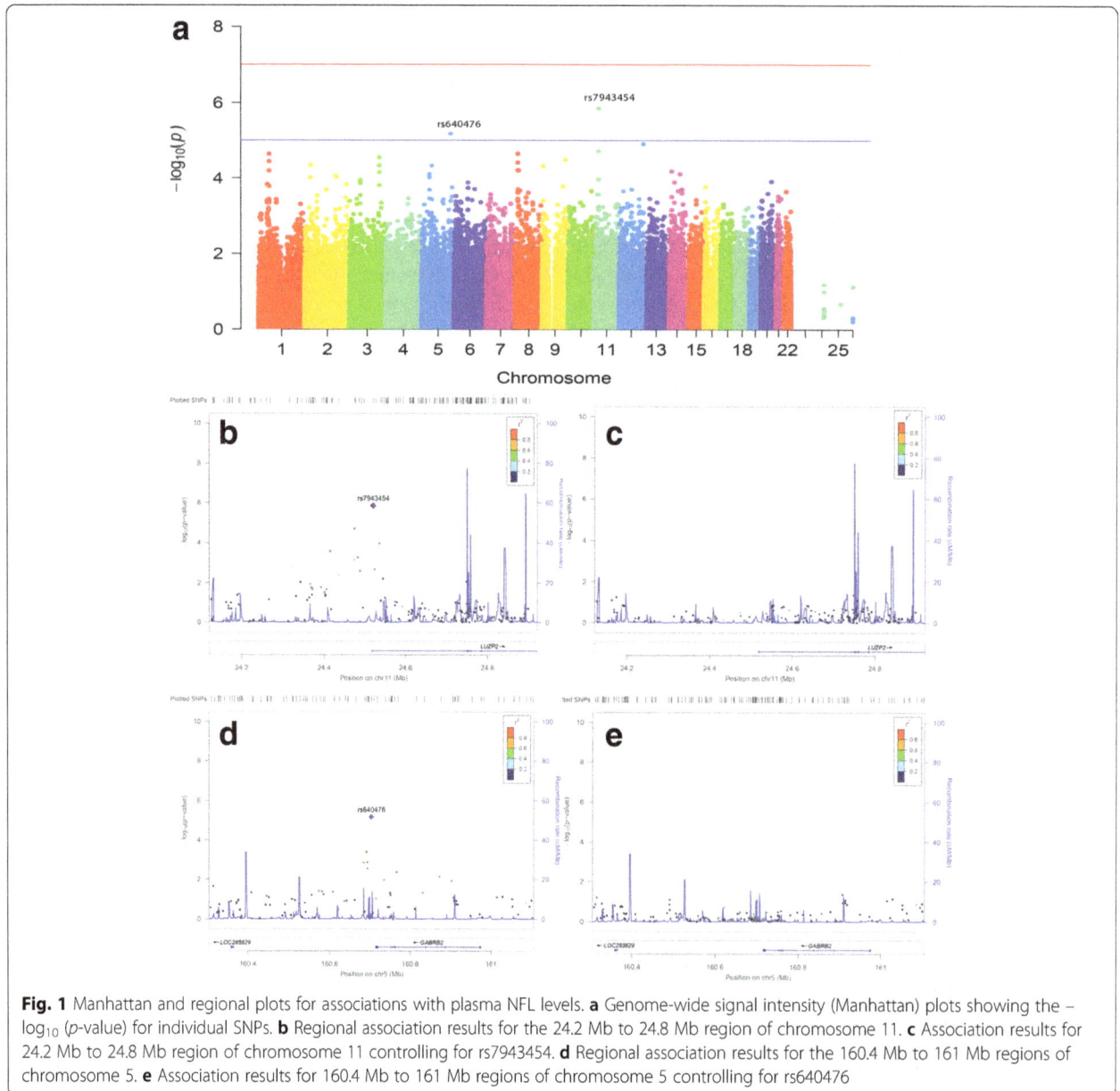

Fig. 1 Manhattan and regional plots for associations with plasma NFL levels. **a** Genome-wide signal intensity (Manhattan) plots showing the −log$_{10}$ (p-value) for individual SNPs. **b** Regional association results for the 24.2 Mb to 24.8 Mb region of chromosome 11. **c** Association results for 24.2 Mb to 24.8 Mb region of chromosome 11 controlling for rs7943454. **d** Regional association results for the 160.4 Mb to 161 Mb regions of chromosome 5. **e** Association results for 160.4 Mb to 161 Mb regions of chromosome 5 controlling for rs640476

for AD [13]. The IGAP research was divided into a discovery step (stage 1) and a replication step (stage 2). We checked the two loci associated with plasma NFL in IGAP database in the stage 1 meta-analysis and identified rs7943454 as a risk locus for AD (P = 0.03476).

Table 2 Top SNPs associated with plasma NFL levels (P values < 10^{-5})

CHR	SNP	MAF	Closest Gene	SNP Type/Location	P values
11	rs7943454	0.460	*LUZP2*	intron	1.39 × 10^{-6}
5	rs640476	0.297	*GABRB2*	intergenic	6.71 × 10^{-6}

Abbreviations: CHR chromosome, LUZP2 leucine zipper protein 2, MAF minor allele frequency, SNP single nucleotide polymorphism, GABRB2 gamma-aminobutyric acid type A receptor beta2 subunit

The minor allele of rs7943454 (T) increased the onset risk of AD 1.547-fold in our analysis (odds ratio = 1.547, confidence interval 95% = 1.018–2.351).

Impact of rs7943454 on brain structure

Several cortical areas including middle temporal gyrus, posterior cingulate, precuneus, parahippocampal gyrus, and hippocampus were chosen as the ROI of the AD related MRI measures analysis. We analyzed the association of rs7943454 with AD related brain structures in a linear model using age, gender, education years, *APOE ε4* status and intracranial volume (ICV) as covariates. There was no regional cortical volume associated with rs7943454 at baseline in the hybrid population (AD, MCI, and HC subjects)

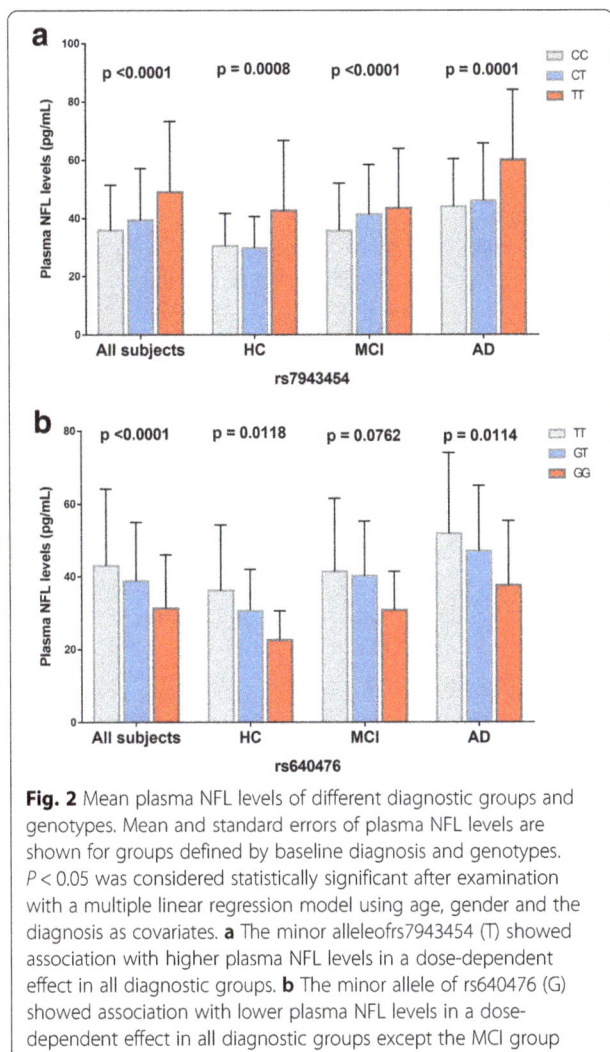

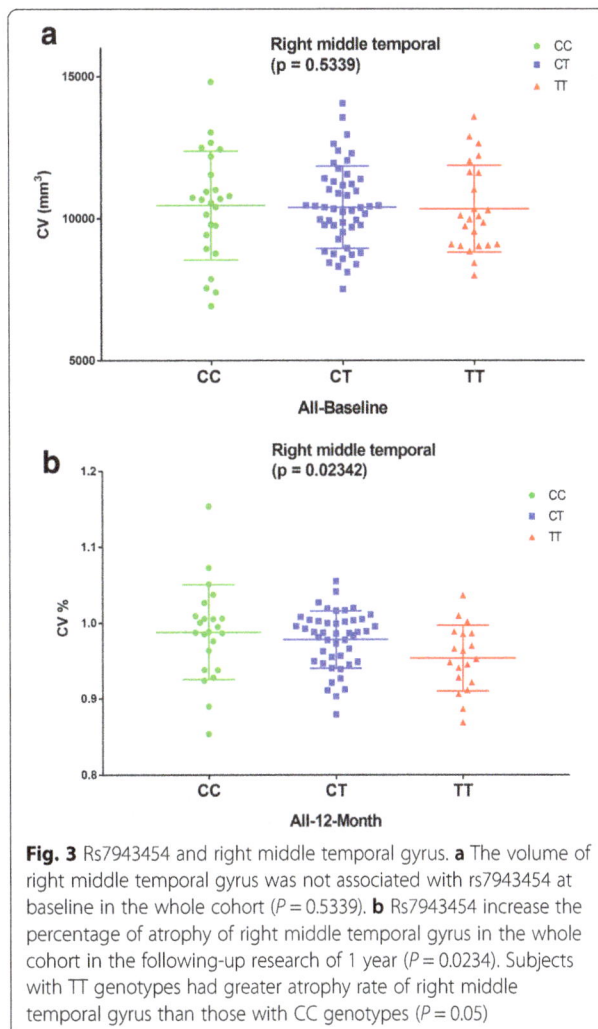

Fig. 2 Mean plasma NFL levels of different diagnostic groups and genotypes. Mean and standard errors of plasma NFL levels are shown for groups defined by baseline diagnosis and genotypes. $P < 0.05$ was considered statistically significant after examination with a multiple linear regression model using age, gender and the diagnosis as covariates. **a** The minor alleleofrs7943454 (T) showed association with higher plasma NFL levels in a dose-dependent effect in all diagnostic groups. **b** The minor allele of rs640476 (G) showed association with lower plasma NFL levels in a dose-dependent effect in all diagnostic groups except the MCI group

Fig. 3 Rs7943454 and right middle temporal gyrus. **a** The volume of right middle temporal gyrus was not associated with rs7943454 at baseline in the whole cohort ($P = 0.5339$). **b** Rs7943454 increase the percentage of atrophy of right middle temporal gyrus in the whole cohort in the following-up research of 1 year ($P = 0.0234$). Subjects with TT genotypes had greater atrophy rate of right middle temporal gyrus than those with CC genotypes ($P = 0.05$)

(Fig. 3a). However, rs7943454 increased the percentage of atrophy of right middle temporal gyrus in the hybrid population in the one-year follow-up research ($P = 0.0234$, Fig. 3b). Subjects with TT genotype had greater atrophy rate of right middle temporal gyrus than those with CC genotype (CC: 0.9880 ± 0.0622, CT: 0.9783 ± 0.0377, TT: 0.9537 ± 0.0433) ($P = 0.05$). There was no significant difference in the volume of right middle temporal gyrus between CT genotype and CC genotype or TT genotype.

Discussion

To our knowledge, this study was the first one using plasma NFL as an endophenotype of AD for GWAS. The use of quantitative traits in GWAS has been shown to increase statistical power over case-control designs [8]. We identified two SNPs (rs7943454, rs640476) associated with plasma NFL at suggestive levels. The minor allele (T) of rs7943454 within *LUZP2* increased the onset risk of AD and was associated with atrophy of right middle temporal gyrus in the entire cohort of the one-

year longitudinal study. The use of plasma NFL as an endophenotype of AD for GWAS enabled us to identify a novel AD candidate gene in addition to examining the influence of well-known AD genes on AD biomarkers. We also found the minor allele (T) of rs7943454 in *LUZP2* was associated with higher plasma NFL levels in a dose-dependent fashion. In contrast, the minor allele (G) of rs640476 near *GABRB2* was associated with lower plasma NFL at suggestive levels in a dose-dependent effect in all diagnostic groups except the MCI group.

Plasma NFL showed significant increase in AD patients than in MCI and healthy controls ($P < 0.001$). Similar with CSF NFL, plasma is not disease-specific and even more marked increases are found in several other neurodegenerative disorders. Increasing evidence indicates that plasma NFL is a potential biomarker for the progression of AD but not for the diagnosis [4, 14–16]. Plasma NFL is noninvasive and has diagnostic accuracy for AD in the same range as established CSF biomarkers [3]. Plasma NFL may be widely used as a biomarker in clinical studies and drug development of AD, although there is still a long way to go. The elevated NFL levels in plasma also indicate that the degeneration of large-caliber axons plays an important role in the progression of AD [14].

The variation rs7943454 is located on chromosome 11p14.3 within *LUZP2* region. *LUZP2* is a leucine zipper protein coding gene that has been reported to be deleted in some patients with Wilms tumor-Aniridia-Genitourinary anomalies-mental Retardation (WAGR) syndrome [17]. It has also been reported that *LUZP2* was associated with prostate cancer and hypereosinophilic syndrome [18, 19]. The function of *LUZP2* is still unclear and inhibition of its expression did not show any obvious abnormal phenotypes in mice [20]. Rs7943454 in *LUZP2* has been reported as a risk locus of AD in IGAP, which has been validated in our analysis. The minor allele (T) of rs7943454 increased plasma NFL levels in a dose-dependent fashion and was associated with atrophy of right middle temporal gyrus in the hybrid population. Neuroimaging changes occur years before cognitive decline and middle temporal gyrusis identified as a critical region of memory that changes in the early stage of AD, followed by progressive neocortical damage. Atrophy of middle temporal gyrus is now considered to be a valid diagnostic marker in the early stage of AD [21]. Our study showed that the minor allele (T) of rs7943454 increased the atrophy rate of right middle temporal gyrus in the one-year follow-up study and the C-allele remarkably prevented its atrophy. This result further proved that rs7943454 was associated with the onset risk of AD and *LUZP2* may be a new susceptibility gene of AD. However, we didn't find any relation between rs7943454 and right middle temporal gyrus in subgroups due to the limited sample size.

The variation rs640476 is located on chromosome 5 q34, the intergenic region between *GABRB2* (gamma-aminobutyric acid type A receptor beta2 subunit) and *LOC285629* (also known as *LINC02159*, long intergenic non-protein coding RNA 2159). *GABRB2* is the gene coding β2 subunit of γ-aminobutyric acid receptor type A (GABAA receptor), which is the major mediator of fast inhibitory synaptic transmission in the central nervous system. Mutations in *GABRB2* genes have been reported to be associated with intellectual disability and epilepsy [22, 23]. A missense mutation in *GABRB2* was also reported to be associated with early myoclonic encephalopathy [24]. Mutations in *GABRB2* may reduce the expression of GABAA receptor and change the channel function, which could perturb GABA ergic inhibition in the brain. Disruption of excitatory-inhibitory (E/I) balance may be an important mechanism contributing to AD cognitive decline. Interestingly, despite vast neuronal loss in AD patients, GABA ergic neurons and receptors are relatively spared [25]. We have conducted

a linkage disequilibrium analysis in order to annotate the identified functional variants. We found five loci which has strong linkage disequilibrium with rs7943454 (rs1509601: $r^2 = 0.81$, D' = 1; rs7927899: $r^2 = 0.81$, D' = 1; rs6484052: $r^2 = 0.99$, D' = 1; rs6484053: $r^2 = 0.8$, D' = 0.98; rs4922682: $r^2 = 0.91$, D' = 0.96). All these loci are also located in an intron region. We detected only one locus which has strong linkage disequilibrium with rs640476 (rs587875: $r^2 = 0.98$, D' = 1) and was also in an intergenic region.

Replication studies with independent, larger samples will be important to confirm these findings. In this study, we used a stringent MAF threshold (MAF > 0.20) and stringent Bonferroni corrections. These restrictions can improve statistical power to avoid false positive result but may miss less common SNPs. The modest number of subjects restricts stratified analyses for the three diagnostic groups. Besides, a two-year follow-up may be too short to observe the influence of rs7943454 on brain structure changes.

Conclusions

In summary, we identified that two SNPs (rs7943454 in *LUZP2* and rs640476 near *GABRB2*) were associated with plasma NFL at suggestive levels. Rs7943454 in *LUZP2* was associated with the onset risk of AD and atrophy of right middle temporal gyrus in the whole cohort. Using endophenotype-based approach, we identified rs7943454 as a new AD risk locus.

Abbreviations

AD: Alzheimer disease; ADNI: Alzheimer's Disease Neuroimaging Initiative; ANOVA: One-way analysis of variance; *APOE*: Apolipoprotein E; Aβ: amyloid-β; CSF: Cerebrospinal fluid; *GABRB2*: Gamma-aminobutyric acid type A receptor beta2 subunit; GWAS: Genome-wide association study; ICV: Intracranial volume; IGAP: The International Genomics of Alzheimer's Disease Project; *LUZP2*: Leucine zipper protein 2 gene; MAF: Minimum minor allele frequencies; MCI: Mild cognitive impairment; MRI: Magnetic resonance imaging; NFL: Neurofilament light; NFT: Neurofibrillary tangles; PET: Positron emission tomography; p-tau: Phosphorylated tau; t-tau: Total-tau; QC: Quality control; ROI: Regions of interest; SD: Standard deviations; SNPs: Single nucleotide polymorphisms; WAGR: Wilms tumor-Aniridia-Genitourinary anomalies-mental Retardation

Acknowledgements

The authors thank scientists contributed in developing the clinical and genetic resources necessary to collect these data and complete this project. The authors also gratefully thank the efforts of hundreds of individuals whose help and participation made this work possible. Data were obtained from the Alzheimer's Disease Neuroimaging Initiative (ADNI) database (adni.loni.usc.edu).

Funding

Data collection and sharing for this project was funded by the Alzheimer's Disease Neuroimaging Initiative (ADNI) (National Institutes of Health Grant U01 AG024904) and DOD ADNI (Department of Defense award number W81XWH-12-2-0012). ADNI is funded by the National Institute on Aging, the National Institute of Biomedical Imaging and Bioengineering, and through generous contributions from the following: AbbVie, Alzheimer's Association; Alzheimer's Drug Discovery Foundation; Araclon Biotech; BioClinica, Inc.; Biogen; Bristol-Myers Squibb Company; CereSpir, Inc.; Cogstate; Eisai Inc.; Elan Pharmaceuticals, Inc.; Eli Lilly and Company; EuroImmun; F. Hoffmann-La Roche Ltd. and its affiliated company Genentech, Inc.; Fujirebio; GE Healthcare; IXICO Ltd.; Janssen Alzheimer Immunotherapy Research & Development, LLC.; Johnson & Johnson Pharmaceutical Research & Development LLC.; Lumosity; Lundbeck; Merck & Co., Inc.; Meso Scale Diagnostics, LLC.; NeuroRx Research; Neurotrack Technologies; Novartis Pharmaceuticals Corporation; Pfizer Inc.; Piramal Imaging; Servier; Takeda Pharmaceutical Company; and Transition Therapeutics. The Canadian Institutes of Health Research is providing funds to support ADNI clinical sites in Canada. Private sector contributions are facilitated by the Foundation for the National Institutes of Health (www.fnih.org). The grantee organization is the Northern California Institute for Research and Education, and the study is coordinated by the Alzheimer's Therapeutic Research Institute at the University of Southern California. ADNI data are disseminated by the Laboratory for Neuro Imaging at the University of Southern California. This work was supported by grants from the Taishan Scholars Program of Shandong Province (ts201511109 and tsqn20161079), Qingdao Key Health Discipline Development Fund, Qingdao Outstanding Health Professional Development Fund, and Qingdao Innovation and Entrepreneurship Leading Talent Program.

Authors' contributions

JQL, XZY, LT, WAC and JTY: design and conceptualization, analysis and interpretation of the data, drafting and revision of the manuscript. HYL: experimental implementation, data collection and analysis. JQL: experimental implementation, data analysis and revision of the manuscript. XPC: revision of the manuscript. All authors have read and approved the manuscript.

Ethics approval and consent to participate

Regional ethical committees of all participating institutions approved the ADNI (https://adni.loni.usc.edu/wp-content/uploads/how_to_apply/ADNI_Acknowledgement_List.pdf). All study participants or authorized representatives provided written informed consent. Ethics approval was obtained from the institutional review boards of each institution involved: Oregon Health and Science University; University of Southern California; University of California—San Diego; University of Michigan; Mayo Clinic, Rochester; Baylor College of Medicine; Columbia University Medical Center; Washington University, St. Louis; University of Alabama at Birmingham; Mount Sinai School of Medicine; Rush University Medical Center; Wien Center; Johns Hopkins University; New York University; Duke University Medical Center; University of Pennsylvania; University of Kentucky; University of Pittsburgh; University of Rochester Medical Center; University of California, Irvine; University of Texas Southwestern Medical School; Emory University; University of Kansas, Medical Center; University of California, Los Angeles; Mayo Clinic, Jacksonville; Indiana University; Yale University School of Medicine; McGill University, Montreal-Jewish General Hospital; Sunnybrook Health Sciences, Ontario; U.B.C.Clinic for AD & Related Disorders; Cognitive Neurology—St. Joseph's, Ontario; Cleveland Clinic Lou Ruvo Center for Brain Health; Northwestern University; Premiere Research Inst (Palm Beach Neurology); Georgetown University Medical Center; Brigham and Women's Hospital; Stanford University; Banner Sun Health Research Institute; Boston University; Howard University; Case Western Reserve University; University of California, Davis—Sacramento; Neurological Care of CNY; Parkwood Hospital; University of Wisconsin; University of California, Irvine—BIC; Banner Alzheimer's Institute; Dent Neurologic Institute; Ohio State University; Albany Medical College; Hartford Hospital, Olin Neuropsychiatry Research Center; Dartmouth-Hitchcock Medical Center; Wake Forest University Health Sciences; Rhode Island Hospital; Butler Hospital; UC San Francisco; Medical University South Carolina; St. Joseph's Health Care Nathan Kline Institute; University of Iowa College of Medicine; Cornell University; and University of South Florida: USF Health Byrd Alzheimer's Institute.

Competing interests

The authors declare that they have no competing interests.

Author details

[1]Department of Neurology, Qingdao Municipal Hospital, Qingdao University, No.5 Donghai Middle Road, Qingdao 266071, Shandong Province, China. [2]Department of Neurology, Weihaiwei People's Hospital, Weihai, China. [3]Clinical Research Center, Qingdao Municipal Hospital, Qingdao University, Qingdao, China. [4]Department of Neurology, The First Affiliated Hospital of Wenzhou Medical University, Nanbaixiang Road, Wenzhou 325000, Zhejiang Province, China.

References

1. Alzheimer's Assoc. 2015 Alzheimer's disease facts and figures. Alzheimer's Dement. 2015;11(3):332–84.
2. Yu JT, Tan L, Hardy J. Apolipoprotein E in Alzheimer's disease: an update. Annu Rev Neurosci. 2014;37:79–100.
3. Mattsson N, Andreasson U, Zetterberg H, Blennow K. Alzheimer's disease neuroimaging I: Association of Plasma Neurofilament Light with Neurodegeneration in patients with Alzheimer disease. JAMA Neurol. 2017;74(5):557–66.
4. Gaiottino J, Norgren N, Dobson R, Topping J, Nissim A, Malaspina A, Bestwick JP, Monsch AU, Regeniter A, Lindberg RL, et al. Increased neurofilament light chain blood levels in neurodegenerative neurological diseases. PLoS One. 2013;8(9):e75091.
5. Wang HF, Wan Y, Hao XK, Cao L, Zhu XC, Jiang T, Tan MS, Tan L, Zhang DQ, Tan L, et al. Bridging integrator 1 (BIN1) genotypes mediate Alzheimer's disease risk by altering neuronal degeneration. J Alzheimers Dis. 2016; 52(1):179–90.
6. Chen J, Yu JT, Wojta K, Wang HF, Zetterberg H, Blennow K, Yokoyama JS, Weiner MW, Kramer JH, Rosen H, et al. Genome-wide association study identifies MAPT locus influencing human plasma tau levels. Neurology. 2017;88(7):669–76.
7. Kim S, Swaminathan S, Shen L, Risacher SL, Nho K, Foroud T, Shaw LM, Trojanowski JQ, Potkin SG, Huentelman MJ, et al. Genome-wide association study of CSF biomarkers Abeta1-42, t-tau, and p-tau181p in the ADNI cohort. Neurology. 2011;76(1):69–79.
8. Cruchaga C, Kauwe JS, Harari O, Jin SC, Cai Y, Karch CM, Benitez BA, Jeng AT, Skorupa T, Carrell D, et al. GWAS of cerebrospinal fluid tau levels identifies risk variants for Alzheimer's disease. Neuron. 2013;78(2):256–68.
9. Weiner MW, Veitch DP, Aisen PS, Beckett LA, Cairns NJ, Green RC, Harvey D, Jack CR, Jagust W, Liu E, et al. The Alzheimer's disease neuroimaging initiative: a review of papers published since its inception. Alzheimers Dement. 2013;9(5):e111–94.
10. Rohrer JD, Woollacott IO, Dick KM, Brotherhood E, Gordon E, Fellows A, Toombs J, Druyeh R, Cardoso MJ, Ourselin S, et al. Serum neurofilament light chain protein is a measure of disease intensity in frontotemporal dementia. Neurology. 2016;87(13):1329–36.
11. Desikan RS, Segonne F, Fischl B, Quinn BT, Dickerson BC, Blacker D, Buckner RL, Dale AM, Maguire RP, Hyman BT, et al. An automated labeling system for subdividing the human cerebral cortex on MRI scans into gyral based regions of interest. NeuroImage. 2006;31(3):968–80.
12. Jack CR Jr, Bernstein MA, Fox NC, Thompson P, Alexander G, Harvey D, Borowski B, Britson PJ, LW J, Ward C, et al. The Alzheimer's disease neuroimaging initiative (ADNI): MRI methods. J Magn Reson Imaging. 2008;27(4):685–91.
13. Lambert JC, Ibrahim-Verbaas CA, Harold D, Naj AC, Sims R, Bellenguez C, DeStafano AL, Bis JC, Beecham GW, Grenier-Boley B, et al. Meta-analysis of

74,046 individuals identifies 11 new susceptibility loci for Alzheimer's disease. Nat Genet. 2013;45(12):1452–8.

14. Zetterberg H, Skillback T, Mattsson N, Trojanowski JQ, Portelius E, Shaw LM, Weiner MW, Blennow K. Alzheimer's disease neuroimaging I: association of cerebrospinal fluid Neurofilament light concentration with Alzheimer disease progression. JAMA Neurol. 2016;73(1):60–7.

15. Mattsson N, Insel PS, Palmqvist S, Portelius E, Zetterberg H, Weiner M, Blennow K, Hansson O. Alzheimer's disease neuroimaging I: cerebrospinal fluid tau, neurogranin, and neurofilament light in Alzheimer's disease. EMBO Mol Med. 2016;8(10):1184–96.

16. Olsson B, Lautner R, Andreasson U, Ohrfelt A, Portelius E, Bjerke M, Holtta M, Rosen C, Olsson C, Strobel G, et al. CSF and blood biomarkers for the diagnosis of Alzheimer's disease: a systematic review and meta-analysis. Lancet Neurol. 2016;15(7):673–84.

17. Fischbach BV, Trout KL, Lewis J, Luis CA, Sika M. WAGR syndrome: a clinical review of 54 cases. Pediatrics. 2005;116(4):984–8.

18. Kjeldsen E. A novel acquired cryptic three-way translocation t(2;11;5)(p21.3; q13.5;q23.2) with a submicroscopic deletion at 11p14.3 in an adult with hypereosinophilic syndrome. Exp Mol Pathol. 2015;99(1):50–5.

19. Zhao J, Zhao Y, Wang L, Zhang J, Karnes RJ, Kohli M, Wang G, Huang H. Alterations of androgen receptor-regulated enhancer RNAs (eRNAs) contribute to enzalutamide resistance in castration-resistant prostate cancer. Oncotarget. 2016;7(25):38551–65.

20. Wu M, Michaud EJ, Johnson DK. Cloning, functional study and comparative mapping of Luzp2 to mouse chromosome 7 and human chromosome 11p13-11p14. Mamm Genome. 2003;14(5):323–34.

21. Frisoni GB, Fox NC, Jack CR Jr, Scheltens P, Thompson PM. The clinical use of structural MRI in Alzheimer disease. Nat Rev Neurol. 2010;6(2):67–77.

22. Srivastava S, Cohen J, Pevsner J, Aradhya S, McKnight D, Butler E, Johnston M, Fatemi A. A novel variant in GABRB2 associated with intellectual disability and epilepsy. Am J Med Genet A. 2014;164A(11):2914–21.

23. Hirose S. Mutant GABA(a) receptor subunits in genetic (idiopathic) epilepsy. Prog Brain Res. 2014;213:55–85.

24. Ishii A, Kang JQ, Schornak CC, Hernandez CC, Shen W, Watkins JC, Macdonald RL, Hirose S. A de novo missense mutation of GABRB2 causes early myoclonic encephalopathy. J Med Genet. 2017;54(3):202–11.

25. Rissman RA, Mobley WC. Implications for treatment: GABAA receptors in aging, Down syndrome and Alzheimer's disease. J Neurochem. 2011; 117(4):613–22.

7

Comprehensive off-target analysis of dCas9-SAM-mediated HIV reactivation via long noncoding RNA and mRNA profiling

Yonggang Zhang[1,2†], Gustavo Arango[3†], Fang Li[1], Xiao Xiao[1], Raj Putatunda[1], Jun Yu[1], Xiao-Feng Yang[1], Hong Wang[1], Layne T. Watson[3,4], Liqing Zhang[3*] and Wenhui Hu[1,5*] (iD)

Abstract

Background: CRISPR/CAS9 (epi)genome editing revolutionized the field of gene and cell therapy. Our previous study demonstrated that a rapid and robust reactivation of the HIV latent reservoir by a catalytically-deficient Cas9 (dCas9)-synergistic activation mediator (SAM) via HIV long terminal repeat (LTR)-specific MS2-mediated single guide RNAs (msgRNAs) directly induces cellular suicide without additional immunotherapy. However, potential off-target effect remains a concern for any clinical application of Cas9 genome editing and dCas9 epigenome editing. After dCas9 treatment, potential off-target responses have been analyzed through different strategies such as mRNA sequence analysis, and functional screening. In this study, a comprehensive analysis of the host transcriptome including mRNA, lncRNA, and alternative splicing was performed using human cell lines expressing dCas9-SAM and HIV-targeting msgRNAs.

Results: The control scrambled msgRNA (LTR_Zero), and two LTR-specific msgRNAs (LTR_L and LTR_O) groups show very similar expression profiles of the whole transcriptome. Among 839 identified lncRNAs, none exhibited significantly different expression in LTR_L vs. LTR_Zero group. In LTR_O group, only TERC and scaRNA2 lncRNAs were significantly decreased. Among 142,791 mRNAs, four genes were differentially expressed in LTR_L vs. LTR_Zero group. There were 21 genes significantly downregulated in LTR_O vs. either LTR_Zero or LTR_L group and one third of them are histone related. The distributions of different types of alternative splicing were very similar either within or between groups. There were no apparent changes in all the lncRNA and mRNA transcripts between the LTR_L and LTR_Zero groups.

Conclusion: This is an extremely comprehensive study demonstrating the rare off-target effects of the HIV-specific dCas9-SAM system in human cells. This finding is encouraging for the safe application of dCas9-SAM technology to induce target-specific reactivation of latent HIV for an effective "shock-and-kill" strategy.

Keywords: Genome editing, CRISPR, Off-target, RNA sequencing, Transcriptome, HIV, Latency, Shock and kill

Background

Recently, CRISPR/Cas9 genome editing technology has been rapidly developed and attracted extensive attention in biomedical research, with preclinical examples and potential clinical trials in genetic diseases, cancer biology, and infectious diseases [1–7]. Simultaneously, the catalytically-deficient Cas9 (dCas9) epigenome editing technology has emerged as a novel platform for the manipulation of cellular or viral gene regulation by incorporating monoplex or multiplex transcriptional activators or repressors [8–19]. Cas9-mediated genome editing technology has been utilized to excise the HIV-1 provirus via HIV-specific multiplex single guide RNAs (sgRNAs) in cultured HIV latent cell lines [20–22], primary T cells [22, 23], and HIV transgenic rodents [24, 25]. The dCas9 epigenome editing technology [8–11, 19] is also used to reactivate the latent HIV-1 provirus using HIV long terminal repeat (LTR)-specific sgRNAs [26–29]. A rapid and robust reactivation of the HIV latent reservoir by

---

* Correspondence: lqzhang@cs.vt.edu; whu@temple.edu
†Yonggang Zhang and Gustavo Arango contributed equally to this work.
³Department of Computer Science, Virginia Tech, Blacksburg, VA 24060, USA
¹Center for Metabolic Disease Research, Temple University Lewis Katz School of Medicine, 3500 N Broad Street, Philadelphia, PA 19140, USA
Full list of author information is available at the end of the article

dCas9-synergistic activation mediator (SAM) via MS2-mediated sgRNAs (msgRNAs) [30] directly induces cellular suicide without additional immunotherapy [31], which might be a novel, practical, and specific method for the "shock and kill" strategy to cure HIV/AIDS. The dCas9-SAM approach also induces specific activation of endogenous viral restriction factors that affect virus replication [32].

In addition to transcriptional activation, the dCas9 property is also extensively repurposed for transcriptional repression and DNA (de)methylation [12, 33–35]. These epigenome-editing approaches can alter the epigenetic code of the target region, and thus offer a durable manipulation of many genes important in infectious diseases, cancer, and chronic noninfectious diseases [12, 36]. Modification of an individual chromatin mark may suppress target gene expression in most cases [36]. However, permanent silencing of target genes in all cell types may require a combination of several epigenetic effectors [12].

Potential off-target effect remains a critical concern for any clinical application of this technology. Several promising strategies have been developed to mitigate any potential off-target responses, such as the sgRNA design optimization [37–42], transcriptome analysis [28, 30], and functional screening after dCas9 treatment [43]. For the parent Cas9 genome editing system, increasing experimental data suggests that the genome editing is highly specific [20, 44–48]. Newly developed unbiased profiling techniques further validate the high specificity of this Cas9/sgRNA technology [49–54]. In vivo off-target effects are expected to be low due to epigenetic protection [55, 56]. Specifically for dCas9 technology, the frequency of off-target binding to essential (functional) exons would also be very low [57]. Further mRNA-seq analysis confirmed the specificity of this dCas9-SAM technology [28, 30].

Our previous studies analyzed the exogenous viral DNA against the host genome for the best scores of efficiency and specificity [20, 21, 31]. In TZM-bI cells expressing the HIV LTR-driven luciferase reporter without the viral genome itself [58], the dCas9-SAM technology with HIV LTR-specific msgRNAs induced potent reactivation of the HIV reporter, but did not influence the cell growth/proliferation [31], supporting the absence of off-target effects by the dCas9-SAM technology [27, 28, 59]. The aim of this study is to further explore the dCas9-SAM-related potential off-target effects by generating deep sequence coverage of the entire transcriptome, comprehensively analyzing mRNAs, lncRNAs, alternative splicing, genetic mutations including single-nucleotide polymorphisms (SNPs) and indels (insertions and deletions) in TZM-bI cells stably expressing dCas9-SAM and HIV-specific msgRNAs. These analyses are important for safety considerations during the

potential clinical application of dCas9 epigenome editing technology [60].

Methods

Experimental design and RNA sample preparation

The HeLa cell-derived TZM-bl cell line stably expressing higher levels of CD4 and CCR5 was obtained from Dr. John C. Kappes through the NIH AIDS Reagent Program, Division of AIDS, NIAID, NIH. It was generated by introducing separate integrated copies of the luciferase and ß-galactosidase genes under control of the HIV-1 LTR promoter. To establish the dCas9-SAM stable expression cell line (designated TZMb-6465 cell line), TZM-bI cells were transduced with pMSCV-dCas9-BFP (puromycin) retroviral vector (Addgene, plasmid #46912) [10], and Lenti-MS2-p65-HSF1 (hygromycin) lentiviral vector (Addgene, plasmid #61426) [30]. After 2 days, cells were subcultured and selected with puromycin (2 μg/ml) and hygromycin (200 μg/ml). After 2 weeks of selection culture, the TZMb-6465 cells were transduced with msgRNA-expressing empty control lentiviral vector (Addgene, Plasmid #61427) [30], HIV-1 LTR_L msgRNA-expressing lentivirus or LTR_O msgRNA-expressing lentivirus. Six samples were prepared: two replicates for the LTR_L editing (LTR_L1 and LTR_L2), two replicates for the LTRO editing (LTR_O1 and LTR_O2), and two replicates for control (LTR_Zer1 and LTR_Zer2). After four days, cells were subjected to total RNA extraction using the Direct-Zol RNA MiniPrep Kit (Genesee Scientific, Catalog number: 11–330). The 4-day post-infection time point was based on the sufficient msgRNA expression and potent LTR-target reactivation [31] while minimizing the possible confounding factor resulting from the indirect downstream effects of any potential off-targets, if they existed. The RNAs were preserved with RNAstable LD (Sigma, Catalog number: 53201–013) and shipped to Novogene Bioinformatics Institute (https://en.novogene.com/) for total RNA sequencing and bioinformatics analysis. The RNA integrity was verified by 1% agarose gel electrophoresis and Agilent 2100. The RNA purity was checked using a NanoPhotometer® spectrophotometer (IMPLEN, CA, USA) and the DNA concentration was measured using Qubit® DNA Assay Kit in Qubit® 2.0 Fluorometer (Life Technologies, CA, USA).

Library construction and sequencing

The RNA quality control (QC) was done using Trimmomatic with default settings, and this step discarded less than 3% of the RNA reads, and the results were shown in Additional file 1: Table S1. After RNA QC, rRNAs were removed by using the Epicentre Ribo-Zero™ Kit. The purified RNAs were first fragmented randomly into short fragments of 150~200 bp by addition of a fragmentation buffer, then cDNA synthesis was performed using random hexamers. After the first strand was synthesized, a custom second strand synthesis buffer (Illumina), dNTPs (dUTP, dATP, dGTP and dCTP) and DNA polymerase I were added to synthesize the second strand, then followed by purification by AMPure XP beads, terminal repair, polyadenylation, sequencing adapter ligation, size selection, and degradation of the second strand U-contained cDNA by the USER enzyme. The strand-specific cDNA library was generated after the final PCR enrichment. The concentration of the library was first quantified by Qubit2.0, then diluted to 1 ng/ul, and the insert size was checked by Agilent 2100 and further quantified by qPCR (library concentration > 2 nM). The libraries were then subjected to HiSeq sequencing according to the concentration and the expected data volume.

Sequence analysis

About 60 GB of RNA sequencing data was generated for all six samples. Original RNA-Seq reads contain adapters and low quality reads that needed to be filtered out. To ensure the quality of the analysis, the sequence adapters (Oligonucleotide sequences for TruSeq™ RNA and DNA Sample Prep Kits) were removed from reads using Trimmomatic [61, 62]. Then all the trimmed reads with more than 10% ambiguous bases (N) were also removed. Finally, low quality reads with a Phred score less than 20 were removed. Additional file 1: Table S1 shows the distribution of quality reads across the L, O, and Zero samples. High quality sequences are mapped to the human genome (hg38) using TopHat2 with default parameters [63]. Overall, approximately 89% of the raw reads were mapped to the human genome (detailed mapping results are shown in Additional file 1: Table S2 and Additional file 2: Figure S1). Mapped reads were then assigned to known types of RNA using the program HTSeq with the union model (see Additional file 1: Table S3 for the distribution of mapped reads in different categories of known RNAs). To quantify the transcript abundance, the FPKM metric (number of fragments per kilobase of transcript sequence per million mapped reads) was used, which considers both the sequencing depth and the transcript length. In order to measure the reliability of the experiments through biological replicates, the Pearson correlation coefficient (R^2) was calculated between all pairs of the L, O, and Zero samples. A correlation coefficient close to one indicates high similarity of gene expression profiles.

LncRNA analysis

The detailed workflow for identifying long noncoding RNAs (lncRNAs) is shown in Additional file 2: Figure S2b. First, *cufflinks* with default parameters was used to assemble the mapped reads into transcripts and quantify transcript expression (including isoforms).

Candidate long noncoding RNAs (lncRNAs) were then classified into three categories (lncRNAs, intronic lncRNAs, and antisense lncRNAs) through five filtering steps (Additional file 2: Figure S2b): (1) assembled transcripts from *cufflinks* were merged using *cuffcompare* and the merged transcripts selected if they appeared in more than one sample, (2) only transcripts with more than 200 bps and two exons were kept, (3) only those transcripts that have ≥3× coverage for at least two exons were kept, (4) transcripts with high coverage were then removed if they matched known non-lncRNAs and non-mRNA (e.g., rRNA, tRNA, snRNA, snoRNA, etc), and (5) the remaining transcripts were then removed if they matched known mRNAs. The final collection of RNAs was the candidate set of lncRNAs, intronic lncRNAs, and antisense lncRNAs. Additional file 2: Figure S3 shows the number of transcripts that were filtered in each step. After all of the five filtering steps, a total of 1615 transcripts were left in the six pooled samples.

To finally determine if a transcript is a lncRNA, four popular methods for coding potential analysis were applied: (1) CPC (Coding-Potential Calculator) [64] computes the coding potential of a transcript by matching it to the NCBI nr database using BLASTX and scoring it using a support vector machine, (2) CNCI (Coding-Non-Coding Index) distinguishes protein-coding and noncoding transcripts independent of known annotations and predicts the coding or noncoding potential based solely on the features of nucleotide triplets, (3) transcripts were translated into proteins and matched to known protein domains in Pfam [65] using HMMER3 [66] where a matched sequence is considered as having coding potential, whereas others are considered as noncoding, and (4) PhyloCSF (Phylogenetic Codon Substitution Frequency) uses genome-wide mammalian sequence alignments to calculate the coding potential of transcripts.

Functions of the lncRNAs were identified by predicting their protein-coding target genes in both a *cis*- and *trans*- manner. The *cis*-acting target prediction assumes that the function of a lncRNA is determined by its adjacent protein coding genes, and in this study, coding genes within ±100 kb of the lncRNAs were considered as *cis*-acting targets. The *trans*-acting targets were predicted based on co-expressed genes, and only those genes that had Pearson correlation coefficients greater than 0.95 with the lncRNAs were selected.

mRNA analysis

Differentially expressed mRNAs were determined using *cuffdiff* with default parameters [67]. A network analysis of protein-protein interactions for the differentially expressed mRNAs was also conducted using the STRING database [68]. If the target genes (such as the expressed mRNAs) were not found in the database, a BLASTX search was done with an E-value of 1e-10 to identify potential protein-protein interactions.

SNP and indel variant calling

To examine whether the dCas9-SAM technology has an effect on genetic mutations, for example, resulting in different sets of SNPs and indel mutations due to the editing, SNPs and indels were called and compared for the six samples. Specifically, SAMtools [69] and Picard [https://broadinstitute.github.io/picard/] were used to preprocess the mapped reads. SNPs and indel variants were called using the GATK2 toolkit [70]. To quantify the similarity between the sets of SNPs and indel mutations in the samples, the Jaccard Index,

$$J = \frac{|S_1 \cap S_2|}{|S_1 \cup S_2|},$$

where $|S|$ denotes the size of set S, S_1 is the set of SNPs/indels in one sample, and S_2 is the set of SNPs/indels in another sample, is calculated for all 15 pairs of sample comparisons. The Jaccard index ranges from 0 to 1, the higher it is, the more similarity in the sets of SNPs/indels between two samples, with 0 indicating that two samples have entirely different sets of SNPs/indels and 1 indicating that two samples have the same set of SNPs/indels.

Alternative splicing

Alternative splicing (AS) was analyzed by first classifying AS events into 12 types as illustrated in Additional file 2: Figure S4 using ASprofile [71]. Then expression levels of alternatively spliced genes were estimated using the probabilistic framework MISO (Mixture of Isoforms) [72]. MISO uses a Bayesian statistical model to give a more accurate estimate of the expression level indicated by the number of reads that covers different isoforms or exons. Differential expression of isoforms was then determined by the Bayes factor (BF) that computes the odds of differential regulation occurring. The higher the BF, the more likely the isoforms/exons are differentially regulated. A cutoff BF = 10 was applied to select the isoforms/exons that were significantly differentially regulated between conditions [72]. Five major AS events, (1) A3SS (alternative 3′ splice sites), (2) A5SS (alternative 5′ splice sites), (3) MXE (mutually exclusive exons), (4) RI (retained intron), and (5) SE (skipped exon), were analyzed.

Statistics

All the statistical tests, including Steiger's test, two proportion z-test, and Chi-square tests were performed in R.

Results

Very similar expression profiles at the whole transcriptome level among the three conditions

In previous studies, 16 msgRNAs targeting the U3 region of the HIV LTR were screened for their efficiency in guiding dCas9-SAM to activate HIV promoter activity [31]. Two targeting sites, LTR_L (– 165/– 145 bp from the transcription start site) and LTR_O (– 112/– 92 bp from the transcription start site) surrounding the enhancer region (Fig. 1a), were identified for robust reactivation of HIV-1 provirus in various types of human cells [31]. These two hotspots were verified in other studies [26–29]. To determine if the dCas9-SAM system mediated by these two hotspots affects the host cells' transcriptomes, the total RNAs from TZM-bI cells stably expressing the dCas9-SAM system plus msgRNA targeting LTR_L or LTR_O were prepared for lncRNA and mRNA sequencing. The empty msgRNA carrying scrambled target sequence was used as the control (LTR_Zero). The TZM-bI cell line was used because it harbors integrated HIV-1 LTR promoter but does not contain HIV-1 proviral DNA that may produce viral proteins leading to potential effects on the host transcriptome [58], complicating the analysis. A total of 600,451,484 raw reads were generated after read quality control and cleanup, of which 97.4% clean reads were kept for downstream analyses (see Additional file 1: Table S1 for details). The clean reads were then mapped to the human reference genome hg38 by Tophat2 [63]. More than 89% of the reads were mapped for all six samples (see Additional file 1: Table S2 for details) and distributions of the mapped reads in the genome are shown in Additional file 2: Figure S1.

The distribution of the transcript expression levels under different conditions (L, O, and Zero) was analyzed by the mean fragments per kilobase of transcript per million mapped reads (FPKM) of the two replicates for each condition (Fig. 1b). It is clear that the expression distributions of all the transcripts among the three conditions are highly similar, except for the LTR-driven reporter genes luciferase and ß-galactosidase (see Additional file 1: Table S3), which is consistent with the increased luciferase activity in the LTR-targeting groups [31]. The square of the Pearson correlation coefficient (R^2) for all the transcripts among the samples and replicates was assessed, for which $R^2 > 0.92$ was considered good quality [73, 74]. Here, the correlations for all pairs of samples fell within the range of 0.9961 to 0.9993 (Fig. 1c). Samples of the same conditions (i.e., the duplicates for each condition) have significantly higher correlation coefficients than those for samples from different conditions (Steiger's test, $p < 0.05$) [75].

Further analysis of the RNA types using HTSeq with the union model identified similar statistical analysis of the mapped reads (Table 1). Of all the reads that were mapped to RNAs, the majority of those reads, ranging

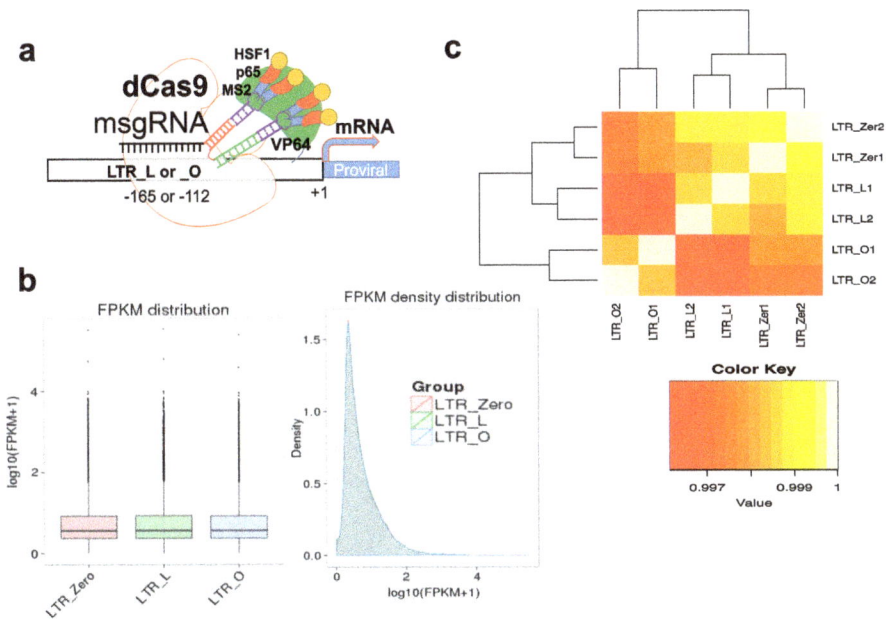

Fig. 1 No difference in the entire RNA transcripts among the three experimental conditions. **a** Diagram showing the HIV proviral activation by the dCas9-SAM system with msgRNAs targeting LTR_L or LTR_O. **b** Box plot and density plot for the distribution of transcript expression levels measured by FPKM (averaged within replicates) of the three conditions. The plotted region of the box plot represents the maximum, upper quartile, median, lower quartile, and minimum, respectively, from top to bottom. **c** Hierarchical clustering of samples based on Pearson correlation coefficient of transcript expression levels for all the pairwise comparisons of the samples

from 88.74 to 89.42%, were mapped to protein coding regions, 1.71 to 2.03% to lncRNA, 3.59 to 4.76% to miscellaneous RNAs, 0.53 to 0.56% to processed transcripts, and 0.5 to 0.55% to antisense RNAs.

Very similar expressions of lncRNAs among the three conditions

Altogether, 1615 transcripts were identified as candidate lncRNAs (see Additional file 2: Figures S2 and S4 for details). These candidate lncRNAs were then subjected to four coding potential prediction methods. A total of 839 lncRNAs were predicted by all the methods (Fig. 2a) and were therefore used in all the subsequent analyses.

As shown in Fig. 2b, there was no clear clustering of samples from the same condition: LTR_L2 showed higher similarity to LTR_Zer2 than to LTR_L1, and LTR_O2 showed higher similarity to LTR_Zer1 than to LTR_O1. Among the 839 lncRNAs, 38 were identified to be differentially expressed for the L vs. Zero comparison at a p-value < 0.05, but none remained significant for the adjusted p-values controlling the false discovery rate (FDR) at 0.10 due to multiple testing. 40 lncRNAs were differentially expressed for the O vs. Zero comparison at p-value < 0.05, but only one lncRNA, TERC, remained statistically significant for the adjusted p-values; 53 were differentially expressed for the L vs. O comparison, but only two lncRNAs, TERC and SCARNA2, remained significant for the

adjusted p-values. Interestingly, the lncRNA TERC showed differential expression levels for all pairwise comparisons of the three conditions (albeit not significant for the L vs. Zero comparison at the adjusted p-value), with the highest expression level under condition L, > 2-fold increase compared to condition O, and a 1.5-fold increase compared to the control (LTR_Zero). The lncRNA SCARNA2 showed the lowest expression level under condition O, followed by increased expression for the control condition (~ 1.4 fold), and condition L (~ 1.7 fold).

Differentially expressed mRNAs

Altogether, 142,791 mRNAs were compared for differential expression among groups. With a false discovery rate of 0.10, four genes (DSC3, EGF, TRIM26, FHDC1, see Additional file 1: Table S5) were differentially expressed between the L and Zero samples, 24 genes were differentially expressed between the O and Zero samples (Additional file 1: Table S5), and 63 genes were differentially expressed between the L and O samples (Additional file 1: Table S5). Gene Ontology analysis revealed no statistically significant enrichment of any specific categories (results not shown). Comparison of the genes across these three lists of differentially expressed genes for the three pairwise comparisons showed that only one gene, TRIM26, was

Table 1 Distribution of mapped reads in different categories of RNAs in the six samples

Sample_name	LTR_Zer1	LTR_Zer2	LTR_L1	LTR_L2	LTR_01	LTR02
3prime_overlapping_ncrna	159 (0.00%)	180 (0.00%)	160 (0.00%)	171 (0.00%)	180 (0.00%)	160 (0.00%)
IG_C_gene	0 (0.00%)	2 (0.00%)	1 (0.00%)	0 (0.00%)	3 (0.00%)	1 (0.00%)
IG_C_pseudogene	0 (0.00%)	0 (0.00%)	0 (0.00%)	0 (0.00%)	0 (0.00%)	0 (0.00%)
IG_D_gene	0 (0.00%)	0 (0.00%)	0 (0.00%)	0 (0.00%)	0 (0.00%)	0 (0.00%)
IG_J_gene	0 (0.00%)	0 (0.00%)	0 (0.00%)	0 (0.00%)	0 (0.00%)	0 (0.00%)
IG_J_pseudogene	0 (0.00%)	0 (0.00%)	0 (0.00%)	0 (0.00%)	0 (0.00%)	0 (0.00%)
IG_V_gene	4 (0.00%)	2 (0.00%)	1 (0.00%)	3 (0.00%)	1 (0.00%)	4 (0.00%)
IG_V_pseudogene	0 (0.00%)	0 (0.00%)	3 (0.00%)	1 (0.00%)	0 (0.00%)	1 (0.00%)
Mt_rRNA	1318 (0.00%)	1488 (0.00%)	1734 (0.00%)	1496 (0.00%)	1342 (0.00%)	1779 (0.01%)
Mt_tRNA	644 (0.00%)	637 (0.00%)	692 (0.00%)	784 (0.00%)	603 (0.00%)	668 (0.00%)
TEC	5415 (0.01%)	5636 (0.01%)	5036 (0.01%)	5747 (0.01%)	5685 (0.02%)	5276 (0.02%)
TR_C_gene	32 (0.00%)	21 (0.00%)	23 (0.00%)	29 (0.00%)	36 (0.00%)	26 (0.00%)
TR_D_gene	0 (0.00%)	0 (0.00%)	0 (0.00%)	0 (0.00%)	0 (0.00%)	0 (0.00%)
TR_J_gene	0 (0.00%)	0 (0.00%)	0 (0.00%)	0 (0.00%)	0 (0.00%)	0 (0.00%)
TR_J_pseudogene	0 (0.00%)	0 (0.00%)	0 (0.00%)	0 (0.00%)	0 (0.00%)	0 (0.00%)
TR_V_gene	0 (0.00%)	0 (0.00%)	0 (0.00%)	1 (0.00%)	0 (0.00%)	0 (0.00%)
TR_V_pseudogene	0 (0.00%)	0 (0.00%)	2 (0.00%)	2 (0.00%)	0 (0.00%)	2 (0.00%)
antisense	191,551 (0.52%)	204,790 (0.53%)	178,062 (0.50%)	205,243 (0.50%)	201,319 (0.54%)	189,642 (0.55%)
known_ncrna	0 (0.00%)	0 (0.00%)	1 (0.00%)	0 (0.00%)	1 (0.00%)	1 (0.00%)
lincRNA	738,731 (2.00%)	761,611 (1.97%)	706,213 (1.98%)	702,871 (1.71%)	742,207 (1.99%)	702,377 (2.03%)
miRNA	2479 (0.01%)	2557 (0.01%)	3497 (0.01%)	3299 (0.01%)	1525 (0.00%)	1430 (0.00%)
misc_RNA	1,612,667 (4.37%)	1,593,547 (4.12%)	1,627,962 (4.57%)	1,960,500 (4.76%)	1,343,420 (3.59%)	1,244,791 (3.59%)
non_coding	0 (0.00%)	0 (0.00%)	0 (0.00%)	0 (0.00%)	0 (0.00%)	0 (0.00%)
polymorphic_pseudogene	319 (0.00%)	355 (0.00%)	320 (0.00%)	369 (0.00%)	333 (0.00%)	312 (0.00%)
processed_pseudogene	10,437 (0.03%)	10,705 (0.03%)	9812 (0.03%)	11,241 (0.03%)	10,275 (0.03%)	8946 (0.03%)
processed_transcript	196,988 (0.53%)	213,355 (0.55%)	194,373 (0.55%)	229,395 (0.56%)	203,313 (0.54%)	192,191 (0.55%)
protein_coding	32,728,357 (88.74%)	34,372,393 (88.92%)	31,562,319 (88.65%)	36,554,719 (88.74%)	33,423,746 (89.42%)	30,949,051 (89.36%)
pseudogene	147 (0.00%)	166 (0.00%)	145 (0.00%)	153 (0.00%)	172 (0.00%)	167 (0.00%)
rRNA	32 (0.00%)	44 (0.00%)	38 (0.00%)	62 (0.00%)	46 (0.00%)	44 (0.00%)
sense_intronic	1015 (0.00%)	1032 (0.00%)	1070 (0.00%)	1071 (0.00%)	1035 (0.00%)	1021 (0.00%)
sense_overlapping	14,067 (0.04%)	15,375 (0.04%)	12,765 (0.04%)	14,949 (0.04%)	15,117 (0.04%)	14,014 (0.04%)
snRNA	3417 (0.01%)	3214 (0.01%)	2915 (0.01%)	3858 (0.01%)	3149 (0.01%)	3236 (0.01%)

Table 1 Distribution of mapped reads in different categories of RNAs in the six samples (Continued)

Sample_name	LTR_Zer1	LTR_Zer2	LTR_L1	LTR_L2	LTR_01	LTR02
snoRNA	160 (0.00%)	172 (0.00%)	136 (0.00%)	149 (0.00%)	197 (0.00%)	170 (0.00%)
transcribed_processed_pseudogene	25,420 (0.07%)	26,038 (0.07%)	24,532 (0.07%)	28,196 (0.07%)	25,315 (0.07%)	23,318 (0.07%)
transcribed_unitary_pseudogene	0 (0.00%)	0 (0.00%)	0 (0.00%)	0 (0.00%)	0 (0.00%)	0 (0.00%)
transcribed_unprocessed_pseudogene	72,052 (0.20%)	77,671 (0.20%)	69,487 (0.20%)	79,027 (0.19%)	78,124 (0.21%)	73,283 (0.21%)
translated_processed_pseudogene	0 (0.00%)	0 (0.00%)	0 (0.00%)	0 (0.00%)	0 (0.00%)	0 (0.00%)
translated_unprocessed_pseudogene	1 (0.00%)	0 (0.00%)	0 (0.00%)	1 (0.00%)	0 (0.00%)	0 (0.00%)
unitary_pseudogene	7892 (0.02%)	8444 (0.02%)	7147 (0.02%)	8507 (0.02%)	8233 (0.02%)	7525 (0.02%)
unprocessed_pseudogene	12,070 (0.03%)	12,228 (0.03%)	11,432 (0.03%)	12,660 (0.03%)	12,177 (0.03%)	11,856 (0.03%)
Others	1,257,539 (3.41%)	1,342,963 (3.47%)	1,185,376 (3.33%)	1,370,001 (3.33%)	1,299,971 (3.48%)	1,201,876 (3.47%)

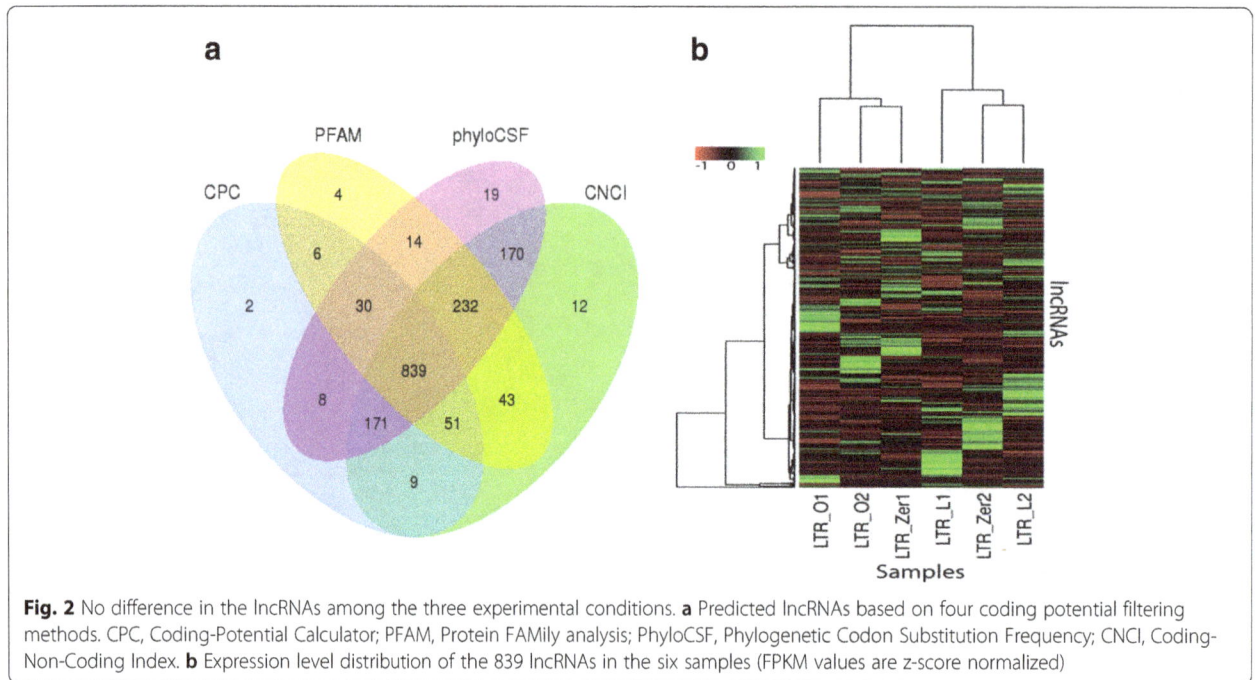

Fig. 2 No difference in the lncRNAs among the three experimental conditions. **a** Predicted lncRNAs based on four coding potential filtering methods. CPC, Coding-Potential Calculator; PFAM, Protein FAMily analysis; PhyloCSF, Phylogenetic Codon Substitution Frequency; CNCI, Coding-Non-Coding Index. **b** Expression level distribution of the 839 lncRNAs in the six samples (FPKM values are z-score normalized)

more robustly down regulated in the L samples (FPKM = ~ 1.4) than in both the O (FPKM = ~ 4.5) and Zero (FPKM = ~ 3.9) samples (all pairwise comparisons are statistically significant). REPS2 was significantly upregulated in both the O and L samples compared to the Zero control, but only showed a statistical significance in the O vs. Zero sample comparison for the adjusted p-value; in the L vs. Zero sample comparison, although the p-value was significant, the adjusted p-value was not. There were 21 genes differentially expressed in the O samples compared with either the L or Zero samples (but not between the L and Zero samples, Table 2). Interestingly, all these 21 genes were significantly downregulated in the O samples as compared to those in both the L and Zero samples. Also interesting was that one third of these genes were histone related: HIST1H2AB, HIST1H2AD, HIST1H2AM, HIST1H4J, HIST2H2AC, HIST2H2BF, HIST2H3D. This result suggestsed that there were no apparent upregulated changes from Zero to LTR_L in all mRNA transcripts. However, LTR_O significantly downregulated some genes. Since the dCas9-SAM was expected to activate the mRNA expression of any potential off-target genes, these downregulated genes might not be directly related to the action of the dCas9-SAM activation system. However, these downregulated genes were specific for the msgRNA LTR_O, and histone-related genes were the most striking, perhaps implying that LTR_O-mediated LTR transcription activation may exhaust some histone proteins. It

was unlikely that LTR_O induced direct suppression of several histone genes, unless the enriched transcriptional activator (VP64, p65, HSF1) by the dCas9-SAM via LTR_O msgRNA might suppress histone genes by interacting with their transcriptional complex. It was also possible that LTR_O affected some genes such as TERC and REPS2 that might negatively regulate the expression of these histone genes.

SNP and indel analysis

To examine whether the dCas9-SAM epigenome editing had an effect on the rate of genetic mutations, SNPs and indel variants in all the samples were identified using GATK2 [70]. Totally, there were 733,334 SNPs and 36,715 indels identified in the six samples. The Jaccard index was computed for each pair of samples where the number of reads that supported the called SNPs and indels was greater than or equal to 20. Figure 3 showed the Jaccard index matrix and clustering result of the six samples for both SNPs and indels. The Jaccard index was high for all sample comparisons, ranging from 0.895 (O_2 vs. L_1) to 0.925 (Z_2 vs. L_2) for SNPs, and from 0.889 (O_2 vs. L_1) to 0.925 (Z_2 vs. L_2) for indels. The clustering result revealed no clear grouping within the same conditions (that is, L samples grouped together, O samples grouped together, or control samples grouped together), suggesting that there were no systematic differences in SNP and indel variations between different editing conditions.

Table 2 21 genes that are significantly downregulated in the O samples as compared to the Zero and L samples

Genes	LTR_O_FPKM	LTR_Zero_FPKM	log₂(fold)	LTR_L_FPKM	log₂(fold)
HNRNPAB	6.55	38.66	− 2.56	43.94	−2.75
PTP4A2	3.62	20.44	−2.50	23.02	−2.67
B4GALT2	2.07	6.02	−1.54	6.07	−1.55
C4orf48	4.99	11.81	−1.24	11.15	−1.16
TPGS1	3.36	7.16	−1.09	8.80	−1.39
HPCAL1	4.01	8.33	−1.05	8.39	−1.06
SLBP	10.55	20.53	−0.96	20.64	−0.97
CITED4	3.56	6.79	−0.93	7.66	−1.11
HIST2H2BF	97.90	175.32	− 0.84	176.52	− 0.85
TMEM160	8.40	14.67	−0.80	16.45	−0.97
HIST2H2AC	444.08	750.59	−0.76	850.05	−0.94
C17orf89	57.82	95.66	−0.73	109.36	−0.92
IER5L	6.61	10.87	−0.72	13.23	−1.00
CEBPD	16.45	26.54	−0.69	29.57	−0.85
HIST2H3D	248.87	400.31	−0.69	425.10	−0.77
HIST1H2AB	336.25	536.04	−0.67	587.46	−0.80
HIST1H2AM	468.32	743.47	−0.67	809.48	−0.79
MIF	128.97	200.45	−0.64	247.69	−0.94
HIST1H4J	1102.07	1656.42	−0.59	1819.34	−0.72
CYBA	179.61	268.40	−0.58	308.07	−0.78
HIST1H2AD	722.53	1057.74	−0.55	1177.36	−0.70

Very similar distribution of alternative splicing events among the three groups

Alternative splicing is an important means for increasing the diversity of transcripts and proteins. In fact, a majority of mammalian genes have around 2~12 mRNA isoforms, with some having a few thousand isoforms [76]. Therefore, characterizing the off-target effects of dCas9 epigenome editing is incomplete without considering how alternative splicing might be affected among different groups as compared to the control. To investigate in detail how isoforms or exons might be affected, alternative splicing events were first classified into 12 types as illustrated in Additional file 2: Figure S4 using ASprofile [71]. The number of each type of alternative splicing event for the six samples was shown in Fig. 4 (also see Additional file 1: Table S6). The total number of alternative splicing events ranged from 297,334 to 298,098 with the two LTR_O samples (O1: 298, 098; O2: 297,999) having the highest number of alternative splicing events, followed by LTR_Zer2 (297,789), LTR_L2 (297,763), LTR_Zer1 (297,580), and LTR_L1 (297,334). The distribution of different types of alternative splicing was very similar among the six samples, and there was no significant difference either within or between groups (all

the pairwise Chi-square tests' p-values are greater than 0.98).

To further examine whether isoforms produced by alternative splicing differed in expression level among the three groups, the MISO (mixture-of-isoforms) model [72] was used to determine the isoforms that differentiate the groups. MISO uses a Bayesian statistical model to estimate the expression level of different isoforms/exons and identifies differentially regulated isoforms by the Bayes factor (BF) that calculates the odds of differential regulation of isoforms or exons. Five major types of alternative splicing events, alternative 3′ splice sites (A3SS), alternative 5′ splice sites (A5SS), mutually exclusive exons (MXE), retained intron (RI), and skipped exon (SE), were analyzed and compared among the three groups. Table 3 showed the genes that exhibited significant differential isoform regulation between the group comparisons. Figure 5 showed an example of the TOPORS gene exhibiting significant differential exon skipping in LTR_O samples compared to the Zero samples. Altogether, there were not many differential isoform regulations between the groups. For example, of the 7244 A3SS events compared between the L samples and Zero samples, only seven (< 0.1%) had significant differential isoform regulation. In fact, the percentage of

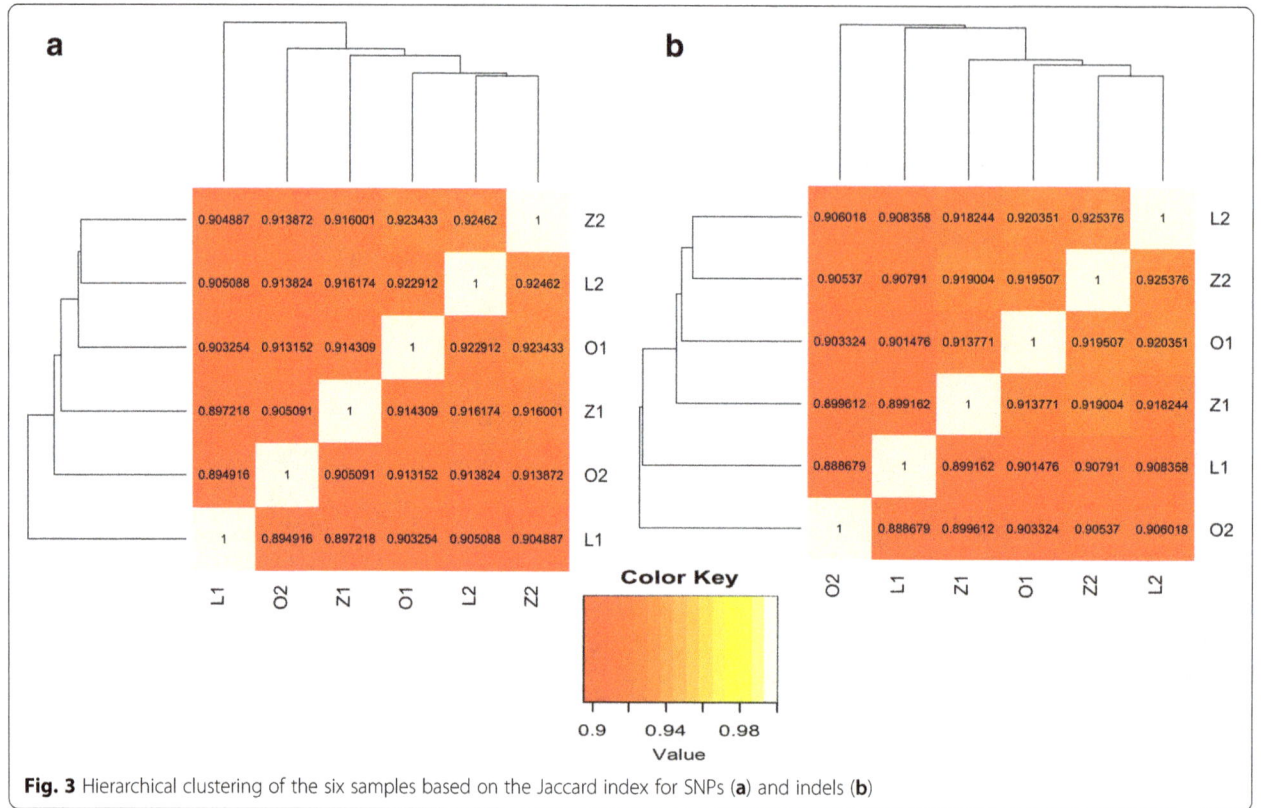

Fig. 3 Hierarchical clustering of the six samples based on the Jaccard index for SNPs (**a**) and indels (**b**)

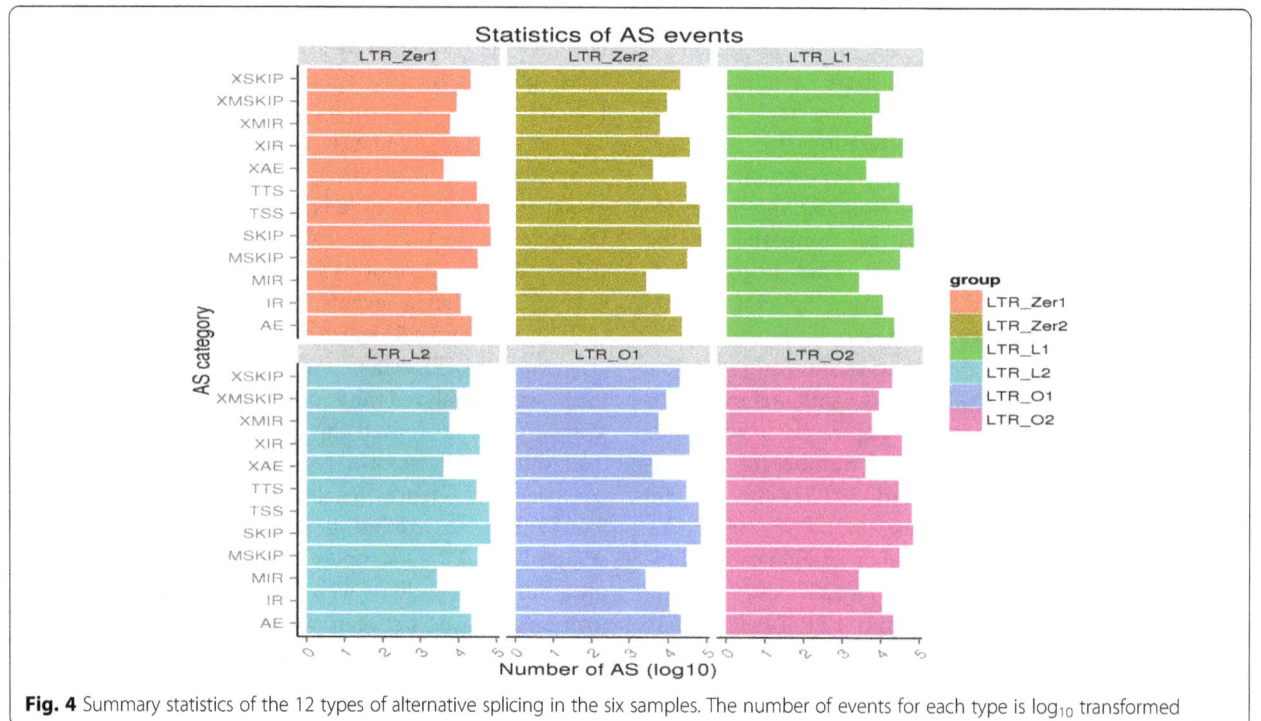

Fig. 4 Summary statistics of the 12 types of alternative splicing in the six samples. The number of events for each type is log₁₀ transformed

Table 3 Comparison of differential isoform regulation between the three groups. The genes in bold font are those shared by two pairwise comparisons. The numbers in parenthesis are the number of events considered for the particular group comparison

AS types	L vs. Zero	O vs. Zero	L vs. O
A3SS (# of events)	(7244)	(7143)	(7239)
	C8orf22	ANKRD11	BMP1
	CLSPN	C11orf48	NFAT5
	COBLL1	CNOT2	**OCEL1**
	DAK	GNB2L1	ORMDL1
	JOSD1	SETMAR	ST5
	OCEL1	YWHAB	ZNF84
	PIH1D1	ZNF587	
A5SS (# of events)	(5399)	(5350)	(5407)
	C17orf70	ANGPT1	HILPDA
	MTMR2	CLEC2D	NBPF11
	NOC2L	LAMA4	NDUFV2
	RP5-1198O20.4	NAA60	NT5C
	SMARCC2	SLC50A1	OXLD1
	TWF1	**TYSND1**	RP4-583P15.15
	ZNF30		SRRM1
			TBC1D7
			TYSND1
			VPS52
			chr1:32336239:32335947
MXE (# of events)	(4959)	(4946)	(5006)
	CNOT1	**CNOT1**	AKIRIN1
	DBNL	EIF4G2	DDHD2
	DPY30	HMGN1	DEK
	MPPE1	PTRH1	DPP3
	PLA2G6	**RPS6KC1**	ELMOD3
	SPDL1	TMBIM4	MPV17L
	TMBIM6	**TMEM116**	**RPS6KC1**
	UQCC1	chr7:143284899:143284974:+@chr7:143285348	TCTN1
	WBP1		**TMEM116**
RI (# of events)	(4109)	(4057)	(4084)
	CENPV	**BAX**	**BAX**
	MRRF	CAPRIN2	FANCI
	RP11-5A19.5	CDK5RAP3	HSD17B4
	RPRD2	**CENPV**	MTA1
	SMTN	GPS2	TAB3
		IMPDH2	
		QARS	
		SERAC1	

Table 3 Comparison of differential isoform regulation between the three groups. The genes in bold font are those shared by two pairwise comparisons. The numbers in parenthesis are the number of events considered for the particular group comparison *(Continued)*

AS types	L vs. Zero	O vs. Zero	L vs. O
SE (# of events)	(25,942)	(25,835)	(25,969)
	C2CD5	**AC013394.2**	**AC013394.2**
	CDC42BPA	AGPAT2	AC124789.1
	DCTD	**ATG7**	ARID1B
	DSC3	**B3GALNT2**	ATG10
	GRB10	**BCL2L12**	**ATG7**
	HMGN1	CENPU	**B3GALNT2**
	KCTD17	CMTR2	BBS1
	LINC00570	GABPB2	**BCL2L12**
	MIPOL1	**HMGN1**	BTBD7
	MRPL52	IMMP1L	CD320
	NCSTN	KDM6A	CD59
	NUMB	KLHL5	DCTD
	PDE4DIP	**MAPK9**	LINC00472
	PXK	**MRPL52**	**MAPK9**
	RAB40B	**PTK2**	MIR4435-1HG
	SCMH1	SETD8	**PTK2**
	SPATA20	SMURF2P1	RHBDD1
	TMEM139	**SP3**	RP4-717I23.3
	TTC23	**TBL1XR1**	RPS6KB2
	ZNF138	TINF2	**SP3**
	ZSCAN21	**TMEM139**	ST20-MTHFS
		TMEM189	**TBL1XR1**
		TOPORS	**TOPORS**
		TRIP6	UBE2I
		UBE2I	YDJC
		VWA9	ZNF639
		ZNF584	ZNF678
	chr7:143284899:143284974		

significant differential isoform regulations between groups for the three pairwise comparisons (L vs. Zero, O vs. Zero, L vs. O) ranged from 0.097 to 0.111% for A3SS, from 0.130 to 0.2% for A5SS, from 0.180 to 0.181% for MXE, from 0.122 to 0.197% for RI, and from 0.081 to 0.112% for SE. Taken together, less than 0.2% of the alternative splicing events considered showed differential isoform regulations between the groups, suggesting no genome-wide systematic alternative splicing changes occurred due to the dCas9 editing. Moreover, comparison of the list of genes with differential isoform regulation to

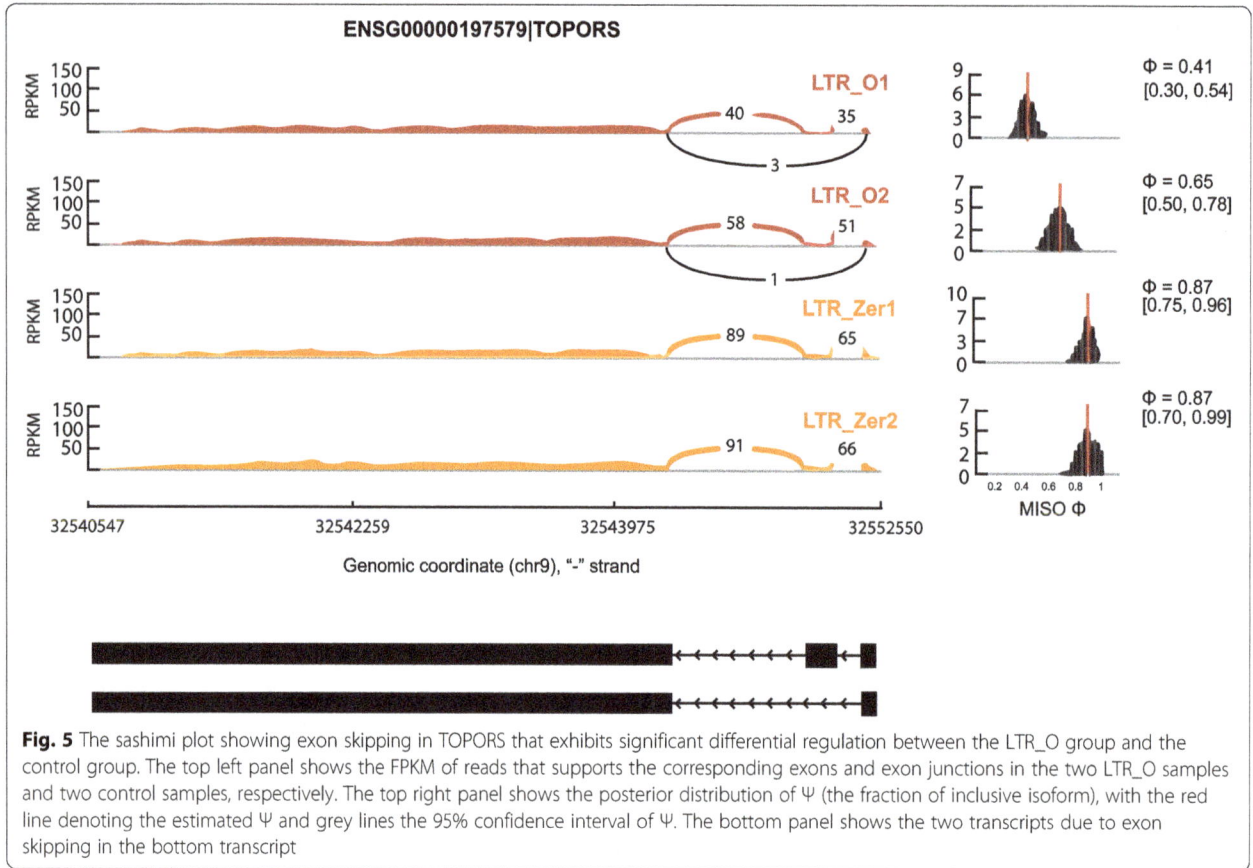

Fig. 5 The sashimi plot showing exon skipping in TOPORS that exhibits significant differential regulation between the LTR_O group and the control group. The top left panel shows the FPKM of reads that supports the corresponding exons and exon junctions in the two LTR_O samples and two control samples, respectively. The top right panel shows the posterior distribution of Ψ (the fraction of inclusive isoform), with the red line denoting the estimated Ψ and grey lines the 95% confidence interval of Ψ. The bottom panel shows the two transcripts due to exon skipping in the bottom transcript

the list of differentially expressed genes (Additional file 1: Table S5) showed that only DSC3 had differential exon regulation between the L and Zero samples, and DSC3 was also significantly downregulated in the L samples compared to the Zero samples.

Discussion

Determining off-target effects from CRISPR/Cas9-based genome editing in a thorough and highly sensitive manner has been a great challenge in the field [6, 77–79]. Apart from ongoing extensive work in optimizing the technology to minimize off-target cleavage [39, 80–82], serious effort has also been devoted to examining the off-target effects resulting in changes at the levels of genomes and transcriptomes [50, 52, 83–89]. In particular, the specificity of the dCas9-SAM system itself has been validated by mRNA-seq analysis [17, 28, 30], although the dCas9-VP160 alone (in the absence of sgRNA) has been shown to reactivate latent HIV-1 in U1 cells [90]. Here, deep sequencing of transcriptomes of human cells after epigenome (transcriptional) editing by HIV-specific msgRNA/dCas9-SAM was performed, and a comprehensive analysis was done to examine any potential off-target effects of the HIV-targeted msgRNA/dCas9--SAM on the mRNA transcription, lncRNA expression,

alternative splicing, as well as genetic mutations including SNPs and indels.

Off-target effect on the overall mRNA expression level

In terms of mRNA expression, if there were significant off-target effects, many genes would be upregulated in the O and L samples compared to the control group (the genes that are upregulated could differ between the O and L samples), but only a handful of the host genes showed significant difference, most of which were actually downregulated (Additional file 1: Table S5). Specifically, of the 28 genes showing a statistically significant difference, only two, HDGF and REPS2, were significantly upregulated in the O samples compared to the control group. Four genes were found differentially expressed in the L group vs. Zero group comparison, but all of them were downregulated in the L group compared to the Zero group (the control group). It is puzzling that most of the differentially expressed genes were significantly downregulated in the dCas9-SAM editing system (O and L samples) compared to the control group. This phenomenon has not yet been reported anywhere in the literature.

The 12~ 14-bp target sequence near the protospacer-adjacent motif (PAM) region (NGG) is critical for the specificity of Cas9 genome editing [91, 92]. In silico off-target effect prediction for LTR_L and LTR_O was done by blasting > 14-bp target + NGG against the human genome/transcripts as we described previously [20, 21, 23], then comparing the list of potential off-target gene locations with the genes identified in Additional file 1: Table S5. There is no overlap between the two lists, suggesting that genes that show significant expression difference between the two dCas9-SAM edited groups and the control group may not be the direct result of the potential off-target effect.

Off-target effects on alternative splicing

Comparison with 12 types of alternative splicing events reveals no statistically significant differences between the edited groups (L and O) and the control group (Fig. 4). Moreover, a detailed expression analysis of isoforms caused by five major types of alternative splicing shows only a small number of differential isoform regulations between groups (< 0.2%, Table 3), further suggesting that there are no pronounced genome-wide alternative splicing changes occurring due to the dCas9-SAM editing. DSC3 is the only gene that shows both significant differential exon regulation and expression level differences between the edited group (L) and the control group, but contrary to expectations, is significantly downregulated. Previous studies show about 47~74% of alterative splicing events show variation among different human tissues and 10~30% of alternative splicing events show variation among individuals [93]. Therefore, comparatively, the level of variation in alternative splicing detected among the three groups (L, O, and control) is 2~3 orders of magnitude lower. Although the level of genetic variation among the samples is also lower (less than one order of magnitude, see results on SNPs and indel comparison), these comparisons nonetheless suggest that the off-target effect due to the dCas9 epigenome editing does not include any noticeable changes at the genome-wide alternative splicing level. Since alternative splicing is an important mechanism for increasing transcript and protein diversity [76, 94], and fine-tuning gene expression and function, any off-target effect caused by dCas9 editing could conceivably create undesirable consequences that in turn limit dCas9 usage. The current finding is thus very encouraging for the safe application of dCas9 epigenome editing to reactivate the silent HIVs for their ultimate elimination.

Off-target effect on lncRNAs

Long noncoding RNA (lncRNA), transcripts longer than 200 nucleotides that cannot be translated into proteins, are derived from 70~90% of the mammalian genome while mRNAs are transcribed from only 1% of the genome [95]. These lncRNAs have been shown to play important regulatory roles in chromatin reprogramming

and pre- and post-mRNA processing [96–98]. Therefore, any off-target effects on lncRNA expression is also important to consider. Using the pipeline shown in Additional file 2: Figure S2b, 839 lncRNAs (Fig. 2a) were identified in the transcripts and their expression compared in six samples. Results (Fig. 2b) reveal no clear clustering of samples within the same groups and no clear separation among groups. There is no significant lncRNA expression difference between the L group and the control group. Only one lncRNA, TERC, is significantly downregulated in the O samples compared to the control samples. In fact, TERC has the highest expression level under condition L, followed by the control condition, and then condition O. This expression difference does not seem to be directly linked to any off-target effect, as one would expect TERC lncRNA to have higher expressions in both edited groups (O and L groups) compared to the control group. The observation for lncRNA expression is similar to the observation for mRNA expression, because the handful of mRNAs and lncRNAs tend to be downregulated, contrary to an expectation of elevated expressions in the edited groups due to the potential off-target transcriptional activation effect. It is therefore concluded that there is little, if any, detectable off-target effects on lncRNA transcription. As more studies have shown the involvement of lncRNAs in various diseases and cancer [99–102], our current finding is reassuring, and further supports the safe application of dCas9-SAM epigenome editing. Note that the current finding does not preclude the possibility that the off-target effects could upregulate some unknown genetic elements/factors, which in turn suppress/reduce the expression of the mRNA and lncRNAs identified in the current study.

Off-target effect on SNPs and indels

Off-target-induced mutations are also another important consideration for the safe application of dCas9-SAM system in clinical settings. Although dCas9 itself does not induce indels or SNPs directly due to its lack of endonuclease activity, it is possible that the dCas9-SAM system induces indels indirectly through potential off-target effects on some mutagenic genes. Results (Fig. 3) comparing both SNPs and indels in the six samples did not show any significant off-target effects. Although previous studies have shown that RNA-guided endonuclease mediated genome editing can induce off-target indel mutations [92, 103–106], numerous studies have also shown that off-target mutations can be effectively reduced and possibly eliminated by careful selection of unique target sequences and guide RNA and Cas9 variant optimization [107]. One cautionary note is that since SNPs and indels were identified using RNA-seq data, the current study cannot address whether there is any significant mutagenic effect due to the dCas9 epigenome editing in non-transcribed regions.

Conclusion

To the authors' knowledge, this study is the most comprehensive and exhaustive characterization of the off-target effects on transcriptomes after HIV-targeted dCas9-SAM epigenome editing. Analysis of known types of RNAs reveals no significant difference between transcriptomes of HIV-targeted and non-targeted msgRNA-treated human cells, supporting the contention that msgRNA-directed dCas9-based SAM technology can be safely used to reactivate dormant HIV for an effective "shock-and-kill" strategy to finally eliminate the virus [108]. One caveat with the current study is that there were only two replicates for each group, which limits the statistical power of the study. Future work needs to include more replicates. Additionally, further assessment of the potential off-target effects with the dCas9-SAM system in human primary cells and preclinical animal models is warranted.

Additional files

Additional file 1: Table S1. Statistics of RNA-Seq quality reads. **Table S2.** Mapping results. **Table S3.** Validation of dCas9-SAM mRNA and sgRNA expression (transcripts per million). **Table S4.** Distribution of reads in known types of RNAs. **Table S5.** Differentially expressed mRNA transcripts for all the three pairwise comparisons of the samples (O vs Zero, L vs Zero, and O vs L). **Table S6.** Distribution of the 12 types of alternative splicing events across samples.

Additional file 2: Figure S1. Distributions of the mapped reads in the genome for the six samples. **Figure S2.** Workflow charts for RNA-seq analysis. (a) Library construction. (b) lncRNA filtering by four pipelines to predict candidate lncRNAs based on their structures and noncoding features. **Figure S3.** Statistics of lncRNA filtering. Horizontal axis represents the filtering step and vertical axis represents the number of remaining transcripts after the filtering step. **Figure S4.** Illustration of 12 types of alternative splicing events analyzed by ASprofile (Picture taken from Florea L, Song L, Salzberg SL: Thousands of exon skipping events differentiate among splicing patterns in sixteen human tissues. *F1000Res* 2013, 2:188).

Abbreviations

A3SS: Alternative 3' splice sites; AS: Alternative splicing; BF: Bayes factor; dCas9: dead CRISPR-associated protein 9; FDR: False discovery rate; FPKM: Fragments per kilobase of transcript per million mapped reads; lncRNA: long noncoding RNA; LTR: Long terminal repeat; MISO: Mixture of isoforms; msgRNA: MS2-mediated single guide RNA; MXE: Mutually exclusive exons; PAM: Protospacer-adjacent motif; RI: Retained intron; SAM: Synergistic activation mediator; SE: Skipped exon; SNP: Single-nucleotide polymorphism

Acknowledgements

We acknowledge Dr. Xiaoxue Jiang and Dr. Wenjie Wei for bioinformatics analysis.

Funding

This work was supported by National Institutes of Health (R01NS087971 and R01DK075964 to W.H. and VT open access subvention fund to L.Z.). The funders had no role in study design, data collection and analysis, decision to publish, or preparation of the manuscript.

Authors' contributions

WH, YZ, LZ and HW conceived and designed the experiments. YZ, FL, XX, RP and JY performed the experiments, acquired/discussed the data and reviewed/edited the manuscript. GA, WH, LZ, LTW and XY analyzed/interpreted the data, prepared figures and extensively edited the manuscript. WH, LZ, YZ, HW and LTW supervised the study, drafted and revised the manuscript. All authors read and approved the final manuscript.

Competing interests

The authors declare that they have no competing interests.

Author details

[1]Center for Metabolic Disease Research, Temple University Lewis Katz School of Medicine, 3500 N Broad Street, Philadelphia, PA 19140, USA. [2]Center for Stem Cell Research and Application, Institute of Blood Transfusion, Chinese Academy of Medical Sciences & Peking Union Medical College (CAMS & PUMC), Chengdu 610052, China. [3]Department of Computer Science, Virginia Tech, Blacksburg, VA 24060, USA. [4]Department of Mathematics, Department of Aerospace and Ocean Engineering, Virginia Tech, Blacksburg, VA 24060, USA. [5]Department of Pathology and Laboratory Medicine, Temple University Lewis Katz School of Medicine, 3500 N Broad Street, Philadelphia, PA 19140, USA.

References

1. Sander JD, Joung JK. CRISPR-Cas systems for editing, regulating and targeting genomes. Nat Biotechnol. 2014;32(4):347–55.
2. Vasileva EA, Shuvalov OU, Garabadgiu AV, Melino G, Barlev NA. Genome-editing tools for stem cell biology. Cell Death Dis. 2015;6:e1831.
3. Sanchez-Rivera FJ, Jacks T. Applications of the CRISPR-Cas9 system in cancer biology. Nat Rev Cancer. 2015;15(7):387–95.
4. Riordan SM, Heruth DP, Zhang LQ, Ye SQ. Application of CRISPR/Cas9 for biomedical discoveries. Cell Bioscience. 2015;5:33.
5. Saayman S, Ali SA, Morris KV, Weinberg MS. The therapeutic application of CRISPR/Cas9 technologies for HIV. Expert Opin Biol Ther. 2015;15(6):819–30.
6. Mali P, Yang L, Esvelt KM, Aach J, Guell M, DiCarlo JE, Norville JE, Church GM. RNA-guided human genome engineering via Cas9. Science. 2013; 339(6121):823–6.
7. Thakore PI, Black JB, Hilton IB, Gersbach CA. Editing the epigenome: technologies for programmable transcription and epigenetic modulation. Nat Methods. 2016;13(2):127–37.
8. Agne M, Blank I, Emhardt AJ, Gabelein CG, Gawlas F, Gillich N, Gonschorek P, Juretschke TJ, Kramer SD, Louis N, et al. Modularized CRISPR/dCas9 effector toolkit for target-specific gene regulation. ACS Synth Biol. 2014; 3(12):986–9.
9. Maeder ML, Linder SJ, Cascio VM, Fu Y, Ho QH, Joung JK. CRISPR RNA-guided activation of endogenous human genes. Nat Methods. 2013;10(10): 977–9.
10. Gilbert LA, Larson MH, Morsut L, Liu Z, Brar GA, Torres SE, Stern-Ginossar N, Brandman O, Whitehead EH, Doudna JA, et al. CRISPR-mediated modular RNA-guided regulation of transcription in eukaryotes. Cell. 2013;154(2):442–51.
11. Cheng AW, Wang H, Yang H, Shi L, Katz Y, Theunissen TW, Rangarajan S, Shivalila CS, Dadon DB, Jaenisch R. Multiplexed activation of endogenous genes by CRISPR-on, an RNA-guided transcriptional activator system. Cell Res. 2013;23(10):1163–71.
12. Amabile A, Migliara A, Capasso P, Biffi M, Cittaro D, Naldini L, Lombardo A. Inheritable silencing of endogenous genes by hit-and-run targeted epigenetic editing. Cell. 2016;167(1):219–32. e214

13. Chavez A, Tuttle M, Pruitt BW, Ewen-Campen B, Chari R, Ter-Ovanesyan D, Haque SJ, Cecchi RJ, Kowal EJ, Buchthal J, et al. Comparison of Cas9 activators in multiple species. Nat Methods. 2016;13(7):563–7.

14. Chavez A, Scheiman J, Vora S, Pruitt BW, Tuttle M, E PRI, Lin S, Kiani S, Guzman CD, Wiegand DJ, et al. Highly efficient Cas9-mediated transcriptional programming. Nat Methods. 2015;12(4):326–8.

15. Qi LS, Larson MH, Gilbert LA, Doudna JA, Weissman JS, Arkin AP, Lim WA. Repurposing CRISPR as an RNA-guided platform for sequence-specific control of gene expression. Cell. 2013;152(5):1173–83.

16. Black JB, Adler AF, Wang HG, D'Ippolito AM, Hutchinson HA, Reddy TE, Pitt GS, Leong KW, Gersbach CA. Targeted epigenetic remodeling of endogenous loci by CRISPR/Cas9-based transcriptional activators directly converts fibroblasts to neuronal cells. Cell Stem Cell. 2016;19(3):406–14.

17. Thakore PI, D'Ippolito AM, Song L, Safi A, Shivakumar NK, Kabadi AM, Reddy TE, Crawford GE, Gersbach CA. Highly specific epigenome editing by CRISPR-Cas9 repressors for silencing of distal regulatory elements. Nat Methods. 2015;12(12):1143–9.

18. Hilton IB, D'Ippolito AM, Vockley CM, Thakore PI, Crawford GE, Reddy TE, Gersbach CA. Epigenome editing by a CRISPR-Cas9-based acetyltransferase activates genes from promoters and enhancers. Nat Biotechnol. 2015;33(5):510–7.

19. Perez-Pinera P, Kocak DD, Vockley CM, Adler AF, Kabadi AM, Polstein LR, Thakore PI, Glass KA, Ousterout DG, Leong KW, et al. RNA-guided gene activation by CRISPR-Cas9-based transcription factors. Nat Methods. 2013;10(10):973–6.

20. Hu W, Kaminski R, Yang F, Zhang Y, Cosentino L, Li F, Luo B, Alvarez-Carbonell D, Garcia-Mesa Y, Karn J, et al. RNA-directed gene editing specifically eradicates latent and prevents new HIV-1 infection. Proc Natl Acad Sci U S A. 2014;111(31):11461–6.

21. Yin C, Zhang T, Li F, Yang F, Putatunda R, Young WB, Khalili K, Hu W, Zhang Y. Functional screening of guide RNAs targeting the regulatory and structural HIV-1 viral genome for a cure of AIDS. AIDS. 2016;30(8):1163–74.

22. Kaminski R, Chen Y, Salkind J, Bella R, Young WB, Ferrante P, Karn J, Malcolm T, Hu W, Khalili K. Negative feedback regulation of HIV-1 by gene editing strategy. Sci Rep. 2016;6:31527.

23. Kaminski R, Chen Y, Fischer T, Tedaldi E, Napoli A, Zhang Y, Karn J, Hu W, Khalili K. Elimination of HIV-1 genomes from human T-lymphoid cells by CRISPR/Cas9 gene editing. Sci Rep. 2016;6:22555.

24. Kaminski R, Bella R, Yin C, Otte J, Ferrante P, Gendelman HE, Li H, Booze R, Gordon J, Hu W, et al. Excision of HIV-1 DNA by gene editing: a proof-of-concept in vivo study. Gene Ther. 2016;23(8–9):690–5.

25. Yin C, Zhang T, Qu X, Zhang Y, Putatunda R, Xiao X, Li F, Xiao W, Zhao H, Dai S, et al. In Vivo Excision of HIV-1 Provirus by saCas9 and Multiplex Single-Guide RNAs in Animal Models. Mol Ther. 2017;25:1168–86.

26. Bialek JK, Dunay GA, Voges M, Schafer C, Spohn M, Stucka R, Hauber J, Lange UC. Targeted HIV-1 latency reversal using CRISPR/Cas9-derived transcriptional activator systems. PLoS One. 2016;11(6):e0158294.

27. Limsirichai P, Gaj T, Schaffer DV. CRISPR-mediated activation of latent HIV-1 expression. Mol Ther. 2016;24(3):499–507.

28. Saayman SM, Lazar DC, Scott TA, Hart JR, Takahashi M, Burnett JC, Planelles V, Morris KV, Weinberg MS. Potent and targeted activation of latent HIV-1 using the CRISPR/dCas9 activator complex. Mol Ther. 2016;24(3):488–98.

29. Ji H, Jiang Z, Lu P, Ma L, Li C, Pan H, Fu Z, Qu X, Wang P, Deng J, et al. Specific reactivation of latent HIV-1 by dCas9-SunTag-VP64-mediated guide RNA targeting the HIV-1 promoter. Mol Ther. 2016;24(3):508–21.

30. Konermann S, Brigham MD, Trevino AE, Joung J, Abudayyeh OO, Barcena C, Hsu PD, Habib N, Gootenberg JS, Nishimasu H, et al. Genome-scale transcriptional activation by an engineered CRISPR-Cas9 complex. Nature. 2015;517(7536):583–8.

31. Zhang Y, Yin C, Zhang T, Li F, Yang W, Kaminski R, Fagan PR, Putatunda R, Young WB, Khalili K, et al. CRISPR/gRNA-directed synergistic activation mediator (SAM) induces specific, persistent and robust reactivation of the HIV-1 latent reservoirs. Sci Rep. 2015;5:16277.

32. Bogerd HP, Kornepati AV, Marshall JB, Kennedy EM, Cullen BR. Specific induction of endogenous viral restriction factors using CRISPR/Cas-derived transcriptional activators. Proc Natl Acad Sci U S A. 2015;112(52):E7249–56.

33. Liu XS, Wu H, Ji X, Stelzer Y, Wu X, Czauderna S, Shu J, Dadon D, Young RA, Jaenisch R. Editing DNA methylation in the mammalian genome. Cell. 2016;167(1):233–47. e217

34. Choudhury SR, Cui Y, Lubecka K, Stefanska B, Irudayaraj J. CRISPR-dCas9 mediated TET1 targeting for selective DNA demethylation at BRCA1 promoter. Oncotarget. 2016;7:46545–56.

35. McDonald JI, Celik H, Rois LE, Fishberger G, Fowler T, Rees R, Kramer A, Martens A, Edwards JR, Challen GA. Reprogrammable CRISPR/Cas9-based system for inducing site-specific DNA methylation. Biol Open. 2016;5(6):866–74.

36. Kungulovski G, Jeltsch A. Epigenome editing: state of the art, concepts, and perspectives. Trends Genet. 2016;32(2):101–13.

37. Wolt JD, Wang K, Sashital D, Lawrence-Dill CJ. Achieving plant CRISPR targeting that limits off-target effects. Plant Genome. 2016;9(3)

38. Ma J, Koster J, Qin Q, Hu S, Li W, Chen C, Cao Q, Wang J, Mei S, Liu Q, et al. CRISPR-DO for genome-wide CRISPR design and optimization. Bioinformatics. 2016;32(21):3336–8.

39. Chari R, Yeo NC, Chavez A, Church GM. sgRNA scorer 2.0: a species-independent model to predict CRISPR/Cas9 activity. ACS Synth Biol. 2017;6:902–4.

40. Cradick TJ, Qiu P, Lee CM, Fine EJ, Bao G. COSMID: a web-based tool for identifying and validating CRISPR/Cas off-target sites. Mol Ther Nucleic Acids. 2014;3:e214.

41. Wang Y, Liu KI, Sutrisnoh NB, Srinivasan H, Zhang J, Li J, Zhang F, Lalith CRJ, Xing H, Shanmugam R, et al. Systematic evaluation of CRISPR-Cas systems reveals design principles for genome editing in human cells. Genome Biol. 2018;19(1):62.

42. Bae S, Park J, Kim JS. Cas-OFFinder: a fast and versatile algorithm that searches for potential off-target sites of Cas9 RNA-guided endonucleases. Bioinformatics. 2014;30(10):1473–5.

43. Tsai SQ, Joung JK. Defining and improving the genome-wide specificities of CRISPR-Cas9 nucleases. Nat Rev Genet. 2016;17(5):300–12.

44. Zuckermann M, Hovestadt V, Knobbe-Thomsen CB, Zapatka M, Northcott PA, Schramm K, Belic J, Jones DT, Tschida B, Moriarity B, et al. Somatic CRISPR/Cas9-mediated tumour suppressor disruption enables versatile brain tumour modelling. Nat Commun. 2015;6:7391.

45. Smith C, Gore A, Yan W, Abalde-Atristain L, Li Z, He C, Wang Y, Brodsky RA, Zhang K, Cheng L, et al. Whole-genome sequencing analysis reveals high specificity of CRISPR/Cas9 and TALEN-based genome editing in human iPSCs. Cell Stem Cell. 2014;15(1):12–3.

46. Veres A, Gosis BS, Ding Q, Collins R, Ragavendran A, Brand H, Erdin S, Cowan CA, Talkowski ME, Musunuru K. Low incidence of off-target mutations in individual CRISPR-Cas9 and TALEN targeted human stem cell clones detected by whole-genome sequencing. Cell Stem Cell. 2014;15(1):27–30.

47. Yang L, Grishin D, Wang G, Aach J, Zhang CZ, Chari R, Homsy J, Cai X, Zhao Y, Fan JB, et al. Targeted and genome-wide sequencing reveal single nucleotide variations impacting specificity of Cas9 in human stem cells. Nat Commun. 2014;5:5507.

48. Sung K, Park J, Kim Y, Lee NK, Kim SK. Target specificity of Cas9 nuclease via DNA rearrangement regulated by the REC2 domain. J Am Chem Soc. 2018;140:7778–81.

49. Ran FA, Cong L, Yan WX, Scott DA, Gootenberg JS, Kriz AJ, Zetsche B, Shalem O, Wu X, Makarova KS, et al. In vivo genome editing using Staphylococcus aureus Cas9. Nature. 2015;520(7546):186–91.

50. Tsai SQ, Zheng Z, Nguyen NT, Liebers M, Topkar VV, Thapar V, Wyvekens N, Khayter C, Iafrate AJ, Le LP, et al. GUIDE-seq enables genome-wide profiling of off-target cleavage by CRISPR-Cas nucleases. Nat Biotechnol. 2015;33(2):187–97.

51. Frock RL, Hu J, Meyers RM, Ho YJ, Kii E, Alt FW. Genome-wide detection of DNA double-stranded breaks induced by engineered nucleases. Nat Biotechnol. 2015;33(2):179–86.

52. Martin F, Sanchez-Hernandez S, Gutierrez-Guerrero A, Pinedo-Gomez J, Benabdellah K. Biased and unbiased methods for the detection of off-target cleavage by CRISPR/Cas9: an overview. Int J Mol Sci. 2016;17(9):1507.

53. Shi L, Tang X, Tang G. GUIDE-Seq to detect genome-wide double-stranded breaks in plants. Trends Plant Sci. 2016;21(10):815–8.

54. Cho GY, Schaefer KA, Bassuk AG, Tsang SH, Mahajan VB. Crispr Genome Surgery in the Retina in Light of Off-Targeting. Retina. 2018;38:1443–55.

55. Hay EA, Khalaf AR, Marini P, Brown A, Heath K, Sheppard D, MacKenzie A. An analysis of possible off target effects following CAS9/CRISPR targeted deletions of neuropeptide gene enhancers from the mouse genome. Neuropeptides. 2017;64:101–7.

56. Cao J, Wu L, Zhang SM, Lu M, Cheung WK, Cai W, Gale M, Xu Q, Yan Q. An easy and efficient inducible CRISPR/Cas9 platform with improved specificity for multiple gene targeting. Nucleic Acids Res. 2016;44(19):e149.

57. Boyle EA, Andreasson JOL, Chircus LM, Sternberg SH, Wu MJ, Guegler CK, Doudna JA, Greenleaf WJ. High-throughput biochemical profiling reveals sequence determinants of dCas9 off-target binding and unbinding. Proc Natl Acad Sci U S A. 2017;114(21):5461–6.

58. Geonnotti AR, Bilska M, Yuan X, Ochsenbauer C, Edmonds TG, Kappes JC, Liao HX, Haynes BF, Montefiori DC. Differential inhibition of human immunodeficiency virus type 1 in peripheral blood mononuclear cells and TZM-bl cells by endotoxin-mediated chemokine and gamma interferon production. AIDS Res Hum Retrovir. 2010;26(3):279–91.

59. Hui L, Rao WW, Yu Q, Kou C, Wu JQ, He JC, Ye MJ, Liu JH, Xu XJ, Zheng K, et al. TCF4 gene polymorphism is associated with cognition in patients with schizophrenia and healthy controls. J Psychiatr Res. 2015;69:95–101.

60. Brocken DJW, Tark-Dame M, Dame RT. dCas9: a versatile tool for epigenome editing. Curr Issues Mol Biol. 2017;26:15–32.

61. Williams CR, Baccarella A, Parrish JZ, Kim CC. Trimming of sequence reads alters RNA-Seq gene expression estimates. BMC Bioinformatics. 2016;17:103.

62. Bolger AM, Lohse M, Usadel B. Trimmomatic: a flexible trimmer for Illumina sequence data. Bioinformatics. 2014;30(15):2114–20.

63. Kim D, Pertea G, Trapnell C, Pimentel H, Kelley R, Salzberg SL. TopHat2: accurate alignment of transcriptomes in the presence of insertions, deletions and gene fusions. Genome Biol. 2013;14(4):R36.

64. Kong L, Zhang Y, Ye ZQ, Liu XQ, Zhao SQ, Wei L, Gao G. CPC: assess the protein-coding potential of transcripts using sequence features and support vector machine. Nucleic Acids Res. 2007;35(Web Server issue):W345–9.

65. Finn RD, Coggill P, Eberhardt RY, Eddy SR, Mistry J, Mitchell AL, Potter SC, Punta M, Qureshi M, Sangrador-Vegas A, et al. The Pfam protein families database: towards a more sustainable future. Nucleic Acids Res. 2016;44(D1):D279–85.

66. Yap CK, Eisenhaber B, Eisenhaber F, Wong WC. xHMMER3x2: utilizing HMMER3's speed and HMMER2's sensitivity and specificity in the glocal alignment mode for improved large-scale protein domain annotation. Biol Direct. 2016;11(1):63.

67. Trapnell C, Roberts A, Goff L, Pertea G, Kim D, Kelley DR, Pimentel H, Salzberg SL, Rinn JL, Pachter L. Differential gene and transcript expression analysis of RNA-seq experiments with TopHat and cufflinks. Nat Protoc. 2012;7(3):562–78.

68. von Mering C, Jensen LJ, Snel B, Hooper SD, Krupp M, Foglierini M, Jouffre N, Huynen MA, Bork P. STRING: known and predicted protein-protein associations, integrated and transferred across organisms. Nucleic Acids Res. 2005;33(Database issue):D433–7.

69. Li H, Handsaker B, Wysoker A, Fennell T, Ruan J, Homer N, Marth G, Abecasis G, Durbin R. Genome project data processing S: the sequence alignment/map format and SAMtools. Bioinformatics. 2009;25(16):2078–9.

70. McKenna A, Hanna M, Banks E, Sivachenko A, Cibulskis K, Kernytsky A, Garimella K, Altshuler D, Gabriel S, Daly M, et al. The genome analysis toolkit: a MapReduce framework for analyzing next-generation DNA sequencing data. Genome Res. 2010;20(9):1297–303.

71. Florea L, Song L, Salzberg SL. Thousands of exon skipping events differentiate among splicing patterns in sixteen human tissues. F1000Res. 2013;2:188.

72. Katz Y, Wang ET, Airoldi EM, Burge CB. Analysis and design of RNA sequencing experiments for identifying isoform regulation. Nat Methods. 2010;7(12):1009–15.

73. Kang Y, Norris MH, Zarzycki-Siek J, Nierman WC, Donachie SP, Hoang TT. Transcript amplification from single bacterium for transcriptome analysis. Genome Res. 2011;21(6):925–35.

74. Li W, Turner A, Aggarwal P, Matter A, Storvick E, Arnett DK, Broeckel U. Comprehensive evaluation of AmpliSeq transcriptome, a novel targeted whole transcriptome RNA sequencing methodology for global gene expression analysis. BMC Genomics. 2015;16:1069.

75. Steiger JH. Tests for comparing elements of a correlation matrix. Psychol Bull. 1980;87(2):245.

76. Roy B, Haupt LM, Griffiths LR. Review: alternative splicing (AS) of genes as an approach for generating protein complexity. Curr Genomics. 2013;14(3):182–94.

77. Cong L, Ran FA, Cox D, Lin S, Barretto R, Habib N, Hsu PD, Wu X, Jiang W, Marraffini LA, et al. Multiplex genome engineering using CRISPR/Cas systems. Science. 2013;339(6121):819–23.

78. Jinek M, East A, Cheng A, Lin S, Ma E, Doudna J. RNA-programmed genome editing in human cells. Elife. 2013;2:e00471.

79. Jinek M, Chylinski K, Fonfara I, Hauer M, Doudna JA, Charpentier E. A programmable dual-RNA-guided DNA endonuclease in adaptive bacterial immunity. Science. 2012;337(6096):816–21.

80. Havlicek S, Shen Y, Alpagu Y, Bruntraeger MB, Zufir NB, Phuah ZY, Fu Z, Dunn NR, Stanton LW. Re-engineered RNA-guided FokI-nucleases for improved genome editing in human cells. Mol Ther. 2017;25(2):342–55.

81. Kleinstiver BP, Pattanayak V, Prew MS, Tsai SQ, Nguyen NT, Zheng Z, Joung JK. High-fidelity CRISPR-Cas9 nucleases with no detectable genome-wide off-target effects. Nature. 2016;529(7587):490–5.

82. Maggio I, Goncalves MA. Genome editing at the crossroads of delivery, specificity, and fidelity. Trends Biotechnol. 2015;33(5):280–91.

83. Kuscu C, Arslan S, Singh R, Thorpe J, Adli M. Genome-wide analysis reveals characteristics of off-target sites bound by the Cas9 endonuclease. Nat Biotechnol. 2014;32(7):677–83.

84. Kim D, Bae S, Park J, Kim E, Kim S, Yu HR, Hwang J, Kim JI, Kim JS. Digenome-seq: genome-wide profiling of CRISPR-Cas9 off-target effects in human cells. Nat Methods. 2015;12(3):237–43. 231 p following 243

85. Wang X, Wang Y, Wu X, Wang J, Wang Y, Qiu Z, Chang T, Huang H, Lin RJ, Yee JK. Unbiased detection of off-target cleavage by CRISPR-Cas9 and TALENs using integrase-defective lentiviral vectors. Nat Biotechnol. 2015;33(2):175–8.

86. Gaj T, Staahl BT, Rodrigues GM, Limsirichai P, Ekman FK, Doudna JA, Schaffer DV. Targeted gene knock-in by homology-directed genome editing using Cas9 ribonucleoprotein and AAV donor delivery. Nucleic Acids Res. 2017;45:e98.

87. Polstein LR, Perez-Pinera P, Kocak DD, Vockley CM, Bledsoe P, Song L, Safi A, Crawford GE, Reddy TE, Gersbach CA. Genome-wide specificity of DNA binding, gene regulation, and chromatin remodeling by TALE- and CRISPR/Cas9-based transcriptional activators. Genome Res. 2015;25(8):1158–69.

88. Liszczak GP, Brown ZZ, Kim SH, Oslund RC, David Y, Muir TW. Genomic targeting of epigenetic probes using a chemically tailored Cas9 system. Proc Natl Acad Sci U S A. 2017;114(4):681–6.

89. Kim D, Kim J, Hur JK, Been KW, Yoon SH, Kim JS. Genome-wide analysis reveals specificities of Cpf1 endonucleases in human cells. Nat Biotechnol. 2016;34(8):863–8.

90. Kim V, Mears BM, Powell BH, Witwer KW. Mutant Cas9-transcriptional activator activates HIV-1 in U1 cells in the presence and absence of LTR-specific guide RNAs. Matters (Zur). 2017;2017

91. Ran FA, Hsu PD, Lin CY, Gootenberg JS, Konermann S, Trevino AE, Scott DA, Inoue A, Matoba S, Zhang Y, et al. Double nicking by RNA-guided CRISPR Cas9 for enhanced genome editing specificity. Cell. 2013;154(6):1380–9.

92. Hsu PD, Scott DA, Weinstein JA, Ran FA, Konermann S, Agarwala V, Li Y, Fine EJ, Wu X, Shalem O, et al. DNA targeting specificity of RNA-guided Cas9 nucleases. Nat Biotechnol. 2013;31(9):827–32.

93. Wang ET, Sandberg R, Luo S, Khrebtukova I, Zhang L, Mayr C, Kingsmore SF, Schroth GP, Burge CB. Alternative isoform regulation in human tissue transcriptomes. Nature. 2008;456(7221):470–6.

94. Matlin AJ, Clark F, Smith CW. Understanding alternative splicing: towards a cellular code. Nat Rev Mol Cell Biol. 2005;6(5):386–98.

95. Lee JT. Epigenetic regulation by long noncoding RNAs. Science. 2012;338(6113):1435–9.

96. Affymetrix ETP, Cold Spring Harbor laboratory ETP: post-transcriptional processing generates a diversity of 5′-modified long and short RNAs. Nature 2009, 457(7232):1028–1032.

97. Millan MJ. Linking deregulation of non-coding RNA to the core pathophysiology of Alzheimer's disease: an integrative review. Prog Neurobiol. 2017;156:1–68.

98. Matsui M, Corey DR. Non-coding RNAs as drug targets. Nat Rev Drug Discov. 2017;16(3):167–79.

99. Faghihi MA, Modarresi F, Khalil AM, Wood DE, Sahagan BG, Morgan TE, Finch CE, St Laurent G 3rd, Kenny PJ, Wahlestedt C. Expression of a noncoding RNA is elevated in Alzheimer's disease and drives rapid feed-forward regulation of beta-secretase. Nat Med. 2008;14(7):723–30.

100. Ronchetti D, Manzoni M, Agnelli L, Vinci C, Fabris S, Cutrona G, Matis S, Colombo M, Galletti S, Taiana E, et al. lncRNA profiling in early-stage chronic lymphocytic leukemia identifies transcriptional fingerprints with relevance in clinical outcome. Blood Cancer J. 2016;6(9):e468.

101. Malik B, Feng FY. Long noncoding RNAs in prostate cancer: overview and clinical implications. Asian J Androl. 2016;18(4):568–74.

102. Niknafs YS, Han S, Ma T, Speers C, Zhang C, Wilder-Romans K, Iyer MK, Pitchiaya S, Malik R, Hosono Y, et al. The lncRNA landscape of breast cancer reveals a role for DSCAM-AS1 in breast cancer progression. Nat Commun. 2016;7:12791.

103. Fu Y, Foden JA, Khayter C, Maeder ML, Reyon D, Joung JK, Sander JD. High-frequency off-target mutagenesis induced by CRISPR-Cas nucleases in human cells. Nat Biotechnol. 2013;31(9):822–6.

104. Tycko J, Myer VE, Hsu PD. Methods for optimizing CRISPR-Cas9 genome editing specificity. Mol Cell. 2016;63(3):355–70.

105. Kim D, Kim S, Kim S, Park J, Kim JS. Genome-wide target specificities of CRISPR-Cas9 nucleases revealed by multiplex Digenome-seq. Genome Res. 2016;26(3):406–15.

106. Pattanayak V, Lin S, Guilinger JP, Ma E, Doudna JA, Liu DR. High-throughput profiling of off-target DNA cleavage reveals RNA-programmed Cas9 nuclease specificity. Nat Biotechnol. 2013;31(9):839–43.

107. Cho SW, Kim S, Kim Y, Kweon J, Kim HS, Bae S, Kim JS. Analysis of off-target effects of CRISPR/Cas-derived RNA-guided endonucleases and nickases. Genome Res. 2014;24(1):132–41.

108. Darcis G, Van Driessche B, Van Lint C. HIV latency: should we shock or lock? Trends Immunol. 2017;38(3):217–28.

8

Circulating miRNome profiling in Moyamoya disease-discordant monozygotic twins and endothelial microRNA expression analysis using iPS cell line

Haruto Uchino[1†], Masaki Ito[1*†]⬤, Ken Kazumata[1], Yuka Hama[2], Shuji Hamauchi[1], Shunsuke Terasaka[1], Hidenao Sasaki[2] and Kiyohiro Houkin[1]

Abstract

Background: Moyamoya disease (MMD) is characterized by progressive stenosis of intracranial arteries in the circle of Willis with unknown etiology even after the identification of a Moyamoya susceptible gene, RNF213. Recently, differences in epigenetic regulations have been investigated by a case-control study in MMD. Here, we employed a disease discordant monozygotic twin-based study design to unmask potential confounders.

Methods: Circulating genome-wide microRNA (miRNome) profiling was performed in MMD-discordant monozygotic twins, non-twin-MMD patients, and non-MMD healthy volunteers by microarray followed by qPCRvalidation, using blood samples. Differential plasma-microRNAs were further quantified in endothelial cells differentiated from iPS cell lines (iPSECs) derived from another independent non-twin cohort. Lastly, their target gene expression in the iPSECs was analyzed.

Results: Microarray detected 309 plasma-microRNAs in MMD-discordant monozygotic twins that were also detected in the non-twin cohort. Principal component analysis of the plasma-microRNA expression level demonstrated distinct 2 groups separated by MMD and healthy control in the twin- and non-twin cohorts. Of these, differential upregulations of hsa-miR-6722-3p/− 328-3p were validated in the plasma of MMD (absolute log2 expression fold change (logFC) > 0.26 for the twin cohort; absolute logFC > 0.26, $p < 0.05$, and q < 0.15 for the non-twin cohort). In MMD derived iPSECs, hsa-miR-6722-3p/− 328-3p showed a trend of up-regulation with a 3.0- or higher expression fold change. Bioinformatics analysis revealed that 41 target genes of miR-6722-3p/− 328-3p were significantly down-regulated in MMD derived iPSECs and were involved in STAT3, IGF-1-, and PTEN-signaling, suggesting a potential microRNA-gene expression interaction between circulating plasma and endothelial cells.

Conclusions: Our MMD-discordant monozygotic twin-based study confirmed a novel circulating microRNA signature in MMD as a potential diagnostic biomarker minimally confounded by genetic heterogeneity. The novel circulating microRNA signature can contribute for the future functional microRNA analysis to find new diagnostic and therapeutic target of MMD.

Keywords: Circulating microRNA, Moyamoya disease, Discordant monozygotic twins, iPS cells, Endothelial cells

* Correspondence: masakiitou-nsu@umin.ac.jp
†Haruto Uchino and Masaki Ito contributed equally to this work.
[1]Department of Neurosurgery, Hokkaido University Graduate School of Medicine, North 15 West 7, Sapporo 0608638, Japan
Full list of author information is available at the end of the article

Background

Moyamoya disease (MMD) is a rare cerebrovascular disorder with unknown cause, characterized by progressive occlusion of the internal carotid arteries and their main branches in the circle of Willis along with the development of an abnormal collateral network known as "moyamoya vessels" [1]. The predominant histopathological feature of MMD is fibrocellular thickening of the intima and attenuation of the media in the affected arterial wall [2–4]. Emerging next generation studies revealed novel genetic aspects of MMD including disease susceptible polymorphisms across the genome in diverse ethnicities [5–7]. In particular, identification of RNF213 gene as a MMD-susceptible gene provided cutting edge impact on MMD research [8, 9]. Endothelial cell (EC) dysfunction has been demonstrated in vitro using iPS cell lines with an RNF213 gene polymorphism (i.e., rs112735431) [10–12], although the primary histopathological features were not reproduced in the intracranial cerebral arteries of RNF213 knock-out mice or in transgenic mice overexpressing RNF213 [11, 13–15].

Recently, several case-control studies have investigated the association between microRNA and MMD upon a non-twin cohort basis [16–18]. MicroRNAs constitute short non-coding RNAs that negatively regulate gene expression at a post-transcriptional level [19]. As they are stable in the sera/plasma and can regulate multiple genes, circulating microRNAs are expected to represent potential diagnostic and prognostic biomarkers of several diseases including stroke [19–21]. Moreover, epigenetic disease studies can particularly benefit from disease-discordant monozygotic twin study design by controlling many potential confounders such as genetic factors, age, and sex [20].

We, therefore, conducted circulating genome-wide microRNA (miRNome) profiling in cohorts of MMD-discordant monozygotic twins, non-twin MMD cases, and healthy controls to unmask potential confounders from a previously reported microRNA signature in MMD [16, 17]. We further studied endothelial microRNA expression using iPS cell lines of another independent non-twin cohort as an in vitro MMD model. Using a published endothelial transcriptome microarray dataset, which has been studied in the exact same cohort, microRNA-gene expression network was analyzed. Understanding the circulating microRNA signature from a discordant monozygotic twin-based study may be invaluable for providing novel insights toward blood biomarker discovery. Furthermore, insights from plasma and endothelial microRNA expression relationships may contribute to provide a potential therapeutic target of MMD.

Methods

A total of 27 Japanese individuals, including 13 patients with MMD and 14 healthy individuals were included. Two subjects with MMD had participated in previous linkage studies [22, 23]. MMD was diagnosed by magnetic resonance angiography (MRA) or catheter angiography in the Department of Neurosurgery at Hokkaido University Hospital or the referral hospitals between 1987 and 2011 based on the published guideline [24]. Quasi-Moyamoya disease was excluded in this study. We used angiographical stages evaluated according to the MRA stage grading system [25] at the closest timing of blood sampling for analysis. The normal control group consisted of healthy volunteers without any recorded or family history of neurological diseases, including MMD. All normal healthy controls were recruited at the Department of Neurology Hokkaido University Graduate School of Medicine, except for one unaffected MMD-discordant monozygotic twin. In the circulating miRNome microarray study, a pair of MMD-discordant monozygotic twins and a non-twin cohort (nine unrelated subjects with MMD and 10 healthy controls) were included. In the experiment using endothelial cells derived from iPS cell line (iPSECs), another independent non-twin cohort (three patients with MMD and three healthy controls) was recruited, comprising exactly same individuals participated in our previous in vitro iPSEC study [12]. Demographics and clinical features of all study participants were summarized in Table 1.

Detailed methods for blood sample and iPSEC collection/ purification, RNA isolation or extraction from plasma or iPSECs, microRNA expression microarray and quantitative real-time polymerase chain reaction (qPCR) analysis, bioinformatics analysis for microRNA-gene expression network and molecular pathway analysis, as well as statistics were provided in supplementary materials and methods (see Additional file 1: Supplementary materials and methods). In brief, differential plasma-microRNA expression microarray analysis was performed in MMD-discordant twin and in non-twin cohorts, respectively. In MMD-discordant monozygotic twins, a set of differential plasma-microRNAs was identified that exhibited a greater than 0.26-absolute expression log fold change between the affected and non-affected monozygotic twins. In the non-twin cohort, a set of differential plasma-microRNAs was identified that exhibited a greater than 0.26-absolute expression log fold change and a less than 0.05 p-value computed by unpaired t-test corrected by Welch's method between MMD and controls followed by multiple testing correction using Storey's Bootstrapping false discovery rate (FDR) method (q value < 0.15). Raw data of the microarray experiments can be accessed through the National Center for Biotechnology Information Gene Expression Omnibus (NCBI GEO accession number GSE100488).

Results

Circulating miRNome profiling demonstrated distinct 2 groups separated by MMD and healthy control

We recruited a pair of MMD-discordant monozygotic twins with familial occurrence of MMD as shown in Fig. 1a

Table 1 Demographics and clinical features of the study participants

	Age (y)		Sex	Disease type	Disease stage	Familial MMD	EC/IC bypass	Comorbidity	Brain lesion	rs112735431 (RNF213)
	at sampling	at onset								
			Circulating miRNome microarray analysis							
			MMD-Discordant Monozygotic Twins							
Affected Twin	12	3	F	TIA	3	Yes	Yes	No	No	AG
Non-affected Twin	12	–	F	–	–	Yes	–	No	No	AG
			Non-Twin cohort							
MMD, n = 9	49.7 ± 5.4	37.3 ± 7.3	66.7%	All TIA	3	56.0%	100%	11%	67%	All AG
Control, n = 10	51.7 ± 3.6	–	70%	–	–	0%	0%	0%	–	All GG
P-value	0.75		1.0							
			iPSEC-microRNA and gene expression analysis							
MMD, n = 3	41.0 ± 3.6	39.1 ± 4.0	67%	All TIA	3	TIA	67%	33%	0%	All AG
Control, n = 3	50.0 ± 2.0	–	0%	–	–	0%	0%	0%	–	All GG

Disease stage indicates MRA grade of the advanced hemisphere if a difference between hemispheres exists. Comorbidity observed in study participants was hypertension. Age (years) was expressed as the mean ± SEM and Disease stage was expressed as median in the non-twin cohort. *F* female, EC/IC bypass: extracranial-intracranial bypass, *TIA* transient ischemic attack. A: minor and G: major allele for rs112735431 of the *RNF213* gene

to conduct disease-discordant monozygotic twin-based circulating miRNome profiling. Although familial occurrence of MMD comprises approximately 15% of reported cases in Japan, MMD-discordant monozygotic twins are extremely rare [3]. MRAs (Fig. 1b-c) demonstrated bilateral occlusion of ICAs with developed moyamoya vessels in the affected twin (II-3 in the pedigree tree), whereas ICAs of the non-affected twin (II-2) were intact. Genome-wide microRNA expression microarray (SurePrint® G3 Human miRNA microarray (Release 21.0, Agilent)) detected 309 plasma-microRNAs (12.1% of 2549 detectable microRNAs) in this pair of MMD-discordant monozygotic twins. Of these, 151 microRNAs were up-regulated and 36 were down-regulated in the affected compared to the non-affected twin (imposed threshold for expression log2-fold change (logFC); 0.26) (Fig. 1d). The detection rate of plasma-microRNA was higher than that reported in the manufacturer's application note, and comparable with that in a previous publication studying circulating microRNA in MMD using the same microarray platform [16]. The top five up-regulated plasma-microRNAs in the affected twin were hsa-miR-150-5p (logFC: 2.2), hsa-let-7a-5p (logFC: 2.1), hsa-miR-122-5p (logFC: 2.0), hsa-miR-4419b (logFC: 1.7), and hsa-miR-126-3p (logFC: 1.6), whereas the top five down-regulated plasma-microRNAs were hsa-miR-144-3p (logFC: – 2.1), hsa-miR-8073 (logFC: – 1.5), hsa-miR -6741-5p (logFC: – 1.4), hsa-miR-1237-3p (logFC: – 1.1), and hsa-miR-33b-3p (logFC: – 1.0).

Using the same microarray platform, we studied circulating miRNome profiles in nine Japanese patients with MMD and 10 unrelated healthy individuals as a non-twin cohort, identifying 546 plasma-microRNAs with detection call (21.4% of 2549 detectable microRNAs). Because microRNAs detected in the twins were predominantly detected in the non-twin cohort (Fig. 2a), we performed a principal component analysis for the 309 plasma-microRNA level in the discordant twins and the non-twin cohort together (Fig. 2b) and identified distinct 2 clusters. One cluster included the affected monozygotic twin and patients with MMD from the non-twin cohort. The other included non-affected monozygotic twins and healthy controls. Component 2 (Y-axis) was the main component separating MMD and non-MMD control. Top 30 microRNAs with higher absolute PCA scores for each microRNA for the component 2 were listed, showing top 30 plasma microRNAs contributing group segregation between MMD and control (Please see Additional file 2: Table S1). This result suggested that the circulating microRNA expression pattern was associated with MMD even in the MMD-discordant monozygotic twins. Because pediatric monozygotic twins share genetic variants predominantly [20] and many life style environments, differential microRNAs may contribute to the discordance of MMD in the monozygotic twins with fewer confounders relative to a general non-twin based case-control study.

Differential microRNA expression analysis highlighted 17 plasma-microRNAs in MMD

Based on the distinct circulating microRNA profile associated with MMD, we next performed differential microRNA expression analysis between MMD and healthy controls in the MMD-discordant monozygotic twin and non-twin cohorts using microarray dataset. In the MMD-discordant monozygotic twins, we found 187 differential plasma-microRNAs (151 up-regulated and 36 down-regulated in the affected twin; imposed threshold: absolute logFC > 0.26; Fig. 3a), whereas in the non-twin cohort, we found 49 differential plasma-microRNAs (30 up-regulated and 19 down-regulated in MMD; imposed threshold: absolute logFC > 0.26, $p < 0.05$,

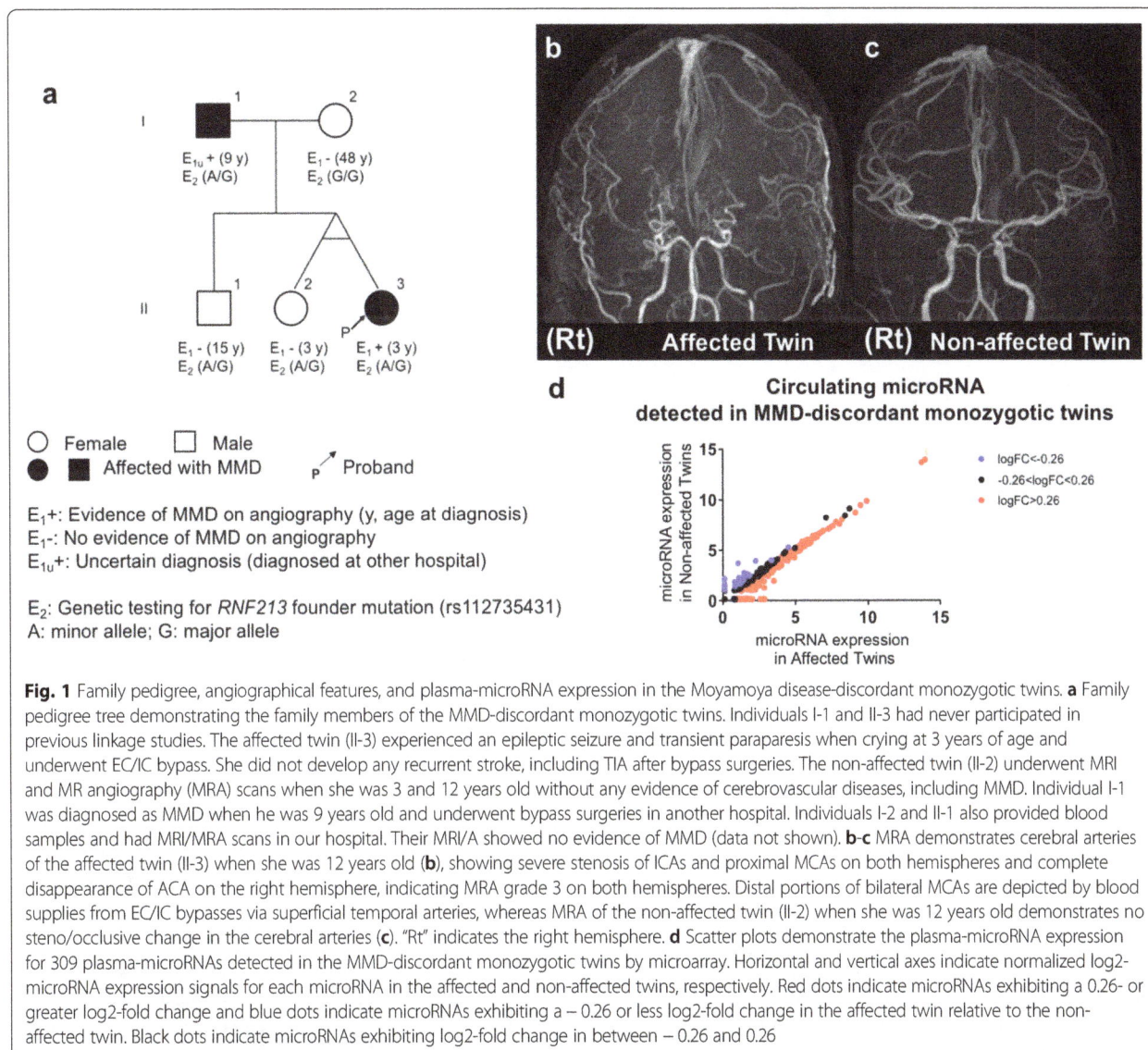

Fig. 1 Family pedigree, angiographical features, and plasma-microRNA expression in the Moyamoya disease-discordant monozygotic twins. **a** Family pedigree tree demonstrating the family members of the MMD-discordant monozygotic twins. Individuals I-1 and II-3 had never participated in previous linkage studies. The affected twin (II-3) experienced an epileptic seizure and transient paraparesis when crying at 3 years of age and underwent EC/IC bypass. She did not develop any recurrent stroke, including TIA after bypass surgeries. The non-affected twin (II-2) underwent MRI and MR angiography (MRA) scans when she was 3 and 12 years old without any evidence of cerebrovascular diseases, including MMD. Individual I-1 was diagnosed as MMD when he was 9 years old and underwent bypass surgeries in another hospital. Individuals I-2 and II-1 also provided blood samples and had MRI/MRA scans in our hospital. Their MRI/A showed no evidence of MMD (data not shown). **b-c** MRA demonstrates cerebral arteries of the affected twin (II-3) when she was 12 years old (**b**), showing severe stenosis of ICAs and proximal MCAs on both hemispheres and complete disappearance of ACA on the right hemisphere, indicating MRA grade 3 on both hemispheres. Distal portions of bilateral MCAs are depicted by blood supplies from EC/IC bypasses via superficial temporal arteries, whereas MRA of the non-affected twin (II-2) when she was 12 years old demonstrates no steno/occlusive change in the cerebral arteries (**c**). "Rt" indicates the right hemisphere. **d** Scatter plots demonstrate the plasma-microRNA expression for 309 plasma-microRNAs detected in the MMD-discordant monozygotic twins by microarray. Horizontal and vertical axes indicate normalized log2-microRNA expression signals for each microRNA in the affected and non-affected twins, respectively. Red dots indicate microRNAs exhibiting a 0.26- or greater log2-fold change and blue dots indicate microRNAs exhibiting a − 0.26 or less log2-fold change in the affected twin relative to the non-affected twin. Black dots indicate microRNAs exhibiting log2-fold change in between − 0.26 and 0.26

$q < 0.15$; Fig. 3b). From these independent sets of differential plasma-microRNAs, we identified 17 plasma-microRNAs that overlapped between the twin and non-twin cohorts. We confirmed that these plasma-microRNAs were consistently up- (12 microRNAs) or down-regulated (five microRNAs) in the affected monozygotic twin and patients with MMD in the non-twin cohort (Table 2). Of note, 12 microRNAs, including hsa-miR-6722-3p, hsa-miR-328, and hsa-miR-150 were found in the top 30 microRNA list correlated with MMD based on the principal component analysis (Please see Additional file 2: Table S1).

A total of 8586 messenger RNAs (mRNAs) were predicted as "target genes" of these 17 differential microRNAs by the IPA® tool and miRmap web interface [26]. We further filtered these 8586 genes and obtained 1069 target gene names according to the IPA knowledge-based disease or function terms, including "Cardiovascular diseases",

"Neurological diseases", and "Vascular physiology" as relevant genes associated with MMD. Table S2 shows the number of target genes for each of the 17 differential microRNAs in detail (see Additional file 3: Table S2).

These 1069-target genes included genes known to be associated with MMD [3, 4, 27], such as RNF213, fibroblast growth factors (FGF2, 7, 14, and 17), hepatocyte growth factor (HGF), platelet derived growth factor B (PDGFB), tumor transforming growth factor beta receptors (TGFBR1 and 2), tumor necrosis factor superfamily member genes (TNFSF4 and 12), and vascular endothelial growth factor A (VEGF A). Notably, hsa-miR-6722-3p can regulate multiple MMD-related genes including RNF213, FGF2 (also known as basic FGF), insulin like growth factor 1 receptor (IGF1R), as well as kinase insert domain receptor (KDR, also known as VEGFR2). Whereas, hsa-328-3p can regulate corticotropin releasing hormone (CRH),

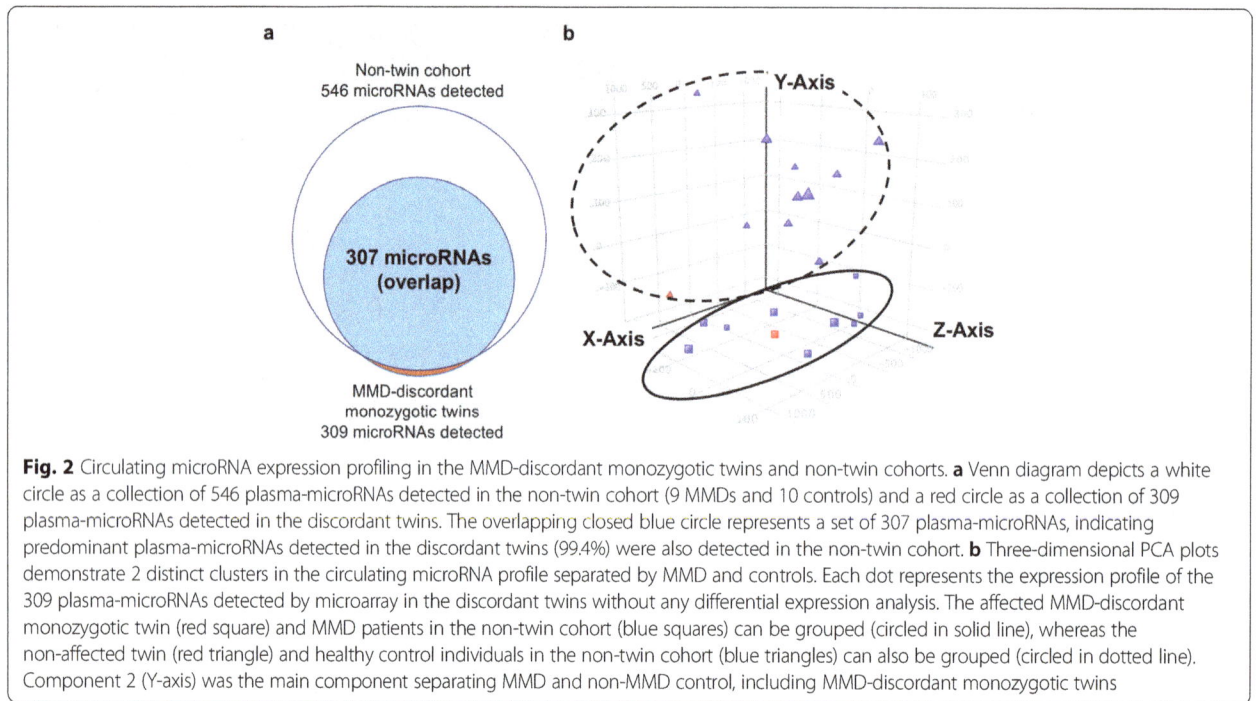

Fig. 2 Circulating microRNA expression profiling in the MMD-discordant monozygotic twins and non-twin cohorts. **a** Venn diagram depicts a white circle as a collection of 546 plasma-microRNAs detected in the non-twin cohort (9 MMDs and 10 controls) and a red circle as a collection of 309 plasma-microRNAs detected in the discordant twins. The overlapping closed blue circle represents a set of 307 plasma-microRNAs, indicating predominant plasma-microRNAs detected in the discordant twins (99.4%) were also detected in the non-twin cohort. **b** Three-dimensional PCA plots demonstrate 2 distinct clusters in the circulating microRNA profile separated by MMD and controls. Each dot represents the expression profile of the 309 plasma-microRNAs detected by microarray in the discordant twins without any differential expression analysis. The affected MMD-discordant monozygotic twin (red square) and MMD patients in the non-twin cohort (blue squares) can be grouped (circled in solid line), whereas the non-affected twin (red triangle) and healthy control individuals in the non-twin cohort (blue triangles) can also be grouped (circled in dotted line). Component 2 (Y-axis) was the main component separating MMD and non-MMD control, including MMD-discordant monozygotic twins

protein kinase, cGMP-dependent type I (PRKG1), progesterone receptor (PGR), and others, which are known to be associated with vascular endothelial cell or smooth muscle cell function.

qPCR verification of hsa-miR-328-3p and − 6722-3p in the plasma and iPSECs

To validate the results from microarray analysis, we performed real-time qPCR for the plasma-microRNAs of interest using a modified $\Delta\Delta CT$ method [28]. Thus, from the 17 differential microRNAs highlighted by the plasma-microRNA microarray analysis (Table 2), we quantified the relative expression level of hsa-miR-150-5p, − 328-3p, − 6722-3p, and − 718 using plasma samples of the non-twin cohort because these microRNAs were more up-regulated in the affected MMD-discordant twins, more significantly up-regulated in patients with MMD in the non-twin cohort, or have target genes relevantly related to MMD (see the rationale for this selection in Additional file 1: Supplementary materials and methods). We confirmed that hsa-miR-150-5p, − 328-3p, and − 6722-3p were significantly up-regulated in the plasma of MMD ($p < 0.05$) (Fig. 4a), which was consistent with the microarray result. Conversely, hsa-miR-718 was not amplified by

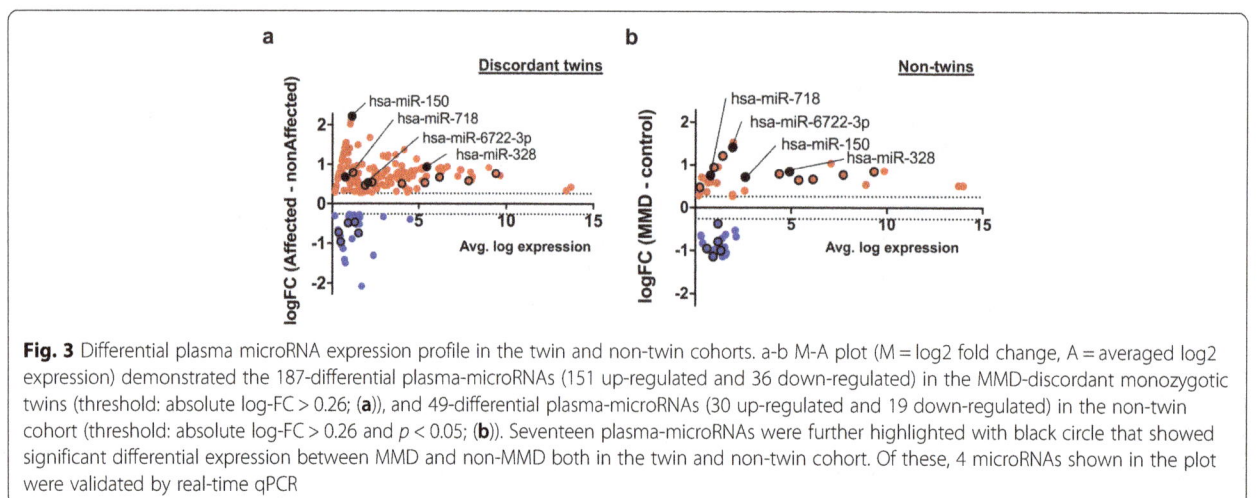

Fig. 3 Differential plasma microRNA expression profile in the twin and non-twin cohorts. a-b M-A plot (M = log2 fold change, A = averaged log2 expression) demonstrated the 187-differential plasma-microRNAs (151 up-regulated and 36 down-regulated) in the MMD-discordant monozygotic twins (threshold: absolute log-FC > 0.26; (**a**)), and 49-differential plasma-microRNAs (30 up-regulated and 19 down-regulated) in the non-twin cohort (threshold: absolute log-FC > 0.26 and $p < 0.05$; (**b**)). Seventeen plasma-microRNAs were further highlighted with black circle that showed significant differential expression between MMD and non-MMD both in the twin and non-twin cohort. Of these, 4 microRNAs shown in the plot were validated by real-time qPCR

Table 2 Differential plasma-microRNAs from discordant monozygotic twin-based study

MicroRNA ID	Discordant twins	Non-twin cohort		
	Log2 fold change	Log2 fold change	p value	q value
hsa-miR-150	2.218	0.714	0.28	0.123
hsa-miR-328	0.931	0.845	0.028	0.123
hsa-miR-3610	0.786	0.475	0.019	0.105
hsa-miR-6089	0.765	0.850	0.005	0.045
hsa-miR-718	0.669	0.749	0.030	0.128
hsa-miR-3665	0.665	0.665	0.023	0.120
hsa-miR-6800-5p	0.576	0.769	0.004	0.042
hsa-miR-762	0.540	1.215	0.009	0.060
hsa-miR-6850-5p	0.528	0.646	0.031	0.128
hsa-miR-6722-3p	0.527	1.415	0.001	0.038
hsa-miR-940	0.503	0.791	0.002	0.038
hsa-miR-4532	0.464	0.940	0.024	0.121
hsa-miR-7845-5p	−0.468	−1.004	0.002	0.038
hsa-miR-623	−0.491	−0.797	0.027	0.123
hsa-miR-595	−0.726	−0.958	0.005	0.045
hsa-miR-6737-3p	−0.746	−0.373	0.000	0.019
hsa-miR-4481	−0.965	−1.136	0.002	0.038

Table listed 17 differential microRNAs that were consistently up- or down-regulated in the affected monozygotic twin and patients with MMD in the non-twin cohort. Log2 fold change indicates relative plasma-microRNA expression level in MMD to control

real-time qPCR presumably due to low abundance in the plasma samples analyzed in this study, which was suggested by lower expression signal in the microarray result (Fig. 3b). Although Fig. 4a indicated that there were 2 types of the miR-328-3p and 150-5p plasma expression pattern (elevated and non-elevated), these 4 elevated samples did not match each other. There was no common trend in these elevated samples.

To investigate the expression levels of these microRNAs in the ECs of MMD, we employed an in vitro MMD-iPSEC

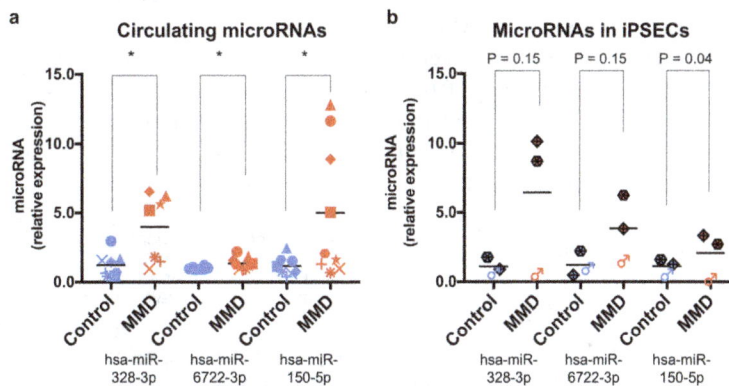

Fig. 4 Quantification of microRNA expression in the plasma and iPSECs. **a** Column scatter graphs demonstrating relative plasma-microRNA expression levels for hsa-miR-328-3p (left), − 6722-3p (middle), and 150-5p (right), quantified by real-time PCR in the non-twin cohort (MMD $n = 9$; red dots, control $n = 8$; blue dots). There was a significant difference in each plasma-microRNA expression level between MMD and control groups (hsa-miR-328-3p, 4.0 ± 0.9 and 1.2 ± 0.3, $p = 0.011$; hsa-miR-6722-3p, 1.4 ± 0.1 and 1.0 ± 0.03, $p = 0.049$, hsa-miR-150-5p, 5.0 ± 1.6 and 1.2 ± 0.2, $p = 0.043$, respectively. *$p < 0.05$). Data represent the mean ± SEM. **b** Column scatter graphs demonstrating relative iPSEC-microRNA expression levels for hsa-miR-328-3p (left), − 6722-3p (middle), and 150-5p (right), quantified by real-time PCR in another non-twin cohort (MMD $n = 3$; red dots, control n = 3; blue dots, please refer to Table 1). There was a trend of difference in the respective hsa-miR-328-3p and − 6722-3p expression levels in iPSECs between MMD and control groups (hsa-miR-328-3p, 6.5 ± 3.0 and 1.1 ± 0.3, $p = 0.15$; hsa-miR-6722-3p, 3.8 ± 1.4 and 1.2 ± 0.5, $p = 0.15$). Conversely, no trend of difference was observed in hsa-miR-150-5p between MMD and control groups (2.1 ± 1.0 and 1.1 ± 0.3, $p = 0.40$, respectively). Data represents as mean ± SEM. Each individual data was plotted by same color and same shape code

model, comprising differentiated and cultured ECs from iPS cell lines derived from another independent non-twin cohort (Table 1). The purity of iPSECs were confirmed by FACS plot (Please see Additional file 4: Figure S1). We found a trend of up-regulation of hsa-miR-328-3p and – 6722-3p in the iPSECs derived from MMD with a 3.0- or higher expression fold change, although it did not reach statistical significance by t-test due to small sample size. Whereas, there was no trend of difference in hsa-miR-150-5p expression level in iPSECs between MMD and the control ($p = 0.40$) (Fig. 4b).

MicroRNA-gene expression network analysis suggests a regulatory role of hsa-miR-328-3p/− 6722-3p involving biological pathways in endothelial cells of MMD

Based on the results from qPCR validations, hsa-miR-328-3p and – 6722-3p were identified as differential microRNAs of MMD, which may be associated with the phenotypic discordance in the MMD-discordant monozygotic twins. As these microRNAs showed a significant upregulation in the plasma in MMD and a trend of differential up-regulation in the MMD-iPSECs, we interrogated the regulatory role of hsa-miR-328-3p/− 6722-3p in their target gene expression. Based on the aforementioned target gene prediction, 327 target genes of hsa-miR-328-3p/− 6722-3p were identified (287 for hsa-miR-6722-3p and 48 for hsa-miR-328-3p) (please see Additional file 3: Table S2). We analyzed an experimentally validated microarray dataset from our previous publication that investigated gene expression profile in the iPSECs derived from the same MMD and healthy control individuals ($n = 3$, respectively, Table 1) as well as differentiated/cultured under identical conditions [12]. Of these 327 target genes, 41 genes (12.5%) were significantly down-regulated (logFC range – 2.0 to – 0.6, $p < 0.05$, $q < 0.15$), and 14 genes (4.3%) were significantly up-regulated (log-FC: range 0.6 to 2.6, $p < 0.05$, $q < 0.15$) in MMD-iPSECs. The gene list was presented in the Additional file 5: Table S3. This result suggested that significant down-regulation of these 41 genes might be associated with epigenetic regulation of the up-regulated hsa-miR-328-3p and – 6722-3p in MMD-iPSECs.

We annotated these 41 down-regulated genes in the MMD-iPSECs using IPA tool. Thus, the least five genes down-regulated in the MMD-iPSECs were ADAM metallopeptidase domain 12 (ADAM12, log-FC: – 2.0), cyclin dependent kinase 6 (CDK6, log-FC: – 2.0), additional sex combs like 3, transcriptional regulator (ASXL3, log-FC: – 1.9), pappalysin 1 (PAPPA, also known as insulin-like growth factor-dependent IGF binding protein-4 protease, log-FC: – 1.8), and RNF213 (log-FC: – 1.6). IPA canonical pathway analysis for these 41 down-regulated genes demonstrated the top three canonical pathways, namely the signal transducer and activator of transcription 3 (STAT3)

pathway, insulin-like growth factor 1 (IGF-1) signaling, and phosphatase and tensin homolog (PTEN) signaling, which are known angiogenesis and vascular homeostasis-related pathways (Fig. 5). In addition, these genes were also involved in autophagy, extracellular signal regulated kinase 5 (ERK5) signaling, phagosome maturation, and the inflammasome pathway, which comprise inflammation or infection-related signaling pathways.

Discussion

We conducted circulating genome-wide microRNA profiling in MMD using a disease-discordant monozygotic twins-based design to discover a less confounded microRNA signature. Result was validated in an independent non-twin MMD cohort. Thus, our strategy could reduce the effect of many possible confounders (i.e., genetic heterogeneity) affecting the findings from a general non-twin-based case-control study. We observed that plasma-microRNA expression profiling could clearly separate MMD and healthy control in the MMD-discordant monozygotic twin- and the non-twin cohort. From differential microRNA expression analysis between MMD and controls, a novel 17 differential plasma-microRNAs signature was identified, since 16 of these plasma-microRNAs have not been reported in the previous exploratory study for circulating microRNA signature in MMD using non-twin based study design [16, 17]. We have successfully validated differential upregulation of hsa-miR-6722-3p/− 328-3p/− 150-5p in the plasma of MMD patients. We also found a trend of upregulation of hsa-miR-6722-3p/− 328-3p in MMD-iPSECs. Furthermore, some of their predicted target genes were significantly downregulated in MMD-iPSECs, suggesting a role of epigenetic regulation of circulating

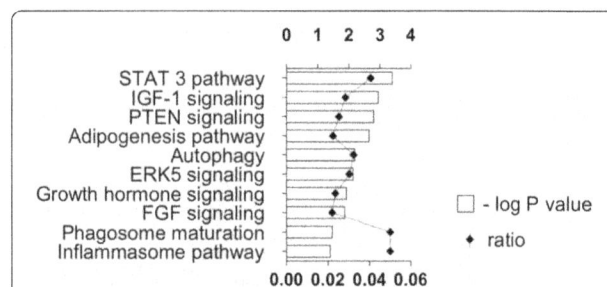

Fig. 5 Top 10 canonical pathways involved by the 41 significantly down-regulated genes in MMD-iPSECs. Graph showing the top 10 canonical pathways from IPA® pathway analysis involved by the 41 significantly down-regulated genes in MMD-iPSECs that were predicted as target genes of significantly up-regulated hsa-miR-328-3p and – 6722-3p in MMD-iPSECs. The ratio expresses the number of differentially down-regulated genes in our dataset over the total number of genes in each canonical pathway based on the IPA knowledge database (represented in the lower X axis). P values for the significance of each pathway were computed based on the number of genes involved in the pathway by using Fisher's exact test, and negatively log10 transformed (represented in the upper X axis)

microRNA in endothelial cells in MMD. This is the first observation of possible microRNA-gene expression network between the plasma and endothelial cells in MMD.

Circulating microRNA signature in MMD in comparison with that from a previous non-twin-based case-control study

Dai et al. first reported 94 differential circulating micro-RNAs in Chinese Han MMD compared to ethnicity-matched normal controls [16] using the same microarray platform. Zhao et al. next specifically analyzed serum microRNA let-7 family expression in the sera of MMD as a regulator of the RNF213 gene [17]. Because both studies employed a general non-twin-based study design and found circulating microRNA signatures as candidates for blood biomarkers in MMD, we considered that our MMD-discordant monozygotic twin-based design could provide additional insights to their findings. In particular, the MMD-discordant monozygotic twins that participated in the present study shared age, sex, ethnicity, and an RNF213 founder mutation polymorphism (rs112735431). Moreover, the affected twin was clinically stable without recurrent transient ischemic attack (TIA), recent surgery (approximately 9 years prior to blood sampling), or ischemic parenchymal lesion. Therefore, the distinct circulating microRNA profile detected in the discordant twins could likely explain the phenotypic discordance between MMD and non-MMD with minimal confounders. Notably, our group and Dai et al. both demonstrated that hsa-miR-595 constituted a differentially down-regulated plasma-microRNA in MMD [16]. Future study to analyze the functional role of hsa-miR-595 in MMD with different subsets of Asian ethnicity may provide important insights to understand the epigenetic aspects of MMD. However, we also identified numerous discrepancies in the results of circulating microRNA signature in MMD between the two publications. Several possible reasons for this discrepancy exist in addition to the difference in study design. First, the plasma sample processing for the array experiment fundamentally differed between studies. Dai et al. pooled plasma samples from 10 individuals with MMD and controls and undertook two microarray experiments for the two plasma pools, whereas we performed microarray experiments using 21 individual (non-pooled) samples. This difference might affect the cluster analysis used to detect the difference of microRNA profile between MMD and control. Second, the imposed threshold to determine differential microRNA in MMD is different. Third, the subgroup of ethnicity in study participants was also different (Japanese or Chinese-Han). As some differences have been observed in the genetic and epidemiological features of MMD in Chinese Han and Japanese or Korean patients [29], this may result in a difference in the circulating microRNA signature. Future work expanding the study population

toward non-Asian MMD would also be invaluable to address the inter-ethnic difference/variability of clinical MMD phenotype [30].

Plasma and iPSEC microRNA expression and gene regulation in MMD

The differential up-regulation of hsa-mir-6722-3p and −328-3p in the plasma of MMD was validated in this study. As well, there was a trend of elevated expression of those microRNAs in the iPSECs (3.0- or higher fold change in MMD compared to healthy control), suggesting possible association in the microRNA expression between circulating plasma and endothelial cells in MMD. Although the functional role of circulating microRNAs is often unclear, they are considered to be secreted actively from cells and involved in inter-cellular communications [31]. From the target gene analysis, a set of 41 genes was confirmed as targets of the up-regulated hsa-mir-6722-3p and − 328-3p in MMD-iPSECs and these genes were further experimentally demonstrated to exhibit significant down-regulation in MMD-iPSECs from the same host with exactly the same differentiation/cultural conditions from our previous publication [12]. The molecular types of the 41 gene products include enzyme (i.e., RNF213), growth factor (i.e., FGF), ion channel, kinase, peptidase, phosphatase, transcription regulator (i.e., STAT3), transmembrane receptor (i.e., IGF1R), and transporter (see Additional file 5: Table S3). IPA canonical pathway analysis revealed that these 41 down-regulated genes were involved in angiogenesis, vascular homeostasis-related signaling/pathways (STAT-3 pathway, IGF-1 signaling, and PTEN signaling), or inflammatory-related biological pathways (ERK signaling, inflammasome pathway). These facts suggest a possible plasma microRNA-endothelial gene expression network as an epigenetic regulation of endothelial biological function of MMD. For example, endothelial STAT3 plays a key role in angiogenesis and extracellular matrix remodeling [32]. IGF-1 has been shown to protect vascular function by promoting nitric oxide production from the endothelium and vascular smooth muscle cells [33]. PTEN plays critical roles for vascular homeostasis by regulating signals via multiple vascular growth factors and responses to shear stress via integrins [34, 35]. Taken together, these 41 down-regulated genes in MMD-iPSECs may play a role in endothelial biological functions via the microRNA-gene expression network in MMD. In addition, these 41 genes were also suggested to be involved in other inflammatory-related pathways. A recent study reported that pro-inflammatory cytokines activated the transcription of RNF213, the product of which plays a role in ECs for proper gene expression in response to inflammatory signals from environments [36]. Our data thus provide additional insights into the potential network of RNF213 gene expression regulation via up-regulated hsa-miR-6722-3p/− 328-3p in MMD.

There are several limitations in this study. First, the sample size was small and limited to the Japanese population. Second, this cross-sectional study sampled plasma at a single time point after development of MMD. Third, the disease type of MMD was limited to TIA-type MMD. Fourth, the differentially expressed plasma-microRNAs in MMD that have not been validated by qPCR should be quantified to verify the microarray result, since we have set less stringent cutoff calling to determine differential plasma-microRNAs in the microarray experiment. Finally, functional validation of the differential plasma-microRNAs was lacking not only in the iPSECs but in other cell types, including vascular smooth muscle cells and circulating immune cells (i.e., monocytes, T lymphocytes, and vascular progenitor cells). Addressing these limitations would be invaluable to consolidate the circulating microRNA signature as a blood biomarker in MMD and potentially uncover disease etiology. Although there are many challenges in the clinical trial designs for rare diseases [37], we think it is necessary to conduct a validation study of the present study with the adequate sample size calculation in an independent cohort.

Conclusions

This study demonstrated a distinct circulating microRNA expression profile in MMD through a unique MMD-discordant monozygotic twin-based study design. A plasma-microRNA dataset presented in this study can provide a seed to discover blood biomarker for MMD with minimal possible confounders. Furthermore, to our knowledge, this is the first study showing that the microRNA-gene expression network may play a role in epigenetic regulation of endothelial function via angiogenesis, vascular homeostasis, and inflammatory-related pathways as a potential therapeutic target for MMD.

Additional files

Additional file 1: Supplementary Materials and Methods. Details supporting the main methods in the manuscript body are provided necessary to comprehend the results.

Additional file 2: Table S1. A list of microRNAs with respective top 15 and least 15 PCA scores. A list of microRNAs with respective top 15 and least 15 PCA scores (correlation value) for each microRNA for the component 2 (Y-axis) were provided, which separated MMD and control, based on the principal component analysis for the 309 plasma-microRNAs (Please see Fig. 2b).

Additional file 3: Table S2. Number of filtered target genes and target gene symbols for each of 17 differential circulating microRNAs in MMD, predicted by microRNA Target Filter implemented in IPA® (QIAGEN) and the miRmap web interface. The target genes were filtered based on their biological function analyzed using "Bioprofiler" implemented in IPA® (QIAGEN). As there is some overlap across microRNAs with respect to their target genes, so the total number of target genes at the bottom of the list is not a simple summation of each number of target genes.

Additional file 4: Figure S1. FACS plot to confirm the purity of iPSECs. The purity of the iPSECs after 5–6 times passages was confirmed as high as 91–97% in all clones using anti-CD31 antibody with the FACS.

Additional file 5: Table S3. The 41 target genes of hsa-miR-6722-3p/ 328-3p that were significantly down-regulated in MMD-iPSECs. Expression log2 fold change (log2 FC), p-value, and q-value were obtained from our previous publication (Hamauchi et al. 2016 [12]). Molecule type for each gene was obtained from the IPA tool.

Abbreviations

CRH: corticotropin releasing hormone; FGF: fibroblast growth factor; HGF: hepatocyte growth factor; IGF1R: insulin like growth factor 1 receptor; iPSECs: endothelial cells differentiated from iPS cell line; KDR: kinase insert domain receptor; logFC: log2-fold change; miRNome: Circulating genome-wide microRNA; MMD: Moyamoya diease; MRA: magnetic resonance angiography; mRNA: messenger RNA; PDGFB: platelet derived growth factor beta; qPCR: quantitative polymerase chain reaction; TGFBR: tumor transforming growth factor beta receptor; TNFSF: tumor necrosis factor superfamily member genes; VEGFA: vascular endothelial growth factor A; PRKG1: protein kinase, cGMP-dependent type I; PGR: progesterone receptor; ADAM12: ADAM metallopeptidase domain 12; CDK6: cyclin dependent kinase 6; ASXL3: additional sex combs like 3 transcriptional regulator; PAPP A: pappalysin 1; STAT3: signal transducer and activator of transcription 3; IGF-1: insulin-like growth factor 1; PTEN: phosphatase and tensin homolog; ERK5: extracellular signal regulated kinase 5; TIA: transient ischemic attack

Acknowledgements

The authors are grateful to patients and their families for their participation in this study. We express appreciation to all the doctors and secretaries for their patient recruitment, treatment, technical, and/or clerical assistance. We also express appreciation to Dr. Michelle Y Cheng, Ph.D. (Department of Neurosurgery, Stanford University School of Medicine) for the technical support for English writing and critical comment to the manuscript. We are also thankful to Dr. Izumi Yanatori, Ph.D. for the critical comments regarding the manuscript (Department of Biochemistry, Stanford University School of Medicine). We also would like to thank Editage (www.editage.jp) for English language editing service.

Funding

This work was supported in part by a grant from the Japanese Ministry of Health, Labor and Welfare for the project of the Research Committee on Spontaneous Occlusion of the Circle of Willis (Moyamoya disease), the Mihara award (2012) from Charitable Trust Mihara Cerebrovascular Disorder Research Promotion Fund (to K.H), and a research grant (2014) from SENSHIN Medical Research Foundation (to K.H).

Authors' contributions

HU performed experiments, analyzed data including completion of the statistical analysis, discussed results, drafted the manuscript and revised the original manuscript. MI designed research, acquired clinical information, assisted in experiments, analyzed data including completion of the statistical analysis, discussed results, listed affiliations, drafted the manuscript and revised the original manuscript. KK treated patients, acquired clinical information, and discussed results. YH assisted in experiments and discussed results. SH assisted in experiments and discussed results. ST assisted in linkable anonymizing and discussed results. HS supervised research, recruited normal healthy control volunteers, and discussed results. KH designed and supervised research, treated patients, acquired clinical information, and discussed results. All authors have read and approved this manuscript.

Competing interests

HU, YH, ST, HS: Nothing to report relating to this study. MI received research fellowship from SENSHIN Medical Research Foundation fellowship for research abroad (2015). SH received a grant funded by Grant-in-Aid for Scientific Research (Grant Number 17 K1662007). KK received a grant funded by Grant-in-Aid for Scientific Research (Grant Number JP15K1028605) and research support from Nihon Medi-Physics Co., Ltd. KH serves on the executive editorial board of Neurologia Medico-Chirurgica and the editorial board of the Journal of Stroke & Cerebrovascular Diseases.

Author details

[1]Department of Neurosurgery, Hokkaido University Graduate School of Medicine, North 15 West 7, Sapporo 0608638, Japan. [2]Department of Neurology, Hokkaido University Graduate School of Medicine, Sapporo, Japan.

References

1. Suzuki J, Takaku A. Cerebrovascular "moyamoya" disease. Disease showing abnormal net-like vessels in base of brain. Arch Neurol. 1969;20:288–99.
2. Masuda J, Ogata J, Yutani C. Smooth muscle cell proliferation and localization of macrophages and T cells in the occlusive intracranial major arteries in moyamoya disease. Stroke. 1993;24:1960–7.
3. Kuroda S, Houkin K. Moyamoya disease: current concepts and future perspectives. Lancet Neurol. 2008;7:1056–66.
4. Houkin K, Ito M, Sugiyama T, Shichinohe H, Nakayama N, Kazumata K, et al. Review of past research and current concepts on the etiology of moyamoya disease. Neurol Med Chir (Tokyo). 2012;52:267–77.
5. Shoemaker LD, Clark MJ, Patwardhan A, Chandratillake G, Garcia S, Chen R, et al. Disease Variant Landscape of a Large Multiethnic Population of Moyamoya Patients by Exome Sequencing. G3 Genes|Genomes|Genetics. 2016;6:41–9.
6. Mukawa M, Nariai T, Onda H, Yoneyama T, Aihara Y, Hirota K, et al. Exome sequencing identified CCER2 as a novel candidate gene for Moyamoya disease. J Stroke Cerebrovasc Dis. 2017;26:150–61.
7. Cecchi AC, Guo D, Ren Z, Flynn K, Santos-Cortez RLP, Leal SM, et al. RNF213 rare variants in an ethnically diverse population with Moyamoya disease. Stroke. 2014;45:3200–7.
8. Kamada F, Aoki Y, Narisawa A, Abe Y, Komatsuzaki S, Kikuchi A, et al. A genome-wide association study identifies RNF213 as the first Moyamoya disease gene. J Hum Genet. 2011;56:34–40.
9. Liu W, Morito D, Takashima S, Mineharu Y, Kobayashi H, Hitomi T, et al. Identification of RNF213 as a susceptibility gene for Moyamoya disease and its possible role in vascular development. PLoS One. 2011;6:e22542.
10. Hitomi T, Habu T, Kobayashi H, Okuda H, Harada KH, Osafune K, et al. Downregulation of Securin by the variant RNF213 R4810K (rs112735431, G>A) reduces angiogenic activity of induced pluripotent stem cell-derived vascular endothelial cells from moyamoya patients. Biochem Biophys Res Commun. 2013;438:13–9.
11. Kobayashi H, Matsuda Y, Hitomi T, Okuda H, Shioi H, Matsuda T, et al. Biochemical and functional characterization of RNF213 (Mysterin) R4810K, a susceptibility mutation of Moyamoya disease, in angiogenesis in vitro and in vivo. J Am Heart Assoc. 2015;4:e002146.
12. Hamauchi S, Shichinohe H, Uchino H, Yamaguchi S, Nakayama N, Kazumata K, et al. Cellular functions and gene and Protein expression profiles in endothelial cells derived from Moyamoya disease-specific iPS cells. PLoS One. 2016;11:e0163561.
13. Sonobe S, Fujimura M, Niizuma K, Nishijima Y, Ito A, Shimizu H, et al. Temporal profile of the vascular anatomy evaluated by 9.4-T magnetic resonance angiography and histopathological analysis in mice lacking RNF213: a susceptibility gene for moyamoya disease. Brain Res. 2014;1552: 64–71.
14. Ito A, Fujimura M, Niizuma K, Kanoke A, Sakata H, Morita-Fujimura Y, et al. Enhanced post-ischemic angiogenesis in mice lacking RNF213; a susceptibility gene for moyamoya disease. Brain Res. 2015;1594:310–20.
15. Sonobe S, Fujimura M, Niizuma K, Fujimura T, Furudate S, Nishijima Y, et al. Increased vascular MMP-9 in mice lacking RNF213. Neuroreport. 2014;25:1442–6.
16. Dai D, Lu Q, Huang Q, Yang P, Hong B, Xu Y, et al. Serum miRNA signature in Moyamoya disease. PLoS One. 2014;9:e102382.

17. Zhao S, Gong Z, Zhang J, Xu X, Liu P, Guan W, et al. Elevated serum MicroRNA let-7c in Moyamoya disease. J Stroke Cerebrovasc Dis. 2015;24:1709–14.
18. Park YS, Jeon YJ, Lee BE, Kim TG, Choi J-U, Kim D-S, et al. Association of the miR-146aC>G, miR-196a2C>T, and miR-499A>G polymorphisms with moyamoya disease in the Korean population. Neurosci Lett. 2012;521:71–5.
19. Uhlmann S, Mracsko E, Javidi E, Lamble S, Teixeira A, Hotz-Wagenblatt A, et al. Genome-wide analysis of the circulating miRNome after cerebral ischemia reveals a reperfusion-induced MicroRNA cluster. Stroke. 2017;48:762–9.
20. Castillo-Fernandez JE, Spector TD, Bell JT. Epigenetics of discordant monozygotic twins: implications for disease. Genome Med. 2014;6:60.
21. Mitchell PS, Parkin RK, Kroh EM, Fritz BR, Wyman SK, Pogosova-Agadjanyan EL, et al. Circulating microRNAs as stable blood-based markers for cancer detection. Proc Natl Acad Sci U S A. 2008;105:10513–8.
22. Yamauchi T, Tada M, Houkin K, Tanaka T, Nakamura Y, Kuroda S, et al. Linkage of familial moyamoya disease (spontaneous occlusion of the circle of Willis) to chromosome 17q25. Stroke. 2000;31:930–5.
23. Mineharu Y, Liu W, Inoue K, Matsuura N, Inoue S, Takenaka K, et al. Autosomal dominant moyamoya disease maps to chromosome 17q25.3. Neurology. 2008;70(Issue 24, Part 2):2357–63.
24. Research Committee on the Pathology and Treatment of Spontaneous Occlusion of the Circle of Willis, Health Labour Sciences Research Grant for Research on Measures for Infractable Diseases. Guidelines for diagnosis and treatment of moyamoya disease (spontaneous occlusion of the circle of Willis). Neurol medico-chirurgica. 2012;52:245–66.
25. Houkin K, Nakayama N, Kuroda S, Nonaka T, Shonai T, Yoshimoto T. Novel magnetic resonance angiography stage grading for Moyamoya disease. Cerebrovasc Dis. 2005;20:347–54.
26. Vejnar CE, Zdobnov EM. miRmap: comprehensive prediction of microRNA target repression strength. Nucleic Acids Res. 2012;40:11673–83.
27. Hamauchi S, Shichinohe H, Houkin K. Review of past and present research on experimental models of moyamoya disease. Brain Circ. 2015;1:88.
28. Pfaffl MW. A new mathematical model for relative quantification in real-time RT-PCR. Nucleic Acids Res. 2001;29:e45.
29. Kleinloog R, Regli L, Rinkel GJE, Klijn CJM. Regional differences in incidence and patient characteristics of moyamoya disease: a systematic review. J Neurol Neurosurg Psychiatry. 2012;83:531–6.
30. Hori S, Kashiwazaki D, Yamamoto S, Acker G, Czabanka M, Akioka N, et al. Impact of interethnic difference of collateral Angioarchitectures on prevalence of hemorrhagic stroke in Moyamoya disease. Neurosurgery. 2018; https://doi.org/10.1093/neuros/nyy236.
31. Finn NA, Searles CD. Intracellular and extracellular miRNAs in regulation of angiogenesis signaling. Curr Angiogenes. 2012;4:299–307.
32. Hoffmann CJ, Harms U, Rex A, Szulzewsky F, Wolf SA, Grittner U, et al. Vascular signal transducer and activator of transcription-3 promotes angiogenesis and neuroplasticity long-term after stroke. Circulation. 2015;131:1772–82.
33. Saber H, Himali JJ, Beiser AS, Shoamanesh A, Pikula A, Roubenoff R, et al. Serum insulin-like growth factor 1 and the risk of ischemic stroke: the Framingham study. Stroke. 2017;48:1760–5.
34. Koide M, Ikeda K, Akakabe Y, Kitamura Y, Ueyama T, Matoba S, et al. Apoptosis regulator through modulating IAP expression (ARIA) controls the PI3K/Akt pathway in endothelial and endothelial progenitor cells. Proc Natl Acad Sci. 2011;108:9472–7.
35. Hamada K, Sasaki T, Koni PA, Natsui M, Kishimoto H, Sasaki J, et al. The PTEN/PI3K pathway governs normal vascular development and tumor angiogenesis. Genes Dev. 2005;19:2054–65.
36. Ohkubo K, Sakai Y, Inoue H, Akamine S, Ishizaki Y, Matsushita Y, et al. Moyamoya disease susceptibility gene RNF213 links inflammatory and angiogenic signals in endothelial cells. Sci Rep. 2015;5:13191.
37. Bogaerts J, Sydes MR, Keat N, McConnell A, Benson A, Ho A, et al. Clinical trial designs for rare diseases: studies developed and discussed by the international rare cancers initiative. Eur J Cancer. 2015;51:271–81.

9

Whole exome sequencing in adult-onset hearing loss reveals a high load of predicted pathogenic variants in known deafness-associated genes and identifies new candidate genes

Morag A. Lewis[1,2], Lisa S. Nolan[3], Barbara A. Cadge[3], Lois J. Matthews[4], Bradley A. Schulte[4], Judy R. Dubno[4], Karen P. Steel[1,2†] and Sally J. Dawson[3*† ⓘ]

Abstract

Background: Deafness is a highly heterogenous disorder with over 100 genes known to underlie human non-syndromic hearing impairment. However, many more remain undiscovered, particularly those involved in the most common form of deafness: adult-onset progressive hearing loss. Despite several genome-wide association studies of adult hearing status, it remains unclear whether the genetic architecture of this common sensory loss consists of multiple rare variants each with large effect size or many common susceptibility variants each with small to medium effects. As next generation sequencing is now being utilised in clinical diagnosis, our aim was to explore the viability of diagnosing the genetic cause of hearing loss using whole exome sequencing in individual subjects as in a clinical setting.

Methods: We performed exome sequencing of thirty patients selected for distinct phenotypic sub-types from well-characterised cohorts of 1479 people with adult-onset hearing loss.

Results: Every individual carried predicted pathogenic variants in at least ten deafness-associated genes; similar findings were obtained from an analysis of the 1000 Genomes Project data unselected for hearing status. We have identified putative causal variants in known deafness genes and several novel candidate genes, including *NEDD4* and *NEFH* that were mutated in multiple individuals.

Conclusions: The high frequency of predicted-pathogenic variants detected in known deafness-associated genes was unexpected and has significant implications for current diagnostic sequencing in deafness. Our findings suggest that in a clinic setting, efforts should be made to a) confirm key sequence results by Sanger sequencing, b) assess segregations of variants and phenotypes within the family if at all possible, and c) use caution in applying current pathogenicity prediction algorithms for diagnostic purposes. We conclude that there may be a high number of pathogenic variants affecting hearing in the ageing population, including many in known deafness-associated genes. Our findings of frequent predicted-pathogenic variants in both our hearing-impaired sample and in the larger 1000 Genomes Project sample unselected for auditory function suggests that the reference population for interpreting variants for this very common disorder should be a population of people with good hearing for their age rather than an unselected population.

Keywords: Hearing loss, Whole exome sequencing, Deafness

* Correspondence: sally.dawson@ucl.ac.uk
†Karen P. Steel and Sally J. Dawson contributed equally to this work.
[3]UCL Ear Institute, University College London, WC1X 8EE, London, UK
Full list of author information is available at the end of the article

Background

Hearing loss is one of the most common sensory deficits in the human population, and it has a strong genetic component [1]. However, although more than 140 human non-syndromic hearing impairment loci have been mapped and over 100 genes identified, most underlie childhood deafness or early-onset hearing loss. The vast majority of genes involved in hearing remain unknown, including those associated with adult-onset, age-related progressive hearing loss. Age-related hearing loss (ARHL) affects 1 in 3 people over the age of sixty, often leading to social isolation and depression, is associated with subsequent cognitive decline [2–4] and a predictor of dementia [5]. The heritability of ARHL has been estimated to be between 30 and 50%, similar to other common complex disorders [1, 6, 7].

Although several ARHL genome-wide association studies (GWAS) have been carried out [8–11] and promising candidate genes identified, such as *SIK3* and *ESRRG* [10, 11], only five loci have been associated with hearing status at the genome-wide significance level: *GRM7* [12], *PCDH20* and *SLC28A3* [13], and *ISG20* or *ACAN* and *TRIOBP* [14]. Furthermore, single genes can underlie progressive hearing loss with post-lingual onset, including in middle-age, particularly genes underlying dominantly-inherited deafness [15, 16]. Thus, adult-onset hearing loss may result from either rare Mendelian gene variants with large effect size or multiple variants each making a small contribution to hearing loss. It is also unclear whether these variants are in novel genes involved in maintenance of auditory pathways or whether they are milder variants of the same genes that are mutated in congenital deafness.

Here, we have taken a more in-depth approach than GWAS, using whole-exome sequencing (WES) to study thirty patients carefully selected from a total sample of 1479 patients with a variety of adult-onset hearing loss phenotypes to represent the mixed phenotypes and varied genetic aetiology that might be present in a clinical scenario, targeting specific sub-phenotypes to maximise power to detect shared variants. Our aim was to establish to what extent exome sequencing is an effective and appropriate tool for genetic diagnosis of hearing loss in a clinic setting, where there is usually only a single adult patient involved and family members are not available for segregation analysis. Whole exome and genome sequencing are beginning to be used in this scenario for diagnosis of adult-onset hearing loss with the clinician faced with challenges in evaluating the candidate variants identified. Our results demonstrate the value of targeting well-characterised phenotypic subtypes and cross-species data comparison in exome sequencing analysis, and highlight issues which need to be considered in interpreting genetic variants of unknown pathogenicity in current genetic diagnosis and gene discovery

studies, in particular the finding that many individuals have multiple predicted-pathogenic variants in different genes known to underlie deafness.

Methods

Recruitment of patients

Twenty patients (seven males, thirteen females) with non-syndromic sensorineural adult-onset hearing loss (self-reported age of onset between 20 and 50) were selected from a larger group of 700 patients recruited from the adult hearing aid clinic at the Royal National Throat Nose and Ear Hospital, London, U.K. (described in [17]). The twenty were chosen based on a family history of hearing loss and an age of onset in middle age. Air and bone conduction thresholds at 0.25, 0.5, 1, 2, 4 and 8 kHz and 0.5, 1, 2 and 4 kHz, respectively were measured with masking as indicated according to BSA Recommended Procedures [18] (Additional file 1: Figs. S1, and Additional file 2: Figs. S2). Ethical approval for this project was granted from the Royal Free Local Research Ethics Committee (reference 6202).

A second group of 10 older individuals were selected from the 779 people in the database of the longitudinal study of ARHL being conducted at the Medical University of South Carolina (MUSC) since 1987 (described in [19]). These individuals were selected for the current analyses on the basis of age (> 60 and < 79 years), negative or limited self-reported occupational and recreational noise history, available DNA samples, and audiometric phenotype (five metabolic: 4 females, 1 male; mean age 69.8 years and five sensory: 2 females, 3 males; mean age 68.3 years) (Additional file 3: Fig. S3). The protocols for this study were approved by the Institutional Review Board at MUSC.

All patients were recruited by written informed consent.

Exome sequencing

DNA was submitted for WES using either the Agilent SureSelect Human All Exon V3 kit or a custom library designed by Agilent for human whole exome sequence capture (which predates the SureSelect kit). Sequencing was carried out on either the Illumina Genome Analyzer IIx or Illumina HiSeq 2000 platform as paired-end 54 bp, 75 bp or 76 bp reads according to the manufacturer's protocol.

The data were filtered on quality, Minor Allele Frequency (MAF) in the ExAC non-Finnish European population [20], most severe consequence and predicted pathogenicity using the pipeline shown in Fig. 1 (Fig. 1, Additional file 4: Table S1). Where no data were recorded in ExAC but a MAF was available from the 1000 Genomes European population [21], e.g. for rs1813100, this was used. The impact of filtering on variant number is shown in Additional file 5: Fig. S4. Following filtering,

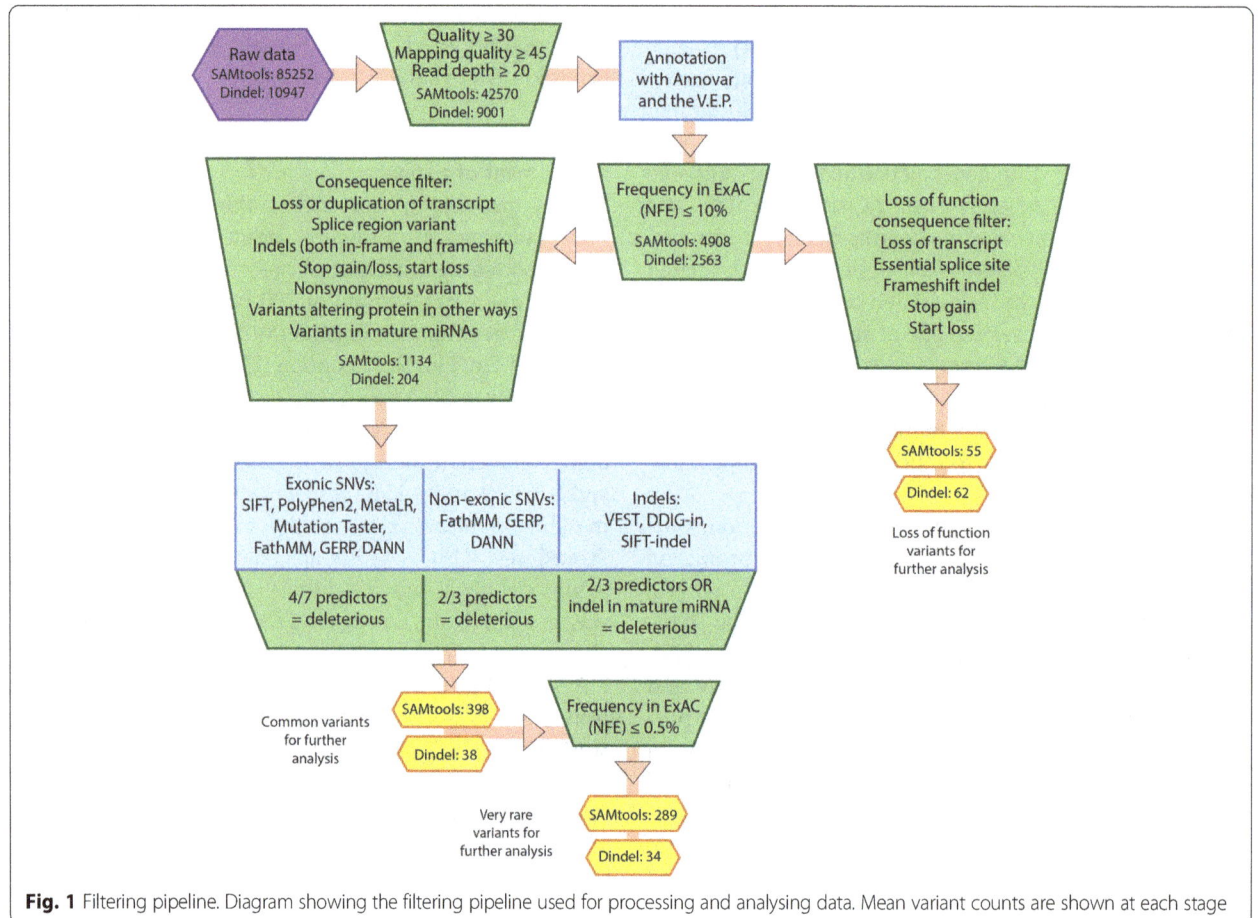

Fig. 1 Filtering pipeline. Diagram showing the filtering pipeline used for processing and analysing data. Mean variant counts are shown at each stage

variants were examined both individually and by gene (using only genes and known miRNAs present in Ensembl, accessed May 2016), and the gene lists analysed to find those mutated genes shared between individuals.

Variant confirmation
Candidate variants were re-sequenced using Sanger sequencing (Source Bioscience). Primers were designed using Primer3 [22] (Additional file 6: Table S2). Sequence data were analysed using Gap4 [23].

1000 Genomes project data
Genotype and annotation data from the 1000 Genomes project [21, 24] were used to create files of gene variants from each of the 2504 individuals sequenced in the project. Variants were processed using the same pipeline (Fig. 1), with the exception of the quality filter (quality of variant call ≥30, read depth ≥ 20, mapping quality ≥45), which was omitted because these variant calls have already been validated and filtered [21].

Results and discussion
In order to determine the possibility of using WES to reveal the genetic basis of adult onset hearing loss in a

typical clinical scenario, we identified 30 individuals with different phenotypic sub-types based on family history, age of onset and audiogram shape from large well characterised cohorts. Twenty patients with family histories were subdivided into ten with probable dominant hearing loss and ten with presumed recessive hearing loss. Ten older adults without a family history of hearing loss were subdivided into five people with a metabolic phenotype of ARHL and five with a sensory phenotype of ARHL based on audiogram shape [19]. These sub-groups are henceforth referred to as *Dominant, Recessive, Metabolic* and *Sensory* respectively.

Because hearing loss is common, we selected a low-stringency allele frequency filter of 10%, to detect common risk variants in our phenotypic sub-groups. We compiled a list of known deafness genes comprising all genes listed in the Hereditary Hearing Loss Homepage [15] plus the human orthologues of all the mouse deafness genes from the Hereditary Hearing Impairment in Mice website (described in [25]); 357 genes in total (Additional file 7: Table S3). Mutant mice continue to be valuable tools for discovering genes required for hearing [25], many of which have subsequently been shown to also underlie deafness in humans, such as *WBP2* [26] and *MIR96* [27, 28].

To identify potential false positives due to platform errors we utilised a list of 507 such genes described for the Illumina Genome Analyser IIx by Fuentes Fajardo et al. [29] (Additional file 8: Table S4). We have not excluded these genes from our analysis but have marked them as "candidates for exclusion" where they occur.

First analysis: Common variants
Here, common variants that were predicted to be pathogenic (≤10% MAF in the non-Finnish European population) were analysed to find genes common within each sub-group.

Known deafness genes in all four sub-groups combined
We first examined known deafness genes in all thirty people together and found that every person had at least ten known deafness genes with one or more predicted pathogenic variants (Fig. 2A, pale blue bars). The same analysis on data from the 1000 Genomes project, which

includes exome sequences from 2504 people with unknown auditory function, produced a very similar distribution of predicted pathogenic variants to the 30 people with adult-onset hearing loss (Fig. 2B). As this high frequency of predicted pathogenic variants was an unexpected finding, we asked if the same pattern of distribution was present in genes known to be involved in retinal disease, another sensory deficit with a large number of single genes known to be involved. We repeated the analysis using 265 retinal disease genes (from RetNet [30, 31], Additional file 9: Table S5) instead of our list of deafness genes. Again, we found a very similar distribution of predicted pathogenic variants in both our thirty patients with hearing loss and in the 2504 samples from the 1000 Genomes project (Fig. 2C, D). We then looked at human dominant deafness genes only (n = 33, Additional file 7: Table S3), where pathogenic variants would be expected to have an effect even when only present in one allele. We found once again a similar

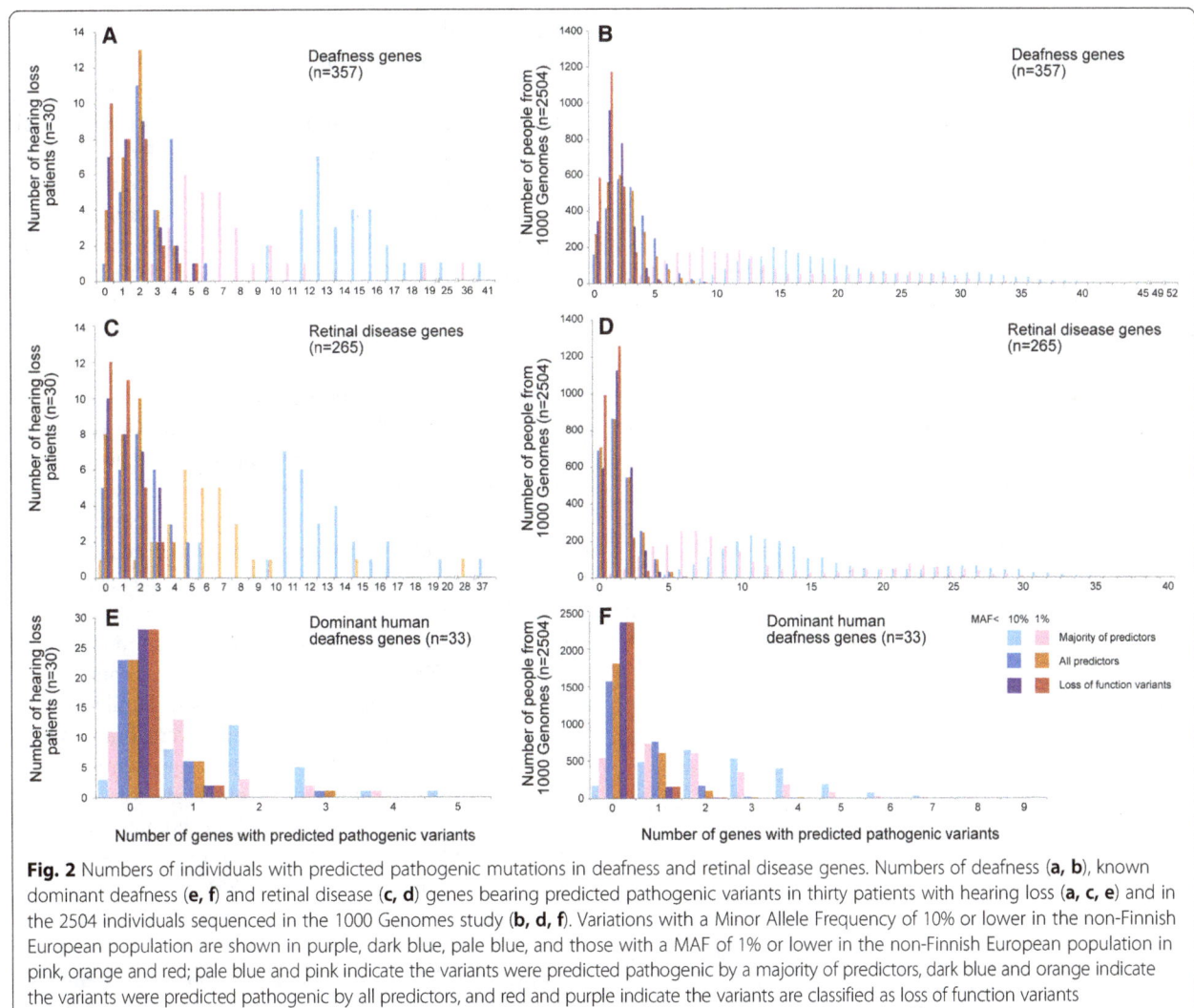

Fig. 2 Numbers of individuals with predicted pathogenic mutations in deafness and retinal disease genes. Numbers of deafness (**a, b**), known dominant deafness (**e, f**) and retinal disease (**c, d**) genes bearing predicted pathogenic variants in thirty patients with hearing loss (**a, c, e**) and in the 2504 individuals sequenced in the 1000 Genomes study (**b, d, f**). Variations with a Minor Allele Frequency of 10% or lower in the non-Finnish European population are shown in purple, dark blue, pale blue, and those with a MAF of 1% or lower in the non-Finnish European population in pink, orange and red; pale blue and pink indicate the variants were predicted pathogenic by a majority of predictors, dark blue and orange indicate the variants were predicted pathogenic by all predictors, and red and purple indicate the variants are classified as loss of function variants

distribution of variants in our thirty patients and the 1000 Genomes samples (Fig. 2E, F) and 27 of our 30 patients had at least one predicted pathogenic variant in a dominant deafness gene (Fig. 2C).

To test whether this finding was due to having too many common variants, we repeated the analysis using a 1% MAF cut-off (instead of 10%), and found the same pattern (Fig. 2, pink bars). We then tested a more stringent filter for pathogenicity, selecting only those variants predicted to be pathogenic by *all* the predictors used instead of the majority of predictors. The distributions were again similar for all groups of people and sets of disease-associated genes with both MAF filters (Fig. 2, dark blue and orange bars for MAF < 10% and MAF < 1% respectively). Finally, we looked for only loss of function variants (loss of transcript, essential splice site, frameshift indel, stop gain or start loss, see Fig. 1), and again observed a similar distribution (Fig. 2, purple and red bars for MAF < 10% and MAF < 1% respectively). Two of our patients and 152 people from the 1000 Genomes project had a loss of function variant in a known human dominant deafness gene (Fig. 2E, F). The two patients were both from the dominant sub-group; one had a single base pair insertion (causing a frameshift) in *MYO6* and the other had a nonsense mutation in *HOMER2*.

Genes common to individual sub-groups

We then looked at individual genes with predicted pathogenic variants (MAF < 10%, predicted by a majority of predictors) present in all members of each sub-group. No known deafness genes were common to any of the sub-groups. We found four other such genes: *TTN* (a candidate for exclusion) bore variants in all ten individuals with recessive hearing loss, *MON1B* was mutated in all five individuals with metabolic deafness (but see later), and the five people with sensory hearing loss all had variants in *NEDD4* and *ZAN* (Table 1).

Implications for WES analyses in common disease

Our common variant analysis has highlighted several potential problems with detecting common variants of small effect size in a common disorder. Although each

Table 1 Genes with common variants (MAF < 10%) in all the members of a subgroup

Gene	Sub-group	Number of variants	Type of variants
TTN	Recessive	22	Non-synonymous
MON1B	Metabolic	1	Frameshift
NEDD4	Sensory	2	Non-synonymous
ZAN	Sensory	7	Six non-synonymous, one in-frame deletion

Details of the four genes found to be mutated in all members of a subgroup. *TTN* (underlined) is a candidate for exclusion

individual had many deafness genes with predicted pathogenic variants, the overall spread didn't look any different to that observed in the 1000 Genomes dataset [21] (Fig. 2). However, the 1000 Genomes data do not exclude people with hearing loss, particularly adult-onset hearing loss which may not be evident at the time of sampling an individual. This highlights the need for good controls in this type of analysis, in both clinics and research; suitable controls in this case might be older adults with good hearing typical of a younger adult. Other exome sequencing projects have reported similar results for age-related macular degeneration [32] and in the ExAC data an abundance of rare, functional variants were reported in many disease genes [20]. It has been hypothesised that both false pathogenicity reports and incomplete penetrance contribute to this over-reporting, but whatever the reason, putative causative variants must be treated with caution until proof of pathogenicity has been obtained, preferably by functional studies and linkage analysis.

Another factor to consider is whether variants which are rare in the most relevant ethnic populations and passed the MAF filter but are more prevalent in other populations should be retained; 1234 of the 10,482 unique variants in the thirty patients which passed all our filtering steps were present in other ExAC populations at a MAF of more than 10%. To give one extreme example, it is worth considering whether a variant which is present in 60% of the African ExAC population should be included even if it is very rare (0.3%) in the non-Finnish European population, as for a T > C missense variant in *LPP* (chr3:g.188327555 T > C).

Second analysis: Very rare variants

Since the pattern of common variants in our thirty patients with hearing loss did not differ from that observed in the data from the 1000 Genomes project, we then filtered for very rare variants with a minor allele frequency of < 0.5%, predicted to be deleterious to protein function by a majority of predictors to identify any likely causal variants. This is the recommended MAF filter for recessive hearing loss (the recommended MAF for dominant hearing loss is 0.05%) [33]. No individuals from any of the groups, including those with a strong family history consistent with recessive inheritance, were homozygous for a variant in a known deafness gene. Apparently-homozygous variants were found in 29 other genes in only one of the individuals, and two genes bore homozygous variants in multiple people: *SIRPA* (a candidate for exclusion) and *ZAN* (Additional file 10: Table S6).

Many known deafness genes were mutated in multiple samples in the heterozygous state (Table 2); for example, 7 individuals bore variants in *GPR98*. One individual from the dominant group had five predicted variants in

Table 2 Genes with very rare predicted pathogenic variants in more than one person

Number of individuals	Genes					
12	*MON1B*					
11	*TTN*					
8	*ADC*	*NEFH*	*ZAN*			
7	*DNAH2*	**GPR98**	*LRBA*	**PAX2**		
6	*CHD3*	*DNAH3*	*MACF1*	*PTGER4*	*UBE2O*	*NEB*
	WDR19	*ZMIZ2*				
5	*VWA5B1*	*DNAH8*	*HSPG2*	*DNAH1*	*CELSR3*	*PCNX*
	DNAH7	*PKHD1L1*	**TECTA**	*ATG2A*	*ATM*	*RANBP17*
	LRIG3	*DNAH9*	*HECTD4*	*OBSCN*	*VPS13B*	*FAT2*
	LAMA2	*CAPN5*	**CDH23**	*WDR41*		
4	**DMD**	**DUOX2**	**RBPJ**	*USH2A*	**MYO6**	*+52*[a]
3	**COL11A1**	**NAV2**	**CPXM2**	**COL4A4**	**LRP2**	**MYO15A**
	MYH9	**TSPEAR**	**ACAN**	**PCDH15**	**OTOG**	*+160*[a]
2	**WFS1**	**MECOM**	**NTN1**	**GJB2**	**TCOF1**	**COL11A2**
	CELSR1	**SLC9A3R1**	**COL9A1**	**TJP2**	*ALMS1*	**JAG1**
	ATP2B2	**SLC26A4**	**LRIG1**	**LOXHD1**	**CHRNA9**	**RDX**
	CHD7	**NTF3**	**ELMOD3**	**SLC4A7**	**ATP8B1**	**NPC1**
	KARS	**ERCC6**	*+745*[a]			

Details of genes found to be mutated in multiple samples. Known deafness genes are in bold, and candidates for exclusion are underlined.
[a]Number of additional non-deafness genes with variants; only known deafness genes shown for these lists

WFS1 (Fig. 3), and many people bore more than one variant in the same gene, including three individuals from the recessive group who bore two heterozygous variants in a deafness gene (Additional file 11: Table S7). These variants might explain the hearing loss seen in these three patients, but with one exception, without segregation analysis it isn't possible to tell whether the variants are on the same chromosome or were inherited one from each parent. The exception is the two variants in *GPR98* in sample 11,813, which are close enough to fall within the same sequencing read, and can be confirmed to originate from the same chromosome. Furthermore, several very rare variants were also found to be present in more than one individual (Additional file 12: Tables S8 and Additional file 13: Table S9).

When we examined heterozygous variants in all genes, we found several genes bearing rare variants in six or more people (Additional file 13: Table S9). One of particular interest was *NEFH*, which encodes the neurofilament heavy chain and is strongly expressed in the spiral ganglion neurons innervating the inner hair cells [34].

We also examined the eight strongest candidate genes (*PCDH20, GRM7, ESRRG, SIK3, SLC28A3, TRIOBP, ISG20* and *ACAN*) linked to adult hearing ability or ARHL in GWAS [10–14]. Five rare variants were found: a novel deletion predicted to cause a frameshift in *GRM7*, a missense variant in *SIK3*, and three missense variants in *ACAN*, each present in one individual except

for one of the variants in *ACAN*, which is present in two people (Additional file 14: Table S10).

Resequencing

We chose 29 variants for confirmation by Sanger sequencing, covering fourteen genes, for our final quality control step. We focussed on variants in the genes common to phenotype-specific subgroups (*NEDD4, MON1B, ZAN,* Table 1), genes with rare variants in multiple people (*SIRPA, ZAN, MON1B, NEFH, ADC, GPR98, LRBA, PAX2* and *DNAH2*, Table 2 and Additional file 10: Table S6), genes with identical variants in multiple people (*PAX2, RBPJ, MON1B, NEFH,* Additional file 12: Tables S8 and Additional file 13: Table S9), variants in GWAS genes (*GRM7, SIK3,* Additional file 14: Table S10) and *WFS1*, which had 5 variants in one individual (Additional file 11: Table S7). Where genes had multiple predicted variants, we focussed on those present in more than one individual.

Approximately two thirds of our selected variants were confirmed (Table 3 and Additional file 15: Table S11), although the predicted zygosity was not always correct. Most failures were single base pair indels called by Dindel, but three were SNVs called by SAMtools (Table 3). Four additional indels called by Dindel were present but found to be different to the Dindel prediction. For example, eight patients were predicted to bear a single base pair insertion in *NEFH*, which would result in a

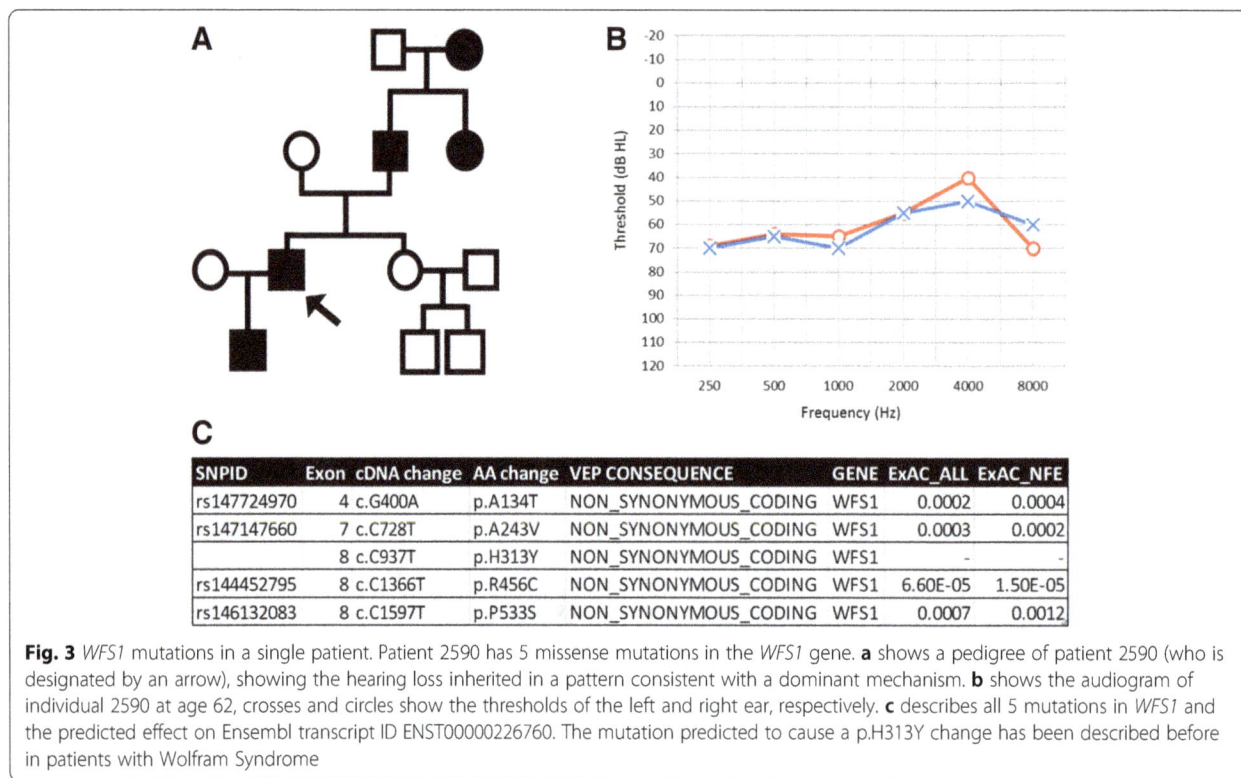

Fig. 3 *WFS1* mutations in a single patient. Patient 2590 has 5 missense mutations in the *WFS1* gene. **a** shows a pedigree of patient 2590 (who is designated by an arrow), showing the hearing loss inherited in a pattern consistent with a dominant mechanism. **b** shows the audiogram of individual 2590 at age 62, crosses and circles show the thresholds of the left and right ear, respectively. **c** describes all 5 mutations in *WFS1* and the predicted effect on Ensembl transcript ID ENST00000226760. The mutation predicted to cause a p.H313Y change has been described before in patients with Wolfram Syndrome

frameshift, but in fact Sanger sequencing detected an 18 bp insertion, which is not a frameshift. This miscalling also leads to incorrect minor allele frequencies being associated with each variant (compare the predicted MAF with the MAF of the confirmed variants in Table 3). None of the confirmed indels were detected by SAMtools, even though it is capable of calling small indels. Our findings suggest that while it is valuable to include Dindel, its output should be used with care in variant calling pipelines. In summary, we found a surprisingly high level of false calls from the exome sequencing, confirming that Sanger sequencing should always be used to verify important variants.

Candidate genes

Eight genes had confirmed variants, including four candidate novel deafness genes; *NEDD4*, *ZAN*, *DNAH2*, and *NEFH*. The four known deafness genes with confirmed variants are *GPR98*, *WFS1*, *GRM7* and *SIK3*.

Details of the 9 predicted variants in *GPR98* are described in Additional file 16: Table S12, including those found in multiple individuals (Table 2), as well as 2 additional variants found in individuals who carry multiple variants in this gene (Additional file 11: Table S7). *GPR98* is a large gene (90 exons encoding 6307 amino acids) encoding a G protein coupled receptor, and frameshift mutations in this gene cause one form of Usher's syndrome,

USH2C, an autosomal recessive disorder [35] causing congenital hearing impairment and retinitis pigmentosa (OMIM #605472). The variants described here in patients without retinitis pigmentosa are heterozygous missense variants, plus one in a splice site (Additional file 14: Table S10), and these are spread throughout the protein from exons 9 to 89. The two missense SNVs we sequenced were confirmed in the three patients predicted to carry them.

All five predicted variants in *WFS1* in individual 2590 were confirmed by resequencing. Mutations in *WFS1* can cause either a dominantly-inherited non-syndromic hearing loss typically affecting the low frequencies (below 2 kHz) or Wolfram Syndrome (OMIM #222300), a recessive neurodegenerative disease which can include mental retardation, childhood diabetes, optic atrophy and deafness which typically is progressive and affects the high frequencies [36]. The family history, medical history and audiogram shape of individual 2590 are consistent with a dominant non-syndromic hearing loss rather than Wolfram Syndrome (Fig. 3). All five mutations are predicted to be pathogenic but only one of the mutations (p.His313Tyr) has been reported previously, in the heterozygous state in 4 families with Wolfram Syndrome [37, 38]. Individuals previously reported with this variant are all deaf, some also had mental retardation but not all, this mutation is reported as a probably pathogenic mutation in the Wolfram Syndrome Mutation Database (https://lovd.euro-wabb.org/home.php?select_db=WFS1).

Table 3 Results of resequencing chosen variants

Gene	Caller	WES Predicted variant	Predicted MAF	Confirmed variant	Patients with variant Heterozygote	Homozygote	Variant ID	MAF	Consequence
NEDD4	Samtools	g.15:56208463A > C	0.0356	g.15:56208463A > C	1D 3S		rs113176671	0.038	Missense
NEDD4	Samtools	g.15:56208933 T > C	0.0992	g.15:56208933 T > C	3D 1S		rs1912403	0.108	Missense
ZAN	Dindel	g.7:100385563delC	–	g.7:100385563_10038597del		3D	rs369526619	0.456[a]	Frameshift deletion
ZAN	Samtools	g.7:100371417G > A	0.0451	g.7:100371417G > A	1M 1R		rs12673041	0.032	Missense
ZAN	Dindel	g.7:100353014_100353016del	0.0548	g.7:100353019_100353021del	2R		rs377643276	–	Inframe deletion
ZAN	Samtools	g.7:100346094G > A	0.0476	g.7:100346094G > A	1D		rs117406702	0.032	Essential splice site
ZAN	Samtools	g.7:100389590C > T	0.0803	g.7:100389590C > T	1S		rs76325149	0.085	Missense, splice site
DNAH2	Samtools	g.17:7736480 T > A	0.0095	g.17:7736480 T > A	1D 1R		rs78354379	0.008	Missense
GPR98	Samtools	g.5:89925039A > C	0.0035	g.5:89925039A > C	2D		rs61744480	0.002	Missense
GPR98	Samtools	g.5:90106415 T > G	0.000015	g.5:90106415 T > G	1R		–	–	Missense
NEFH	Dindel	g.22:29885564_2988556insG	–	g.22:29885568_2988585dup	1R 1S	3D 2R 1S	rs147489453	0.577	Inframe duplication
NEFH	Samtools	g.22:29885016G > A	0.0971	g.22:29885016G > A	2D 1R	1D	rs59371099	0.1	Missense
WFS1	Samtools	g.4:6290798G > A	0.0004	g.4:6290798G > A	1D		rs147724970	0.0002	Missense
WFS1	Samtools	g.4:6296783C > T	0.0002	g.4:6296783C > T	1D		rs147147660	0.00013	Missense
WFS1	Samtools	g.4:6302459C > T	–	g.4:6302459C > T	1D		rs86044563	–	Missense
WFS1	Samtools	g.4:6302888C > T	0.000015	g.4:6302888C > T	1D		–	–	Missense
WFS1	Samtools	g.4:6303119C > T	0.0012	g.4:6303119C > T	1D		rs146132083	0.001	Missense
GRM7	Dindel	g.3:7494306delT	–	g.3:7494272_7494273del	1M		–	–	Frameshift deletion
SIK3	Samtools	g.11:116728913G > A	0.0002	g.11:116728913G > A	1M		rs61738656	0.0002	Missense
MON1B	Dindel	g.16:77228709_77228710insG	–	Failed	n/a	n/a			
ADC	Dindel	g.1:33583668_33583669insG	0.0005	Failed	n/a	n/a			
ADC	Dindel	g.1:33583674_33583675insC	3.24E-05	Failed	n/a	n/a			
PAX2	Dindel	g.10:102587323dupC	4.58E-05	Failed	n/a	n/a			
PAX2	Dindel	g.10:102587329dupG	–	Failed	n/a	n/a			
PAX2	Dindel	g.10:102587333dupC	–	Failed	n/a	n/a			
SIRPA	Dindel	g.20:1895964_1895965del	–	Failed	n/a	n/a			
LRBA	Samtools	g.4:151727540C > A	0.0028	Failed	n/a	n/a			
LRBA	Samtools	g.4:151837565G > T	0.0011	Failed	n/a	n/a			
RBPJ	Samtools	g.4:2426018C > G	0	Failed	n/a	n/a			

Details of variant validation. The number of heterozygous and homozygous patients with each variation is annotated with the subgroups to which each belonged, where "D" stands for the 10 patients with dominantly inherited hearing loss, "R" for the 10 patients with recessive hearing loss, "M" for the 5 patients with a metabolic phenotype and "S" for the 5 patients with a sensory phenotype. Predicted variant MAF is from gnomAD genome data [24]; confirmed variant MAF is from the NHLBI GO Exome Sequencing Project [70]

Both variants in two of the genes linked to hearing loss by previous GWAS reports were confirmed, in two patients from the metabolic subgroup, one with a deletion in *GRM7* and one with a *SIK3* SNV (Table 3). *GRM7* codes for a metabotropic glutamate receptor, and is expressed in the spiral ganglion and the cochlear and vestibular hair cells in the mouse [12]. The variant was predicted to be a deletion of a T, but we found instead a deletion of TG 34 bp 5′ of the prediction and 22 bp 5′ of the acceptor splice site for exon 6 (transcript ENST00000357716), which makes it an intronic variant and unlikely to affect protein function. *SIK3* is a salt-inducible kinase, and is also expressed in the mouse spiral ganglion and cochlear hair cells, although only in young mice [11]. The contribution of these heterozygous variants to the hearing loss of the patients bearing them is unclear.

NEDD4 is a particularly interesting novel candidate; it is known to be widely expressed in the cochlear duct [39], and the encoded protein is a ubiquitin ligase that binds to and ubiquitylates the products of several deafness genes, including *WBP2* [40] and *KCNQ1* [41], both of which are implicated in sensorineural deafness in humans and mice [26, 42–44] (Fig. 4). It is involved in AMPA receptor ubiquitination, playing a critical role in AMPA receptor trafficking in rat neurons [45]. The two variants are both missense, one resulting in a substitution of arginine for serine in exon 1, and the other is a substitution of valine for methionine towards the start of exon 1. Patients bearing these variants are all heterozygotes, and fall into the dominant and sensory subgroups.

NEFH, the neurofilament heavy chain, is expressed in the rat cochlear nucleus [46] and the spiral ganglion

neurons [34]. It is known to bind to OTOF [47], which is involved in deafness in humans and mice [48–50], and its expression is affected by several other deafness genes (Fig. 4). We confirmed an 18 bp duplication (rs147489453) in eight people (homozygotes and heterozygotes, from the recessive, sensory and dominant subgroups), and a missense variant (rs59371099) in four people (heterozygotes and one homozygote, from the dominant and recessive subgroups) (Table 3). Four people carried both variants, three from the dominant subgroup and the one individual from the recessive subgroup who was heterozygous for both. The other two patients from the recessive subgroup with a variant in *NEFH* were homozygous for the 18 bp duplication (Table 3). Both variants are in the last exon of *NEFH* (exon 4), which has only one isoform. The 18 bp duplication is predicted to duplicate six amino acids in a low complexity region. The missense variant results in a substitution of lysine, which is positively charged, for glutamate, which is negatively charged, which may affect protein function, but without functional studies it is hard to predict what difference either variant would make to the function of the protein.

ZAN is a multiple-domain transmembrane protein found on the apical region of the sperm head [51], which functions to bind the sperm to the zona pellucida [52]. The MAM domains, D domains, EGF-like domains and mucin-like domains it contains all play a role in adhesion in other proteins, typically in cell-cell or cell-extracellular matrix binding [51]. Although ZAN is thought to be testis-specific, it may also be involved in cell-cell adhesion in the organ of Corti. Variants in *ZAN*

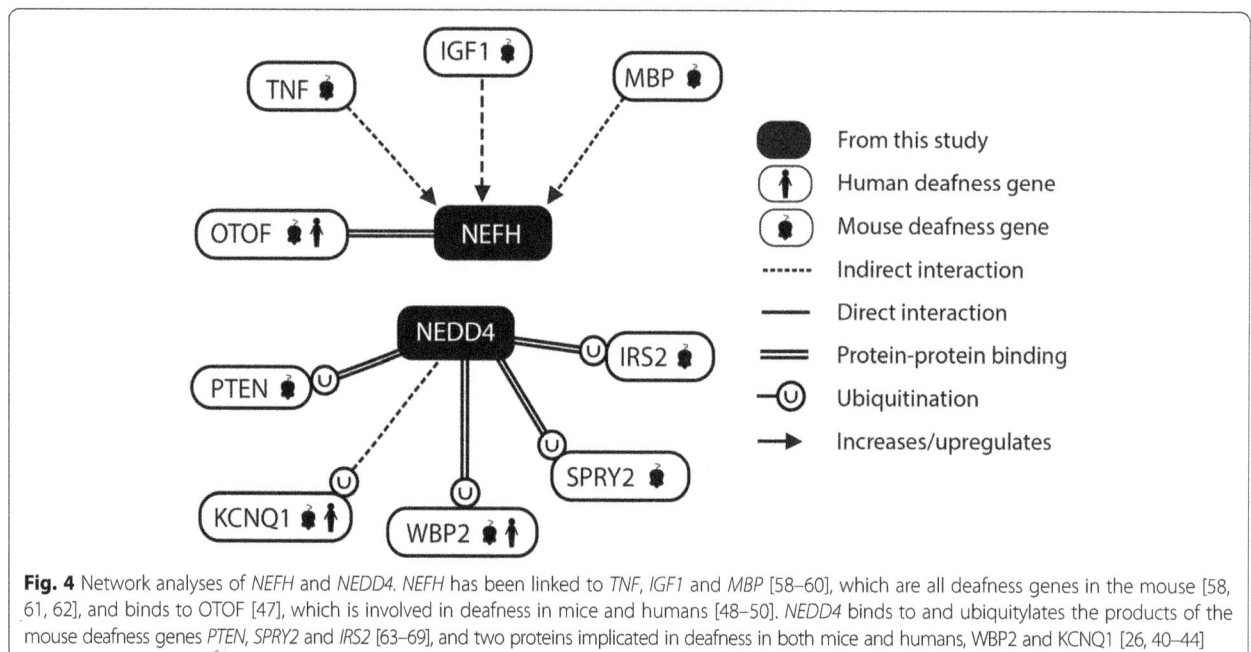

Fig. 4 Network analyses of *NEFH* and *NEDD4*. *NEFH* has been linked to *TNF*, *IGF1* and *MBP* [58–60], which are all deafness genes in the mouse [58, 61, 62], and binds to OTOF [47], which is involved in deafness in mice and humans [48–50]. *NEDD4* binds to and ubiquitylates the products of the mouse deafness genes *PTEN*, *SPRY2* and *IRS2* [63–69], and two proteins implicated in deafness in both mice and humans, WBP2 and KCNQ1 [26, 40–44]

were found in patients from each subgroup, all in the heterozygote state except for three dominant patients who were homozygous for a 35 bp deletion (g.7:100385563_100385597del).

DNAH2 is an axonemal dynein heavy chain, about which very little is known. Six missense variants, one intronic splice site SNV and one single base pair insertion were predicted in seven patients (MAF < 0.5%), and six further missense variants with a MAF < 10% were predicted in 5 patients, of which we have confirmed one missense variant present in the heterozygous state in two patients from the dominant and recessive subgroups.

Expression and mouse mutations of novel candidate deafness genes

We examined the expression of our novel candidate deafness genes using the gEAR portal [53], which displays data from the mouse organ of Corti at postnatal day (P)0 [54] – P7 [55], and found that both *Nedd4* and *Zan* were detected during this period. *Nedd4* is expressed at reasonably high levels in sensory cells, and only slightly lower levels in non-sensory cells, in accordance with previous publications [39]. *Zan* has very little expression in the hair cells but is strongly expressed in the supporting cells at P0 [54]. *Nefh* is expressed in the neurons under the inner hair cells [34], and is commonly used as a neuronal marker [26]. *Dnah2* is expressed in the cochlear duct at P0, but not as strongly as *Zan* or *Nedd4*.

There are several mouse lines bearing mutations in *Nedd4*, *Zan*, and *Nefh*, but the only mouse line with a variant in *Dnah2* has a large inversion on chromosome 11 covering 1898 genes. No hearing phenotype has been reported for any of the mutant alleles of these genes (as recorded in the Mouse Genome Informatics database [56]), but these mice may not have been tested for auditory function.

Conclusions

Our analysis has identified several candidate variants and genes for involvement in adult-onset progressive hearing loss, in particular variants in *NEFH* and *NEDD4*. It is perhaps surprising that our relatively small sample size of thirty individuals was able to identify good candidate variants and genes. By targeting our approach to specific phenotypic subtypes within large, well-characterised patient cohorts based on audiogram shape, family history and similar age of onset, we have sought to increase power to detect causal genetic variants. In addition, by cross-referencing our data in the filtering pipeline with data from the mouse we were able to prioritise the strongest candidate variants.

The two strongest candidates from our analysis, the variants in *NEDD4* and *NEFH*, should be followed up in larger cohorts and by functional studies to confirm whether they are causal mutations.

Our study also highlights the potential pitfalls of using targeted sequencing to diagnose the cause of adult-onset hearing loss in a typical clinical scenario, where relatives are not available for segregation analysis especially on a gene by gene basis. Of the 30 individuals WES was only able to identify the likely causal mutation in one individual with five WFS1 variants. For the remaining patients the variants identified are of uncertain pathogenicity without further validation. Interpretation of these variants in single individuals is extremely challenging given that even when we limited our analysis to dominantly-inherited human deafness genes, 2334 of the 2504 individuals in the 1000 Genomes Project data carried at least one predicted pathogenic variant in a known dominant human deafness gene. These findings reveal the need for allele frequency databases from carefully-selected controls with good hearing for their age rather than the existing unselected general population controls in studies of highly-prevalent disorders such as hearing loss. Here, we have explored the use of WES in undiagnosed individuals, based on our results it would be interesting to pursue a similar study in individuals who have received a genetic diagnosis to ascertain the number of other predicted pathogenic variants that are present in deafness genes. Furthermore, our study demonstrates that confirmation of candidate variants by Sanger sequencing is always a necessary step. Our findings further suggest that for diagnostics in a clinical situation, novel candidate variants identified by sequencing should be investigated by family analysis if possible, to look for segregation. Without these additional steps, our data suggest that it is not possible to determine with confidence the causative mutation responsible for a patient's hearing impairment from exome sequence alone. Even with these secondary steps great caution should be exercised in interpreting predicted disease-causing variants, given our findings of the incidence of such variants in every genome.

Additional files

Additional file 1: Figure S1. showing the audiograms of each participant in the recessive patient group.

Additional file 2: Figure S2. showing the audiograms of each participant in the dominant patient group.

Additional file 3: Figure S3. showing the audiograms of each participant in the metabolic and sensory patient groups.

Additional file 4: Table S1. which lists the software prediction tools used to call and annotate variants, with relevant references.

Additional file 5: Figure S4. and legend detailing counts at each filtering step for common variant analysis.

Additional file 6: Table S2. detailing primers used for confirming selected variants.

Additional file 7: Table S3. listing genes reported to underlie deafness in humans and/or mice.

Additional file 8: Table S4. and lists candidates for exclusion - genes with predicted pathogenic variants in many exome projects or across multiple families exhibiting a variety of phenotypes. This list consists of the genes in Supplementary Tables S1 and S2 from [29].

Additional file 9: Table S5. and lists human retinal disease genes, from RetNet [30].

Additional file 10: Table S6. listing individuals homozygous for very rare variants in any gene.

Additional file 11: Table S7. listing individuals with more than one very rare mutation in the same gene.

Additional file 12: Table S8. giving details of the single very rare variants in known deafness genes found in multiple samples.

Additional file 13: Table S9. giving details of genes with identical variants found in more than one person.

Additional file 14: Table S10. detailing very rare mutations in GWAS candidates.

Additional file 15: Table S11. which contains further details of the validated variants listed in Table 3.

Additional file 16: Table S12. giving details of very rare mutations identified in GPR98.

Abbreviations

ARHL: Age-related hearing loss; EGA: European Genome-Phenome Archive; GWAS: Genome-wide association studies; MAF: Minor allele frequency; MUSC: Medical University of South Carolina; WES: Whole-exome sequencing

Acknowledgements

We thank Carol Scott, Wellcome Trust Sanger Institute, for help and support with the exome sequencing study and variant calling pipeline.

Funding

This work was supported by the following: the Medical Research Council, the Wellcome Trust [grant numbers 098051; 100669 to KPS]; National Institutes of Health/National Institute on Deafness and Other Communication Disorders [grant number P50 DC000422]; the South Carolina Clinical & Translational Research Institute, the Medical University of South Carolina [grant numbers NIH/NCATS UL1 TR000062 and UL1 TR001450]; the Haigh Fellowship in Age Related Deafness and Deafness Research UK, now Action on Hearing Loss [grant number 444:UEI:SD to SJD]. The London ARHL Cohort collection was initiated by funding from Research into Ageing [grant number 223 to SJD]; Teresa Rosenbaum Golden Charitable Trust, Telethon Foundation [grant number GGP09037]. The funders played no part in the design of the study or the collection, analysis and interpretation of the data, or the writing of the manuscript.

Authors' contributions

LJM, BAS, JRD were involved in sample selection and interpretation of the USA patient data regarding the audiological findings. SJD, LSN and BAC were involved in recruitment of UK patients and LSN and BAC produced the patient database and selected patients for sequencing. DNA purification of UK samples was done by LSN. MAL analysed the variant calls and carried out the common variant analysis. The rare variant analysis was done by SJD. SJD and KPS designed the experiments. The manuscript was written by SJD, MAL and KPS, and all authors read, edited and approved the final version.

Competing interests

The authors declare that they have no competing interests.

Author details

[1]Wolfson Centre for Age-Related Diseases, King's College London, WC2R 2LS, London, UK. [2]Wellcome Trust Sanger Institute, Hinxton, Cambridge CB10 1SA, UK. [3]UCL Ear Institute, University College London, WC1X 8EE, London, UK. [4]Medical University of South Carolina, Charleston, SC 29425, USA.

References

1. Gates GA, Couropmitree NN, Myers RH. Genetic associations in age-related hearing thresholds. Arch otolaryngol Head Neck Surg. 1999;125:654–9.
2. Fellinger J, Holzinger D, Pollard R. Mental health of deaf people. Lancet. 2012;379:1037–44.
3. Karpa MJ, Gopinath B, Beath K, Rochtchina E, Cumming RG, Wang JJ, et al. Associations between hearing impairment and mortality risk in older persons: the Blue Mountains hearing study. Ann Epidemiol. 2010;20:452–9.
4. Mick P, Kawachi I, Lin FR. The association between hearing loss and social isolation in older adults. Otolaryngol Head Neck Surg. 2014;150:378–84.
5. Livingston G, Sommerlad A, Orgeta V, Costafreda SG, Huntley J, Ames D, et al. Dementia prevention, intervention, and care. Lancet. 2017;390:2673–734.
6. Karlsson KK, Harris JR, Svartengren M. Description and primary results from an audiometric study of male twins. Ear Hear. 1997;18:114–20.
7. Wolber LE, Steves CJ, Spector TD, Williams FM. Hearing ability with age in northern European women: a new web-based approach to genetic studies. PLoS One. 2012;7:e35500.
8. Fransen E, Bonneux S, Corneveaux JJ, Schrauwen I, Di Berardino F, White CH, et al. Genome-wide association analysis demonstrates the highly polygenic character of age-related hearing impairment. Eur J Hum Genet. 2015;23:110–5.
9. Huyghe JR, Van Laer L, Hendrickx JJ, Fransen E, Demeester K, Topsakal V, et al. Genome-wide SNP-based linkage scan identifies a locus on 8q24 for an age-related hearing impairment trait. Am J Hum Genet. 2008;83:401–7.
10. Nolan LS, Maier H, Hermans-Borgmeyer I, Girotto G, Ecob R, Pirastu N, et al. Estrogen-related receptor gamma and hearing function: evidence of a role in humans and mice. Neurobiol Aging. 2013;34:2077 e2071–9.
11. Wolber LE, Girotto G, Buniello A, Vuckovic D, Pirastu N, Lorente-Canovas B, et al. Salt-inducible kinase 3, SIK3, is a new gene associated with hearing. Hum Mol Genet. 2014;23:6407–18.
12. Friedman RA, Van Laer L, Huentelman MJ, Sheth SS, Van Eyken E, Corneveaux JJ, et al. GRM7 variants confer susceptibility to age-related hearing impairment. Hum Mol Genet. 2009;18:785–96.
13. Vuckovic D, Dawson S, Scheffer DI, Rantanen T, Morgan A, Di Stazio M, et al. Genome-wide association analysis on normal hearing function identifies PCDH20 and SLC28A3 as candidates for hearing function and loss. Hum Mol Genet. 2015;24:5655–64.
14. Hoffmann TJ, Keats BJ, Yoshikawa N, Schaefer C, Risch N, Lustig LR. A large genome-wide association study of age-related hearing impairment using electronic health records. PLoS Genet. 2016;12:e1006371.
15. Van Camp G, Smith RJ: Hereditary Hearing Loss Homepage. http://hereditaryhearingloss.org/. Accessed Jan 2016.
16. Van Camp G, Willems PJ, Smith RJ. Nonsyndromic hearing impairment: unparalleled heterogeneity. Am J Hum Genet. 1997;60:758–64.
17. Nolan LS, Cadge BA, Gomez-Dorado M, Dawson SJ. A functional and genetic analysis of SOD2 promoter variants and their contribution to age-related hearing loss. Mech Ageing Dev. 2013;134:298–306.
18. British Society of Audiology: BSA Recommended Procedure: Pure tone air-conduction and bone-conduction threshold audiometry with and without masking. http://www.thebsa.org.uk/resources/. Accessed July 2016.
19. Dubno JR, Eckert MA, Lee FS, Matthews LJ, Schmiedt RA. Classifying human audiometric phenotypes of age-related hearing loss from animal models. J Assoc Res Otolaryngol. 2013;14:687–701.
20. Lek M, Karczewski K, Minikel E, Samocha K, Banks E, Fennell T, et al. Analysis of protein-coding genetic variation in 60,706 humans. bioRxiv. 2015;
21. Auton A, Brooks LD, Durbin RM, Garrison EP, Kang HM, Korbel JO, et al. A global reference for human genetic variation. Nature. 2015;526:68–74.
22. Untergasser A, Cutcutache I, Koressaar T, Ye J, Faircloth BC, Remm M, et al. Primer3--new capabilities and interfaces. Nucleic Acids Res. 2012;40:e115.
23. Bonfield JK, Smith K, Staden R. A new DNA sequence assembly program. Nucleic Acids Res. 1995;23:4992–9.
24. The International Genome Sample Resource: 1000 Genomes data. http://ftp.1000genomes.ebi.ac.uk/vol1/ftp/release/20130502/. Accessed June 2016.
25. Ohlemiller KK, Jones SM, Johnson KR. Application of mouse models to research in hearing and balance. J Assoc Res Otolaryngol. 2016;17:493–523.

26. Buniello A, Ingham NJ, Lewis MA, Huma AC, Martinez-Vega R, Varela-Nieto I, et al. Wbp2 is required for normal glutamatergic synapses in the cochlea and is crucial for hearing. EMBO Mol Med. 2016;8:191–207.

27. Lewis MA, Quint E, Glazier AM, Fuchs H, De Angelis MH, Langford C, et al. An ENU-induced mutation of miR-96 associated with progressive hearing loss in mice. Nat Genet. 2009;41:614–8.

28. Mencia A, Modamio-Hoybjor S, Redshaw N, Morin M, Mayo-Merino F, Olavarrieta L, et al. Mutations in the seed region of human miR-96 are responsible for nonsyndromic progressive hearing loss. Nat Genet. 2009;41:609–13.

29. Fuentes Fajardo KV, Adams D, Mason CE, Sincan M, Tifft C, Toro C, et al. Detecting false-positive signals in exome sequencing. Hum Mutat. 2012;33:609–13.

30. Daiger SP, Rossiter BJF, Greenberg J, Christoffels A, Hide W. Data services and software for identifying genes and mutations causing retinal degeneration. Invest Opthalmol Vis Sci. 1998;39:S295.

31. Daiger SP, Sullivan LS, Bowne SJ: RetNet Retinal Information Network https://sph.uth.edu/retnet/home.htm. Accessed June 2016.

32. Tabor HK, Auer PL, Jamal SM, Chong JX, Yu JH, Gordon AS, et al. Pathogenic variants for Mendelian and complex traits in exomes of 6,517 European and African Americans: implications for the return of incidental results. Am J Hum Genet. 2014;95:183–93.

33. Shearer AE, Eppsteiner RW, Booth KT, Ephraim SS, Gurrola J 2nd, Simpson A, et al. Utilizing ethnic-specific differences in minor allele frequency to recategorize reported pathogenic deafness variants. Am J Hum Genet. 2014;95:445–53.

34. Hafidi A, Despres G, Romand R. Cochlear innervation in the developing rat: an immunocytochemical study of neurofilament and spectrin proteins. J Comp Neurol. 1990;300:153–61.

35. Jacobson SG, Cideciyan AV, Aleman TS, Sumaroka A, Roman AJ, Gardner LM, et al. Usher syndromes due to MYO7A, PCDH15, USH2A or GPR98 mutations share retinal disease mechanism. Hum Mol Genet. 2008;17:2405–15.

36. Cryns K, Sivakumaran TA, Van den Ouweland JM, Pennings RJ, Cremers CW, Flothmann K, et al. Mutational spectrum of the WFS1 gene in Wolfram syndrome, nonsyndromic hearing impairment, diabetes mellitus, and psychiatric disease. Hum Mutat. 2003;22:275–87.

37. Hansen L, Eiberg H, Barrett T, Bek T, Kjaersgaard P, Tranebjaerg L, et al. Mutation analysis of the WFS1 gene in seven Danish Wolfram syndrome families; four new mutations identified. Eur J Hum Genet. 2005;13:1275–84.

38. Rohayem J, Ehlers C, Wiedemann B, Holl R, Oexle K, Kordonouri O, et al. Diabetes and neurodegeneration in Wolfram syndrome: a multicenter study of phenotype and genotype. Diabetes Care. 2011;34:1503–10.

39. Zhong SX, Liu ZH. Expression patterns of Nedd4 isoforms and SGK1 in the rat cochlea. Acta Otolaryngol. 2009;129:935–9.

40. Persaud A, Alberts P, Amsen EM, Xiong X, Wasmuth J, Saadon Z, et al. Comparison of substrate specificity of the ubiquitin ligases Nedd4 and Nedd4-2 using proteome arrays. Mol Syst Biol. 2009;5:333.

41. Jespersen T, Membrez M, Nicolas CS, Pitard B, Staub O, Olesen SP, et al. The KCNQ1 potassium channel is down-regulated by ubiquitylating enzymes of the Nedd4/Nedd4-like family. Cardiovasc Res. 2007;74:64–74.

42. Casimiro MC, Knollmann BC, Ebert SN, Vary JC Jr, Greene AE, Franz MR, et al. Targeted disruption of the Kcnq1 gene produces a mouse model of Jervell and Lange-Nielsen syndrome. Proc Natl Acad Sci U S A. 2001;98:2526–31.

43. Lee MP, Ravenel JD, Hu RJ, Lustig LR, Tomaselli G, Berger RD, et al. Targeted disruption of the Kvlqt1 gene causes deafness and gastric hyperplasia in mice. J Clin Invest. 2000;106:1447–55.

44. Neyroud N, Tesson F, Denjoy I, Leibovici M, Donger C, Barhanin J, et al. A novel mutation in the potassium channel gene KVLQT1 causes the Jervell and Lange-Nielsen cardioauditory syndrome. Nat Genet. 1997;15:186–9.

45. Lin A, Hou Q, Jarzylo L, Amato S, Gilbert J, Shang F, et al. Nedd4-mediated AMPA receptor ubiquitination regulates receptor turnover and trafficking. J Neurochem. 2011;119:27–39.

46. Friedland DR, Popper P, Eernisse R, Ringger B, Cioffi JA. Differential expression of cytoskeletal genes in the cochlear nucleus. Anat Rec A Discov Mol Cell Evol Biol. 2006;288:447–65.

47. Duncker SV, Franz C, Kuhn S, Schulte U, Campanelli D, Brandt N, et al. Otoferlin couples to clathrin-mediated endocytosis in mature cochlear inner hair cells. J Neurosci. 2013;33:9508–19.

48. Longo-Guess C, Gagnon LH, Bergstrom DE, Johnson KR. A missense mutation in the conserved C2B domain of otoferlin causes deafness in a new mouse model of DFNB9. Hear Res. 2007;234:21–8.

49. Roux I, Safieddine S, Nouvian R, Grati M, Simmler MC, Bahloul A, et al. Otoferlin, defective in a human deafness form, is essential for exocytosis at the auditory ribbon synapse. Cell. 2006;127:277 89.

50. Yasunaga S, Grati M, Cohen-Salmon M, El-Amraoui A, Mustapha M, Salem N, et al. A mutation in OTOF, encoding otoferlin, a FER-1-like protein, causes DFNB9, a nonsyndromic form of deafness. Nat Genet. 1999;21:363–9.

51. Gao Z, Garbers DL. Species diversity in the structure of zonadhesin, a sperm-specific membrane protein containing multiple cell adhesion molecule-like domains. J Biol Chem. 1998;273:3415–21.

52. Lea IA, Sivashanmugam P, O'Rand MG. Zonadhesin: characterization, localization, and zona pellucida binding. Biol Reprod. 2001;65:1691–700.

53. Hertzano RP, Orvis J. gEAR Portal. https://umgear.org/. Accessed June 2016.

54. Cai T, Jen HI, Kang H, Klisch TJ, Zoghbi HY, Groves AK. Characterization of the transcriptome of nascent hair cells and identification of direct targets of the Atoh1 transcription factor. J Neurosci. 2015;35:5870–83.

55. Scheffer DI, Shen J, Corey DP, Chen ZY. Gene expression by mouse inner ear hair cells during development. J Neurosci. 2015;35:6366–80.

56. The Jackson Laboratory: Mouse Genome Informatics. www.informatics.jax.org. Accessed Sept 2017.

57. EGA Consortium: European Genome-Phenome Archive. http://ega-archive.org. Accessed June 2016.

58. Camarero G, Avendano C, Fernandez-Moreno C, Villar A, Contreras J, de Pablo F, et al. Delayed inner ear maturation and neuronal loss in postnatal Igf-1-deficient mice. J Neurosci. 2001;21:7630–41.

59. Brady ST, Witt AS, Kirkpatrick LL, de Waegh SM, Readhead C, Tu PH, et al. Formation of compact myelin is required for maturation of the axonal cytoskeleton. J Neurosci. 1999;19:7278–88.

60. Zer C, Sachs G, Shin JM. Identification of genomic targets downstream of p38 mitogen-activated protein kinase pathway mediating tumor necrosis factor-alpha signaling. Physiol Genomics. 2007;31:343–51.

61. Fujiyoshi T, Hood L, Yoo TJ. Restoration of brain stem auditory-evoked potentials by gene transfer in shiverer mice. Ann Otolo Rhinol Laryngol. 1994;103:449–56.

62. Oishi N, Chen J, Zheng HW, Hill K, Schacht J, Sha SH. Tumor necrosis factor-alpha-mutant mice exhibit high frequency hearing loss. J Assoc Res Otolaryngol. 2013;14:801–11.

63. Fukushima T, Yoshihara H, Furuta H, Kamei H, Hakuno F, Luan J, et al. Nedd4-induced monoubiquitination of IRS-2 enhances IGF signalling and mitogenic activity. Nat Commun. 2015;6:6780.

64. Edwin F, Anderson K, Patel TB. HECT domain-containing E3 ubiquitin ligase Nedd4 interacts with and ubiquitinates Sprouty2. J Biol Chem. 2010;285:255–64.

65. Wang X, Trotman LC, Koppie T, Alimonti A, Chen Z, Gao Z, et al. NEDD4-1 is a proto-oncogenic ubiquitin ligase for PTEN. Cell. 2007;128:129–39.

66. Trotman LC, Wang X, Alimonti A, Chen Z, Teruya-Feldstein J, Yang H, et al. Ubiquitination regulates PTEN nuclear import and tumor suppression. Cell. 2007;128:141–56.

67. Murillo-Cuesta S, Camarero G, Gonzalez-Rodriguez A, De La Rosa LR, Burks DJ, Avendano C, et al. Insulin receptor substrate 2 (IRS2)-deficient mice show sensorineural hearing loss that is delayed by concomitant protein tyrosine phosphatase 1B (PTP1B) loss of function. Mol Med. 2012;18:260–9.

68. Dong Y, Sui L, Yamaguchi F, Kamitori K, Hirata Y, Hossain MA, et al. Phosphatase and tensin homolog deleted on chromosome 10 regulates sensory cell proliferation and differentiation of hair bundles in the mammalian cochlea. Neuroscience. 2010;170:1304–13.

69. Shim K, Minowada G, Coling DE, Martin GR. Sprouty2, a mouse deafness gene, regulates cell fate decisions in the auditory sensory epithelium by antagonizing FGF signaling. Dev Cell. 2005;8:553–64.

70. (ESP) NGESP: Exome Variant Server. http://evs.gs.washington.edu/EVS/. Accessed July 2018.

10

Association between genetic risk variants and glucose intolerance during pregnancy in north Indian women

Geeti P. Arora[1,2], Peter Almgren[2], Charlotte Brøns[3], Richa G. Thaman[1], Allan A. Vaag[2,3,5], Leif Groop[2,4] and Rashmi B. Prasad[2*] (ID)

Abstract

Background: Gestational diabetes (GDM) is a more common problem in India than in many other parts of the world but it is not known whether this is due to unique environmental factors or a unique genetic background. To address this question we examined whether the same genetic variants associated with GDM and Type 2 Diabetes (T2D) in Caucasians also were associated with GDM in North Indian women.

Methods: Five thousand one hundred pregnant women of gestational age 24–28 weeks from Punjab were studied by a 75 g oral glucose tolerance test (OGTT). GDM was diagnosed by both WHO1999 and 2013 criteria. 79 single nucleotide polymorphisms (SNPs) previously associated with T2D and glycemic traits (12 of them also with GDM) and 6 SNPs from previous T2D associations based on Indian population (some also with European) were genotyped on a Sequenom platform or using Taqman assays in DNA from 4018 women.

Results: In support of previous findings in Caucasian GDM, SNPs at *KCJN11* and *GRB14* loci were nominally associated with GDM1999 risk in Indian women (both $p = 0.02$). Notably, T2D risk alleles of the variant rs1552224 near *CENTD2*, rs11708067 in *ADCY5* and rs11605924 in *CRY2* genes associated with protection from GDM regardless of criteria applied ($p < 0.025$). SNPs rs7607980 near *COBLL1* ($p = 0.0001$), rs13389219 near *GRB14* ($p = 0.026$) and rs10423928 in the *GIPR* gene ($p = 0.012$) as well as the genetic risk score (GRS) for these previously shown insulin resistance loci here associated with insulin resistance defined by HOMA2-IR and showed a trend towards GDM. GRS comprised of 3 insulin secretion loci here associated with insulin secretion but not GDM.

Conclusions: GDM in women from Punjab in Northern India shows a genetic component, seemingly driven by insulin resistance and secretion and partly shared with GDM in other parts of the world. Most previous T2D loci discovered in European studies did not associate with GDM in North India, indicative of different genetic etiology or alternately, differences in the linkage disequilibrium (LD) structure between populations in which the associated SNPs were identified and Northern Indian women. Interestingly some T2D risk variants were in fact indicative of being protective for GDM in these Indian women.

Keywords: Genetics, Risk variant, Gestational diabetes mellitus, Single nucleotide polymorphism, Diagnostic criteria, Insulin resistance, Insulin secretion, Type 2 diabetes mellitus

* Correspondence: rashmi.prasad@med.lu.se
[2]Department of Clinical Sciences, Clinical Research Centre, Lund University, Malmö, Sweden
Full list of author information is available at the end of the article

Background

Gestational Diabetes Mellitus (GDM) has been officially defined as "carbohydrate intolerance" of variable severity with onset or first recognition during pregnancy [1–3] irrespective of treatment and whether or not the condition persists after pregnancy. GDM represents almost 90% of all pregnancies complicated by diabetes [4]. The prevalence of GDM is rapidly increasing, ranging from 2 to 14% depending upon diagnostic criteria [5, 6]. In a study of South Indian women, GDM prevalence varied between 12 and 21% [7] while another study of North Indian women reported a prevalence of 10% using WHO criteria [8]. The hallmark of GDM is increased insulin resistance accompanied by decreased compensatory insulin secretory response. Type 2 diabetes (T2D) is also caused by increased insulin resistance and decreased insulin secretion to compensate for the former. Thus, both T2D and GDM share the same pathophysiology which is influenced by similar risk factors like high body mass index (BMI), history of abnormal glucose intolerance, family history of diabetes, age, and ethnicity [9–11].

A family history of both T2D and GDM is known to increase GDM risk, indicative of a common genetic component underlying both T2D and GDM [12, 13]. Till date, more than 120 T2D risk loci have been confirmed to be associated with T2D [14]. A large proportion of them have also shown association with GDM. T2D risk variants at the *MTNR1B, FTO, TLE1, G6PC2, GCKR, TCF7L2, ADCY5, CDKAL1, TCF2, HNF1B, PPARG, KCNJ11, SLC30A8* loci have previously been associated with GDM in European populations [15–18] whereas variants in the *CDKAL1, CDKN2A/2B, MTNR1B* and *KCNQ1* loci were associated with GDM in Korean women [19, 20].

Some genetic variants are more unique to Indian T2D patients e.g. the *SGCG* (rs9552911) and *TMEM163* (rs998451) variants [21–25]. However, genetic studies of GDM in India are scarce. The SNPs rs7754840 and rs7756992 in the *CDKAL1* gene were associated with GDM in South Indian women [26], while variants in the *HMG20A* (rs7178572) and *HNF4A* (rs4812829) genes were associated with both GDM and T2D [27]. The aim of the present study was to investigate whether a panel of known variants previously associated with GDM and T2D in Indian and European populations are associated with GDM in Punjabi women.

Methods

Study population and phenotyping

Five thousand one hundred pregnant women were recruited by applying a multistage random screening in the State of Punjab in North India for GDM. Pregnant women at gestational week 24–28 were randomly selected and recruited [8, 28]. This was part of a WDF supported project titled "Gestational diabetes in Punjab" with the goal to create and implement sustainable awareness, education, screening, intervention and treatment capacities of diabetes in pregnancy (GDM) within the public and private health care system, as well as in the general population in Punjab. The team included a chief research coordinator, an assistant coordinator, doctors, nurses, lab technicians from all selected sites both in private hospitals and public healthcare system. Approval for screening was obtained from DRME, Chandigarh, India. The recruitment sites included Recruitment sites:, Deep Hospital, Model Town, Ludhiana as the epicenter, Shri Rama Charitable Hospital, Ludhiana, Chawla Hospital, Ludhiana, Iqbal Hospital, Ludhiana, Government Medical Colleges and Hospital, Patiala, Amritsar and Faridkot, PHC Verka, Amritsar, Health Centre Bhadsoan, Patiala, Health Centre Faridkot. The project was approved by Independent ethics committee, Ludhiana in 2009. The ethics committee is registered with Office of Drugs Controller General (India) Directorate General of Health Services with Registration no. ECR/525/Inst/PB/2014.

Information was obtained on age, BMI, family history of diabetes, diet, habitat (urban or rural), education and religion. All information material and written consent forms were provided in 3 languages (Hindi, Punjabi & English) and duly signed by the participants. The study protocol was approved by local Ethical Committees. Glucose was measured in venous plasma samples at fasting and at 2 h after a 75 g glucose challenge using glucometers (Accucheck-Roche Diagnostics). Fasting insulin concentrations were determined with ELISA (Diametra, Milan, Italy; intra- and inter-assay variation of < 5.0 and < 10.0%, respectively). The homeostatic model assessment (HOMA2) was used to quantify insulin resistance (HOMA2-IR) and beta-cell function (HOMA2-B) from fasting insulin and glucose values using the HOMA2 calculator v2.2.3 (http://https://www.dtu.ox.ac.uk/homacalculator/) [29]. GDM was diagnosed according to the WHO1999 (FPG ≥7.0 mmol/l and/or 2-h glucose ≥7.8 mmol/l) and the adapted WHO2013 (FPG ≥5.1 and/or 2-h glucose ≥8.5 mmol/l) criteria (ref). The clinical characteristics of subjects are shown in Table 1.

Genotyping

DNA was extracted from frozen and stored buffy coats using (QIAGEN Autopure LS kits. Six SNPs previously associated with GDM or T2D in India [21, 22, 26, 27, 30] (Additional file 2: Table S1) and 79 SNPs previously associated with T2D in Europe and elsewhere from GWAS studies up to 2012 (some of these also with GDM risk from candidate gene studies in GDM populations) were genotyped in the present study (Additional file 2: Table

Table 1 Study population characteristics

	N	Mean	±SD	N	Mean	±SD	N	Mean	±SD	N	Mean	±SD	N	Mean	±SD
				GDM1999			Controls			GDM2013			Controls		
Age (years)	4018	21.41	3.40	346	21.11	3.59	3672	21.44	3.38	1386	21.68	3.5	2632	21.27	3.34
BMI	4018	24.11	4.34	346	24.28	4.71	3672	24.09	4.30	1386	24.36	4.48	2632	23.97	4.25
Fasting plasma glucose (mmol/l)	4018	4.81	0.76	346	5.53	1.32	3672	4.74	0.65	1386	5.51	0.69	2632	4.44	0.49
Plasma insulin (pmol)	4018	54.25	61.86	346	46.73	42.24	3672	54.96	63.35	1386	52.74	54.44	2632	55.05	65.43
2 h glucose (venous, mmol/l)	4018	6.20	1.37	346	9.15	1.83	3672	5.93	0.92	1386	6.85	1.70	2632	5.86	1.00
homa2_b with steady state glucose and insulin values	3680	104.02	55.71	346	78.01	37.56	3672	106.36	56.49	1386	77.37	38.02	2632	117.92	58.36
homa2_ir with steady state glucose and insulin values	3680	0.97	0.74	346	0.96	0.73	3672	0.97	0.74	1386	1.02	0.79	2632	0.95	0.71

S1) [14] on a Sequenom Mass ARRAY Platform (Sequenom San Diego, CA, USA) PLEX using MALDI-TOF mass spectrometer [31] or Taqman allelic discrimination assays using an ABI Prism 7900 sequence detection system (Applied Biosystems, Foster City, CA, USA). Genotyping was performed at the Lund University Diabetes Centre, Sweden after obtaining permission from ICMR (dated 21 october 2010 and Office of Drugs Controller General (India)(dated 14/12/2010).

Replication genotyping of 6% of the samples showed > 98% concordance. rs6467136, and rs7202877 had a Hardy-Weinberg equilibrium (HWE) p-value of < 0.001 in unaffected women based on WHO1999 criteria and < 0.05 in unaffected women based on WHO2013 criteria and were hence removed from the analysis.

Statistical analyses

Association of selected SNPs with risk of GDM was assessed by logistic regression analysis adjusted for maternal age and BMI and results presented as ORs with 95% confidence intervals (CI). We also tested for associations with fasting and 2-h glucose values as well as with fasting insulin and HOMA2-B and HOMA2-IR (Additional file 2: Table S1) using linear regression analysis with maternal age and BMI as covariates. Individuals with missing data were excluded. Data were logarithmically transformed before analysis. The power to detect association with GDM2013 including 1386 GDM women and 2632 controls at $p < 0.0006$ (0.05/79) (after Bonferroni correction) for a SNP allele frequency of 0.3 and effect size 1.3 was 0.97, which decreased to 0.64 for effect size 1.2 under an additive model. For GDM1999, with 346 GDM and 3672 controls, the corresponding figures were 0.39 and 0.12 respectively. For association with quantitative glucose traits, power to detect association was 1 at alpha 0.05 for and allele frequency of 0.3 [32, 33]. A p-value of ≤0.05 was considered statistically significant on account of the current analyses being replication of previously published associations.

Genetic risk scores for insulin secretion (HOMA-2B) and insulin resistance (HOMA-2IR) were calculated using SNPs previously associated with insulin secretion and insulin resistance. SNPs were assessed for linkage disequilibrium (LD) and for those in high LD (r^2), only one representative SNP was retained. Individual scores were calculated based on number of risk alleles weighed by their effect sizes reported in previous GWAS studies and logistic regression was performed against normalized measures of insulin secretion and insulin resistance.

All calculations were implemented in STATA, plink 1.09 and SPSS v22.0.

Results

Among the 4018 genotyped women, applying the WHO2013 criteria resulted in a total of 1386 women with GDM (34.5%) whereas the number was reduced to 346 (8.6%) when WHO1999 criteria were used. Notably, only 283 (7.0%) women were diagnosed using both GDM 2013 and GDM 1999 criteria (Additional file 1: Figure S1) [34]. This is concordant with our previously published reports on the larger subset of the same population comprising 5100 women [28]. HOMA2-B was lower in GDM women defined by both criteria compared to pregnant normal glucose tolerant women (PNGT). HOMA2-IR was also higher in women with GDM2013 who thereby were more insulin resistant than PNGT (Table 1).

SNPs previously associated with GDM/T2D in India

None of the 8 SNPs previously associated with GDM or T2D in Indian populations was here associated with GDM (Table 2). However, analysis for association with GDM1999 or GDM 2013 against controls who did not satisfy either criterion revealed the nominal association of rs7756992 in *CDKAL1* while rs689 in *INS* showed a trend towards association with GDM2013 (Table 3).

Table 2 Association of previously reported GDM and T2D loci from Indian population based studies with risk of GDM according to both criteria

Genotype	EA	Chr	Gene/nearest gene	Location	OR_WHO1999	lower CI	upper CI	p_who1999	OR_WHO2013	lower CI	upper CI	p_who2013	n
rs998451	A	2	TMEM163	intron	0.987	0.795	1.224	0.902	0.959	0.843	1.09	0.518	3882
rs1799999	A	7	PPP1R3A	missense	0.862	0.728	1.02	0.083	0.997	0.905	1.098	0.953	3890
rs689	A	11	INS	5'UTR	1.077	0.879	1.319	0.474	1.033	0.914	1.167	0.603	3903
rs9552911	A	13	SGCG	intron	1.057	0.83	1.347	0.653	1.017	0.875	1.183	0.824	3890
rs4812829	A	20	HNF4A	intron	1.04	0.871	1.24	0.667	0.988	0.89	1.096	0.814	3801
rs7178572	G	15	HMG20A	intron	0.988	0.832	1.173	0.891	1.017	0.921	1.122	0.743	3541
rs7756992	G	6	CDKAL 1	intron	0.91	0.75	1.1	0.34	0.97	0.87	1.08	0.64	3686
rs7754840	C	6	CDKAL1	intron	0.87	0.72	1.06	0.17	0.96	0.86	1.07	0.51	3721

EA effect allele, *OR_WHO1999* odds ratio based on WHO1999 criteria, *OR_WHO2013* Odds ratio based on WHO2013 criteria, *CI* confidence interval

Previously reported GDM risk loci

Out of 12 selected previously reported GDM risk loci, the T allele of the missense SNP rs5219 in the *KCNJ11* gene was nominally associated with GDM1999 ($p = 0.019$) (Table 4). Contrary to previous reports, the risk allele A of SNP rs11708067 in the *ADCY5* gene showed reduced risk for GDM defined by 2013 ($p = 0.037$) (Table 4) but not by 1999 criteria. The SNP rs2796441 in the *TLE1* gene was associated with decreased insulin secretion ($p = 0.013$) (Additional file 2: Table S2). The rs13266634 at *SLC30A8* locus associated with GDM1999 while SNPs rs5219 in *KCNJ11* and rs11708067 in *ADCY5* associated with GDM2013 nominally when controls satisfying neither GDM diagnosis criteria were considered (Table 3).

Previously reported T2D loci

The risk allele C of SNP rs13389219 in the *GRB14* gene was associated with GDM1999 ($p = 0.022$) (Table 5) but not with GDM2013 ($p = 0.058$) (Table 5). The T2D risk allele T of SNP rs11920090 in the intron of the *SLC2A2* gene was associated with GDM2013 ($p = 0.030$) (Table 5).

Surprisingly, the T2D risk allele A of SNP rs11605924 in the *CRY2* gene was associated with reduced risk of GDM1999 ($p = 0.025$) (Table 5). The same variant associated with GDM1999 in a sensitivity analysis when controls meeting neither GDM diagnosis criteria were considered (Table 3). In support of this, the same allele was also associated with lower 2-h glucose levels ($p = 0.038$) (Additional file 2: Table S3).

Table 3 Association of previously reported GDM loci with risk of GDM according to both criteria

SNP	EA	Chr	Gene/nearest gene	Location	WHO 1999				WHO 2013				n
					OR	CI(lower)	CI(upper)	*p*-value	OR	CI(lower)	CI(upper)	*p*-value	
rs9939609	A	16	FTO	intron	1.04	0.86	1.26	0.67	0.98	0.88	1.10	0.83	3120
rs2796441	G	9	TLE 1	intergenic	0.99	0.84	1.16	0.92	1.07	0.97	1.17	0.15	3905
rs560887	C	2	G6PC2/ABCB11	intron	1.18	0.92	1.52	0.19	1.11	0.96	1.28	0.13	3910
rs11708067	A	3	ADCY5	intron	0.98	0.81	1.18	0.86	0.88	0.79	0.99	**0.037**	3877
rs1111875	C	10	HHEX	intergenic	0.90	0.77	1.06	0.22	1.05	0.96	1.16	0.24	3901
rs10811661	T	9	CDKN2A/2B	intergenic	0.99	0.77	1.26	0.93	1.08	0.94	1.25	0.23	3890
rs4402960	T	3	IGF2BP2	intron	1.02	0.87	1.20	0.77	0.95	0.86	1.04	0.29	3750
rs13266634	C	8	SLC30A8	coding-missense	0.96	0.79	1.17	0.75	0.97	0.87	1.08	0.61	3898
rs7903146	T	10	TCF7L2	Intronic/promoter	1.13	0.95	1.35	0.14	1.01	0.916	1.12	0.76	3543
rs10830963	G	11	MTNR1B	intron	0.89	0.75	1.05	0.20	0.98	0.89	1.08	0.69	3714
rs1801282	C	3	PPARG	Coding-missense	0.86	0.89	1.12	0.22	0.99	0.93	1.08	0.21	3652
rs10010131	G	4	WFS1	intron	1.13	0.95	1.36	0.16	0.99	0.90	1.10	0.99	3843
rs5219	T	11	KCNJ11	coding-missense	1.21	1.03	1.42	**0.019**	1.00	0.90	1.10	0.99	3595

EA effect allele, *OR_WHO1999* odds ratio based on WHO1999 criteria, *OR_WHO2013* Odds ratio based on WHO2013 criteria, *CI* confidence interval
significant *p* values where $p < 0.05$ are indicated in bold

Table 4 Association of previously reported T2D loci with risk of GDM according to both criteria

SNP	EA	Chr	Gene/nearest gene	Location	WHO 1999				WHO 2013				n
					OR	CI(lower)	CI(upper)	p-value	OR	CI(lower)	CI(upper)	p-value	
rs2296172	G	1	MACF1	coding-missense	0.92	0.71	1.20	0.56	1.04	0.89	1.21	0.58	3847
rs340874	C	1	PROX1	intergenic	0.94	0.80	1.11	0.52	0.96	0.87	1.06	0.47	3709
rs7578597	T	2	THADA	coding-missense	0.90	0.72	1.12	0.37	0.92	0.80	1.06	0.27	3710
rs243088	T	2	BCL 11A	intergenic	1.10	0.94	1.29	0.22	1.07	0.97	1.18	0.15	3717
rs7593730	T	2	RBMS1/ITGB6	intronic	1.01	0.84	1.22	0.83	0.99	0.88	1.11	0.93	3906
rs7607980	C	2	COBLL1	coding-missense	0.95	0.73	1.24	0.75	0.95	0.81	1.11	0.52	3885
rs13389219	C	2	GRB14	intergenic	1.25	1.03	1.52	**0.022**	1.11	0.99	1.23	0.058	3829
rs7578326	A	2	KIAA1486/IRS1	intron of uncharacterized LOC646736	0.97	0.80	1.18	0.78	0.98	0.87	1.10	0.79	3600
rs2943641	C	2	IRS1	intergenic	0.92	0.76	1.12	0.43	0.97	0.87	1.09	0.67	3643
rs4675095	A	2	IRS1	intron	1.11	0.87	1.42	0.39	1.04	0.90	1.19	0.58	3817
rs831571	C	3	PSMD6	intergenic	1.02	0.84	1.25	0.77	0.93	0.83	1.05	0.26	3726
rs4607103	C	3	ADAMTS9-AS2	intron	1.14	0.98	1.33	0.08	1.00	0.91	1.09	0.97	3884
rs11920090	T	3	SLC2A2	intron	1.19	0.93	1.51	0.16	1.16	1.01	1.33	**0.03**	3606
rs6815464	C	4	MAEA	intron	1.04	0.83	1.30	0.71	1.03	0.90	1.18	0.64	3722
rs459193	G	5	ANKRD55	intergenic	0.99	0.84	1.16	0.90	1.07	0.97	1.18	0.16	3884
rs4457053	G	5	ZBED3	intron of ZBED3-AS1	1.05	0.86	1.29	0.57	0.95	0.84	1.07	0.45	3579
rs9470794	C	6	ZFAND3	intron	1.07	0.85	1.35	0.51	1.05	0.91	1.21	0.48	3608
rs17168486	T	7	DGKB	intergenic	0.99	0.83	1.17	0.92	0.97	0.88	1.07	0.62	3855
rs2191349	T	7	DGKB/TMEM195	intergenic	1.04	0.88	1.22	0.62	1.00	0.91	1.10	0.95	3903
rs864745	T	7	JAZF1	intron	0.98	0.83	1.16	0.87	1.02	0.92	1.13	0.68	3876
rs4607517	A	7	GCK	intergenic	1.04	0.82	1.32	0.70	1.01	0.88	1.16	0.86	3903
rs17133918	C	7	GRB10	intron	1.03	0.87	1.23	0.67	0.97	0.88	1.08	0.65	3907
rs933360	A	7	GRB10	intron	1.03	0.87	1.22	0.70	1.03	0.93	1.14	0.54	3905
rs6943153	C	7	GRB10	intron	0.86	0.73	1.03	0.11	0.95	0.86	1.05	0.36	3602
rs516946	C	8	ANK1	intron	1.01	0.82	1.23	0.91	1.09	0.97	1.23	0.13	3922
rs896854	T	8	TP53INP1	intron	0.97	0.83	1.14	0.75	0.97	0.88	1.06	0.57	3903
rs7034200	A	9	GLIS3	intron	0.98	0.83	1.15	0.84	1.03	0.93	1.13	0.52	3868
rs13292136	C	9	TLE4 (CHCHD9)	intergenic	0.94	0.75	1.18	0.62	0.98	0.86	1.12	0.79	3706
rs12571751	A	10	ZMIZ1	intron	0.86	0.73	1.01	0.07	0.96	0.87	1.06	0.49	3601
rs553668	A	10	ADRA2A	UTR-3	1.17	0.99	1.39	0.06	1.07	0.97	1.19	0.15	3666
rs10885122	G	10	ADRA2A	intergenic	1.03	0.84	1.27	0.75	1.05	0.93	1.18	0.42	3683
rs163184	G	11	KCNQ1	intron	0.90	0.76	1.07	0.23	1.00	0.90	1.10	0.98	3713
rs2237895	C	11	KCNQ1	intron	0.96	0.81	1.13	0.66	1.01	0.92	1.11	0.79	3682
rs11605924	A	11	CRY2	intron	0.84	0.72	0.97	**0.025**	1.00	0.92	1.10	0.85	3909
rs7944584	A	11	MADD	intron	0.91	0.74	1.13	0.41	1.09	0.96	1.23	0.15	3553
rs174550	T	11	FADS1	intron	0.94	0.76	1.17	0.62	0.96	0.85	1.09	0.56	3908
rs1552224	A	11	CENTD2	intergenic	0.92	0.75	1.13	0.45	0.81	0.72	0.92	**0.001**	3911
rs11063069	G	12	CCND2	intergenic	0.99	0.80	1.23	0.98	1.04	0.91	1.19	0.52	3671
rs10842994	C	12	KLHDC5	intergenic	1.13	0.89	1.44	0.28	0.97	0.84	1.11	0.67	3906
rs1153188	A	12	DCD	intergenic	1.15	0.93	1.42	0.19	1.01	0.89	1.14	0.82	3912
rs1531343	C	12	HMGA2	intron of pseudogene	0.83	0.67	1.03	0.09	0.90	0.80	1.02	0.10	3915
rs7961581	C	12	TSPAN8,LGR5	intergenic	0.91	0.77	1.08	0.31	1.02	0.92	1.13	0.61	3703

Table 4 Association of previously reported T2D loci with risk of GDM according to both criteria *(Continued)*

SNP	EA	Chr	Gene/nearest gene	Location	WHO 1999				WHO 2013				n
					OR	CI(lower)	CI(upper)	p-value	OR	CI(lower)	CI(upper)	p-value	
rs7957197	T	12	OASL/TCF1/HNF1A	intron of QASL	0.87	0.65	1.17	0.37	1.00	0.83	1.21	0.96	3924
rs17271305	G	15	VPS13C	intron	1.02	0.86	1.20	0.81	0.92	0.83	1.02	0.15	3825
rs11071657	A	15	FAM148B	intergenic	1.03	0.87	1.22	0.72	0.92	0.83	1.02	0.13	3897
rs7177055	A	15	HMG20A	intergenic	1.00	0.85	1.17	0.99	0.98	0.89	1.08	0.74	3907
rs35767	G	12	IGF1	nearGene-5	0.88	0.91	1.10	0.19	0.93	0.94	1.06	0.21	3910
rs11634397	G	15	ZFAND6	intergenic	0.89	0.76	1.04	0.16	0.96	0.87	1.06	0.47	3910
rs8042680	A	15	PRC1	intron	0.89	0.76	1.04	0.16	0.99	0.90	1.10	0.95	3887
rs8090011	G	18	LAMA1	intron	0.95	0.81	1.11	0.57	0.93	0.84	1.02	0.13	3911
rs10401969	C	19	SUGP1	intron	0.96	0.72	1.27	0.79	0.86	0.72	1.01	**0.07**	3605
rs8108269	G	19	GIPR	intergenic	1.02	0.85	1.23	0.77	1.07	0.96	1.19	0.16	3508
rs10423928	A	19	GIPR	intron	0.85	0.67	1.08	0.20	1.06	0.93	1.20	0.37	3911
rs6017317	G	20	FITM2-R3HDML-HNF4A	intergenic	0.96	0.81	1.13	0.64	0.98	0.89	1.08	0.72	3758
rs5945326	A	X	DUSP9	intergenic	0.95	0.81	1.12	0.58	1.01	0.92	1.12	0.74	3589

EA effect allele, *OR_WHO1999* odds ratio based on WHO1999 criteria, *OR_WHO2013* Odds ratio based on WHO2013 criteria, *CI* confidence interval
significant p values where p < 0.05 are indicated in bold

The risk allele A of SNP rs1552224 in the *CENTD2* locus was associated with decreased risk of GDM2013 (*p* = 0.001) (Table 5).

Association with insulin secretion and insulin resistance
Twelve SNPs previously associated with insulin secretion were here tested for association with HOMA2-B. The T2D risk allele A of rs11071657 at the *FAM148B* locus was nominally associated with increased insulin secretion (*p* = 0.044) (Table 6). A GRS comprising of 3 previously reported insulin secretion loci with the lowest *p*-values for insulin secretion in the present study associated with insulin secretion in the present study (*p* = 0.008, beta = 0.25, SE = 0.098). GRS for insulin secretion did not associate

with either GDM2013 (*p* = 0.15, beta = − 0.06, SE = 0.045) or GDM1999 (*p* = 0.73, beta = − 0.009, SE = 0.026).

Of 6 SNPs previously associated with measures of insulin resistance, 3 SNPs here associated with HOMA2-IR. The C allele of rs7607980 in the *COBLL1* gene was associated with decreased HOMA2-IR (*p* = 0.0001). The C allele of rs13389219 near *GRB14* (*p* = 0.026) and A allele of rs10423928 in the intron of the *GIPR* gene (*p* = 0.012) showed worse insulin resistance (increased HOMA2-IR; Table 7). Genetic risk scores (GRS) calculated based on the 3 SNPs associated with insulin resistance showed an increase of insulin resistance by 0.07 (SE = 0.145, *p* = 0.006) per allele. GRS for insulin resistance showed a trend towards GDM2013

Table 5 Sensitivity analysis for association of selected risk variants with GDM risk

SNP	EA	Chr	Gene/ nearest gene	Location	WHO 1999					WHO 2013				n
					OR	CI(lower)	CI(upper)	p-value	n	OR	CI(lower)	CI(upper)	p-value	
rs13266634[a]	T	8	SLC30A8	coding-missense	1.24	1.01	1.53	**0.037**	2834	1.049	0.91	1.21	0.50	3837
rs11605924	A	11	CRY2	intron	0.84	0.71	0.99	**0.038**	2833	1.005	0.91	1.10	0.91	3848
rs35767	T	12	IGF1	nearGene-5	1.26	1.00	1.60	0.054	2837	1.15	0.98	1.33	0.07	3848
rs5219[a]	T	11	KCNJ11	coding -missense	1.18	1.00	1.40	0.059	2605	1.00	0.91	1.11	0.91	3539
rs11708067[a]	G	3	ADCY5	intron	1.11	0.86	1.44	0.42	2810	1.25	1.09	1.45	**0.002**	3816
rs689[a]	A	11	INS	Promoter/intron	0.91	0.64	1.29	0.60	2835	0.81	0.65	1.00	0.054	3842
rs8108269	G	19	GIPR	intergenic	1.14	0.94	1.36	0.17	2568	1.12	0.99	1.25	0.059	3449
rs7756992[a]	G	6	CDKAL1	intron	0.96	0.76	1.19	0.69	2670	2.80	1.00	7.87	**0.049**	3626

[a]indicates loci previously associated with GDM / T2D in India or GDM in studies based on the European population
Logistic regression was performed on GDM cases diagnosed according to WHO1999 and WHO2013 criteria against controls who had no GDM diagnosis using either criteria
significant p values where p < 0.05 are indicated in bold

Table 6 Association of selected loci with insulin secretion (HOMA2-B)

SNP	EA	Chr	Gene/nearest gene	Location	Beta	SE	p-value	N
rs340874	C	1	PROX1	intergenic	0.009	0.011	0.388	3395
rs560887	C	2	G6PC2/ABCB11	intron	−0.004	0.016	0.818	3578
rs11708067	A	3	ADCY5	intron	−0.024	0.012	0.053	3556
rs11920090	T	3	SLC2A2	intron	−0.014	0.015	0.361	3301
rs4607517	A	7	GCK	intergenic	0.007	0.012	0.571	3372
rs2191349	T	7	DGKB/TMEM195	intergenic	−0.008	0.011	0.480	3575
rs7034200	A	9	GLIS3	intron	0.002	0.016	0.922	3576
rs10885122	G	10	ADRA2A	intergenic	−0.006	0.010	0.546	3545
rs7944584	A	11	MADD	intron	−0.021	0.013	0.116	3372
rs7903146	T	10	TCF7L2	Intronic/promoter	0.003	0.011	0.798	3240
rs10830963	G	11	MTNR1B	intron	−0.007	0.011	0.473	3398
rs174550	T	11	FADS1	intron	0.011	0.014	0.435	3248
rs7756992	G	6	CDKAL1	intron	0.011	0.014	0.446	3576
rs11071657	A	15	FAM148B	intergenic	−0.023	0.011	**0.044**	3568

significant p values where p < 0.05 are indicated in bold

(p = 0.065, beta = 0.076, SE = 0.04) but not GDM1999 (p = 0.14, beta = 0.023, SE = 0.025).

Discussion

In this large study, we investigated the genetic basis of gestational diabetes mellitus in Punjabi Indian women [15, 16, 19, 27].

Surprisingly, the genetic variants in the *HMG20A* and *HNF4A* genes which previously have been associated with risk of T2D and GDM in South India [27] were not associated with GDM or T2D in Punjabi pregnant women. This could be due to differences in allele frequencies between the North and South Indian populations, which are ethnically quite distinctive populations [35]. The Punjabi Indian population belongs to the "Ancestral North Indians" group and shares genetic similarities with populations from Middle East, Central Asia and to some degree Europe whereas the South Indian population genetically belongs to the distinct "Ancestral South Indian" group [35]. Notably the *CDKAL1* variant associated with GDM only when a sensitivity analysis was performed using controls that had no GDM diagnosis using either GDM1999 or GDM2013 criteria, thus replicating a previous association.

Neither did we observe associations with loci associated with GDM elsewhere including variants in the *CDKAL1* and *MTNR1B* loci, which have been reported to be associated with GDM in South Korea [19]. A sensitivity analysis using controls that had no GDM diagnosis using either criterion revealed the nominal association of variants in *SLC30A8*, *KCNJ11* and *ADCY5*. These largely negative findings could be attributed to population-based differences. Previous studies have indicated differences in anthropometry between Indian and

European populations, with the former manifesting a "thin-fat" phenotype [36]. Subsequently, it is possible that since most T2D loci were identified in European ancestry cohorts, the negative findings could reflect differences in tagging SNPs due to differences haplotypes between populations. On the other hand, the underlying etiology of GDM could also be different genetically. While the study population is the largest GDM study till date, this might lack sufficient power to detect genome-wide significance levels of association with an unstable phenotype. The effect sizes of previously reported T2D loci were low, generally under odds ratios of 1.2, therefore the study was not sufficiently powered to demonstrate association of SNPs with such low effect sizes. Alternately, considering the lack of consensus for GDM diagnosis criteria worldwide, it is plausible that this could be due to different thresholds that might apply for the Indian population.

Notably, T2D risk variants in the *CRY2* (WHO1999), *CENTD2* (WHO2013) and the *ADCY5* (WHO2013) genes were here protective for GDM. *CRY2* encodes for the cryptochrome protein involved in the regulation of the circadian clock. Risk allele carriers of the rs11708067 SNP in *ADCY5* has previously been shown to reduce *ADCY5* expression in pancreatic beta cells and important for coupling glucose to insulin secretion in human islets [37]. It has been previously shown that T2D risk alleles show extreme directional differentiation across various populations, with T2D risk alleles decreasing in frequency along human migration into East Asia [38]. Such flip-flops of risk alleles may be explained by population differences, possibly due to genetics or environment. Alternately, such "flip-flop" associations have also been attributed to multi-locus effects as shown from

Table 7 Association with HOMA-IR selected loci: insulin resistance SNPs

SNP	EA	Chr	Gene/nearest gene	Location	Beta	SE	p-value	N
rs2943641	C	2	IRS1	intergenic	−0.001	0.014	0.923	3337
rs4675095	A	2	IRS1	intron	−0.028	0.017	0.102	3500
rs4607517	A	7	GCK	intergenic	0.018	0.018	0.299	3576
rs7607980	C	2	COBLL1	coding-missense	0.070	0.019	**0.0001**	3557
rs13389219	C	2	GRB14	intergenic	0.029	0.013	**0.026**	3518
rs10423928	A	19	GIPR	intron	0.041	0.016	**0.012**	3585

significant p values where p < 0.05 are indicated in bold

theoretical modeling studies demonstrating that the direction of allelic effect may flip when tested allele is inversely correlated with another risk allele at another locus, or positively correlated with a protective allele at another locus [39].

A HWE threshold of < 0.001 in unaffected individuals based in either criteria was set as a cut-off; SNPs showing significant deviations from HWE should be interpreted with caution, since these could be indicative of population substructures, inbreeding or selection. The current study only comprises genotyping data from candidate SNPs which do not provide sufficient coverage of the genome to detail population stratification or inbreeding. HWE could also be indicative of actual association. A serious problem in the study of the genetics of GDM is the implementation of different criteria, since some women could be classified as controls based on different criteria. For SNP rs5219 in *KCNJ11* (HWE p = 0.004, WHO1999; HWE p = 0.01, WHO2013) and rs11605924 in *CRY2* (HWE p = 0.007 WHO1999 and HWE p = 0.06, WHO2013), HWE values were nominally significant for the same criteria where an association was observed; these findings need to be replicated in independent cohorts.

Of 6 loci previously associated with insulin resistance, here 3 also showed an association with HOMA2-IR and a trend towards significance for GDM2013 but not GDM1999 including SNPs rs7607980 in the *COBLL1* gene [40], rs13389219 near *GRB14* and rs10423928 in the *GIPR* gene indicating that some of the genetic basis seem to be driven by previously reported insulin resistance loci. Similarly, a GRS with the 3 variants with the lowest p-values for insulin secretion associated with insulin secretion but not GDM2013 or GDM1999.

Taken together, the results demonstrate that GDM in women from Punjab in Northern India shows a genetic component, partially shared with GDM in other parts of the world, and seems to be driven by both insulin resistance and secretion. However, the direction of the effect can differ; some T2D risk variants were indicative of being protective for GDM in these Indian women.

Conclusions

GDM in women from Punjab in Northern India shows a genetic component shared with T2D. This genetic basis is seemingly driven by a complex interplay between insulin secretion and sensitivity during pregnancy and is at least partly shared with GDM in other parts of the world. Interestingly some of the T2D risk variants in *ADCY5* and *CRY2* were protective against GDM. Most of the previous T2D loci discovered in European studies did not associate with GDM in North India. Interestingly some T2D risk variants were in fact indicative of being protective for GDM in these Indian women. This could be attributed to different genetic etiology or differences in the LD structure between populations in which the associated SNPs were identified and Northern Indian women. GWAS or whole genome sequencing will be interesting to further unravel the genetic basis of GDM in India.

Abbreviations
GDM: Gestational diabetes mellitus; GRS: Genetic risk score; GWAS: Genome wide association study; HOMA2: Homeostatic model assessment; HOMA2-B: Homeostatic model assessment for insulin secretion; HOMA2-IR: Homeostatic model assessment for insulin resistance; LD: Linkage disequilibrium; OGTT: Oral glucose tolerance test; SNP: Single nucleotide polymorphism; T2D: Type 2 diabetes

Acknowledgements
We wish to thank the World Diabetes Foundation for providing a database in Punjab, India and Mr. Raman Gautam for coordinating screening and sampling, Dr. Baldeep and his team from Deep Hospital, Ludhiana, India for providing the infrastructure for the study and the government health authorities of Punjab for supporting the study. We gratefully acknowledge Gabriella Gremsperger, Maria Sterner, Malin Neptin and Jasmina Kravic for their technical assistance, sampling and organization of data. Finally, we thank all the participating pregnant women in the study.

Funding
Funding was received from the World Diabetes Foundation, Denmark, the Danish Strategic Research Council, Novo Nordisk Foundation, the Augustinus Foundation, Center for Physical Activity Research and by Deep Hospital and Ved Nursing Home and Eye Hospital, Ludhiana, India, Sydvästra Skånes Diabetesförening, the Swedish Research Council, Hospital Region of Region Skåne, the Swedish Research Council Networking Grant and the European Research Council.

Authors' contributions

GPA, PA, CB and RPB researched data, and reviewed/edited the manuscript. GPA, RT, RPB, and AAV acquired data. RPB, GPA, AAV, RT, LG contributed to study design and reviewed/edited the manuscript. LG and AAV contributed to the discussion and extensively reviewed/edited the manuscript. All authors have read and approved the manuscript. RPB wrote the manuscript. RPB and LG take responsibility for the contents of the article.

Competing interests

AAV is employed at the Translational Research and Early Clinical Development, Cardiovascular and Metabolic Research, AstraZeneca, Mölndal, Sweden, On behalf of all the authors, Dr. Prasad B has nothing to disclose.

Author details

[1]Deep Hospital, Ludhiana, Punjab, India. [2]Department of Clinical Sciences, Clinical Research Centre, Lund University, Malmö, Sweden. [3]Department of Endocrinology (Diabetes and Metabolism), Rigshospitalet, Copenhagen, Denmark. [4]Finnish Institute of Molecular Medicine (FIMM), Helsinki University, Helsinki, Finland. [5]Cardiovascular and Metabolic Disease (CVMD) Translational Medicine Unit, Early Clinical Development, IMED Biotech Unit, AstraZeneca, Gothenburg, Sweden.

References

1. Freinkel N. Banting Lecture 1980. Of pregnancy and progeny. Diabetes. 1980;29(12):1023–35.
2. Freinkel N. Gestational diabetes 1979: philosophical and practical aspects of a major public health problem. Diabetes Care. 1980;3(3):399–401.
3. National Diabetes Data Group. Classification and diagnosis of diabetes mellitus and other categories of glucose intolerance. Diabetes. 1979;28(12): 1039–57.
4. Engelgau MM, et al. The epidemiology of diabetes and pregnancy in the U. S., 1988. Diabetes Care. 1995;18(7):1029–33.
5. Jovanovic L, Pettitt DJ. Gestational diabetes mellitus. JAMA. 2001;286(20): 2516–8.
6. Metzger BE. Summary and recommendations of the third international workshop-conference on gestational diabetes mellitus. Diabetes. 1991; 40(Suppl 2):197–201.
7. Kalra S, Malik S, John M. Gestational diabetes mellitus: a window of opportunity. Indian J Endocrinol Metab. 2011;15(3):149–51.
8. Arora GP, et al. Prevalence and risk factors of gestational diabetes in Punjab, North India: results from a population screening program. Eur J Endocrinol. 2015;173(2):257–67.
9. Kim C, et al. Does frank diabetes in first-degree relatives of a pregnant woman affect the likelihood of her developing gestational diabetes mellitus or nongestational diabetes? Am J Obstet Gynecol. 2009;201(6):576 e1–6.
10. Robitaille J, Grant AM. The genetics of gestational diabetes mellitus: evidence for relationship with type 2 diabetes mellitus. Genet Med. 2008; 10(4):240–50.
11. Buchanan TA, Xiang AH. Gestational diabetes mellitus. J Clin Invest. 2005; 115(3):485–91.
12. Martin AO, et al. Frequency of diabetes mellitus in mothers of probands with gestational diabetes: possible maternal influence on the predisposition to gestational diabetes. Am J Obstet Gynecol. 1985;151(4):471–5.
13. Williams MA, et al. Familial aggregation of type 2 diabetes and chronic hypertension in women with gestational diabetes mellitus. J Reprod Med. 2003;48(12):955–62.
14. Prasad RB, Groop L. Genetics of type 2 diabetes-pitfalls and possibilities. Genes (Basel). 2015;6(1):87–123.
15. Lauenborg J, et al. Common type 2 diabetes risk gene variants associate with gestational diabetes. J Clin Endocrinol Metab. 2009;94(1):145–50.
16. Huopio H, et al. Association of risk variants for type 2 diabetes and hyperglycemia with gestational diabetes. Eur J Endocrinol. 2013;169(3):291–7.
17. Mao H, Li Q, Gao S. Meta-analysis of the relationship between common type 2 diabetes risk gene variants with gestational diabetes mellitus. PLoS One. 2012;7(9):e45882.
18. Cho YM, et al. Type 2 diabetes-associated genetic variants discovered in the recent genome-wide association studies are related to gestational diabetes mellitus in the Korean population. Diabetologia. 2009;52(2):253–61.
19. Kwak SH, et al. A genome-wide association study of gestational diabetes mellitus in Korean women. Diabetes. 2012;61(2):531–41.
20. Kim JY, et al. Melatonin receptor 1 B polymorphisms associated with the risk of gestational diabetes mellitus. BMC Med Genet. 2011;12:82.
21. Saxena R, et al. Genome-wide association study identifies a novel locus contributing to type 2 diabetes susceptibility in Sikhs of Punjabi origin from India. Diabetes. 2013;62(5):1746–55.
22. Tabassum R, et al. Genome-wide association study for type 2 diabetes in Indians identifies a new susceptibility locus at 2q21. Diabetes. 2013;62(3): 977–86.
23. Kooner JS, et al. Genome-wide association study in individuals of south Asian ancestry identifies six new type 2 diabetes susceptibility loci. Nat Genet. 2011;43(10):984–9.
24. Radha V, et al. Role of genetic polymorphism peroxisome proliferator-activated receptor-gamma2 Pro12Ala on ethnic susceptibility to diabetes in south-Asian and Caucasian subjects: evidence for heterogeneity. Diabetes Care. 2006;29(5):1046–51.
25. Abate N, et al. ENPP1/PC-1 K121Q polymorphism and genetic susceptibility to type 2 diabetes. Diabetes. 2005;54(4):1207–13.
26. Kanthimathi S, et al. Identification of genetic variants of gestational diabetes in south Indians. Diabetes Technol Ther. 2015;17(7):462–7.
27. Kanthimathi S, et al. Association of recently identified type 2 diabetes gene variants with gestational diabetes in Asian Indian population. Mol Gen Genomics. 2017;292(3):585–91.
28. Arora GP, et al. Insulin secretion and action in north Indian women during pregnancy. Diabet Med. 2017;34(10):1477–82. https://doi.org/10.1111/dme. 13428.
29. Levy JC, Matthews DR, Hermans MP. Correct homeostasis model assessment (HOMA) evaluation uses the computer program. Diabetes Care. 1998;21(12): 2191–2.
30. Sokhi J, et al. Association of genetic variants in INS (rs689), INSR (rs1799816) and PP1G.G (rs1799999) with type 2 diabetes (T2D): a case-control study in three ethnic groups from north-West India. Mol Gen Genomics. 2016;291(1): 205–16.
31. Gabriel S, Ziaugra L, Tabbaa D. SNP genotyping using the Sequenom MassARRAY iPLEX platform. Curr Protoc Hum Genet. 2009;60:2–12. Chapter 2: p. Unit 2 12
32. Skol AD, et al. Joint analysis is more efficient than replication-based analysis for two-stage genome-wide association studies. Nat Genet. 2006;38(2):209–13.
33. Purcell S, Cherny SS, Sham PC. Genetic power calculator: design of linkage and association genetic mapping studies of complex traits. Bioinformatics. 2003;19(1):149–50.
34. Been LF, et al. A low frequency variant within the GWAS locus of MTNR1B affects fasting glucose concentrations: genetic risk is modulated by obesity. Nutr Metab Cardiovasc Dis. 2012;22(11):944–51.
35. Reich D, et al. Reconstructing Indian population history. Nature. 2009; 461(7263):489–94.
36. Yajnik CS. Early life origins of insulin resistance and type 2 diabetes in India and other Asian countries. J Nutr. 2004;134(1):205–10.
37. Hodson DJ, et al. ADCY5 couples glucose to insulin secretion in human islets. Diabetes. 2014;63(9):3009–21.
38. Chen R, et al. Type 2 diabetes risk alleles demonstrate extreme directional differentiation among human populations, compared to other diseases. PLoS Genet. 2012;8(4):e1002621.
39. Lin PI, et al. No gene is an island: the flip-flop phenomenon. Am J Hum Genet. 2007;80(3):531–8.
40. Mancina RM, et al. The COBLL1 C allele is associated with lower serum insulin levels and lower insulin resistance in overweight and obese children. Diabetes Metab Res Rev. 2013;29(5):413–6.

11

Burden of de novo mutations and inherited rare single nucleotide variants in children with sensory processing dysfunction

Elysa Jill Marco[1,2,3*], Anne Brandes Aitken[1], Vishnu Prakas Nair[1], Gilberto da Gente[1], Molly Rae Gerdes[1], Leyla Bologlu[6], Sean Thomas[4] and Elliott H. Sherr[1,3,5]

Abstract

Background: In children with sensory processing dysfunction (SPD), who do not meet criteria for autism spectrum disorder (ASD) or intellectual disability, the contribution of de novo pathogenic mutation in neurodevelopmental genes is unknown and in need of investigation. We hypothesize that children with SPD may have pathogenic variants in genes that have been identified as causing other neurodevelopmental disorders including ASD. This genetic information may provide important insight into the etiology of sensory processing dysfunction and guide clinical evaluation and care.

Methods: Eleven community-recruited trios (children with isolated SPD and both biological parents) underwent WES to identify candidate de novo variants and inherited rare single nucleotide variants (rSNV) in genes previously associated with ASD. Gene enrichment in these children and their parents for transmitted and non-transmitted mutation burden was calculated. A comparison analysis to assess for enriched rSNV burden was then performed in 2377 children with ASD and their families from the Simons Simplex Collection.

Results: Of the children with SPD, 2/11 (18%), were identified as having a de novo loss of function or missense mutation in genes previously reported as causative for neurodevelopmental disorders (MBD5 and FMN2). We also found that the parents of children with SPD have significant enrichment of pathogenic rSNV burden in high-risk ASD candidate genes that are inherited by their affected children. Using the same approach, we confirmed enrichment of rSNV burden in a large cohort of children with autism and their parents but not unaffected siblings.

Conclusions: Our findings suggest that SPD, like autism, has a genetic basis that includes both de novo single gene mutations as well as an accumulated burden of rare inherited variants from their parents.

Keywords: Sensory Processing Disorder, Autism, Neurodevelopment, Genetics, MBD5, FMN2

Background

Sensory processing dysfunction (SPD) affects 5–16% of children and can contribute to long-term impairments in cognition, social development, and family well-being [1–3]. Additionally, hyper and hypo-sensitivity to sound and touch has recently been added to the symptom cluster for Autism Spectrum Disorders (ASD) in the most recent Diagnostic and Statistical Manual, DSM-5

* Correspondence: elysa.marco@ucsf.edu
[1]Department of Neurology, University of California, San Francisco, 675 Nelson Rising Lane, San Francisco, CA 9415, USA
[2]Department of Psychiatry, University of California, San Francisco, 401 Parnassus Ave, San Francisco, CA 94143, USA
Full list of author information is available at the end of the article

[4]. We have recently shown that children with SPD, who do not meet criteria for ASD, have measurable differences in white matter microstructure predominantly in the posterior brain regions, which are critical to sensory perception and processing [5]. We have further demonstrated overlap between these brain findings in children with SPD and children with ASD, suggesting that there is not only a phenotypic overlap between SPD and ASD, but that there may be a mechanistic connection as well [6]. However, in our study, children with ASD have broader neural disruption, including key white matter tracts that subserve language, emotional memory, and processing. Approaches to address ASD mechanisms have

included deep genetic analyses, including whole exome sequencing (WES), demonstrating that loss of function de novo mutations occur in genes that play important roles in neurodevelopmental pathophysiology. This type of rigorous approach to investigate the genetics of SPD remains to be undertaken, despite the growing recognition that SPD can present both as an isolated neurodevelopmental concern as well as a co-morbid condition for children who meet criteria for other behaviorally described conditions in the DSM-5 such as ASD, attention deficit disorders, and anxiety [7–10].

There are, however, some suggestions as to the genetic architecture of SPD. Numerous genetically mediated neurodevelopmental disorders have been reported to show increased sensory sensitivity, including triplet repeat disorders (e.g. Fragile X), chromosomal copy number variations (e.g. Williams syndrome), and single gene disorders (e.g. ARHGEF9) [11–13]. In addition, large population-based twin studies suggest that sensory over-responsivity (SOR) shows moderate heritability across sensory domain with 38% of auditory SOR and 52% of tactile SOR attributed to genetic factors [14].

The search for genes that explain the observed heritability in cognitive and behavioral disorders has been challenging. Despite that, recent WES with large ASD cohorts have shown that loss of function mutations in certain genes occur in 10–15% of patients with a frequency that provides strong statistical evidence for causality in ASD [15]. There is also evidence that ASD patients carry an oligogenic or polygenic combination of variations in "high-risk" neurodevelopment genes, each variant making either a large or small contribution to the phenotype [16, 17]. In fact, it is now posited that as many as 1000 genes can confer risk for ASD [18].

WES technology allows for the investigation of both de novo mutations and inherited risk polymorphisms when sequencing is performed for the index patient and his/her parents. In cohorts of children with intellectual disability or global developmental delay, the diagnostic rate using WES for de novo single gene etiologies was estimated to be 33% [19]. In an initial study of 238 families where only one member has autism, Sanders, et al. 2012 identified 16 loss of function mutations in probands, including nonsense, splice site and frame shift mutations [20]. In a follow up study, integrating both copy number variations and de novo loss of function mutations from WES, Sanders, et al. 2015 report 65 high-risk autism genes which show enrichment in protein-protein interactions and suggest two main sub-networks: chromatin regulation and synaptic control [21]. In this preliminary study, we sought to identify de novo loss of function mutations in children who presented with SPD to investigate monogenic etiologies. We further aimed to test whether there is an increased burden of inherited (or transmitted) rare Single Nucleotide Variants (rSNV) in high- and moderate- risk ASD genes when compared to non-transmitted rare variants in both our preliminary SPD cohort and in the larger ASD family cohort from the Simons Simplex Collection. We hypothesize that, as there are phenotypic and brain structure similarities in children with ASD or SPD, there may also be an overlap in genetic etiologies.

Methods

This genetic cohort study aims to establish the occurrence of de novo missense and loss of function mutations in children with community diagnosed SPD. We further aimed to determine if there is a higher burden of transmitted rSNV in children with SPD and their parents in high and moderate-risk genes associated with ASD.

Characteristics of participants

SPD cohort

We recruited 11 children (7 boys and 4 girls) with SPD and their biologic mother and father. Children were recruited from our existing Sensory Neurodevelopment and Autism Program (SNAP) cohort for whom we have neuroimaging, cognitive, and sensory processing characterization (see Table 1 for demographics). Informed consent was obtained from participants and parents, with assent of all participants from 12 to 18 years of age in accordance with the UCSF Institutional Review Board protocol. Inclusion criteria consist of a "Sensory Processing Disorder" diagnosis made by a community occupational therapist and a score on the Sensory Profile in the "Definite Difference" range (< 2% probability in a typically developing cohort) in one or more of the sensory domains (auditory, visual, oral/olfactory, tactile, vestibular, or multisensory

Table 1 Probands demographics

	SPD cohort +/− Standard deviation [range]
Age	9.8 years +/− 1.3 [8–11]
VCI	121.5 +/− 11.6 [100–138]
PRI	111.5 +/− 16.7 [79–131]
SSP Total	116.4 +/− 18.0 [95–145]
Ethnicity	
Caucasian	8
Hispanic	0
Asian	0
Multiracial/Other	2
Unknown/Declined	1

VCI Verbal Comprehension Index of the Wechsler Intelligence Scale for Children-IV (WISC-IV), *PRI* Perceptual Reasoning Index WISC-IV, *SSP* Short Sensory Profile

processing). The Sensory Profile (Dunn, 1999) is a parent-report questionnaire that characterizes sensory experiences, behavior, and their functional impact. The domain scores were collectively used for differentiation of SPD and typically developing children. Higher scores indicate greater dysfunction. Subjects were excluded if they met research criteria for ASD which begins with screening using the parent report measure, the Social Communication Questionnaire (SCQ- ASD cut-off at 15), and confirmed using the direct assessment measure, the Autism Diagnostic Observation Schedule (ADOS); if they had cognitive impairment as defined as a full scale or performance IQ less than 70; or if they had a brain malformation on MRI, history of stroke or encephalitis, head injury with loss of consciousness > 15 min, multiple sclerosis, movement disorders, psychiatric disorders (e.g. bipolar disorder or schizophrenia), current history of pacemaker, ferromagnetic matter in body, claustrophobia or significant medical illness, premature delivery (gestational age < 36 weeks), or previously diagnosed genetic etiology for their neurodevelopmental condition.

ASD cohort

We included 2377 families (male, $n = 2049$) with ASD from the Simons Simplex Collection (SSC) [22] including 1786 quads and 591 trios. The SSC is overseen by SFARI (Simons Foundation Autism Research Initiative) in collaboration with 12 university-affiliated research clinics. Parents consented and children assented as required by each local institutional review board. Participants were de-identified before data distribution. This resource includes individuals (confirmed to have ASD) and their nuclear family members, with recruitment limited to families in which only a single individual has met research criteria for ASD, including first cousins. The nuclear family also includes an unaffected sibling. Families were excluded if there was intellectual disability or schizophrenia in a sibling or parent. Each proband was evaluated with a detailed battery of assessments including the ADOS; [23])and the Autism Diagnostic Interview-Revised (ADI-R; [24]).

Description of biologic materials
Sample collection

Upon consent to participate in this study, families were directed to the UCSF pediatric phlebotomy lab or a local lab of their choice to obtain ~ 8 ml of whole blood in an ACD tube for processing by the UCSF Genome Core Facility.

DNA preparation

DNA was isolated using the Qiagen Gentra Puregene system. DNA quality was confirmed by standard 260/280 ratios and agarose gel visual inspection. Prior to library generation and exome sequencing, DNA was tested for purity and size using the Agilent Bioanalyzer.

WES

The DNA was fragmented using a Covaris E220 ultra sonicator to a size range of 350-450 bases. After fragmentation, the DNA was processed using the Agilent library preparation kit following the manufacturer's protocol. Exome sequencing was performed using the Nimblegen Human SeqCap EZ Exome (v3.0) kit according to the manufacturer's protocol. This kit targets genes from CCDS.2, Vega, Gencode and Ensembl in addition to microRNA's from miRBase and snoRNABase, for a total of over 20,000 genes and 64 Mb of covered genomic region. This yields an average of > 60× coverage overall for the sequenced bases.

Rare single nucleotide variants (rSNV) analytic pipeline

Our variant analysis follows 'The Broad Institute's Best Practices' guidelines for discovering putative variants and utilizes the Genome Analysis Toolkit (GATK; software version 2014.2-3.1.7-10) in combination with BWA-mem, Picard Tools, and SAM Tools [25–28]. After aligning the DNA read sequences to the GRCh37 reference build using BWA-mem, Picard Tools is used to identify and remove PCR duplicates, add read group information, and sort alignment files using modules Mark Duplicates, SortSam, and AddOrReplaceReadGroups respectively. Subsequently, GATK modules RealignerTarget Creator is used to identify putative indels and IndelRealigner is used to realign around those intervals. Base recalibration is performed using the GATK modules BaseRecalibrator in combination with PrintReads to produce sample specific BAM files. Variant calling is performed using GATK HaplotypeCaller in combination with CombineGVCFs module to produce sample specific gVCF files. These individual patient/parent files are combined, annotated, and genotyped over intervals of interest using GenotypeGVCFs to produce a single project specific VCF file of variants. GATK modules, VariantRecalibrator and ApplyRecalibration are used to add a VQSLOD score (confidence score that estimates the probability that the variant is a true positive) using HapMap 3.3, the Omni 2.5 SNP BeadChip, 1000 Genome, and Mills indels as training sets.

The resulting VCF file is then stored in a MySQL database table with separate rows for each variant and columns representing VCF file format required headers. Each variant in the database is annotated against a reference transcript. For variants falling within coding regions, codon affect is assessed with nonsynonymous identified variants further analyzed using Polyphen-2 for predictive damage. All variants are cross-referenced against public and private datasets to assess population frequency. These include data from the Exome Sequencing Project and 1000 Genomes. Variants are further annotated against UCSC genome tracks as well as external location specific or gene specific datasets. The resulting relational database permits complex initial filtering of variants by protein consequence (synonymous, nonsynonymous, stop, and frameshifts), location (within gene boundaries, exon, boundaries, and splice sites), and confidence score (VQSLOD, polyphen, SIFT, RVIS). Once a subset of variants is identified, sample genotype information can be processed to assess inheritance pattern.

Determination of variant significance

For de novo analysis, variants were required to be missense, indel, or within 3 base pairs of a splice site, have a VQSLOD score greater than 0, and be below a population frequency of 1% (as determined by 1000 Genomes and the Exome Variant Server). In addition, affected genotype quality (GQ) should be greater than 85 and have a minimum of 10 reads with at least 3 showing the alternate variant. Both parents are required to have a GQ greater than 50 and no more than 3 reads showing the alternate variant. For inheritance analysis given computational limitations, we limited our scope to missense variants within ASD or the Coronary Artery Disease (CAD) comparision genes which had a VQSLOD greater than 2 and a population frequency below 1% [29]. Gene lists are included in Additional files 1 and 2. For each gene group, variants were separated into subgroups of transmitted (passed from parent to child) or non-transmitted (not passed from parent to child).

Variant confirmation

De novo variants were first directly examined by inspection of the aligned reads in the proband and both parents using the integrated genomics viewer (IGV). Sanger sequencing using well-established approaches confirmed candidates that remained after this inspection.

Statistical analysis

De novo analysis

All variants were compared to parental samples to determine if they were de novo or inherited from the biological mother or father. We investigated the biological relevance of the affected genes based on human and animal literature reported in the Online Mendelian Inheritance in Man database.

Enrichment analysis

Statistical analysis of enrichment for transmitted and non-transmitted rSNV was conducted using a set of 76

high probability candidate genes linked to ASD from SFARI Gene 2.0 (AutDB) [30]. These high-risk genes were determined using the SFARI Gene database. This database utilizes a human curated biological approach, linking information on autism candidate genes within its original Human Gene Module to corresponding data within diverse modules such as Animal Model, Protein Interaction, Gene Scoring, and Copy Number Variant. Each ASD risk gene is classified in a specific category using a set of annotation rules developed by an advisory board. Seventy-six genes from AutDB (date pull 05.21.15) were determined to be "probably damaging" and were included in the high-risk ASD gene set whereas 292 were categorized as possibly damaging and included as moderate-risk ASD gene set (see Additional files 1 and 2.)

Assuming random draws from the genome, the probability of drawing a mutation from the gene set can be calculated as the sum of transcript lengths in the gene set divided by the total length of the assayed transcriptome. To determine the probability that each individual exhibits a mutation enrichment in a designated gene set (e.g., high-risk autism gene set or moderate-risk autism gene set), the number of gene set-specific mutations was compared to the expected distribution as modeled by the binomial distribution and parameterized by the length-corrected draw probability described above. The resulting probability describes the gene set enrichment score for that individual. To obtain a population level probability, each individual probability was converted into a z-score equivalent, and a Chi Square test was performed with a number of degrees of freedom equal to the number of individuals in the cohort - 1. This overall Chi Square probability describes the population enrichment of mutations in the relevant set of genes. For the ASD/CAD analysis of SSC samples, the analysis was performed as described above, except for computational reasons related to processing data for 8917 samples, a list of 580 CAD genes were used as the background instead of the entire genome.

Results

De novo mutation analysis

We conducted WES in 11 SPD trios. Given the limitation of power with this sample size, we have chosen to conduct this initial analysis by focusing on de novo loss of function and missense mutations. We identified 12 candidate genes with de novo loss of function and/or missense variants in our 11 SPD probands. Among these genes, there were two (18%) de novo mutations (one each, nonsense and missense) in neurodevelopment candidate genes: MBD5 and FMN2. The nonsense mutation in MBD5 leads to a premature termination of the protein at serine 318 (S318X). The missense in FMN2 leads to a proline to leucine amino acid substitution (P927L), which is predicted to have a damaging effect. Based on standards and guidelines for interpretation of sequence variants, the MBD5 de novo loss of function mutation would be considered pathogenic with a very strong evidence of pathogenicity [31]. The FMN2 is also predicted to be pathogenic- however given that it is reported in the ExAC database, the formal clinical interpretation would be a "variant of unclear significance." Nine additional mutations were identified (Table 2). The changes in MBD5, FMN2, DNAH9, KLHL33, MCM2, PFDN6, and SLCO2B1 were confirmed by Sanger sequencing.

Enrichment of rare single nucleotide variants in ASD associated genes

Experiment 1: Burden of rSNV in children with SPD and their parents

Given the literature suggesting strong heritability of sensory over-responsivity and the co-occurrence of sensory processing dysfunction in autism, we sought to determine whether there was a greater than chance inheritance of rSNV from amongst the high and moderate risk ASD candidate genes. We found that the children with SPD show trend level enrichment of inherited high risk ASD rSNV ($p < 0.068$, approximately 1/14 chance of false positive) with all individual children showing the same direction of rSNV burden (i.e. each child inherited greater than 50% of the available deleterious rare alleles in the high probability ASD genes) for this gene set. By contrast, these 11 children did not show an increase burden of variants in the moderate-risk ASD gene set ($p = 0.966$).

Based on the increased burden of inherited rSNV in high risk ASD genes in children with SPD, we sought to explore the burden of variants from amongst the high- and moderate- risk ASD genes in their parents—including variants that were passed to their affected children (transmitted) and those that were not (non-transmitted). The data suggests that parents of children with SPD have a significant enrichment of transmitted variants in the

high-risk ASD genes ($p = < 2.4e\text{-}10$) which exceeds the association for non-transmitted high probability ASD genes ($p = < 0.058$) or transmitted moderate-risk ASD genes ($p < 0.942$; Fig. 1.)

Experiment 2: Burden of rSNV in children with ASD, their parents and unaffected siblings

Based on finding an enriched burden of inherited rare genetic variants, specifically in the high- but not moderate-risk ASD genes in our small SPD cohort, we aimed to determine if this finding was also evident in a large simplex cohort of children with ASD and their parents. In a group of children with ASD, with parents and siblings who do not meet criteria for ASD, we found that the parents and the affected child with ASD show an enhanced burden of inherited/transmitted variants in high-risk candidate ASD genes relative to genes from an unrelated condition, coronary artery disease. By contrast, the unaffected siblings do not show this increase in high-risk candidate ASD genes variants that were transmitted to the proband. Additionally, unaffected parents and siblings do not show an increase in the number of variants in non-transmitted high-risk candidate ASD genes (Fig. 2a). In comparison with the small SPD cohort, the large SSC ASD cohort shows a greater range of variant burden than the SPD cohort. Finally, the SPD cohort has equivalent or greater burden of genetic variants in high-risk ASD genes relative to the ASD group (Fig. 2b).

Discussion

There is growing interest in the etiology of sensory processing dysfunction for individuals with social communication challenges meeting DSM-5 criteria for ASD. This stems in part from the fact that in the current version of the DSM, "hyper- or hyporeactivity to sensory input or unusual interests in sensory aspects of the environment" is now included in the ASD phenotypic criteria. There

Table 2 De novo variance in children with SPD

	PolyPhen2 HVAR score	Mutation type	AA position	AA change	Chromosome position	Base change
MBD5	–	Stop	318	S- > Stop	149,226,465	TCA - > TAA
FMN2	.86	Missense	947	P- > L	240,370,952	CCT - > CTT
DNAH9	.88	Missense	2716	R- > W	11,696,904	CGG - > TGG
KLHL33	.96	Missense	263	R- > W	20,898,048	CGG - > TGG
PFDN6	.99	Missense	62	P- > L	33,258,152	CCG - > CTG
SLCO2B1	1.0	Missense	651	L- > P	74,915,513	CTG - > CCG
MCM2	0	Missense	636	P- > L	127,337,968	CCG - > CTG
TULP4	.06	Missense	1456	G- > R	158,925,061	GGG - > AGG
SPTYD1	.003	Missense	135	N- > S	18,637,417	AAT - > AGT

AA Amino acid, S Serine, P Proline, L Leucine, R Arginine, W Tryptophan, G Glycine, N Asparagine

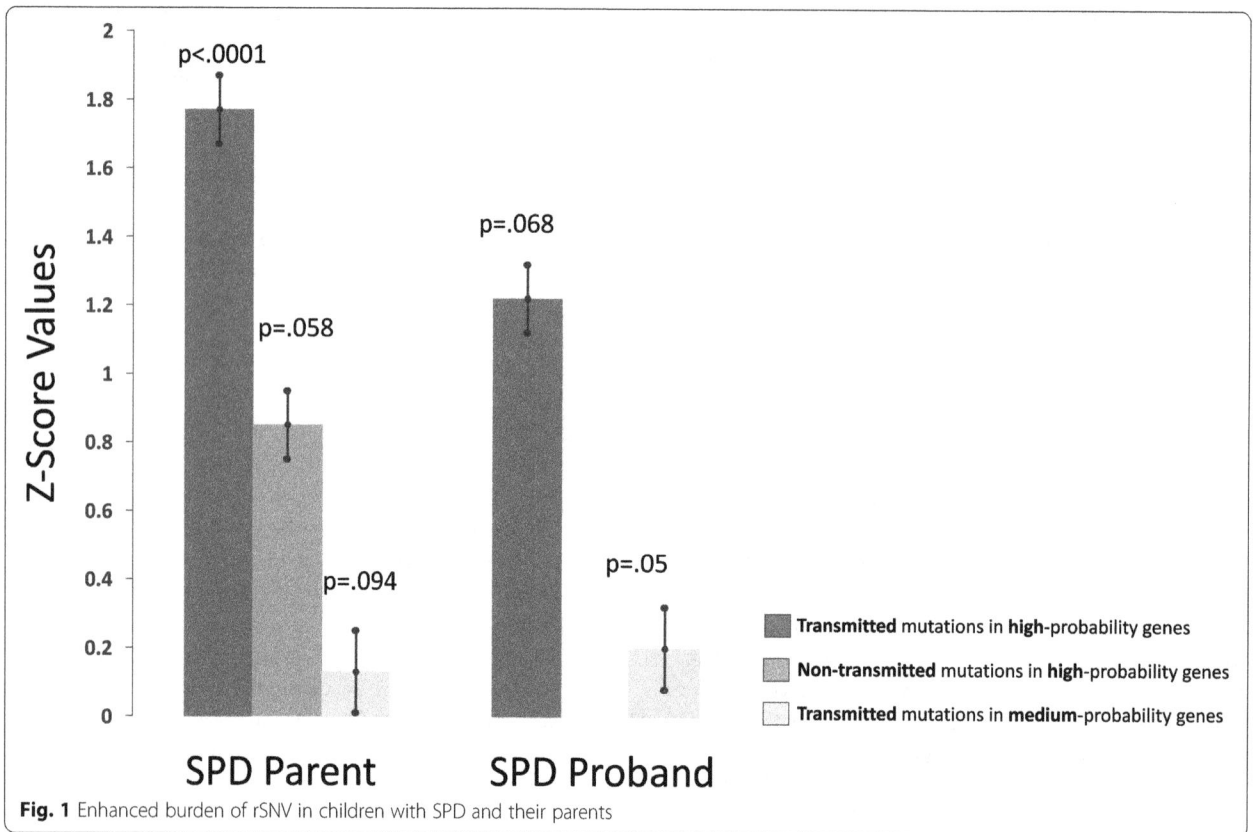

Fig. 1 Enhanced burden of rSNV in children with SPD and their parents

are, however, many individuals who are over-responsive to sensory input but do not have the degree of social or communication challenges that meet an ASD label. These individuals are currently being lumped under the category of Sensory Processing Disorder or SPD. With an estimated 10–15% of children with an ASD label currently being reported to have disease associated variants identified via WES, we sought to investigate the occurrence of de novo missense/nonsense mutations in ASD candidate genes in children with SPD. Furthermore, we sought to investigate whether children with SPD and their parents would show an increased burden of deleterious rSNV in high and moderate-risk ASD candidate genes. Herein, we report that 18% of our sample has a pathogenic de novo missense/nonsense mutation in genes previously associated with neurodevelopmental disorders. We further show that there is an enhanced rate of rare inherited variants in high-risk ASD genes transmitted from parent to affected child in SPD and ASD patients, but not in unaffected ASD siblings.

In this report, WES has identified a stop codon mutation in MBD5 that likely causes premature truncation and nonsense mediated decay of the protein from one of the two alleles leading to haploinsufficiency. Methyl-CpG-binding domain 5 (MBD5) is a gene located at 2q23.1. This gene, reviewed by

Mullegama, et al. 2016, is believed to contribute to DNA methylation and through that to potentially be involved in cell division, growth, and differentiation however further research is indicated to better understand the role of this protein [32]. Haploinsufficiency is believed to impact the expression of downstream genes such as upregulation of CF4 and UBE3A, and down regulation of MEF2C, EHMT1, RAI1 in a dose sensitive fashion [33]. Loss of function mutations in MBD5 are highly likely to be pathogenic given that the probability of loss of function intolerance is 1.00 [34].

MBD5, also referred to as mental retardation autosomal dominant 1 and now given the name MBD5-Associated Neurodevelopmental Disorder (MAND), was originally described in the context of the 2q23.1 microdeletion syndrome thought to be an Angelman Syndrome mimic. Clinically, affected individuals are variably affected by intellectual disability, motor delay, and severe speech impairment. The language deficits, social challenges and stereotypies seen in affected individuals can result in the affected child meeting criteria for autism [35, 36]. Additionally, children may have seizures, sleep disorders, and attentional challenge and some individuals will show mild craniofacial and skeletal anomalies [33, 37]. In the review article by Hodge et al. 2014, they summarize the phenotype for individuals in the literature with either

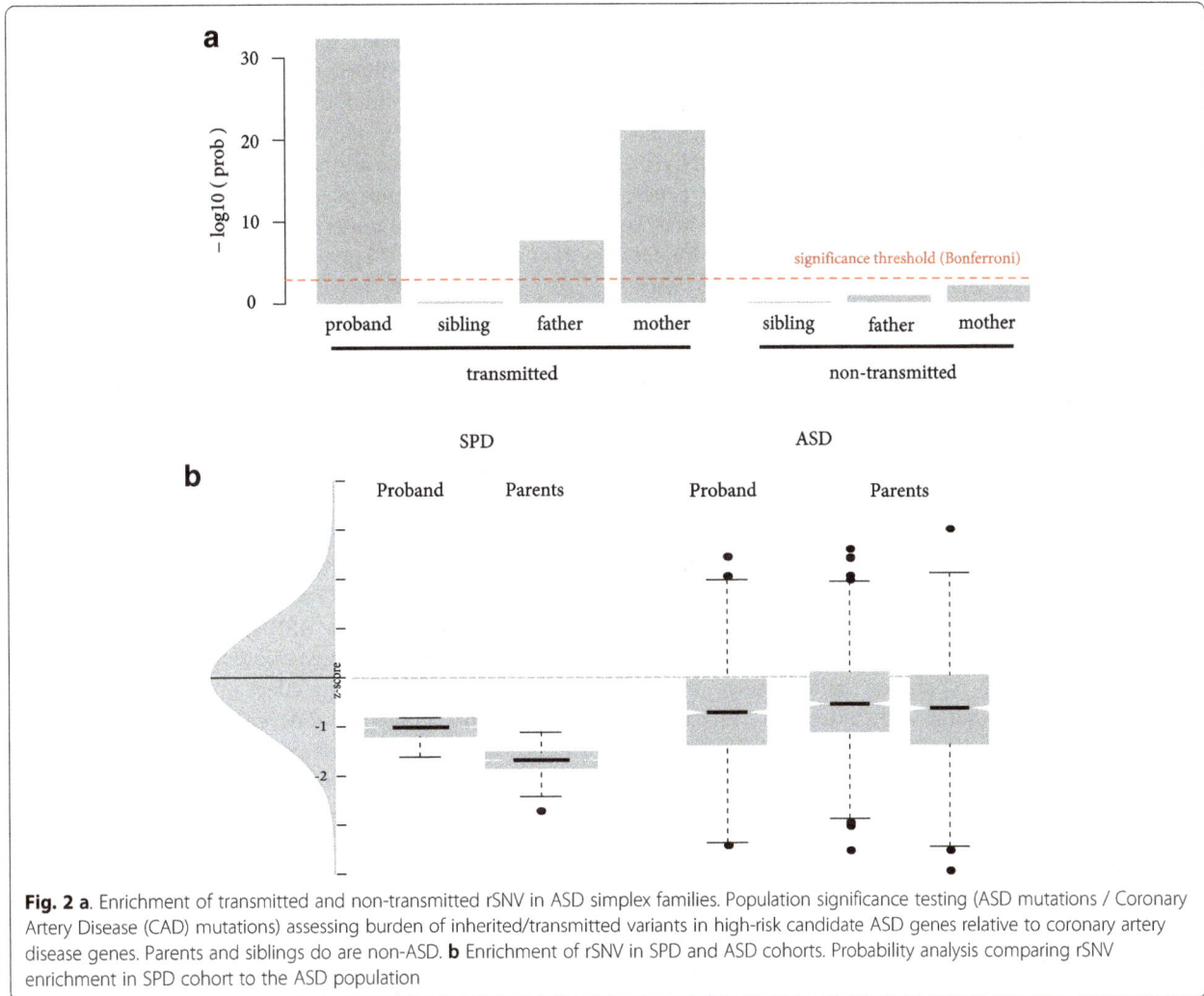

Fig. 2 a. Enrichment of transmitted and non-transmitted rSNV in ASD simplex families. Population significance testing (ASD mutations / Coronary Artery Disease (CAD) mutations) assessing burden of inherited/transmitted variants in high-risk candidate ASD genes relative to coronary artery disease genes. Parents and siblings do are non-ASD. **b** Enrichment of rSNV in SPD and ASD cohorts. Probability analysis comparing rSNV enrichment in SPD cohort to the ASD population

point mutations in the MBD5 gene or microdeletions containing MBD5. In their summary table, they include reports of sensory integration disorder (SID) which is a label frequently used in the occupational therapy community. In children with MBD5 point mutations, there is no comment on SID, however SID is reported in 2/3 (66%) children with 2q23.1 microdeletions [33]. So while, sensory over-responsivity to either sound or touch was a key clinical inclusion phenotype in our cohort, it is not always considered in the current genetic literature and thus difficult to know the extent to which it affects children with single gene disorders.

The female patient in this study first presented to our SNAP clinic at age 11 years due to prominent sensory dysfunction affecting her auditory, vestibular, visual, tactile, and oral systems (classified as 2 standard deviations below average on the Sensory Profile [38]). On evaluation by a pediatric geneticist, no dysmorphic features were noted and she is normocephalic with a head circumference at the 44th percentile. On evaluation by a licensed community pediatric neuropsychologist (L.D.) using the Wechsler Intelligence Scale for Children-4th edition (WISC IV), she had a verbal comprehension index of 121, Perceptual Reasoning Index of 86, and a working memory index of 99. These scores are all in the average to above average range but highlight a relative challenge in the perceptual measures. While verbal conceptual skills are a strength, multiple aspects of motor control are a significant concern with poor articulation and dysgraphia leading to severe school based challenges. In addition, while socially alert, interested and driven, she has challenges with interpretation of non-verbal social cues as well as heightened distractibility affecting sustained focus and selective attention. Specifically, she meets cut-off criteria for combined Inattentive/Hyperactive subtype on the Vanderbilt ADHD Diagnostic Parent Rating Scale [39]. These challenges contribute to a lack of social finesse that has led to difficulty with maintaining age appropriate friendships. However on evaluation in the lab, in the community, and at school, she did not meet the social communication criteria for an autism spectrum disorder.

Of the nine genes with missense mutation leading to amino acid substitution, six were considered potentially damaging to the protein structure: FMN2, DNAH9, KLHL33, MCM2, PFDN6, SLCO2B1. Of these genes, only Formin 2 (FMN2) has been previously reported to be associated with neurodevelopmental impairment. FMN2, located at chromosome 1q43, is one of 15 members of the formin homology protein family and is thought to play a role in actin cytoskeleton organization and cellular polarity. FMN2 has received the designation: mental retardation, autosomal recessive 47. In addition to the literature implicating mutations of FMN2 with autosomal recessive inheritance, there are reports of heterozygous deletion involving FMN2 in two additional reports in patients with neurodevelopmental impairment [40, 41]. Law, et al. 2014 reports that FMN2 localizes to the dendrites and likely alters synaptic density in a mouse model that has demonstrated challenges with fear-learning [42]. Affected patients were reported to have challenges with cognition and speech out of proportion to their motor difficulties. In the existing literature, there is no report of associated dysmorphic features and in one family there were rare complex partial seizures. There is no mention of sensory processing ability or challenges in the extant literature.

The male patient in this study with the FMN2 missense mutation first presented to SNAP research at 9 years of age. The patient had sensory dysfunction affecting his auditory, vestibular, tactile, multisensory and oral systems (classified as 2 standard deviations below average on the Sensory Profile [38]). The patient had a verbal comprehension index of 116, Perceptual Reasoning Index of 115, and a working memory index of 94 as assed using the WISC IV. He did not meet ASD cut-off scoring using the ADOS Assessment. Finding these two, highly penetrant de novo mutations in SPD patients who do not meet criteria for ASD suggests that de novo mutations may be found as the primary etiology in a significant percentage (up to 18%) of children with a sensory-first presentation.

While it has long been recognized that triplet repeat and single gene disorders, such as Fragile X or SHANK2, and more recently copy number variation disorders, such as 16p11.2 deletion, are associated with neurodevelopmental conditions; there has also been substantial interest in whether a cumulative burden of rare single nucleotide variants, either inherited or de novo, can result in a clinical condition such as ASD or SPD. In this study, we looked first at our SPD pediatric cohort with the hypothesis that these affected children would have a higher burden of inherited rSNV in high- or moderate-

risk ASD genes relative to the expected mutation rate. We found that, despite the small number of individuals in this pilot SPD cohort, there was indeed a trend level increase in transmitted rSNV in high-risk ASD candidate genes but not moderate-risk ASD genes. This result has two main implications. This finding suggests, first, that the SPD phenotype and the ASD phenotype may have shared genetic underpinnings in a "high value" gene set, as of now only 76 genes. Second, the phenotype may also result from an accumulation of multiple changes each with a smaller effect size, hence polygenic (and thus inherited from parents). Given that in the ASD literature, parents have been reported to show an increase in sensory processing behavioral differences, we investigated the burden of rSNV in the parents of our probands with SPD [43, 44].

Despite the small number of individuals in the cohort, there was a robust increase in the transmitted high risk ASD gene rSNV for parents of children with SPD. There was no increase in rSNV for either transmitted or non-transmitted moderate-risk ASD genes. This finding supports the importance of investigating the role of variant burden in SPD with a large effect in a small sample, and also highlights a potential difference in causality between the high and moderate-risk candidate genes. This robust increase in burden of variants in the parents is interesting given that the ASD literature suggests increased sensory differences in parents of affected individuals. In this SPD cohort, there are a couple of explanations that merit further exploration. First, it is possible that SPD parents themselves are affected by sensory processing dysfunction that is similar to their children's. Second, one must consider that the probands have additional variants contributing to their clinical symptomatology that we are not measuring in the exonic DNA meriting a whole genome approach. Finally, it may not be simply the additive burden of the variants but rather a particular combination of variants in specific genes that may work in an epistatic fashion to contribute to sensory processing dysfunction.

We chose to further investigate the relationship between rSNV burden in affected children with SPD and their parents by applying this analysis to a cohort of children also known to have an increased prevalence of sensory difference, those with ASD. In the SSC ASD family cohort, we were also able to increase our statistical power both by the sheer number of ASD families and by the inclusion of an unaffected sibling in the family cluster. We thus investigated whether children with ASD from the SSC and their unaffected siblings and parents have a higher burden of rSNV that were transmitted to the identified proband with ASD. As predicted, the affected child when compared to his or her parents, but not the unaffected sibling, shows an increase in transmitted rSNV from the high-risk ASD gene set. After stringent Bonferroni correction, neither the unaffected siblings nor the parents showed a significant burden of non-transmitted rSNV. These findings underscore the importance of inherited variants in ASD, even in families recruited for an increased likelihood of de novo variants. In one recent genome-wide ASD study, children with ASD show a "nominal difference" in rare inherited nonsense/splice site mutations when compared to their unaffected siblings [45]. Similarly, a study including 3871 ASD cases investigating the interplay of common and rare variants, reports that 5% of the ASD cohort has de novo loss of function mutation in a set of 107 autosomal genes involved in synaptic formation, transcriptional regulation, and chromatin remodeling pathways. However, this study did not show an association for inherited missense variants, so these variants were not included in their Transmission And De novo Associated (TADA) analysis [46]. De Rubeis et al., 2014 suggest that while the de novo loss of function (LOF) mutations confer the largest effect on risk, by including de novo missense SNV and transmitted LOF variants, they were able to double their gene discovery rate and suggest that ASD genes show "a strong constraint against variation." Future genetic investigation to determine whether there are genes specific to sensory challenges, specifically SOR, and genes more specific to language and social differences would greatly contribute to our understanding of neurodevelopment and neurodevelopmental disorders.

There are limitations to this work, which bear mentioning. This work needs to be replicated in a much larger independent sample, despite the provocative findings in this initial cohort. In future investigations, direct assessment of auditory and tactile SOR phenotype in parents and children with isolated SPD and ASD/SPD is warranted. Finally, bringing direct sensory phenotyping in a broader cohort of children with neurodevelopmental concerns with their parents and siblings in conjunction with genetic investigation will deepen our understanding of the contributing genetic variations, both monogenic and polygenic.

Conclusions

In this study, we find a rough estimate of 18% de novo, disease-associated, single gene mutations in a cohort of children identified on the basis of a sensory processing dysfunction. Furthermore, we find that this pediatric sensory cohort and their parents, similar to an autism cohort, show an enrichment of rare single nucleotide variants in genes previously reported to be associated with autism and neurodevelopmental delay. This small-scale study suggests that SPD results from genetically coded, brain based differences, with monogenic and

polygenic contributions. It highlights the need for additional genetic research in SPD and the importance of a thorough genetic evaluation in children presenting with sensory processing dysfunctions, regardless of the additional neurodevelopmental concerns.

Abbreviations
ADOS: Autism Diagnostic Observation Schedule; ASD: Autism Spectrum Disorder; CAD: Coronary Artery Disease; DSM: Diagnostic and Statistical Manual; FMN2: Formin 2; GATK: Genome Analysis Toolkit; GQ: Genotype quality; ID: Intellectual disability; LOF: Loss of function; MBD-5: Methyl-CpG-binding domain 5; rSNV: Rare Single Nucleotide Variants; SCQ: Social Communication Questionnaire; SFARI: Simons Foundation Autism Research Initiative; SNAP: Sensory Neurodevelopment and Autism Program; SNV: Single Nucleotide Variants; SPD: Sensory processing dysfunction; SSC: Simons Simplex Collection; UCSF: University of California, San Francisco; WES: Whole exome sequencing

Acknowledgements
We thank the Simons Simplex Collection (SSC) investigators and the Simons foundation for data provided in this manuscript. We are grateful to all of the families at the participating SSC sites, as well as the principal investigators (A. Beaudet, R. Bernier, J. Constantino, E. Cook, E. Fombonne, D. Geschwind, R. Goin-Kochel, E. Hanson, D. Grice, A. Klin, D. Ledbetter, C. Lord, C. Martin, D. Martin, R. Maxim, J. Miles, O. Ousley, K. Pelphrey, B. Peterson, J. Piggot, C. Saulnier, M. State, W. Stone, J. Sutcliffe, C. Walsh, Z. Warren, E. Wijsman). Approved researchers can obtain the SSC population dataset described in this study by applying at https://www.sfari.org/resource/sfari-base/ appreciate obtaining access to phenotypic data on SFARI Base.

Funding
This work was supported by grants from the Wallace Research Foundation to EJM and EHS and gifts from the Mickelson and Brody Family Foundation, the Gates Family Foundation, and generous support through gifts large and small to our UCSF Sensory Neurodevelopment and Autism Program (SNAP). EHS was supported in part by a grant from the NINDS; 2R01NS058721.

Authors' contributions
EJM contributed concept formation, data collection and analysis, and manuscript preparation. ABA collected data as well as contributing to manuscript preparation. VPN analyzed the data. GdG conducted genetic data processing and analysis along and contributed to manuscript preparation. LB collected data and contributed to manuscript oversight. MRG contributed to manuscript preparation and submission. ST contributed to the biostatistical design and performed primary analysis on the rSNV data. He also contributed to the manuscript preparation. EHS aided in original concept formation, statistical approach, data interpretation and manuscript preparation. All authors have read and approved the manuscript.

Competing interests
The authors declare that they have no competing interests.

Author details
[1]Department of Neurology, University of California, San Francisco, 675 Nelson Rising Lane, San Francisco, CA 9415, USA. [2]Department of Psychiatry, University of California, San Francisco, 401 Parnassus Ave, San Francisco, CA 94143, USA. [3]Department of Pediatrics, University of California, San Francisco, 550 16th Street, Box 0110, San Francisco, CA 94143, USA. [4]Department of Biostatistics & Epidemiology, University of California, San Francisco, 550 16th Street, 2nd Floor, Box #0560, San Francisco, CA 94158-2549, USA. [5]Institute of Human Genetics, University of California, San Francisco, 513 Parnassus Avenue, S965, San Francisco, CA 94143-0794, USA. [6]San Francisco, CA, USA.

References

1. Ahn RR, Miller LJ, Milberger S, et al. Prevalence of parents' perceptions of sensory processing disorders among kindergarten children. Am J Occup Ther [Internet]. 2004;58:287–93. Available from: http://www.ncbi.nlm.nih.gov/pubmed/15202626

2. Ben-Sasson A, Carter AS, Briggs-Gowan MJ. Sensory over-responsivity in elementary school: prevalence and social-emotional correlates. J Abnorm Child Psychol. 2009;37:705–16.

3. Ben-Sasson A, Soto TW, Heberle AE, et al. Early and Concurrent Features of ADHD and Sensory Over-Responsivity Symptom Clusters. J Atten Disord [Internet]. 2015; Available from: http://jad.sagepub.com/content/early/2014/08/01/1087054714543495.full.pdf+html.

4. American Psychiatric Association. Task Force on DSM-V. Diagnostic and Statistical Manual of Mental Disorders: DSM-5. Arlington: American Psychiatric Publishing; 2013.

5. Owen JP, Marco EJ, Desai S, et al. Abnormal white matter microstructure in children with sensory processing disorders. Neuroimage Clin. 2013;2:844–53.

6. Chang YS, Owen JP, Desai SS, et al. Autism and sensory processing disorders: Shared white matter disruption in sensory pathways but divergent connectivity in social-emotional pathways. PLoS One. 2014;9.

7. Baranek GT, David FJ, Poe MD, et al. Sensory experiences questionnaire: discriminating sensory features in young children with autism, developmental delays, and typical development. J Child Psychol Psychiatry Allied Discip [Internet]. 2006;47:591–601. Available from: http://doi.wiley.com/10.1111/j.1469-7610.2005.01546.x. [cited 19 Jul 2017]

8. Suarez MA. Sensory processing in children with autism spectrum disorders and impact on functioning. Pediatr Clin N Am. 2012;59(1):203–14.

9. Ghanizadeh A. Sensory processing problems in children with ADHD, a systematic review. Psychiatry Investig [Internet]. 2011;8:89–94. Available from: http://www.pubmedcentral.nih.gov/articlerender.fcgi?artid=3149116&tool=pmcentrez&rendertype=abstract

10. Engel-Yeger B, Dunn W. The relationship between sensory processing difficulties and anxiety level of healthy adults. Br J Occup Ther. 2011;74:210–6.

11. Miller LJ, McIntosh DN, McGrath J, et al. Electrodermal responses to sensory stimuli in individuals with fragile X syndrome: a preliminary report. Am J Med Genet. 1999;83:268–79.

12. Marco EJ, Abidi FE, Bristow J, et al. ARHGEF9 disruption in a female patient is associated with X linked mental retardation and sensory hyperarousal. J Med Genet [Internet]. 2008;45:100–5. Available from: http://www.ncbi.nlm.nih.gov/pubmed/17893116. [cited 25 May 2013]

13. Zarchi O, Attias J, Gothelf D. Auditory and visual processing in Williams syndrome. Isr J Psychiatry Relat Sci. 2010;47:125–31.

14. Keuler MM, Schmidt NL, Van Hulle CA, et al. Sensory overresponsivity: prenatal risk factors and temperamental contributions. J Dev Behav Pediatr [Internet]. 2011;32:533–41. Available from: http://www.pubmedcentral.nih.gov/articlerender.fcgi?artid=3163729&tool=pmcentrez&rendertype=abstract. [cited 4 Sept 2013]

15. Iossifov I, O'Roak BJ, Sanders SJ, et al. The contribution of de novo coding mutations to autism spectrum disorder. Nature [Internet]. 2014;515:216–21. Available from: http://www.nature.com/doifinder/10.1038/nature13908

16. Guo W, Samuels JF, Wang Y, et al. Polygenic risk score and heritability estimates reveals a genetic relationship between ASD and OCD. Eur Neuropsychopharmacol [Internet]. 2017;27:657–66. Available from: http://linkinghub.elsevier.com/retrieve/pii/S0924977X17301931. [cited 24 Aug 2017]

17. Weiner DJ, Wigdor EM, Ripke S, et al. Polygenic transmission disequilibrium confirms that common and rare variation act additively to create risk for autism spectrum disorder. Nat Publ Group [Internet]. 2017;49. Available from: https://www.nature.com/ng/journal/v49/n7/pdf/ng.3863.pdf. [cited 24 Aug 2017]

18. Sanders SJ, He X, Willsey AJ. Insights into autism Spectrum disorder genomic architecture and biology from 71 risk loci. Neuron [Internet]. 2015; 87:1215–33. Available from: http://www.ncbi.nlm.nih.gov/pubmed/26402605. [cited 12 Jul 2017]

19. Yang Y, Muzny DM, Reid JG, Bainbridge MN, Willis A, Ward PA, Braxton A, Beuten J, Xia F, Niu Z, Hardison M, Person R, Bekheirnia MR, Leduc MS, Kirby A, Pham P, Scull J, Wang M, Ding Y, Plon SE, Lupski JR, Beaudet AL, Gibbs RA, Eng CM. Clinical whole-exome sequencing for the diagnosis of mendelian disorders. N Engl J Med. 2013;369(16):1502–11.

20. Sanders SJ, Murtha MT, Gupta AR, et al. De novo mutations revealed by whole-exome sequencing are strongly associated with autism. Nature [Internet]. 2012;485:237–241. Available from: https://doi.org/10.1038/nature10945. [cited 17 Oct 2013].

21. Sanders SJ, He X, Willsey AJ, et al. Insights into Autism Spectrum Disorder Genomic Architecture and Biology from 71 Risk Loci. Neuron. 2015;87(6):1215–33.

22. Krumm N, Turner TN, Baker C, et al. Excess of rare, inherited truncating mutations in autism. Nat Genet. 2015;47:582–8.

23. Lord C, Rutter M, Goode S, et al. Autism diagnostic observation schedule: a standardized observation of communicative and social behavior. J Autism Dev Disord. 1989;19:185–212.

24. Lord C, Rutter M, Le Couteur A. Autism diagnostic interview-revised: a revised version of a diagnostic interview for caregivers of individuals with possible pervasive developmental disorders. J Autism Dev Disord. 1994;24:659–85.

25. Institute B. No Title [Internet]. 2016. Available from: https://software.broadinstitute.org/gatk/best-practices/bp_3step.php?case=GermShortWGS. Accessed 9 Jan 2018.

26. McKenna A, Hanna M, Banks E, et al. The genome analysis toolkit: a MapReduce framework for analyzing next-generation DNA sequencing data. Genome Res. 2010;20:1297–303.

27. DePristo MA, Banks E, Poplin R, et al. A framework for variation discovery and genotyping using next-generation DNA sequencing data. Nat Genet. 2011;43:491–8.

28. Van der Auwera GA, Carneiro MO, Hartl C, Poplin R, Del Angel G, Levy-Moonshine A, Jordan T, Shakir K, Roazen D, Thibault J, Banks E, Garimella KV, Altshuler D, Gabriel S, DePristo MA. From fastQ data to high confidence variant calls: the Genome Analysis Toolkit best practices pipeline. Curr Protoc Bioinformatics. 2013;43:11.

29. Liu H, Liu W, Liao Y, et al. CADgene: a comprehensive database for coronary artery disease genes. Nucleic Acids Res. 2011;39:991–6.

30. Basu SN, Kollu R, Banerjee-Basu S. AutDB: a gene reference resource for autism research. Nucleic Acids Res [Internet]. 2009;37:832–6. Available from: http://autism.mindspec.org/autdb/Welcome.do

31. Richards Chair S, Aziz N, Bick D, et al. Standards and guidelines for the interpretation of sequence variants: a joint consensus recommendation of the American College of Medical Genetics and Genomics and the Association for Molecular Pathology. Available from: https://www.ncbi.nlm.nih.gov/pmc/articles/PMC4544753/pdf/nihms697486.pdf. [cited 29 Mar 2018].

32. Mullegama SV, Elsea SH. Clinical and Molecular Aspects of MBD5-Associated Neurodevelopmental Disorder (MAND). Eur J Hum Genet. 2016;24(9):1376.

33. Hodge JC, Mitchell E, Pillalamarri V, et al. Disruption of MBD5 contributes to a spectrum of psychopathology and neurodevelopmental abnormalities. Mol Psychiatry [Internet]. 2014;19:368–79. Available from: http://www.ncbi.nlm.nih.gov/pubmed/23587880

34. ExAC Browser [Internet]. Available from: http://exac.broadinstitute.org/gene/ENSG00000204406. [cited 4 Sept 2017].

35. Williams SR, Mullegama SV, Rosenfeld JA, et al. Haploinsufficiency of MBD5 associated with a syndrome involving microcephaly, intellectual disabilities, severe speech impairment, and seizures. Eur J Hum Genet [Internet]. 2010; 18:436–41. Available from: https://doi.org/10.1038/ejhg.2009.199

36. Ladha S. Getting to the bottom of autism spectrum and related disorders: MBD5 as a key contributor. Clin Genet. 2012;18(4):363–64.

37. Talkowski ME, Mullegama SV, Rosenfeld JA, et al. Assessment of 2q23.1 microdeletion syndrome implicates MBD5 as a single causal locus of intellectual disability, epilepsy, and autism spectrum disorder. Am J Hum Genet. 2011;89:551–63.

38. Dunn W. Sensory profile user's manual. San Antonio: Psychological Corporation; 1999.

39. Wolraich ML. Psychometric properties of the Vanderbilt ADHD diagnostic parent rating scale in a referred population. J Pediatr Psychol. 2003;28:559–68.

40. Perrone MD, Rocca MS, Bruno I, et al. De novo 911 Kb interstitial deletion on chromosome 1q43 in a boy with mental retardation and short stature. Eur J Med Genet. 2012;55:117–9.

41. Almuqbil M, Hamdan FF, Mathonnet G, et al. De novo deletion of FMN2 in a girl with mild non-syndromic intellectual disability. Eur J Med Genet. 2013;56:686–8.

42. Law R, Dixon-Salazar T, Jerber J, et al. Biallelic truncating mutations in FMN2, encoding the actin-regulatory protein formin 2, cause nonsyndromic autosomal-recessive intellectual disability. Am J Hum Genet. 2014;95:721–8.

43. Donaldson CK, Stauder JEA, Donkers FCL. Increased sensory processing atypicalities in parents of multiplex ASD families versus typically developing and simplex ASD families. J Autism Dev Disord. 2017;47(3):535–48.

44. Glod M, Riby DM, Honey E, Rodgers J. Sensory atypicalities in dyads of children with autism spectrum disorder (ASD) and their parents. Autism Res. 2017;10(3):531–8.

45. Beauvois M, Saillant B, Meininger V, et al. Insights into autism spectrum disorder genomic architecture and biology from 71 risk loci. Neuron [Internet]. 2015;87:1215–33. Available from: https://doi.org/10.1016/j.neuron.2015.09.016

46. De Rubeis S, He X, Goldberg AP, et al. Synaptic, transcriptional and chromatin genes disrupted in autism. Nature [Internet]. 2014;515:209–15. Available from: http://www.nature.com/doifinder/10.1038/nature13772

12

Identification of glioblastoma gene prognosis modules based on weighted gene co-expression network analysis

Pengfei Xu, Jian Yang, Junhui Liu, Xue Yang, Jianming Liao, Fanen Yuan, Yang Xu, Baohui Liu and Qianxue Chen[*]

Abstract

Background: Glioblastoma multiforme, the most prevalent and aggressive brain tumour, has a poor prognosis. The molecular mechanisms underlying gliomagenesis remain poorly understood. Therefore, molecular research, including various markers, is necessary to understand the occurrence and development of glioma.

Method: Weighted gene co-expression network analysis (WGCNA) was performed to construct a gene co-expression network in TCGA glioblastoma samples. Gene ontology (GO) and pathway-enrichment analysis were used to identify significance of gene modules. Cox proportional hazards regression model was used to predict outcome of glioblastoma patients.

Results: We performed weighted gene co-expression network analysis (WGCNA) and identified a gene module (yellow module) related to the survival time of TCGA glioblastoma samples. Then, 228 hub genes were calculated based on gene significance (GS) and module significance (MS). Four genes (OSMR + SOX21 + MED10 + PTPRN) were selected to construct a Cox proportional hazards regression model with high accuracy (AUC = 0.905). The prognostic value of the Cox proportional hazards regression model was also confirmed in GSE16011 dataset (GBM: $n = 156$).

Conclusion: We developed a promising mRNA signature for estimating overall survival in glioblastoma patients.

Keywords: GBM, WGCNA, TCGA, Cox proportional hazards regression module

Background

Glioblastoma multiforme (GBM), the most prevalent and aggressive primary intracranial tumour, displays heterogeneity, rapid proliferation and extensive invasion, with a median survival of approximately 15 months [1, 2]. Therefore, developing appropriate and effective biomarkers to predict prognosis is crucial for glioblastoma patients. Previous genomic analyses of glioblastoma have identified some molecular markers, including epidermal growth factor receptor (EGFR), platelet-derived growth factor receptor alpha (PDGFRA), vascular endothelial growth factor (VEGF), insulin-like growth factor 1 (IGF-1), P53 and isocitrate dehydrogenase 1 (IDH1), and X-linked alpha thalassemia mental retardation syndrome gene (ATRX) [3, 4]. In addition, methylation levels of the promoter of O6methylguanineDNA methyltransferase

(MGMT) are related to sensitivity of temozolomide therapy and the prognosis of patients. The 1p/19q loss is another prognosis marker and indicates a better prognosis [5].

With the development of high-throughput sequencing and bioinformatics, abundant sequencing data provide a remarkable opportunity to detect glioblastoma-associated key genes, networks and pathways. However, identification of these features remains challenging. Weighted gene co-expression network analysis (WGCNA) is a system biology method used for describing the correlation patterns among genes and finding highly correlated modules. In this study, we performed WGCNA for RNASeq data derived from The Cancer Genome Atlas (TCGA) and reconstructed gene co-expression networks. Then, we identified gene modules related to survival and recurrence time. Using Kaplan-Meier survival analysis and multivariate Cox regression analysis, we identified an independent prognostic model. This finding provides new insights into the molecular mechanism of GBM.

---

* Correspondence: chenqx666@whu.edu.cn
Department of Neurosurgery, Renmin Hospital of Wuhan University, 9 Zhangzhidong Road and 238 Jiefang Road, Wuchang, Wuhan, Hubei 430060, People's Republic of China

Methods

Data download and pre-processing

RNA sequencing data (RNA-Seq2 level 3 data) from human glioblastoma samples were obtained from the TCGA data portal (https://portal.gdc.cancer.gov), which contains 152 glioblastoma tissues [3]. These data were updated to January 28, 2016. According to the instructions for WGCNA, fragments per kilobase per million (FPKM) is recommended as the data type for subsequent analysis. As some genes without significant changes in expression between samples will be highly correlated in WGCNA, the 5000 most differentially expressed genes were used in the following WGCNA studies. The clinical metadata of 152 samples were also downloaded and filtered for useful information. Because the clinical data of TCGA database was constantly updated, the survival time of the death patients was more accurate. The age, gender, survival time and recurrence time data of 75 deceased patients were selected and divided into two groups according to the median (Table 1). Subtype data of 152 samples was downloaded from GlioVis database (http: //gliovis.bioinfo.cnio.es/) [6]. The GSE36245, GSE16011 and GSE50161 datasets were included in the study, and both originated from an Affymetrix Human Genome U133 Plus 2.0 Array [7–9]. GSE36245 dataset only contained 46 glioblastoma samples, so it was used to validate whether the modules which are obtained from TCGA database were reproducible. GSE16011 dataset (GBM: $n = 159$) was used to validate whether the Cox proportional hazards regression model was reproducible. GSE50161 dataset (GBM: $n = 34$; Normal control: $n = 13$) contained glioblastoma and normal brain samples and was used to perform difference analysis.

Table 1 Information for 75 glioblastoma patients

TCGA Datasets	
Variables	Case number (N = 75)
Age	
< 59	38
> =59	37
Gender	
Female	55
Male	20
Survival time	
< 448	39
> =448	36
Recurrence time	
< 178	38
> =178	37

Weighted gene co-expression network analysis and module preservation

WGCNA was performed using the R package WGCNA [10]. First, RNASeq data were filtered to reduce outliers. A co-expression similarity matrix was composed of the absolute value of the correlation between the expression levels of transcripts. For an unsigned network, the correlation coefficient between gene i and j was defined as Sij: $Sij = |cor(i,j)|$. The co-expression similarity matrix was then transformed into the adjacency matrix by choosing 7 as a soft threshold (Fig. 1a). A topological matrix was created using the topological overlap measure (TOM) [11, 12]. Finally, we chose the dynamic hybrid cut method, a bottom-up algorithm, to identify co-expression gene modules [13]. To identify the significance of each module, we calculated gene significance (GS) to measure the correlation between genes and sample traits. Module significance (MS) was defined as the average GS within modules and was calculated to measure the correlation between modules and sample traits (age, gender, survival time and recurrence time) [14, 15]. Statistical significance was determined using the correlation P value. The module Preservation function in the WGCNA R package was used to calculate the $Z_{summary}$ to evaluate whether a module was conserved [16].

Hub gene identification and module visualisation

Hub genes were identified using "network screening" within the R package WGCNA [10]. This method identifies genes that have high GS and MS. We selected the q. weighted < 0.01 as a cutoff to obtain the hub genes [17]. The targeted module visualisation was performed using Cytoscape3.5.1. Cytoscape is an open source software for visualising molecular interaction network (http://www.cytoscape.org/index.html) [18].

Functional enrichment analysis

Gene ontology (GO) and pathway-enrichment analysis (Kyoto Encyclopedia of Genes and Genomes (KEGG)) were performed using the R package clusterProfiler (https://guangchuangyu.github.io/clusterProfiler) [19–21]. Enriched ontological terms and pathways with $P < 0.05$ were selected.

Cox proportional hazards regression model

The prognostic value of each hub gene was first assessed by univariate Cox proportional hazards regression. Then, statistically significant genes were used to construct the multivariate Cox regression model as follows: Risk score = (0.2844* expression level of oncostatin M receptor (OSMR)) + (−0.1682* expression level of SRY-Box 21 (SOX21)) + (1.3462* expression level of mediator complex subunit 10 (MED10)) + (0.3776* expression level of protein tyrosine phosphatase, receptor type N (PTPRN)). Glioblastoma samples were divided into high-score and low-score groups based on the

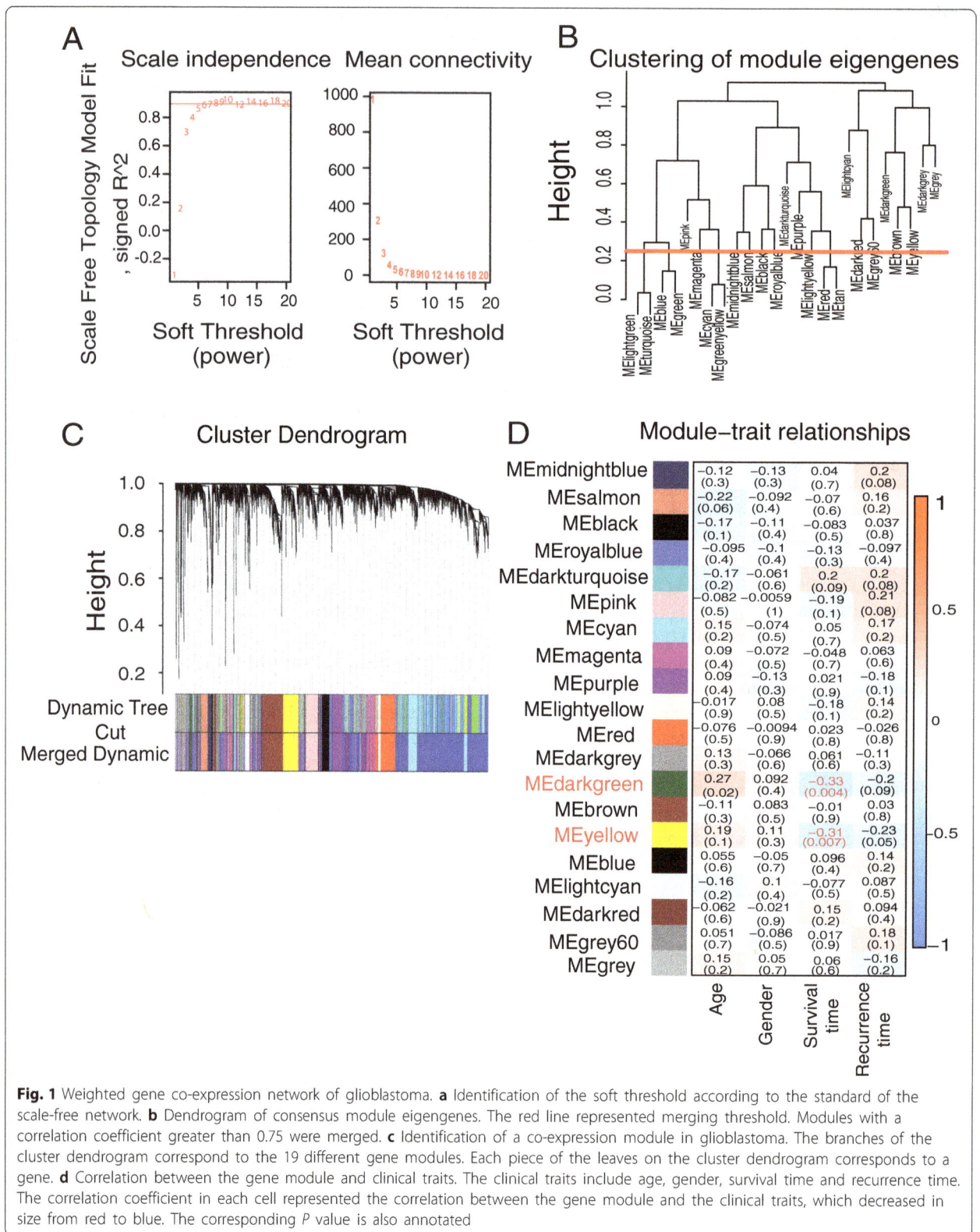

Fig. 1 Weighted gene co-expression network of glioblastoma. **a** Identification of the soft threshold according to the standard of the scale-free network. **b** Dendrogram of consensus module eigengenes. The red line represented merging threshold. Modules with a correlation coefficient greater than 0.75 were merged. **c** Identification of a co-expression module in glioblastoma. The branches of the cluster dendrogram correspond to the 19 different gene modules. Each piece of the leaves on the cluster dendrogram corresponds to a gene. **d** Correlation between the gene module and clinical traits. The clinical traits include age, gender, survival time and recurrence time. The correlation coefficient in each cell represented the correlation between the gene module and the clinical traits, which decreased in size from red to blue. The corresponding *P* value is also annotated

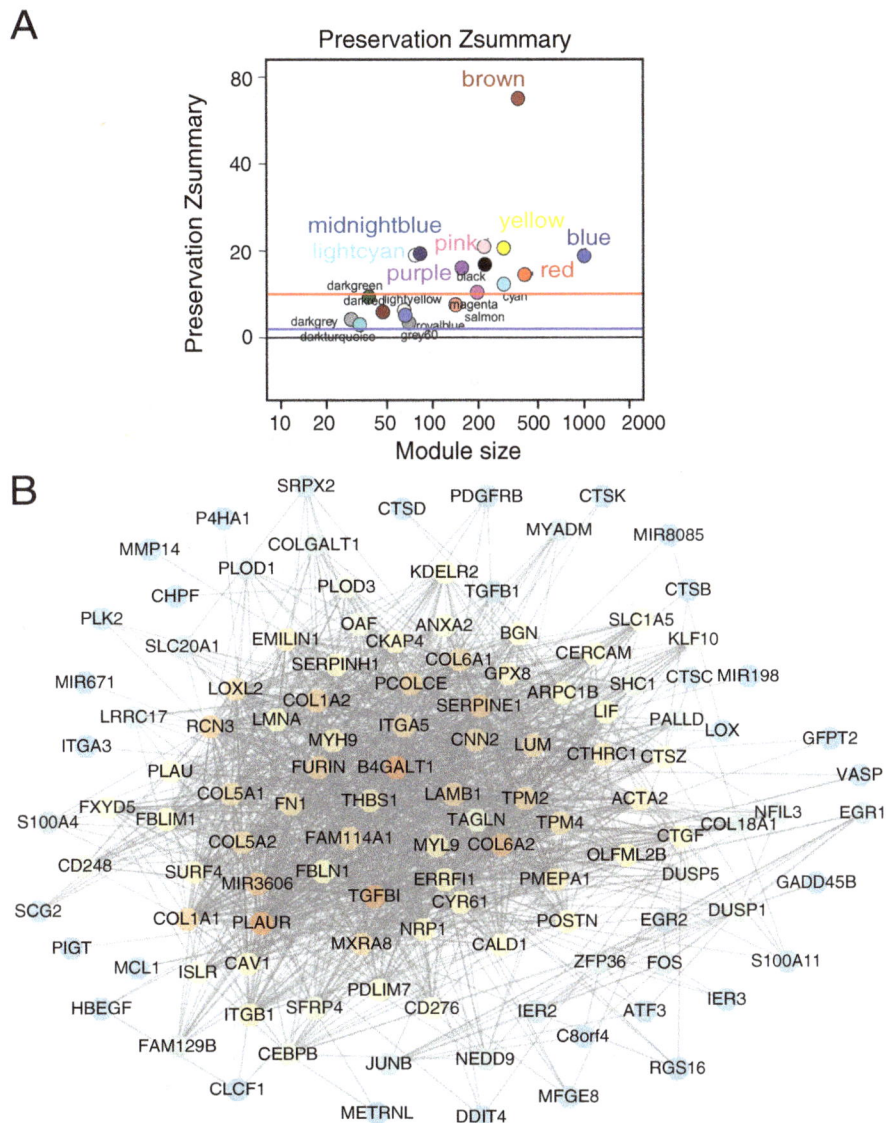

Fig. 2 Module preservation and visualisation. **a** Module preservation statistics of TCGA modules in GEO modules (y - axis) vs module size (x - axis). **b** Visualisation of the gene co-expression network of the yellow module was generated using Cytoscape. Based on weight, not all genes corresponding to each module were represented

median of the risk score. K-M survival curves were generated to assess the prognostic value of the model using the R package "survival" (https://CRAN.R-project.org/package= survival). The receiver operating characteristic curve (ROC) was generated to assess the accuracy of the model with the R package "survivalROC" (https: //CRAN.R-project.org/ package = survivalROC) [22].

Statistical analysis
The Pairwise t tests and Tukey's Honest Significant Difference test were used to perform differentail analysis. All statistical tests and graphing were performed using RStudio (www.rstudio.com) and

GraphPad Prism 7.0. P values < 0.05 were considered statistically significant [23]. Statistical significance was indicated in the figures as follows: $*P < 0.05$, $**P < 0.01$ and $***P < 0.001$.

Results

Pre-processing of TCGA RNA sequencing and clinical data
Glioblastoma RNASeq data were downloaded from TCGA and constructed into a matrix RNASeq with gene symbols as the rows and patient barcodes as the column names. Furthermore, expression estimates in less than 20% of cases were removed, and the top 5000 most differentially expressed genes were used in WGCNA

studies. Simultaneously, the corresponding clinical data were also downloaded to relate co-expression modules to clinical phenotypes. After outliers were removed, we selected data from 75 deceased patients among the 152 samples, including 5000 genes (Table 1).

Gene co-expression network analysis

WGCNA was performed to construct a gene co-expression network to identify biologically meaningful gene modules and better understand the molecular mechanism of glioblastoma. WGCNA defined gene modules as a set of genes with topological overlaps. The specific approach was to establish a hierarchical clustering tree based on dynamic hybrid cut. Each piece of the leaves on this tree corresponded to a gene, and the different gene modules were the branches of the tree. Identification of co-expression modules could facilitate identification of hub genes that drive and maintain important functions. Ultimately, 19 gene modules were

identified. The grey module includes genes that were not assigned to any gene modules (Fig. 1b, c).

Calculation of module-trait correlations in GBMs

To analyse the relationship between gene modules and sample clinical information, we used the module eigengene (ME) as the overall gene expression level of corresponding modules and calculated correlations with clinical phenotypes, such as age, gender, survival time and recurrence time. The yellow and dark green modules were significantly associated with survival time (Fig. 1d and Additional file 1: Table S6).

Module preservation statistics

To validate whether the modules were reproducible (or preserved), we selected 4644 genes which from GSE36245 (GBM: $n = 46$) to construct a weighted gene co-expression network. Then, the $Z_{summary}$ score was calculated to determine module preservation. Modules with a $Z_{summary}$ score > 10 were regarded as preserved [24]. That is, the

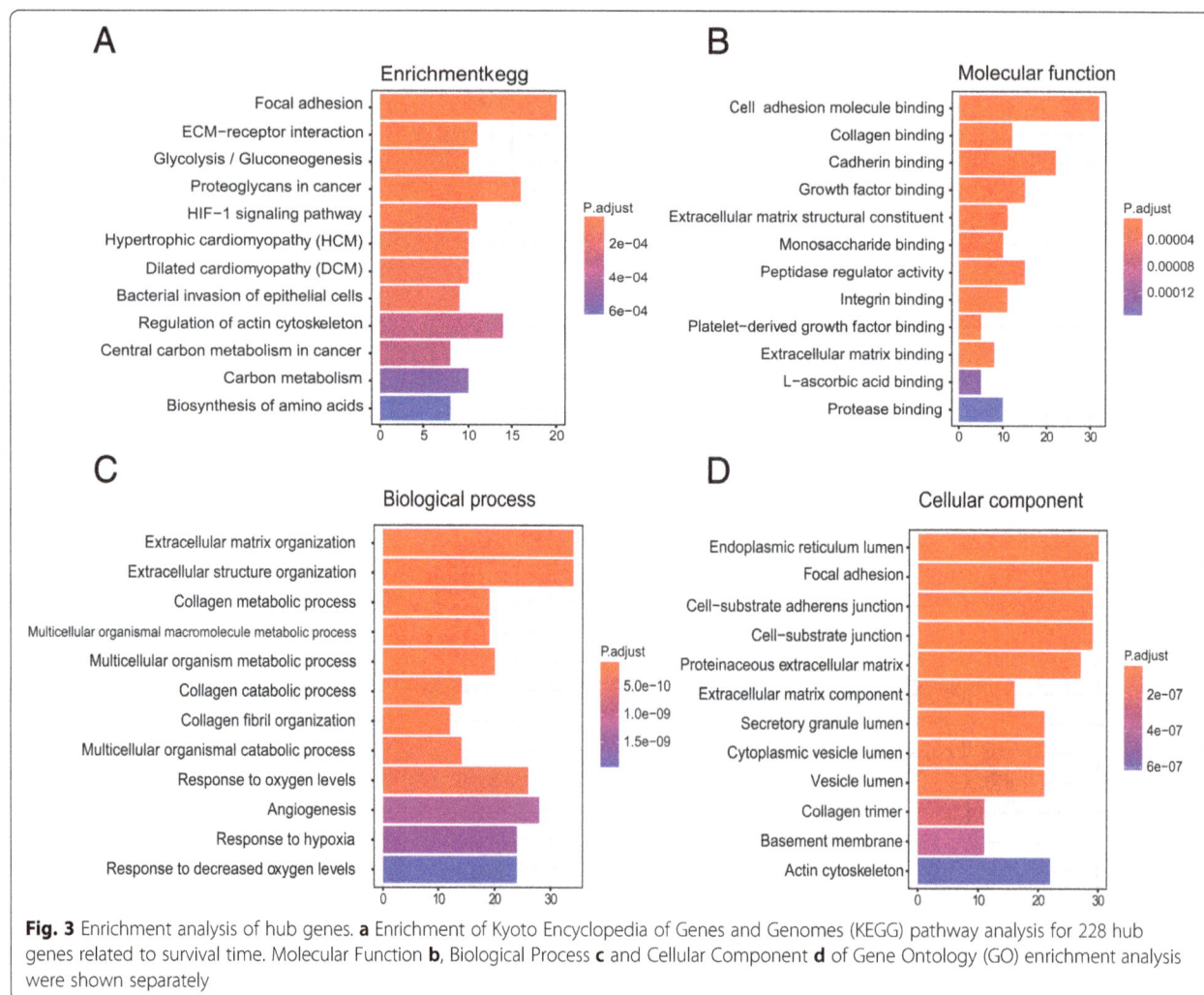

Fig. 3 Enrichment analysis of hub genes. **a** Enrichment of Kyoto Encyclopedia of Genes and Genomes (KEGG) pathway analysis for 228 hub genes related to survival time. Molecular Function **b**, Biological Process **c** and Cellular Component **d** of Gene Ontology (GO) enrichment analysis were shown separately

modules of the TCGA dataset also existed in the network of the Gene Expression Omnibus (GEO) dataset. The 10 modules were highly conserved, including the yellow module, while the dark green module was poorly conserved (Fig. 2a). Thus, we focused on analysis of the yellow module in the follow-up study.

Identification of the hub gene

The function of the WGCNA R package, called network Screening, was used to search for the hub gene in the yellow module. We used the q. weighted < 0.01 and obtained 228 survival-related genes. These intramodular hub genes were centrally located in their respective modules and may thus be critical components within the modules [25].

Module visualisation of network connections

To further depict the expression network of module genes related to survival time, we exported the co-expression network of the yellow module into Cytoscape. The nodes were defined as individual genes in the network, and edges were defined as the interactions between genes. As shown in Figures, the yellow module included 311 nodes and 21,557 edges. The hub genes of the modules were marked as orange nodes (Fig. 2b).

GO and pathway-enrichment analysis of hub genes

To explore the cellular component (CC), molecular function (MF) and biological process (BP), we performed GO enrichment analysis. A total of 228 hub genes were significantly enriched in the following subclasses of GO classification (Fig. 3): focal junction (GO: 0005925, $P = 3.17E - 15$), cell adhesion molecule binding (GO: 0050839, $P = 1.07E - 15$), collagen binding (GO: 0005518, $P = 1.56E - 11$), extracellular matrix organisation (GO: 0030198, $P = 2.67E - 20$), and extracellular structure organisation (GO: 0043062, $P = 1.10E - 21$). KEGG pathway analysis showed that the top enriched terms were focal adhesion (hsa04510, $P = 1.53E - 10$) and ECM-receptor interaction (hsa04512, $P = 1.39E - 07$) based on P value. These results suggest that these genes were closely related to the cell adhesion function (Fig. 3a–d and Additional files 2, 3, 4, 5: Table S2–5).

Construction of the cox proportional hazards regression model based on hub genes and Kaplan-Meier analysis

We further narrowed down and selected the top 20 genes significantly related to survival time by univariate Cox analysis of 228 hub genes (Additional file 6: Table S1). Then, we used the 20 genes to perform multivariate Cox analysis and construct a Cox proportional hazards regression model from 152 glioblastoma patients. The risk score for predicting survival time was calculated with a formula based on the above mentioned four genes: risk score = (0.2844 * expression level of OSMR) + (− 0.1682 *

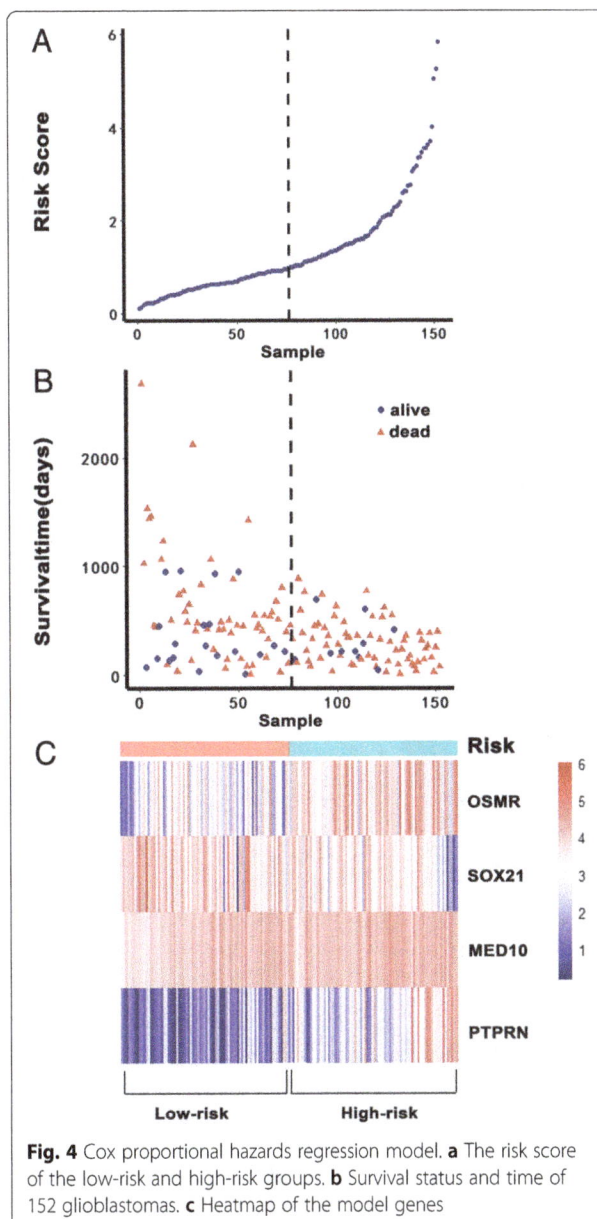

Fig. 4 Cox proportional hazards regression model. **a** The risk score of the low-risk and high-risk groups. **b** Survival status and time of 152 glioblastomas. **c** Heatmap of the model genes

expression level of SOX21) + (1.3462 * expression level of MED10) + (0.3776 * expression level of PTPRN) (Fig. 4a–c). We divided 152 patients into high-risk ($N = 76$) and low-risk ($N = 76$) groups according to the median of the risk score. The five-year survival rate of the high-risk group was significantly poorer than that of the low-risk group (Fig. 5a). The model was reproducible in GSE16011 dataset (Additional file 7: Figure S1 and Additional file 8: Table S7). Elevated expression of OSMR, MED10 and PTPRN was associated with an increased risk score, but SOX21 produced the opposite effect. The area under the ROC curve was 0.905 (Fig. 5c), indicating a higher predictive value. Moreover, K-M curves confirmed that the four

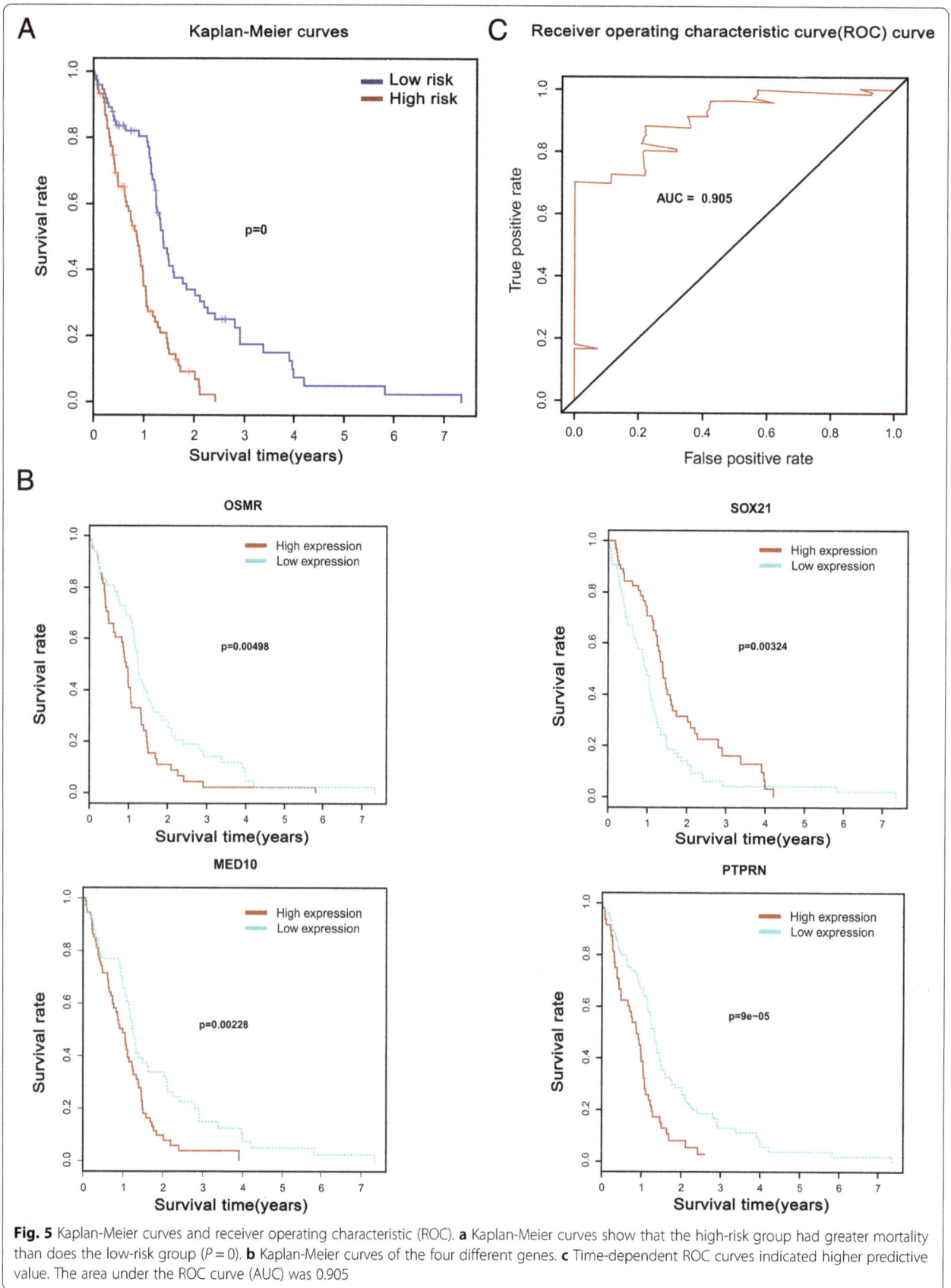

Fig. 5 Kaplan-Meier curves and receiver operating characteristic (ROC). **a** Kaplan-Meier curves show that the high-risk group had greater mortality than does the low-risk group (P = 0). **b** Kaplan-Meier curves of the four different genes. **c** Time-dependent ROC curves indicated higher predictive value. The area under the ROC curve (AUC) was 0.905

genes could function as an independent predictive indicator for the survival of glioblastoma patients (Fig. 5b).

Difference analysis of the four genes

To assess the expression level of the four genes between normal and glioblastoma tissues, we chose the GSE50161 datasets (normal brain tissue = 13, glioblastoma tissue = 34) to perform difference analysis. Interestingly, OSMR ($P = 0.0011$) and PTPRN ($P < 0.0001$) were differentially expressed (Fig. 6a, d), while MED10 ($P = 0.5332$) and SOX21 ($P = 0.2831$) were not (Fig. 6b, c). Subsequently, we assessed the mRNA expression levels of the four genes within each subtype (Classical, Mesenchymal and Proneural) [26]. The results showed that mRNA expression levels of the four genes in proneural subtype were significantly different from the other two subtypes (Fig. 7a). Meanwhile, the four genes had a better prognosis in proneural subtype (Fig. 7b).

Discussion

Due to the diffusely infiltrative nature of glioblastoma, completely removing tumours is difficult, and these tumours also resist radiation therapy and chemotherapy. Thus, molecular studies, including various markers, are necessary to understand gliomagenesis and development. In addition, some molecular markers are important for determining molecular subtypes, identifying individualised treatments and judging clinical prognosis. For instance, overexpression or amplification of EGFR, mutations in IDH1 and IDH2 and phosphatase and tensin homologue (PTEN) mutations contribute to the pathogenesis of glioblastoma [27]. With the rapid development of high-throughput sequencing and bioinformatics methods, exploiting the great potential of RNASeq data requires new analytic approaches that move beyond gene difference analysis.

Instead of relating thousands of genes to a clinical trait, we used a recently developed methodology to construct a weighted gene co-expression network in 75 glioblastoma

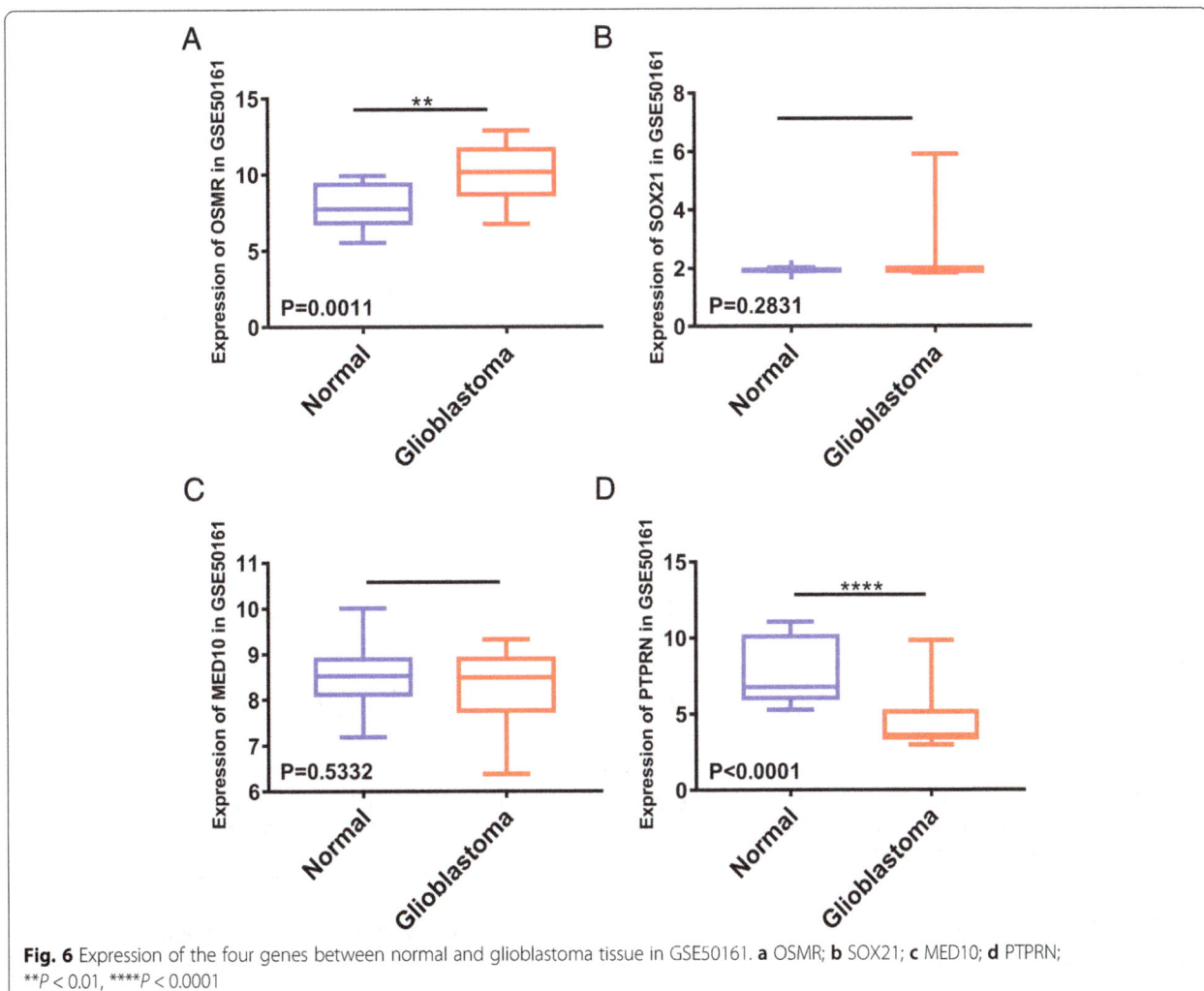

Fig. 6 Expression of the four genes between normal and glioblastoma tissue in GSE50161. **a** OSMR; **b** SOX21; **c** MED10; **d** PTPRN; ******$P < 0.01$, ********$P < 0.0001$

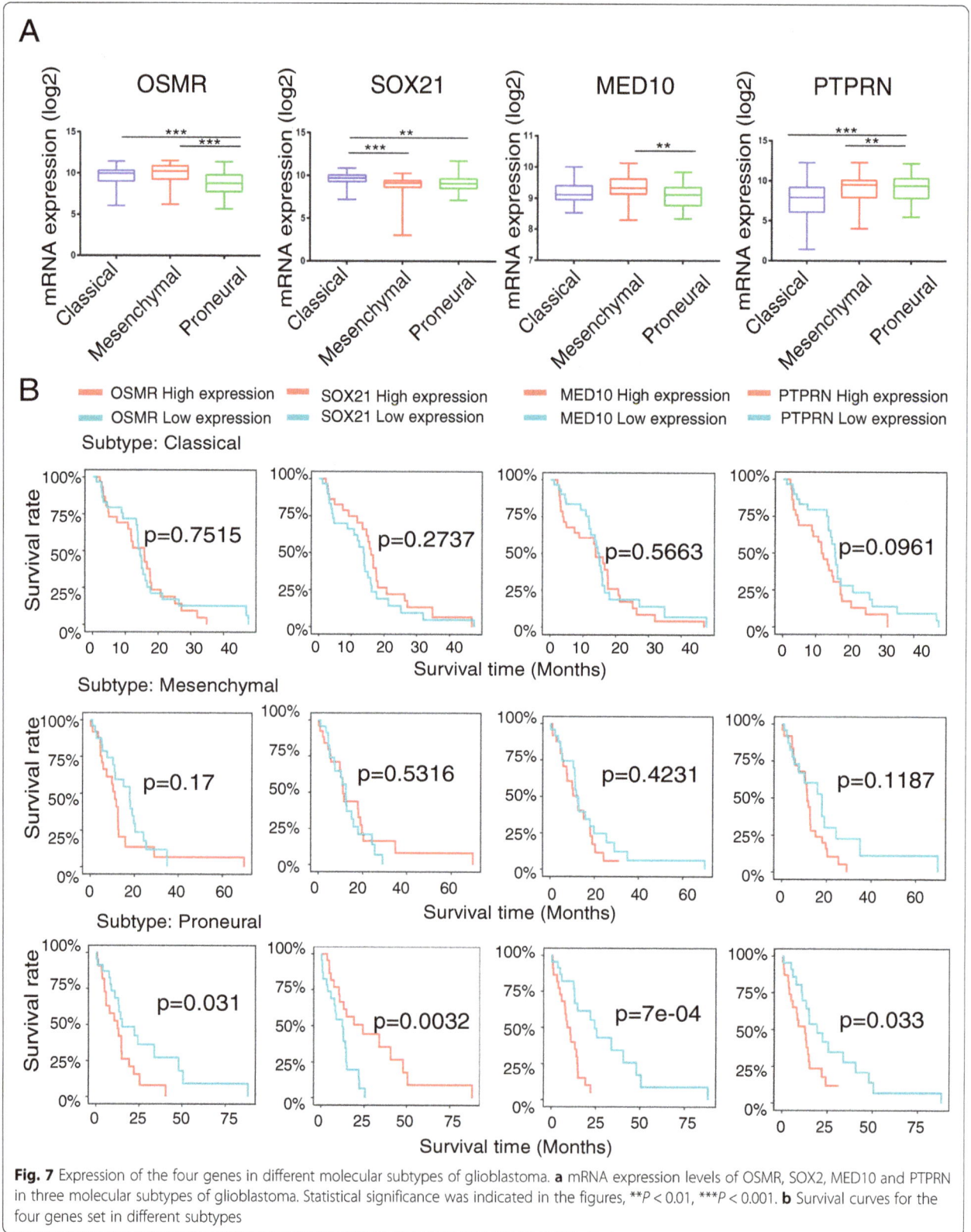

Fig. 7 Expression of the four genes in different molecular subtypes of glioblastoma. **a** mRNA expression levels of OSMR, SOX2, MED10 and PTPRN in three molecular subtypes of glioblastoma. Statistical significance was indicated in the figures, **$P < 0.01$, ***$P < 0.001$. **b** Survival curves for the four genes set in different subtypes

samples from TCGA, revealing survival time-specific modules (yellow, $p < 0.01$). As the most important gene in the module, the hub gene is the main feature of the gene module and closely related to the corresponding clinical information. Thus, we identified 228 intramodular hub genes based on GS and MS. The enrichment analysis of GO and

KEGG showed that adhesion function and adhesion molecules accounted for the highest proportion of hub genes. These results can partly explain why glioblastoma tumours exhibit high invasiveness, and adhesion molecules can play an important role in gliomagenesis. By constructing the Cox proportional hazards regression model, we selected an optimal four-gene model (OSMR + SOX21 + MED10 + PTPRN) for prognosis prediction. Among the genes in this model, OSMR and SOX21 have been previously reported in glioblastoma studies [28–31]. OSMR encodes a member of the type I cytokine receptor family. OSMR forms a complex with EGFRvIII, the most common EGFR mutation that occurs in glioblastoma, and regulates glioblastoma tumour growth. Overexpression of OSMR and low methylation level was reported to have a poor survival time in GBM [28]. According to our research and previous reports [29], expression level of OSMR was higher in mesenchymal and classical subtypes than proneural subtype. SOX21, the counteracting partner of SOX2, functions as a tumour suppressor during gliomagenesis by negatively regulating SOX2 [30, 31]. Currently, MED10 is known only as a component of the coactivator for DNA-binding factors that activate transcription via RNA polymerase II. The protein encoded by PTPRN is a member of the protein tyrosine phosphatase family and may be involved in cancer initiation and progression [32]. However, MED10 and PTPRN have not been previously reported in glioblastoma-related studies. Each gene was confirmed to have independent prognostic significance. The difference analyses were performed in the GSE50161 datasets. Although MED10 ($P = 0.5332$) and SOX21 ($P = 0.2831$) exhibited no differential expression in glioblastoma and normal tissues, they may exhibit differential expression between glioblastoma and low-grade glioma. Thus, further studies are needed.

WGCNA used a statistical method to make the gene network consistent with the scale-free distribution; the resulting gene modules are more in line with biological phenomena and can be more finely divided. To date, there are a few similar studies on glioblastoma. Aoki K used the Cox proportional hazards regression model to investigate the effects of genetic alterations in 308 diffuse lower-grade gliomas (LGGs) and verified the results using the dataset from TCGA. The authors reported that IDH mutation, 1p19q deletion, Notch homologue 1 (NOTCH1) mutations and phosphoinositide-3-kinase regulatory subunit 1 (PIK3R1) mutations were significantly associated with poor prognosis in LGGs [33]. However, glioblastomas were not examined. Horvath S adopted WGCNA to detect oncogenic modules and confirm abnormal spindle-like microcephaly-associated protein (ASPM) as a potential molecular target in glioblastoma [34]. Yu X used protein expression data of development process of macaque rhesus brain and RNA-seq data of GBM to identify several prognostic genes [35]. Similarly, Xiang Y applied WGCNA and K-means algorithm in gene

expression data of GBM obtained from the TCGA database and found some prognosis sub-networks [36]. But, compared to the K-mean clustering method, WGCNA can construct a gene co-expression network to identify the hub genes associated with trait-related modules directly. Whether the two methods are used simultaneously was reasonable needed to further research. In addition, similar studies using WGCNA to predict prognostic molecules are rare. These results indicate that further analysis of this module may provide more clues to understand the occurrence and development of glioma. However, this study has some limitations. First, we did not validate the prognostic value of the four-gene model due to the lack of survival data in the GEO datasets. Thus, prediction of prognosis using the four-gene model needs further verification. Second, we selected only 5000 genes for analysis in WGCNA. These transcript changes can not represent all the genetic changes in glioblastomas. By increasing the number of genes in the study, we can find more molecular targets and key pathways. Third, these results were only detected using bioinformatics analysis and needed further experimental verification. Overall, our study provide a new perspective to identify the potential molecules and therapeutic targets for glioblastoma.

Conclusions

In conclusion, in this study we performed a WGCNA approach with GBM RNA-seq data from TCGA database to reveal a survival time-specific module. We also constructed a Cox proportional hazards regression model and identified four independent prognostic factors (OSMR, SOX21, MED10 and PTPRN). Although the specific mechanism remained to be studied, these genes could be considered as risk factors for GBM patients and novel therapeutics.

Abbreviations
ATRX: X - linked alpha thalassemia mental retardation syndrome gene; AUC: Area under the curve; BP: Biological Process; CC: Cellular Component; EGFR: Epidermal growth factor receptor; FPKM: Fragments per kilobase per million; GBM: Glioblastoma multiforme; GEO: Gene Expression Omnibus; GO: Gene Ontology; GS: Gene significance; IDH1: Isocitrate dehydrogenase 1; IDH2: Isocitrate dehydrogenase 2; IGF-1: Insulin-like growth factor 1; KEGG: Kyoto Encyclopedia of Genes and Genomes; MED10: Mediator complex subunit 10; MF: Molecular Function; MGMT: O6methylguanine DNA methyltransferase; MS: Module significance; OSMR: Oncostatin M receptor; PDGFRA: Platelet-derived growth factor receptor alpha; PTPRN: Protein tyrosine phosphatase, receptor type N; ROC: Receiver operating characteristic curve; SOX21: SRY (sex determining region Y)-box 21; TCGA: The Cancer Genome Atlas; TOM: Topological overlap measure; VEGF: Vascular endothelial growth factor precursor; WGCNA: Weighted Gene Co-expression Network Analysis

Acknowledgements
We gratefully acknowledge the TCGA project organizers as well as all study participants for making data and results available. Meanwhile, we would like to thank Sturm D and Donson AM.

Funding
The present study was supported by grants from the National Science Foundation of China (nos. 81572489).

Authors' contributions

P-FX designed the study, analysed the data, performed computational coding. J-AY, J-HL, XY, J-ML collected the data. P-FX, F-EY, Y X, B-HL, and Q-XC involved in drafting the manuscript and revising it critically for important intellectual content. All authors agreed to be accountable for all aspects of the work and approved the final manuscript.

Competing interests

The authors declare that they have no competing interests.

References

1. Omuro A, DeAngelis LM. Glioblastoma and other malignant gliomas: a clinical review. JAMA. 2013;310(17):1842–50.
2. Alifieris C, Trafalis DT. Glioblastoma multiforme: pathogenesis and treatment. Pharmacol Ther. 2015;152:63–82.
3. Verhaak RG, Hoadley KA, Purdom E, Wang V, Qi Y, Wilkerson MD, Miller CR, Ding L, Golub T, Mesirov JP, et al. Integrated genomic analysis identifies clinically relevant subtypes of glioblastoma characterized by abnormalities in PDGFRA, IDH1, EGFR, and NF1. Cancer Cell. 2010;17(1):98–110.
4. Network TC. Corrigendum: comprehensive genomic characterization defines human glioblastoma genes and core pathways. NATURE. 2013;494(7438):506.
5. Westphal M, Lamszus K. Circulating biomarkers for gliomas. NAT REV NEUROL. 2015;11(10):556–66.
6. Bowman RL, Wang Q, Carro A, Verhaak RG, Squatrito M. GlioVis data portal for visualization and analysis of brain tumor expression datasets. Neuro-Oncology. 2017;19(1):139–41.
7. Sturm D, Witt H, Hovestadt V, Khuong-Quang DA, Jones DT, Konermann C, Pfaff E, Tonjes M, Sill M, Bender S, et al. Hotspot mutations in H3F3A and IDH1 define distinct epigenetic and biological subgroups of glioblastoma. Cancer Cell. 2012;22(4):425–37.
8. Griesinger AM, Birks DK, Donson AM, Amani V, Hoffman LM, Waziri A, Wang M, Handler MH, Foreman NK. Characterization of distinct immunophenotypes across pediatric brain tumor types. J Immunol. 2013; 191(9):4880–8.
9. Gravendeel LA, Kouwenhoven MC, Gevaert O, de Rooi JJ, Stubbs AP, Duijm JE, Daemen A, Bleeker FE, Bralten LB, Kloosterhof NK, et al. Intrinsic gene expression profiles of gliomas are a better predictor of survival than histology. Cancer Res. 2009;69(23):9065–72.
10. Langfelder P, Horvath S. WGCNA: an R package for weighted correlation network analysis. BMC BIOINFORMATICS. 2008;9:559.
11. Li A, Horvath S. Network neighborhood analysis with the multi-node topological overlap measure. BIOINFORMATICS. 2007;23(2):222–31.
12. Yip AM, Horvath S. Gene network interconnectedness and the generalized topological overlap measure. BMC BIOINFORMATICS. 2007;8:22.
13. Langfelder P, Zhang B, Horvath S. Defining clusters from a hierarchical cluster tree: the dynamic tree cut package for R. BIOINFORMATICS. 2008; 24(5):719–20.
14. Fuller TF, Ghazalpour A, Aten JE, Drake TA, Lusis AJ, Horvath S. Weighted gene coexpression network analysis strategies applied to mouse weight. Mamm Genome. 2007;18(6–7):463–72.
15. Ghazalpour A, Doss S, Zhang B, Wang S, Plaisier C, Castellanos R, Brozell A, Schadt EE, Drake TA, Lusis AJ, et al. Integrating genetic and network analysis to characterize genes related to mouse weight. PLoS Genet. 2006;2(8):e130.
16. Langfelder P, Luo R, Oldham MC, Horvath S. Is my network module preserved and reproducible? PLoS Comput Biol. 2011;7(1):e1001057.
17. Storey JD, Tibshirani R. Statistical significance for genomewide studies. Proc Natl Acad Sci U S A. 2003;100(16):9440–5.
18. Shannon P, Markiel A, Ozier O, Baliga NS, Wang JT, Ramage D, Amin N, Schwikowski B, Ideker T. Cytoscape: a software environment for integrated models of biomolecular interaction networks. Genome Res. 2003;13(11): 2498–504.
19. Yu G, Wang LG, Yan GR, He QY. DOSE: an R/bioconductor package for disease ontology semantic and enrichment analysis. BIOINFORMATICS. 2015; 31(4):608–9.
20. Ashburner M, Ball CA, Blake JA, Botstein D, Butler H, Cherry JM, Davis AP, Dolinski K, Dwight SS, Eppig JT, et al. Gene ontology: tool for the unification of biology. The Gene Ontology Consortium NAT GENET. 2000;25(1):25–9.
21. Yu G, Wang LG, Han Y. He QY: clusterProfiler: an R package for comparing biological themes among gene clusters. OMICS. 2012;16(5):284–7.
22. Tang RX, Chen WJ, He RQ, Zeng JH, Liang L, Li SK, Ma J, Luo DZ, Chen G. Identification of a RNA-Seq based prognostic signature with five lncRNAs for lung squamous cell carcinoma. ONCOTARGET. 2017;8(31):50761–73.
23. Loraine AE, Blakley IC, Jagadeesan S, Harper J, Miller G, Firon N. Analysis and visualization of RNA-Seq expression data using RStudio, bioconductor, and integrated genome browser. Methods Mol Biol. 2015;1284:481–501.
24. He D, Liu ZP, Chen L. Identification of dysfunctional modules and disease genes in congenital heart disease by a network-based approach. BMC Genomics. 2011;12:592.
25. Goh KI, Cusick ME, Valle D, Childs B, Vidal M, Barabasi AL. The human disease network. Proc Natl Acad Sci U S A. 2007;104(21):8685–90.
26. Wang Q, Hu B, Hu X, Kim H, Squatrito M, Scarpace L, DeCarvalho AC, Lyu S, Li P, Li Y, et al. Tumor evolution of Glioma-intrinsic gene expression subtypes associates with immunological changes in the microenvironment. Cancer Cell. 2017;32(1):42–56.
27. Garrett-Bakelman FE, Melnick AM. Differentiation therapy for IDH1/2 mutant malignancies. Cell Res. 2013;23(8):975–7.
28. Wang W, Zhao Z, Wu F, Wang H, Wang J, Lan Q, Zhao J. Bioinformatic analysis of gene expression and methylation regulation in glioblastoma. J Neuro-Oncol. 2018;136(3):495–503.
29. Natesh K, Bhosale D, Desai A, Chandrika G, Pujari R, Jagtap J, Chugh A, Ranade D, Shastry P. Oncostatin-M differentially regulates mesenchymal and proneural signature genes in gliomas via STAT3 signaling. NEOPLASIA. 2015; 17(2):225–37.
30. Caglayan D, Lundin E, Kastemar M, Westermark B, Ferletta M. Sox21 inhibits glioma progression in vivo by forming complexes with Sox2 and stimulating aberrant differentiation. Int J Cancer. 2013;133(6):1345–56.
31. Ferletta M, Caglayan D, Mokvist L, Jiang Y, Kastemar M, Uhrbom L, Westermark B. Forced expression of Sox21 inhibits Sox2 and induces apoptosis in human glioma cells. Int J Cancer. 2011;129(1):45–60.
32. Frankson R, Yu ZH, Bai Y, Li Q, Zhang RY, Zhang ZY. Therapeutic targeting of oncogenic tyrosine phosphatases. Cancer Res. 2017;77(21):5701–5.
33. Aoki K, Nakamura H, Suzuki H, Matsuo K, Kataoka K, Shimamura T, Motomura K, Ohka F, Shiina S, Yamamoto T, et al. Prognostic relevance of genetic alterations in diffuse lower-grade gliomas. Neuro-Oncology. 2018; 20(1):66–77.
34. Horvath S, Zhang B, Carlson M, Lu KV, Zhu S, Felciano RM, Laurance MF, Zhao W, Qi S, Chen Z, et al. Analysis of oncogenic signaling networks in glioblastoma identifies ASPM as a molecular target. Proc Natl Acad Sci U S A. 2006;103(46):17402–7.
35. Yu X, Feng L, Liu D, Zhang L, Wu B, Jiang W, Han Z, Cheng S. Quantitative proteomics reveals the novel co-expression signatures in early brain development for prognosis of glioblastoma multiforme. ONCOTARGET. 2016;7(12):14161–71.
36. Xiang Y, Zhang CQ, Huang K: Predicting glioblastoma prognosis networks using weighted gene co-expression network analysis on TCGA data. BMC BIOINFORMATICS 2012, 13 Suppl 2: S12.

13

Differentially expressed proteins in positive versus negative HNSCC lymph nodes

Alessandra Vidotto[1], Giovana M. Polachini[1], Marina de Paula-Silva[2], Sonia M. Oliani[2], Tiago Henrique[1], Rossana V. M. López[3], Patrícia M. Cury[4], Fabio D. Nunes[5], José F. Góis-Filho[6], Marcos B. de Carvalho[7], Andréia M. Leopoldino[8] and Eloiza H. Tajara[1,9]*

Abstract

Background: Lymph node metastasis is one of the most important prognostic factors in head and neck squamous cell carcinomas (HNSCCs) and critical for delineating their treatment. However, clinical and histological criteria for the diagnosis of nodal status remain limited. In the present study, we aimed to characterize the proteomic profile of lymph node metastasis from HNSCC patients.

Methods: In the present study, we used one- and two-dimensional electrophoresis and mass spectrometry analysis to characterize the proteomic profile of lymph node metastasis from HNSCC.

Results: Comparison of metastatic and non-metastatic lymph nodes showed 52 differentially expressed proteins associated with neoplastic development and progression. The results reinforced the idea that tumors from different anatomical subsites have dissimilar behaviors, which may be influenced by micro-environmental factor including the lymphatic network. The expression pattern of heat shock proteins and glycolytic enzymes also suggested an effect of the lymph node environment in controlling tumor growth or in metabolic reprogramming of the metastatic cell. Our study, for the first time, provided direct evidence of annexin A1 overexpression in lymph node metastasis of head and neck cancer, adding information that may be useful for diagnosing aggressive disease.

Conclusions: In brief, this study contributed to our understanding of the metastatic phenotype of HNSCC and provided potential targets for diagnostic in this group of carcinomas.

Keywords: Head and neck carcinoma, Metastasis, Lymph node, Proteomics

Background

Metastases are the main cause of death in cancer patients [1]. The power of these malignant cells to kill their hosts resides in their ability to leave the primary tumor, disseminate and invade ectopic sites, as well as to exhibit self-renewal and uncontrollable growth, leading to painful and incurable secondary tumors. In recent years, many data have revealed the determining factors mediating this destructive cascade, which include an extensive and growing list of genetic and epigenetic alterations [2].

In the initial steps of metastatization, tumor cell mutations and signals released by the stromal cells may cooperate to reduce cell-cell adhesion and to promote migration of epithelial neoplastic cells [3]. These events are similar to those of an important reversible differentiation program named epithelial-mesenchymal transition (EMT), which occurs during embryogenesis and have also been implicated in tumor invasion and metastasis [4].

As the tumor grows, low oxygen tension stimulates a proangiogenic response [5]. Due to cytokines secreted by neoplastic and stromal cells, endothelial cells from pre-existing blood vessels synthesize proteases, allowing their migration through the stroma [6]. These migrating endothelial cells proliferate and generate new vessels, which can supply oxygen and nutrients to sustain cancer growth and are an important route for metastasis [7]. Lymphatic vessel formation, a common event in various

* Correspondence: tajara@famerp.br
[1]Departamento de Biologia Molecular, Faculdade de Medicina (FAMERP), Av. Brigadeiro Faria Lima, 5416, Vila São Pedro, São José do Rio Preto, SP CEP 15090-000, Brazil
[9]Departamento de Genética e Biologia Evolutiva, Instituto de Biociências, Universidade de São Paulo, R. do Matão, 321, São Paulo, SP CEP 05508-090, Brazil
Full list of author information is available at the end of the article

inflammatory conditions, is also stimulated in some human cancers [8] and evolves to an important route of spread of tumors cells to regional lymph nodes [9].

The lymphatic network is more permissive for metastatic spread than the blood vascular system because (a) the basement membranes of the vessels are incomplete, (b) their capillaries exhibit a single endothelial cell layer not surrounded by pericytes and (c) have intercellular valve-like structures that facilitate the uptake of cells [10]. In addition to the permissive structure, the hydrostatic pressure of the lymphatic system is lower compared to blood circulation, reducing the mechanical challenge [11]. Otherwise, lymph is richer in immune response factors which, although insufficient to destroy tumor cells [12], may play an important role in selecting immune resistance phenotypes [13]. Examples of tumors that frequently metastasize to regional lymph nodes via lymphatic route instead of spreading to distant sites are the head and neck carcinomas (HNSCC) [14], a group of neoplasms nearly always associated with chronic inflammation.

Arrival at a secondary site does not ensure success for most metastatic cells. The processes of extravasation and seeding require specific tumor characteristics and receptive conditions. To increase the chances of a favorable outcome, it has been suggested that target sites are prepared in advance by long-distance interaction with the primary tumor [15, 16]. The pattern of metastatic seeding and colonization is not random and, depending on the primary site, tumor cells spread to particular organ sites more frequently than to others [17].

The mechanisms involved in metastasis organotropism are not completely known but chemokines and their receptors, as well as circulation patterns and structural features of local capillaries should be important contributors for the process [18]. Several critical genes driving organ-specific metastases have been described in different tumors [19, 20]. However, a number of questions remain unanswered. For example, in head and neck carcinomas, regional lymph nodes are the preferential target sites and distant metastases are a late and infrequent finding [21]. Why HNSCCs have this behavior and why small cell carcinomas of the head and neck [22] and several tumors of salivary gland [23], located in the same anatomical site, typically have distant metastases? The answer probably lies in the characteristics of the metastatic cell as well as in its interaction with the microenvironment.

Considering (a) the atypical feature of HNSCC to remain a locoregional disease, (b) the limitations of relapse risk assessment and (c) clinical and histological criteria for the diagnosis of lymph node spread, still the most powerful prognostic factor for these cancers [24], it is urgently necessary to define appropriate biomarkers of the metastatic phenotype for this group of diseases. In the present study, we aimed to characterize the proteomic profile of

lymph node metastasis from HNSCC using one- and two-dimensional electrophoresis and mass spectrometry analysis.

Methods
Tissue samples

Thirty-two samples of lymph nodes (12 non-metastatic or N0 and 20 metastatic or N+) were obtained from patients with surgically resected head and neck squamous cell carcinomas of three anatomical subsites classified according to the 10th edition of the International Classification of Diseases-10: C02 = other and unspecified parts of tongue; C04 = floor of mouth; C32 = larynx. Ten of the lymph node samples were derived from patients with tongue, 13 from floor of the mouth and 9 from larynx carcinomas and their extracted proteins were analyzed by either one-dimensional gel (1-D) or two-dimensional (2-D) gel electrophoresis. An overlapping set of 22 samples was analyzed by Western blot. Immunohistochemical staining was also performed using formalin-fixed, paraffin-embedded blocks (14 lymph nodes and 9 surgical margins) and tissue microarray slides (65 primary tumors) containing samples from C02, C03 (gum), C04, C32 and C06 (other and unspecified parts of mouth) neoplasms. Therefore, two anatomical sites were analyzed: oral cavity (C02, C03, C04, C06 subsites) and larynx (C032).

Surgical specimens were obtained before radio- or chemotherapy by the Head and Neck Genome Project (GENCAPO), a collaborative consortium of research groups from hospitals and universities in São Paulo State, Brazil, whose aim is to develop clinical, genetic and epidemiological analysis of head and neck squamous cell carcinomas.

Immediately after surgery, part of specimen was frozen in liquid nitrogen and stored at − 80 °C, and part was fixed in formalin for immunohistochemistry or routine histopathological examination. Frozen sections of the lymph nodes were analyzed to confirm the presence (N+) or absence (N0) of tumor cells. The primary tumors were classified by the Tumor-Node-Metastases (TNM) system [25]. A full description of the clinicopathological data is provided in Additional file 1.

The study protocol was approved by each institutional review board and by the National Committee on Ethics in Research/CONEP (reference number 1763/05, 18/05/2005). All patients provided written informed consent.

Proteomic approaches
Sample preparation

Sample preparation was performed according to the protocol described by de Marqui et al. [26], with modifications. In brief, lymph node samples were cut into small pieces and washed with 500 μL of lysis buffer containing 7 M urea, 2 M thiourea, 4% CHAPS detergent, 65 mM DTT, and 0.2% carrier ampholytes. The specimens were disrupted by sonication twice for 1 min at 0 °C and vortexed vigorously for approximately 2 min. The lysates were centrifuged at 10,000 g for 3 min at 4 °C. Protein concentration of the resulting supernatant was determined by the Bradford method [27]. The protein samples were stored in aliquots at − 80 °C.

To optimize the experiments with 32 samples in triplicates, lymph node samples were pooled according to the presence or absence of tumor cells and according to the anatomic subsite, namely tongue, floor of the mouth, and larynx (Additional file 2). The 6 pools (A-F) combined equal amounts of protein from each sample, resulting in 100 µg and 1500 µg per pool for one-dimensional gel electrophoresis (1-DE) and two-dimensional gel electrophoresis (2-DE) gels, respectively.

One-dimensional gel electrophoresis (1-DE)

Two protein pools (E and F) of 3 N0 and 6 N+ lymph nodes from larynx carcinomas were analyzed by 1-DE. Under reducing conditions, 100 µg of each protein pool were denatured at 96 °C for 5 min in 5X loading buffer with β-mercaptoethanol and loaded on one-dimensional 12% resolving/5% stacking sodium dodecyl sulfate (SDS) - polyacrylamide gel (PAGE), according to Laemmli [28]. Electrophoresis was carried out on a vertical electrophoresis apparatus (SE 400 Vertical Unit, GE Healthcare, Uppsala, Sweden) at 120 V. Proteins were detected by Coomassie Blue staining, and the molecular mass was estimated using molecular weight standard proteins of 14.4–97 kDa (LMW Calibration Kit for SDS Electrophoresis, GE Healthcare).

Two-dimensional gel electrophoresis (2-DE)

Three protein pools of N0 and three protein pools of N+ lymph nodes from patients with tongue (pools A and B), floor of the mouth (pools C and D) or larynx carcinomas (pools E and F) were analyzed by 2-DE, according to de Marqui et al. [26], with modifications. Proteins were precipitated using ice-cold acetone 100%, and centrifuged at 13,000 g for 5 min at 4 °C. Aliquots containing approximately 1500 µg of protein were diluted with rehydration buffer [8 M urea, 2% w/v CHAPS, 0.6% w/v DTT, 0.5% v/v immobilized linear pH gradient (IPG) buffer pH 3–10, trace of bromophenol blue] to a total volume of 250 µL and loaded onto an IPG strip (13 cm, pH 3–10 L, GE Healthcare).

After isoelectric focusing/IEF (total of 26,500 V-hours at 20 °C, 50 mA/strip) on an IPGphor apparatus (GE Healthcare), IPG strips were incubated in the equilibration solution (6 M urea, 50 mM Tris-HCl pH 8.8, 30% v/v glycerol, 2% w/v SDS, trace of bromophenol blue) containing 1% w/v DTT, followed by incubation in the same solution containing 2.5% w/v iodoacetamide instead of DTT. IPG

strips were sealed on top of 12.5% SDS-polyacrylamide gel 0.5% w/v low-melting agarose in SDS running buffer.

Electrophoresis was performed in a Hoefer SE 600 Ruby vertical electrophoresis unit (GE Healthcare) at 15 mA/gel for 30 min and 30 mA/gel for 7 h at 10 °C. The samples were run in triplicate and the LMW Calibration Kit was used as a molecular mass standard. After Coomassie blue staining, the gels were scanned using an ImageScanner (GE Healthcare) and the images were analyzed using the ImageMaster 2D Platinum software, version 6.0 (GE Healthcare). Gels from N0 and N+ groups of each anatomical subsite were matched to a reference gel. Spot quantification was based on the spot volume as percentage of the total volume of all spots in the gel. For each anatomical subsite, differential image analysis was carried out by matching spots from gel triplicates of each group (N0 and N+). Differences between groups were evaluated statistically by using the Student's t-test with $p < 0.05$ as significant.

In-gel protein digestion and mass spectrometry (MS)

Sequential slices of 1-DE gels and differentially expressed protein spots from 2-DE gels were manually cut out from the gels. The samples were mixed with 50% acetonitrile (ACN)/25 mM ammonium bicarbonate solution and dehydrated with ACN for 15 min. Acetonitrile was discarded and the gel pieces were dried in a vacuum centrifuge for 30 min. Gel pieces were digested with trypsin and incubated for 24 h at 37 °C. Peptides were extracted with 1% trifluoroacetic acid (TFA) for 12 h and 1% TFA/50% ACN for 2 h. The supernatants were mixed and concentrated in a vacuum centrifuge to approximately 5–10 µL.

Digested samples from 1-DE gels were applied to a C18 (100 µm X 100 mm) RP-nanoUPLC (nanoAcquity, Waters, Milford, MA, USA) coupled with a Q-TOF (Quadrupole Ion Trap - Time of Flight) Ultima mass spectrometer (Waters) with nano-electrospray source at a flow rate of 0.6 µL/min. The gradient condition was developed with 0–50% acetonitrile in 0.1% formic acid for 60 min. The instrument was operated in the 'top three' mode and the spectra were acquired using the MassLynx software version 4.1 (Waters). The raw data files were processed to peak list with the Mascot Distiller software, version 2.2.1.0 (Matrix Science, London, UK). Mascot search results were exported to Scaffold software (version 3.06, Proteome Software Inc., Portland, OR, USA) for validation. Protein and peptide identification probabilities were set up at > 95%, with one minimum peptide. The samples were grouped in metastatic and non-metastatic, the spectral counts were normalized and proteins with a fold change ≥2.0 were considered to be differentially expressed. Fold change was calculated by Scaffold software (according to [29]).

After trypsin digestion, the peptide samples from 2-DE gels were placed into matrix solution (10 mg/mL α-cyano-4-hydroxycinnamic acid, 0.1% *v*/v TFA in 50% v/v ACN) in a 1:1 (v:v) ratio, spotted on a stainless steel sample plate and analyzed by a MALDI-Q-TOF (Matrix Assisted Laser Desorption Ionization - Quadrupole Ion Trap - Time of Flight) Premier mass spectrometer (Waters). Mascot Daemon (version 2.2.0, Matrix Science) was used to search the NCBI non-redundant database with the parameters: enzyme, trypsin; allowed number of missed cleavages, 1; fixed modification, carbamidomethylation on cysteine; variable modification, oxidation on methionine; peptide tolerance, 0.1 Da; MS/MS tolerance, 0.1 Da; monoisotopic masses.

Metabolic pathways, associated ontologies and expression data

The set of genes encoding differentially expressed proteins was imported into HNdb [30], a head and neck database that provides information on genes and proteins involved in head and neck squamous cell carcinoma, covering data on genomics, transcriptomics, proteomics, literature citations and also cross-references of external databases. Using this database, the genes were linked to KEGG [31] metabolic pathways, associated ontologies [32], and microarray data [33].

The set of genes was also functionally clustered using DAVID [34, 35], a database for annotation, visualization and integrated discovery. The one-tail Fisher Exact Probability Value was used for gene-enrichment analysis, and Bonferroni and Benjamini–Hochberg corrected *p*-values less than 0.05 were considered significant.

Immunodetection

In order to validate the proteomic findings, a literature search was performed to select candidate targets showing an unclear role in head and neck tumorigenesis or involved in the development and progression of head and neck neoplasms but never evaluated in their lymph node metastasis. Using these criteria, two proteins (epidermal-type fatty acid-binding protein or E-FABP, and annexin A1 or ANXA1) were selected to be validated.

Western blot

The expression of E-FABP was analyzed by Western blot in a subset of 22 individual samples (11 N0 and 11 N+ lymph nodes from 8 tongue, 8 floor of the mouth and 6 larynx carcinomas). The antibodies used were polyclonal primary anti-E-FABP (ab37267, Abcam, Cambridge, MA, USA) diluted 1:500, and monoclonal primary anti-β-actin antibody (A1978 Sigma-Aldrich, Saint Louis, MO, USA) diluted 1:5000. In brief, protein samples (10 μg) were subjected to SDS-PAGE (12% resolving gel with 5% stacking gel) under denaturing conditions at 120 V for 120 min, using a Mini-Protean 3 Cell Electrophoresis

System (BioRad, Hercules, CA, USA). The molecular weight ladder was the PageRuler™ Prestained Protein Ladder (SM0671, Fermentas Life Sciences, Vilnius, Lithuania).

Samples were transferred electrophoretically (90 V for 90 min) to polyvinylidene difluoride (PVDF) membranes (Immobilon-P Membrane, Millipore, Bedford, MA, USA) by using transfer buffer (25 mM Tris, 0.2 M glycine, 20% *v*/v methanol). Antibodies were detected using Western Breeze chromogenic system (Invitrogen, Carlsbad, CA, USA) and the blots were then scanned and analyzed using a Kodak Gel Logic 2200 Digital Imaging System (Carestream Health, Rochester, NY, USA).

Immunohistochemistry

Immunohistochemical analysis of a tissue microarray (TMA) with duplicate tissue cores of 65 primary oral squamous cell carcinoma samples was carried out by a polymer-based immunohistochemistry method using rabbit polyclonal antibody anti-E-FABP (ab37267), at a dilution of 1:500. Nine tissue slides containing archival formalin-fixed, paraffin-embedded tissue (FFPE) sections of surgical margins were used to establish a cut off value level for positivity. After deparaffinization and rehydration in xylene and graded ethanol, the slides were immersed in 10 mM citrate buffer (pH 6.0) and heated in a water bath (97 °C, 20 min) for antigen epitope retrieval. Endogenous peroxidase activity was blocked with methanol containing 3% hydrogen peroxide for 30 min. Specimens were incubated overnight with the primary antibody in a humidity-controlled chamber. The sections were washed twice with PBS and Tween 0.25% at room temperature. Immune complexes were subsequently treated using EnVision+Dual Link System-HRP (K4061, DAKO, Fisher Scientific, Hampton, NH, USA), and DAB (3,3′-diamino-benzidine) in chromogen solution (K3468; DAKO, Fisher Scientific). Counterstaining was performed with Mayer's hematoxylin. Nuclear and cytoplasmatic staining of the epithelial cells was considered specific.

Percentage of positive cells in each TMA spot was scored as follows: 0 or negative (not detectable or detectable in less than 5% of tumor cells), 1 (labeling of more than 5% and less than 10% of tumor cells), 2 (labeling of more than 10% and less than 50% of tumor cells), 3 (labeling of more than 50% and less than 75% of tumor cells), 4 (widely and highly expressed in more than 75% of the tumor cells), at × 400 magnification. The intensity of immunoreaction was scored as negative (0), mild (1), moderate (2) and intense (3). The percentage of positive tumor cells and the staining intensity then were multiplied to produce an E-FABP score for each case. Cases with a final score > 9.4 (the average score from normal tissue) were defined as positive.

Immunohistochemical analysis of 14 lymph node specimens from patients with C02, C04 and C32 tumors was also performed to investigate the expression of annexin

A1. Two-micrometer FFPE sections were processed by deparaffinization, rehydration and antigen epitope retrieval, as described above. Endogenous peroxidase and non-specific epitopes were blocked with 3% hydrogen peroxide and 5% bovine serum albumin in phosphate-buffered saline (BSA-PBS) for 30 min, respectively. The slides were then incubated overnight at 4 °C with rabbit polyclonal anti-ANXA1 (71–3400, Thermo Fisher Scientific, Waltham, MA, USA) at a dilution of 1:2000, in 1% BSA. Some sections were incubated with 1% BSA instead of the primary antibody to provide a negative control of the reaction. After washing, sections were incubated with the secondary biotinylated antibody (959943-B, Thermo Fisher Scientific). Positive staining was detected using a peroxidase-conjugated streptavidin complex and the color was developed using DAB substrate (002014, Thermo Fisher Scientific). Finally, sections were counterstained with hematoxylin and mounted. ANXA1 immunostaining was evaluated by densitometric analysis conducted using an Axioskop 2-Mot Plus Microscope and AxioVision 4.8 software (Carl Zeiss, Jena, Germany) on an arbitrary scale from 0 to 255. Data were expressed as mean ± standard error.

Results

Casuistic

Of the 32 lymph node samples evaluated by 1-DE/MS, 2-DE/MS, 12 were derived from patients with N0 and 20 with N+ tumors classified as: 10 tongue, 13 floor of the mouth and 9 larynx carcinomas (C02, C04, C32, respectively). The samples were combined in six pools and analyzed using 1-DE and/or 2-DE and mass spectrometry (Additional file 2). The mean age of the patients was 60.1 years (range, 45–79 years), and the male/female sex ratio was 9.7:1. Most patients were smokers or former smokers (28/32) and had a history of chronic alcohol consumption (29/32) (Additional file 1).

Proteomic approaches

One- and two-dimensional gel electrophoresis (1-DE and 2-DE)

The 1-DE data validated by Scaffold software allowed the identification of 39 differentially expressed proteins (≥ 2.0-fold change) between N0 and N+ lymph nodes, with over 99% confidence (as per the Scaffold algorithm, at least one unique peptide per protein) (Table 1). Using these parameters, the false discovery rate (FDR) for protein identification was 0.2%. The 2-DE analysis revealed 22 differentially expressed proteins between metastatic and non-metastatic lymph nodes (Student's t test $p < 0.05$). Fourteen proteins were overexpressed and eight underexpressed in metastatic samples compared with non-metastatic ones (Table 2, Fig. 1, Additional file 3). Nine differentially expressed proteins were detected by both 1-DE and 2-DE (Apo-AI, CA-I, GSTP1–1, HspB1, hemoglobin

subunit delta, CK1, profilin-1, TIM, protein S100-A9), four of them (Apo-AI, GSTP1–1, HspB1, CK1) overexpressed by 2-DE and underexpressed by 1-DE (Tables 1 and 2). Therefore, a total of 52 differentially expressed proteins were identified. Some of them exhibited a diverse 2-DE profile in metastasis of tongue, floor of the mouth and larynx carcinomas. For example, Apo-AI only showed differential expression in N+ lymph nodes of floor of the mouth tumors, and calreticulin and PDI in N+ lymph nodes of larynx carcinomas. Differences between C02 and C04, which are derived from the same anatomical subsite (oral cavity), were also observed, such as hemoglobin subunit delta, endoplasmin, LAP-3, Apo-AI, Ig gamma and kappa chains, and CK1 (Table 2).

Metabolic pathways, associated ontologies and expression data

Clustering the set of 52 differentially expressed genes using DAVID, 16 annotation clusters were obtained, 6 of them with Bonferroni and Benjamini–Hochberg corrected p-values < 0.05 (Additional file 4). These clusters were related to regulation of cell-cell adhesion, cellular oxidant detoxification, response to reactive oxygen species, and membrane organization. When analyzed individually by HNdb tools, over and underexpressed proteins showed activities expected for lymph nodes containing metastatic cells, many being associated with angiogenesis, apoptosis, cell growth, cell migration, and development processes (Tables 3 and 4).

Positive scores for gene-to-HNSCC association determined by HNdb hypergeometric test were referred to 30/52 genes encoding these proteins (Additional file 5). Seven out of 52 genes (GSTP1, HSP90B1, HSPB1, PFN1, RAP1A, SFN, YWHAZ) were assigned to KEGG pathways in cancer, cell migration and cell cycle, and in signaling networks involved in proliferation, cellular motility, apoptosis, cell adhesion, angiogenesis and genetic integrity.

Immunodetection

A protein related to invasive phenotype (E-FABP) and a potential cancer marker showing an unanticipated expression profile (annexin A1) were selected for validation by Western blotting and/or immunohistochemical assay. As expected, Western blot analysis revealed high levels of E-FABP in most N+ lymph nodes (10/11) when compared with N0 samples (0/11) (Fig. 2), which was confirmed by pixel density quantification using Image J software. In immunohistochemical assays, 41/65 primary tumor samples were considered positive for E-FABP (Fig. 3). Fisher's exact test was used to estimate statistical difference between E-FABP positivity and clinicopathological parameters. There was no significant association between tumor size ($p = 0.61$), nodal metastasis ($p = 0.80$), pathologic

Table 1 Under and overexpressed proteins identified by one-dimensional gel electrophoresis (1-DE) in metastatic (N+) and non-metastatic (N0) lymph nodes from laryngeal SCC patients. Proteins were separated by one-dimensional gel electrophoresis and identified by Q-TOF MS and Scaffold software according to quantitative value. Thirty-nine proteins with a fold change of at least 2.0 were considered with differential abundance between the categories

Protein name	Gene symbol	UniProt accession	Quantitative value		Fold change	N+
			N+	N0	N+/N0	
Actin, cytoplasmic 1	ACTB	P60709	1	8	0.1	Down
Serum albumin	ALB	P02768	2	14	0.1	Down
Apolipoprotein A-I	APOA1	P02647	0	10	< 2.0	Down
Rho GDP-dissociation inhibitor 1	ARHGDIA	P52565	0	2	< 2.0	Down
Rho GDP-dissociation inhibitor 2	ARHGDIB	P52566	0	4	< 2.0	Down
Flavin reductase (NADPH)	BLVRB	P30043	0	3	< 2.0	Down
Carbonic anhydrase 1	CA1	P00915	0	2	< 2.0	Down
Coactosin-like protein	COTL1	Q14019	0	2	< 2.0	Down
Glyceraldehyde-3-phosphate dehydrogenase	GAPDH	P04406	1	2	0.5	Down
Glutathione S-transferase P	GSTP1	P09211	0	2	< 2.0	Down
Hemoglobin subunit alpha	HBA1/HBA2	P69905	0	28	< 2.0	Down
Hemoglobin subunit beta	HBB	P68871	0	10	< 2.0	Down
Hemoglobin subunit delta	HBD	P02042	0	17	< 2.0	Down
Histone H2A type 1-A	HIST1H2AA	Q96QV6	0	2	< 2.0	Down
Histone H2B type 1-C/E/F/G/I	HIST1H2BG	P62807	0	3	< 2.0	Down
Histone H3.1	HIST1H3A	P68431	0	4	< 2.0	Down
Heat shock protein beta-1	HSPB1	P04792	0	3	< 2.0	Down
Keratin, type II cytoskeletal 1	KRT1	P04264	0	3	< 2.0	Down
Keratin, type I cytoskeletal 9	KRT9	P35527	0	2	< 2.0	Down
Myosin light polypeptide 6	MYL6	P60660	0	2	< 2.0	Down
Protein deglycase DJ-1	PARK7	Q99497	0	3	< 2.0	Down
Profilin-1	PFN1	P07737	0	5	< 2.0	Down
Peptidyl-prolyl cis-trans isomerase A	PPIA	P62937	1	6	0.2	Down
Peroxiredoxin-1	PRDX1	Q06830	1	6	0.2	Down
Peroxiredoxin-2	PRDX2	P32119	0	5	< 2.0	Down
Peroxiredoxin-6	PRDX6	P30041	0	2	< 2.0	Down
Proteasome subunit beta type-5	PSMB5	P28074	0	2	< 2.0	Down
Ras-related protein Rab-10	RAB10	P61026	1	2	0.5	Down
Ras-related protein Rab-5B	RAB5B	P61020	0	2	< 2.0	Down
Ras-related protein Rap-1A	RAP1A	P62834	0	2	< 2.0	Down
Transgelin-2	TAGLN2	P37802	0	2	< 2.0	Down
Triosephosphate isomerase	TPI1	P60174	2	11	0.2	Down
14–3-3 protein beta/alpha	YWHAB	P31946	0	7	< 2.0	Down
14–3-3 protein zeta/delta	YWHAZ	P63104	3	10	0.3	Down
Annexin A1	ANXA1	P04083	4	0	> 2.0	Up
Keratin, type I cytoskeletal 13	KRT13	P13646	3	0	> 2.0	Up
Keratin, type II cytoskeletal 6A	KRT6A	P02538	4	0	> 2.0	Up
Periostin	POSTN	Q15063	2	0	> 2.0	Up
Protein S100-A9	S100A9	P06702	10	0	> 2.0	Up

Table 2 Under and overexpressed proteins identified by two-dimensional gel electrophoresis (2-DE) in metastatic (N+) and non-metastatic (N0) lymph nodes from oral cavity SCC patients. Proteins were separated by two-dimensional electrophoresis and identified by MALDI-Q-TOF MS/MS. Twenty-two proteins were considered with differential abundance between the categories (Student's t test $p < 0.05$). C02, C04, C32 columns correspond to pools from tongue (pools A and B), floor of the mouth (pools C and D) and larynx carcinomas (pools E and F), respectively. N+/N0: abundance ratio

Protein name	Gene symbol	UniProt accession	pI	Mass	Sequence coverage (%)	Score	Queries matched	Area[a]	C02 N+/N0	C04	C32	N+
Carbonic anhydrase 1 or CA-I	CA1	P00915	6.65	28,620	16	116	3	VII	0.4402	0.2033	0.2971	Down
Calreticulin or CRP55	CALR	P27797	4.29	48,283	9	167	3	IX			0.6211	Down
Hemoglobin subunit delta	HBD	P02042	7.97	16,028	19	64	2	IV		0.3906	0.1063	Down
Heat shock protein 90 kDa beta member 1 or endoplasmin	HSP90B1	P14625	4.76	92,696	4	69	3	I	0.4010		0.5364	Down
Cytosol aminopeptidase or LAP-3	LAP3	P28838	6.29	53,006	4	71	3	IX	0.4514		0.6685	Down
Protein disulfide-isomerase or PDI	P4HB	P07237	4.76	57,480	8	201	4	IX			0.6616	Down
Profilin-1	PFN1	P07737	8.48	15,085	10	50	2	IV	0.3568	0.4595	0.6419	Down
Triosephosphate isomerase or TIM	TPI1	P60174	6.51	26,807	8	51	1	VI	0.5020	0.3262	0.3373	Down
Aldo-keto reductase family 1 member B10 or ARL-1	AKR1B10	O60218	7.12	36,226	12	149	3	II	3.7339	2.2564		Up
Apolipoprotein A-I or Apo-AI	APOA1	P02647	5.56	30,759	11	104	3	VI		1.5333		Up
Cystatin-B or CPI-B	CSTB	P04080	7.90	11,224	24	64	2	XI	2.0971	1.9614		Up
Fatty acid-binding protein, epidermal or E-FABP	FABP5	Q01469	6.84	15,366	18	94	2	VIII	4.0016	7.4081	5.5954	Up
Glutathione S-transferase P or GSTP1–1	GSTP1	P09211	5.44	23,438	12	78	2	VI	2.3289	4.0385	2.9731	Up
Heat shock protein beta-1 or HspB1	HSPB1	P04792	5.98	22,826	20	105	3	III	3.2028	4.1256	4.5202	Up
Ig gamma-1 chain C region	IGHG1	P01857	8.46	36,596	9	71	2	X	4.1259		4.3046	Up
Ig kappa chain C region	IGKC	P01834	7.55	26,077	14	48	2	VII		2.5279	2.1303	Up
Keratin, type II cytoskeletal 1 or CK1	KRT1	P04264	8.16	66,018	4	82	2	VII		1.7525	2.0958	Up
Galectin-1 or Gal-1	LGALS1	P09382	5.34	14,917	8	54	1	V	1.8654	2.2229	1.4698	Up
Galectin-7 or Gal-7	LGALS7B	P47929	7.00	14,992	19	73	2	VIII	6.2867	2.5605	2.7244	Up
Protein S100-A7 or psoriasin	S100A7	P31151	6.26	11,433	34	103	3	VIII	6.4075	9.3486	5.3993	Up
Protein S100-A9 or calgranulin-B	S100A9	P06702	5.71	13,291	42	100	3	VIII	4.7500	5.9737	4.9505	Up
14–3–3 protein sigma or stratifin	SFN	P31947	4.64	27,874	15	98	3	III	13.4829	7.3989	27.6468	Up

[a]Areas are numbered as in Additional file 1

TNM classification ($p = 0.37$), pathological grade ($p = 0.20$), lymphatic, and perineural invasion ($p = 1.00$; $p = 0.36$). Overall survival rate was compared with the expression of FABP5 using the Kaplan-Meier method, and the P value for the survival curve, determined by the log-rank test, was not statistically significant in the survival rates between positive and negative tumors ($p = 0.88$).

Immunohistochemical analysis of ANXA1 was carried out on metastatic and non-metastatic lymph node samples. Constitutive ANXA1 expression was observed in the subcapsular sinus of N0 lymph nodes (Fig. 4a). In the N+ samples, its expression was increased, especially in the loose conjunctive tissue, which constitutes the subcapsular sinus, above the external cortex of the lymph node. In these metastatic samples, epithelial cells showed a more intense cytoplasmic expression of ANXA1 compared

to control biopsies (Fig. 4b). No immunostaining was detected in the negative control (Fig. 4c).

ANXA1 was not validated by Western blot. Due to the limited amount of protein from lymph node samples, the detection by immunohistochemistry was prioritized, since it is a more sensitive and specific assay and can be performed on paraffin-embedded sections.

Discussion

In the present study, we investigated the proteomic profile of lymph node metastasis from squamous cell carcinomas of tongue, floor of the mouth and larynx, by using one- and two-dimensional electrophoresis and mass spectrometry analysis. Fifty-two proteins were differentially expressed in metastatic compared with non-metastatic lymph nodes analyzed by 1-DE and 2-DE.

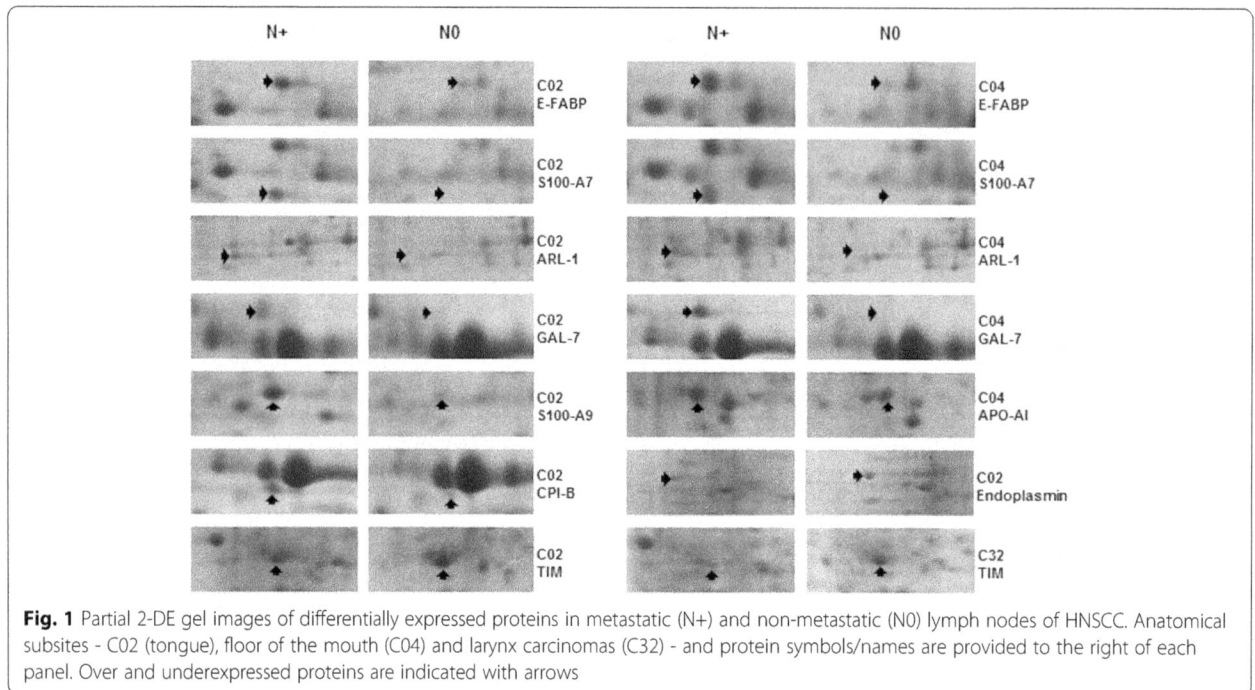

Fig. 1 Partial 2-DE gel images of differentially expressed proteins in metastatic (N+) and non-metastatic (N0) lymph nodes of HNSCC. Anatomical subsites - C02 (tongue), floor of the mouth (C04) and larynx carcinomas (C32) - and protein symbols/names are provided to the right of each panel. Over and underexpressed proteins are indicated with arrows

Western blot and/or immunohistochemical analysis confirmed the results for two representative proteins (E-FABP and annexin A1). Although the performance of 1-DE was better than that of 2-DE, several recent studies using 2-DE technique present consistent results [36–40] and show that it is still an important top-down analytical approach [41]. Anyhow, 1-DE is also unable to completely resolve complex mixtures of proteins.

Some of the over and underexpressed proteins may play an important role in the head and neck tumorigenesis and metastatization processes. For example, aldo-keto reductase ARL-1 is a potential biomarker for non-small cell lung cancer of smokers [42] and, therefore, may be involved in the pathogenesis of tobacco-related cancers [43], including HNSCCs. Other proteins have already been associated with HNSCC by several authors [44–46] and by our group, particularly annexin A1 [47, 48], fatty acid-binding protein E-FABP [49, 50], heat shock protein beta-1 [51, 52], galectin-1 [53, 54], glutathione S-transferase P [55, 56], keratin, type I cytoskeletal 13 [57, 58], peptidyl-prolyl cis-trans isomerase A [59, 60], periostin [61], protein deglycase DJ-1 [62, 63], protein S100A7 [64, 65] and Ras-related protein RAP-1A [66]. In fact, the genes encoding some of these proteins showed the highest scores for gene-to-HNSCC association determined by HNdb hypergeometric test, namely *FABP5, S100A7, ANXA1, LGALS1, PARK7, GSTP1*, with scores ranging from 1.88 to 83. The expression pattern of these proteins was also evaluated using The Human Protein Atlas (https://www.proteinatlas.org), a public database

containing protein expression information based on approximately 700 antibodies combined with transcriptomics data from The Cancer Genome Atlas - TCGA (average fragments per kilobase of transcript per million mapped reads - FPKM) [67]. Because Protein Atlas has very few samples analyzed by immunohistochemistry and joins different subsites of head and neck carcinomas, the data showed low concordance with our findings. Otherwise, our findings showed higher concordance with the average FPKM values, especially for upregulated proteins. Similarly to what our group and other authors (44, 45, 81) observed for ANXA1/annexin A1 in primary tumors, Protein Atlas and TCGA refer a low expression of this protein in primary HNSCC.

Some differences were observed between lymph node samples from dissimilar anatomic subsites, which support a molecular heterogeneity for HNSCC metastasis, also previously reported by us for the primary tumors [68]. The differences in expression of, for example, APO-AI, calreticulin, CK1, endoplasmin, LAP-3, PDI, may affect tumor progression and drug response because these proteins are involved in signaling, cell proliferation, response to hypoxia and oxidative stress.

In regard to the metastasis environment, many questions remain. What proteins are predictive biomarkers for regional metastasis in HNSCC? What features were previously selected and expressed in cells leaving the primary tumor? After arriving in the lymph nodes, what would be the new challenge for tumor cells? Tentative answers to these questions may be exemplified by the findings we

Table 3 Information on biological processes based on Gene ontology. Up-regulated proteins identified by proteomic analysis of positive lymph node samples. Proteins are referenced by their HGNC gene symbol

Biological process	Up-regulated proteins[a]
Angiogenesis	HSPB1
Apoptosis	LGALS1, S100A9, SFN
Anti-apoptosis	ANXA1, GSTP1, HSPB1
Autophagy	S100A9
Cell adhesion	
Cell-cell adhesion	APOA1, POSTN
Cell communication	
Signaling	ANXA1, APOA1, HSPB1, IGHG1, IGKC, LGALS1, S100A7, S100A9, SFN
Cell-cell signaling	S100A9
Cell growth	
Positive regulation of cell growth	S100A9
Cell migration or movement	
Cell motility	ANXA1, HSPB1, S100A9
Cytoskeleton organization	KRT13, S100A9
Developmental process	
System development	GSTP1, POSTN
Cell differentiation	ANXA1
Epidermis development	FABP5, S100A7, SFN
Metabolic process	AKR1B10, APOA1, FABP5, GSTP1
Protein metabolic process	APOA1, CSTB
Lipid metabolic process	APOA1, FABP5
Protein modification process	GSTP1, SFN
Response to stimulus	ANXA1, HSPB1
Defense response	KRT6A, S100A7, S100A9
Inflammatory response	ANXA1, APOA1, S100A9
Immune response	APOA1, IGHG1, IGKC
Response to ROS	GSTP1, S100A7
Transcription	S100A9, SFN
Translation	HSPB1
Transport	APOA1

[a]Name of up-regulated proteins:*AKR1B10* Aldo-keto reductase family 1 member B10, *ANXA1* Annexin A1, *APOA1* Apolipoprotein A-I, *CSTB* Cystatin-B, *FABP5* Fatty acid-binding protein, epidermal, *GSTP1* Glutathione S-transferase P, *HSPB1* Heat shock protein beta-1, *IGHG1* Ig gamma-1 chain C region, *IGKC* Ig kappa chain C region, *KRT6A* Keratin, type II cytoskeletal 6A, *KRT13* Keratin, type I cytoskeletal 13, *LGALS1* Galectin-1, *POSTN* Periostin, *S100A7* Protein S100A7, *S100A9* Protein S100A9, *SFN* 14-3-3 protein sigma

obtained for galectin-1 and psoriasin. These proteins have been shown to be associated with hypoxia [69–71], a common adverse condition faced by metastatic, as well as primary tumor cells. The findings of Chaudary and Hill [72] reinforce the idea that 'hypoxia-related' factors

regulate lymph node metastasis under intermittent hypoxic conditions. According to these authors, lymphatic vessels occur more often only in the periphery of tumors; these regions of acute hypoxia may stimulate the cells to spread through lymphatic vessels, leading to increased lymph node metastasis [73].

Concerning epidermal-type fatty acid-binding protein (E-FABP), our proteomic approach detected that this member of the fatty acid-binding protein family is over-expressed in lymph node metastasis, a result supported by Western blotting experiments in tumor samples. These findings are somewhat in disagreement with those of Uma and collaborators [49], who reported a down-regulation of *FABP5* in metastatic lymph nodes compared to the corresponding primary tumors. These discordant results can be explained by the fact that Uma's group analyzed transcripts while the present work evaluated gene expression at the protein level. General correlations between the levels of RNA and the corresponding proteins have been observed, but even with stringent methods partial or reverse correlations are also detected, probably due to regulatory mechanisms or variable accuracy on the RNA level, as reviewed by Gry and collaborators [74].

However, similarly to our findings, *FABP5*/E-FABP overexpression in HNSCC lymph node metastasis has been observed by others [50, 75]. Increased serum reactivity to E-FABP in HNSCC patients [75], and association of higher E-FABP levels with HPV-positive oral and oropharyngeal carcinomas [76] and with cell proliferation and invasiveness [50] have also been found. In respect to HPV status, our group have previously studied a cohort of more than 1000 HNSCC cases to determine the serological response to oncoproteins of HPV16 and 400 HNSCC cases to investigate HPV16 DNA in tumor samples. The results showed a low prevalence of HPV16 DNA and HPV16 E6 and E6/E7 antibodies in oral and larynx carcinomas [77]. Given that the patients analyzed by the present study represent a subset included in this previous report, we can hypothesize that *FABP5*/E-FABP findings are not related to the HPV status in our cohorts. Regarding other neoplasms, a high expression of E-FABP was detected in tumor tissues, serum [78] and urinary extracellular vesicles from patients with high prostate cancer [79] as well as in cervical cancer tissues, and significantly correlated with lymph node metastasis, lymphovascular space invasion, stage and tumor size [80].

E-FABP is a cytosolic lipid binding protein of epidermal cells that uptakes, binds and transports long chain fatty acids to cell organelles. The study of Bao et al. [81] demonstrated that E-FABP overexpression results in an increase in the levels of fatty acid uptake and transport into the nucleus, and also in tumor-promoting activity. The authors suggested that such tumorigenic activity is due to the activation of the nuclear receptor peroxisome

Table 4 Information on biological processes based on Gene ontology. Down-regulated proteins identified by proteomic analysis of positive lymph node samples. Proteins are referenced by their HGNC gene symbol

Biological process	Down-regulated proteins[a]
Apoptosis	CALR, YWHAB
Regulation of apoptosis	HBA1/2, HBB, P4HB, PRDX2
Anti-apoptosis	ALB, ARHGDIA, HSP90B1, PARK7, PSMB5, YWHAZ
Cell adhesion	ARHGDIA, ARHGDIB
Cell cycle	
Arrest	CALR, PSMB5
Cell communication	
Signaling	ACTB, ARHGDIA, ARHGDIB, CALR, HIST1H3A, HSP90B1, MYL6, PARK7, PSMB5, RAP1A, YWHAB, YWHAZ
Cell migration or movement	ARHGDIA, ARHGDIB, PFN1, PPIA
Cell motility	ACTB
Cell proliferation	
Positive regulation	CALR
Cytoskeleton organization	ARHGDIB, PFN1
Developmental process	ARHGDIB, MYL6
System development	PRDX1
Cell differentiation	CALR, RAP1A, TAGLN2
Epidermis development	KRT9
Metabolic process	ALB, BLVRB, CA1, GAPDH, HBA1/2, HBB, P4HB, PARK7, PSMB5, RAP1A
Protein metabolic process	ACTB, CALR, P4HB, RAP1A
Protein modification process	ACTB, CALR, HBA1/2, HBB, HIST1H3A, HSP90B1, PARK7, PFN1, PPIA, PSMB5, YWHAB
Monosaccharide metabolic process	GAPDH, TPI1
Oxidation-reduction process	HBA1/2, HBB
Response to stimulus	HBA1/2, PARK7, RAP1A
Defense response	COTL1, HIST1H2BG, HIST1H3A
Immune response	ACTB, ARHGDIB, HIST1H2BG, HSP90B1, PSMB5, YWHAB
Response to stress	HSP90B1, P4HB
Response to oxidative stress	HBA1/2, HBB, PARK7, PRDX1, PRDX2, PRDX6
Replication	
DNA replication	CALR, HIST1H3A, PPIA
Senescence	CALR
Transcription	CALR, HIST1H3A, PARK7, PRDX1, PRDX2, PSMB5, YWHAB, YWHAZ
Translation	CALR, GAPDH
Transport	ALB, CA1, HBA1/2, HBB, HBD, HSP90B1, RAB10, RAB5B, RAP1A

[a]Name of down-regulated proteins: *ACTB* Actin, cytoplasmic 1, *ALB* Serum albumin, *ARHGDIA* Rho GDP-dissociation inhibitor 1, *ARHGDIB* Rho GDP-dissociation inhibitor 2, *BLVRB* Flavin reductase (NADPH), *CA1* Carbonic anhydrase 1, *CALR* Calreticulin, *COTL1* Coactosin-like protein, *GAPDH* Glyceraldehyde-3-phosphate dehydrogenase, *HBA1/2* Hemoglobin subunit alpha, *HBB* Hemoglobin subunit beta, *HBD* Hemoglobin subunit delta, *HIST1H2BG* Histone H2B type 1-C/E/F/G/I, *HIST1H3A* Histone H3.1, *HSP90B1* Heat shock protein 90 kDa beta member 1, *KRT9* Keratin, type I cytoskeletal 9, *MYL6* Myosin light polypeptide 6, *P4HB* Protein disulfide-isomerase, *PARK7* Protein deglycase DJ-1, *PFN1* Profilin-1, *PPIA* Peptidyl-prolyl cis-trans isomerase A, *PRDX1* Peroxiredoxin-1, *PRDX2* Peroxiredoxin-2, *PRDX6* Peroxiredoxin-6, *PSMB5* Proteasome subunit beta type-5, *RAB10* Ras-related protein Rab-10, *RAB5B* Ras-related protein Rab-5B, *RAP1A* Ras-related protein Rap-1A, *TAGLN2* Transgelin-2, *TPI1* Triosephosphate isomerase, *YWHAB* 14-3-3 protein beta/alpha, *YWHAZ* 14-3-3 protein zeta/delta

proliferator-activated receptor gamma (PPARγ) by fatty acids resulting in upregulation of genes involved in angiogenesis, apoptosis suppression and invasion.

E-FABP and protein S100-A7, both over-expressed in our N+ samples, stabilize the level of each other, and colocalize in focal adhesion-like structures in response to calcium, possibly as part of a protein complex with an important role in the metastatic process [82]. Abnormal expression of S100 proteins has already been detected in metastasis of colorectal cancers [83] and associated

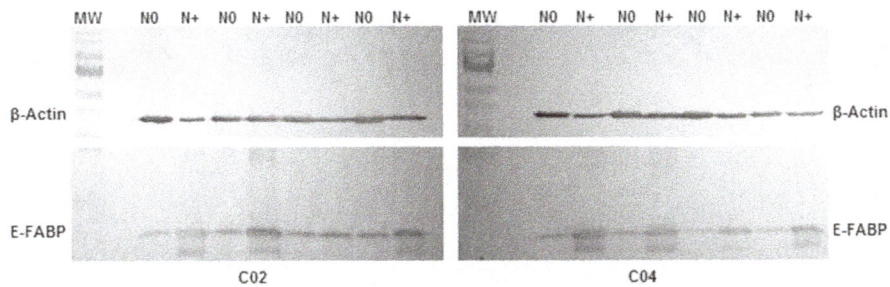

Fig. 2 Immunodetection of E-FABP by Western blot. Representative Western blot illustrating the E-FABP expression in tumor-free (N0) and positive (N+) lymph nodes. β-actin was used as an internal control. MW=PageRuler Prestained Protein Ladder

with lymph node positive tumors and invasive/migratory phenotype [84]. Similar results have been observed for apolipoprotein A-I, which also shows high expression in lymph node metastasis of primary colonic adenocarcinomas [85] and saliva and serum from HNSCC [86].

Some proteins identified by us presented opposite results to those of the literature regarding their expression in cancer cells. For example, endoplasmin and triosephosphate isomerase were found downregulated in our metastatic lymph node samples, and upregulated in tumor samples analyzed by Nomura H et al. [87] and Polachini GM et al. [88], which may be explained by the effect of the lymph node immune environment in modulating tumor growth or in metabolic reprogramming

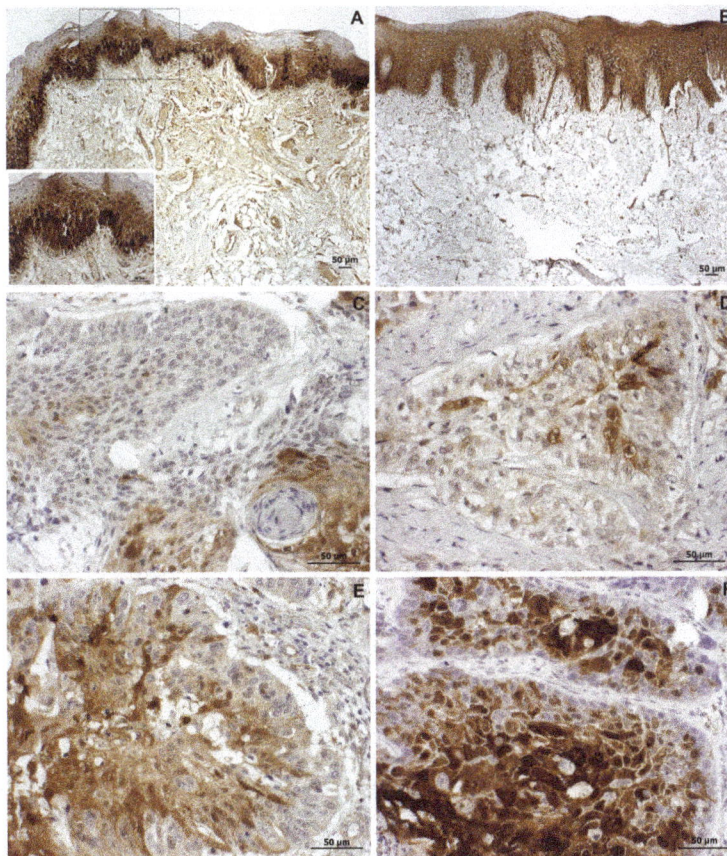

Fig. 3 Immunohistochemical analysis of E-FABP expression in oral squamous cell carcinoma and non-tumoral (margin) samples. **a** Intense positivity of E-FABP in nucleus and cytoplasm of the basal and spinous layer of the normal epithelium, **b** reaching all epithelial layers. Immunolabeling intensity and proportion varied in tumor samples, with (**c**) expression in nests of well differentiated areas, **d** heterogeneous pattern with predominance of low intensity level in tumor cells; and also (**e**) moderate and (**f**) high intensity level of staining in nests. Scale bar indicates 50 μm

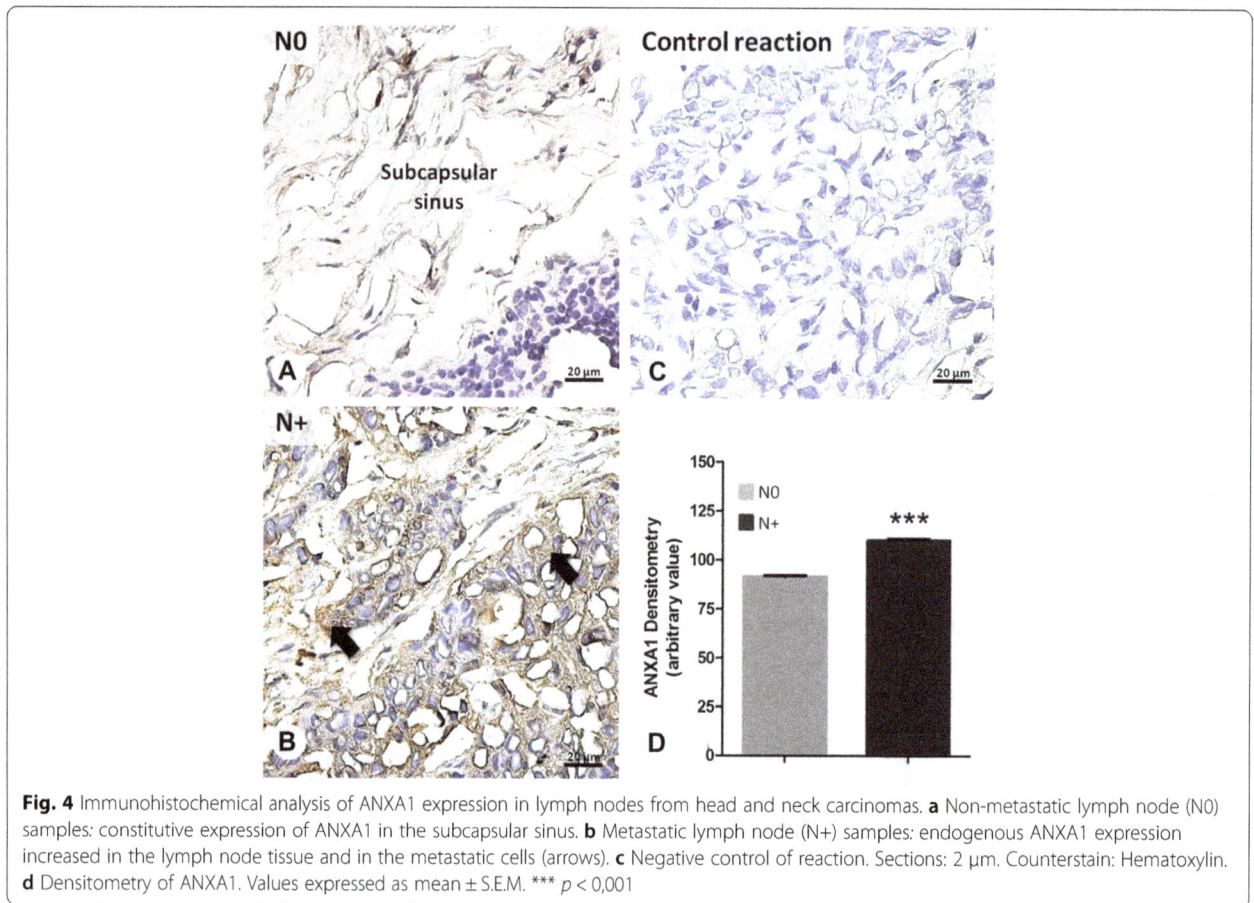

Fig. 4 Immunohistochemical analysis of ANXA1 expression in lymph nodes from head and neck carcinomas. **a** Non-metastatic lymph node (N0) samples: constitutive expression of ANXA1 in the subcapsular sinus. **b** Metastatic lymph node (N+) samples: endogenous ANXA1 expression increased in the lymph node tissue and in the metastatic cells (arrows). **c** Negative control of reaction. Sections: 2 μm. Counterstain: Hematoxylin. **d** Densitometry of ANXA1. Values expressed as mean ± S.E.M. *** $p < 0.001$

of the metastatic cell considering the blood flow, oxygen and nutrient supplies in the secondary site.

Annexin A1, a member of the annexin superfamily, has been observed underexpressed in primary HNSCC studied by us [47] and by others [48, 88]. However, our mass spectrometry and immunohistochemical analyses showed that it is overexpressed in positive lymph nodes. This is the first direct evidence of annexin A1 overexpression in lymph node metastasis of head and neck cancer. Annexin A1 is a protein involved in inflammation [89], apoptosis [90], cell differentiation [91], migration, invasion [92], and signaling [93]. It is a substrate of growth factors and kinases and exhibits abnormal (high or low) levels in several tumors and inflammatory conditions (reviewd by [94–96]. In HNSCC, ANXA1 down-regulation has been associated with poor differentiation and advanced stages [91, 97], but also with early stages, at least in laryngeal tumorigenesis [47]. In breast cancer, ANXA1 is highly expressed and modulates activation of M2 macrophage, which in its turn promotes angiogenesis, tumor progression and adaptive immune response [98]. Increased levels of annexin A1 are also observed in bronchoalveolar lavage fluid and correlated with lymphatic invasion and malignant progression of lung cancer [99]. A similar expression

pattern has been described in hypoxic conditions, when it binds to formyl peptide receptors and induces cell invasion [100]. Thus, the conflicting data between our lymph node samples and previously analyzed primary tumors may indicate a complex annexin A1-cancer relationship, with distinct actions depending on the cell type, as well discussed by Tu Y et al. [101].

At the present time, there are few biomarkers that can predict progression of head and neck carcinomas. Although the lymph node status is still the most important predictor, occult micrometastases may not be detected by the routine histopathological examination of neck dissection specimens. Therefore, markers of a well characterized metastatic phenotype could help to identify reduced numbers of neoplastic cells in lymph nodes or even before homing to and colonizing lymph nodes – the circulating tumor cells (CTCs) - using non-invasive tests. However, the number of CTCs in HNSCC patients is low and enrichment strategies need to be performed to increase CTC concentration and, consequently, to facilitate their detection and characterization [102]. Recently, Kulasinghe and collaborators [103, 104] demonstrate that CTC clusters may actually be an important HNSCC prognostic marker. In vivo and in vitro experiments should validate this finding and probably will help to clarify why lymphatic vessels and regional lymph nodes are the preferential target sites of head and neck carcinoma cells.

Conclusions

The present study has some methodological limitations. First, the number of expressed proteins in complex biological samples is many orders of magnitude greater than the total number of spots visible in 2-DE gels after staining. Therefore, only a small percentage of the total sample proteome is available for comparisons. Second, the usage of pools may miss relevant differences between samples. Third, the methodology of the present study does not allow to determine whether differences between groups are cause or consequence of tumorigenesis, an issue that should be the aim of future analyses, such as the analysis of cells before lymph node colonization - the circulating tumor cells.

Despite methodological limitations, this study provides, for the first time, direct evidence of annexin A1 overexpression in lymph node metastasis of head and neck cancer and adds information that may be useful for diagnosing metastatic disease. The results on the expression of heat shock proteins and enzymes of the glycolytic pathway suggest an effect of the lymph node environment in controlling tumor growth or in metabolic reprogramming of the metastatic cell. In addition, the observation of several proteins with differential expression between lymph node metastasis from tongue, floor of the mouth and larynx carcinomas reinforces the idea that head and neck sites and subsites are dissimilar entities whose behavior may be influenced by micro-environmental factors including the lymphatic network. Taken together, the results from this study contributed to our understanding of the metastatic phenotype of HNSCC and provided novel potential targets for diagnostic in metastatic head and neck squamous cell carcinomas.

Abbreviations

1-DE: One-Dimensional Gel Electrophoresis; 2-DE: Two-Dimensional Gel Electrophoresis; ACN: Acetonitrile; ANXA1: Annexin A1; CHAPS: 3-[(3-Cholamidopropyl) Dimethylammonio]-1-Propanesulfonate Hydrate; DAB: 3,3 Diaminobenzidine; DTT: Dithiothreitol; E-FABP: Fatty Acid-Binding Protein, Epidermal; EMT: Epithelial-Mesenchymal Transition; FDR: False Discovery Rate; FFPE: Formalin-Fixed, Paraffin-Embedded Tissue; HCL: Hydrochloric Acid; HGNC: Hugo Gene Nomenclature Committee; HNSCC: Head and Neck Squamous Cell Carcinoma; KEGG: Kyoto Encyclopedia of Genes and Genomes; MALDI: Matrix Assisted Laser Desorption Ionization; MS: Mass Spectrometry; N + : Lymph Node positive for neoplastic cells.; N0: Lymph Node negative for neoplastic cells; PBS: Phosphate-Buffered Saline; PPARγ: Peroxisome Proliferator-Activated Receptor Gamma; PVDF: Polyvinylidene Difluoride; Q-TOF: Quadrupole Ion Trap - Time Of Flight; SDS: Sodium Dodecyl Sulfate; TFA: Trifluoroacetic Acid; TMA: Tissue Microarray; TNM: Tumor-Node-Metastases

Acknowledgments

We are grateful to Professors Fabio C. Gozzo (University of Campinas/UNICAMP, Brasil) and Adriana F. P. Leme (Brazilian Biosciences National Laboratory/LNBio, CNPEM, Campinas) for their assistance in mass spectrometry analysis. We also thank Edilson Solim for technical support and GENCAPO (Head and Neck Genome Project -http://www.gencapo.famerp.br/) team for the valuable discussions that motivated the present study. Finally, we thank the Mass Spectrometry Laboratory at LNBio for support with the use of mass spectrometers.

Funding

This research was supported by grants from Fundação de Amparo à Pesquisa do Estado de São Paulo/FAPESP (grant number 2004/12054–9), Rede Proteoma do Estado de São Paulo/FAPESP (grant number 2004/14846–0), and Conselho Nacional de Pesquisas/CNPq (grant number 308904/2014–1).

Authors' contributions

AV participated in the design of the study, performed the 1-DE, 2-DE, MS and Western blot experiments, validated the results of 1-DE using the Scaffold software, and contributed to the manuscript preparation. GMP analyzed the 2-DE gel images using the ImageMaster 2D Platinum software, carried out the analysis and interpretation of the data, and preparation of the manuscript. MPS and SMO performed immunohistochemical analysis of ANXA1 expression in lymph node specimens and contributed to data analysis and interpretation. TH identified the metabolic pathways, associated ontologies and expression data related to the differentially expressed proteins and contributed to the interpretation of data. RVML implemented the data bank, supervised clinical data bank collection and performed data cleaning. PMC evaluated the histology and percentage of normal and tumor cells in all lymph nodes analyzed. FDN performed immunohistochemical analysis of E-FABP expression and contributed to data analysis and interpretation. JFGF and MBC recruited participants, performed sample collection and clinical evaluation of the patients. AML performed the Western blot experiments and contributed to data analysis and interpretation. EHT conceived and coordinated the design of the study, evaluated the results, contributed to drafting the manuscript and supervised all the process. All authors critically revised the manuscript, checked the accuracy of the data, and approved the version to be published.

Competing interests

The authors declare that they have no competing interests.

Author details

[1]Departamento de Biologia Molecular, Faculdade de Medicina (FAMERP), Av. Brigadeiro Faria Lima, 5416, Vila São Pedro, São José do Rio Preto, SP CEP 15090-000, Brazil. [2]Departamento de Biologia, Instituto de Biociências, Letras e Ciências Exatas (IBILCE), Universidade Estadual Paulista (UNESP), R. Cristóvão Colombo, 2265, São José do Rio Preto, SP CEP 15054-000, Brazil. [3]Instituto do Câncer de São Paulo Octavio Frias de Oliveira – ICESP, Av. Dr. Arnaldo, 251 - Cerqueira César, São Paulo, SP 01246-000, Brazil. [4]Faculdade Ceres (Faceres), Av. Anísio Haddad, 6751, São José do Rio Preto, SP CEP 15090-305, Brazil. [5]Departamento de Estomatologia, Faculdade de Odontologia, Universidade de São Paulo, Av. Prof. Lineu Prestes, 2227, São Paulo, SP CEP 05508-000, Brazil. [6]Instituto do Câncer Arnaldo Vieira de Carvalho, R. Dr Cesário Mota Jr, 112, São Paulo, SP CEP 01221-020, Brazil. [7]Departamento de Cirurgia de Cabeça e Pescoço, Hospital Heliópolis, R. Cônego Xavier, 276, São Paulo, SP CEP 04231-030, Brazil. [8]Departamento de Análises Clínicas, Toxicológicas e Bromatológicas, Faculdade de Ciências Farmacêuticas, Universidade de São Paulo, Avenida do Café, s/n, Ribeirão Preto, SP CEP 14040-903, Brazil. [9]Departamento de Genética e Biologia Evolutiva, Instituto de Biociências, Universidade de São Paulo, R. do Matão, 321, São Paulo, SP CEP 05508-090, Brazil.

References

1. Sporn MB. The war on cancer. Lancet. 1996;347(9012):1377–81.
2. Nguyen DX, Massague J. Genetic determinants of cancer metastasis. Nat Rev Genet. 2007;8(5):341–52.

3. Yang J, Weinberg RA. Epithelial-mesenchymal transition: at the crossroads of development and tumor metastasis. Dev Cell. 2008;14(6):818–29.

4. Polyak K, Weinberg RA. Transitions between epithelial and mesenchymal states: acquisition of malignant and stem cell traits. Nat Rev Cancer. 2009; 9(4):265–73.

5. Harris AL. Hypoxia--a key regulatory factor in tumour growth. Nat Rev Cancer. 2002;2(1):38–47.

6. Brooks SA, Lomax-Browne HJ, Carter TM, Kinch CE, Hall DM. Molecular interactions in cancer cell metastasis. Acta Histochem. 2009;112:3–25.

7. Blood CH, Zetter BR. Tumor interactions with the vasculature: angiogenesis and tumor metastasis. Biochim Biophys Acta. 1990;1032(1):89–118.

8. Ji RC. Lymph node lymphangiogenesis: a new concept for modulating tumor metastasis and inflammatory process. Histol Histopathol. 2009;24(3):377–84.

9. Zlotnik A. Chemokines in neoplastic progression. Semin Cancer Biol. 2004; 14(3):181–5.

10. Saharinen P, Tammela T, Karkkainen MJ, Alitalo K. Lymphatic vasculature: development, molecular regulation and role in tumor metastasis and inflammation. Trends Immunol. 2004;25(7):387–95.

11. Paduch R. The role of lymphangiogenesis and angiogenesis in tumor metastasis. Cell Oncol (Dordr). 2016;39(5):397–410.

12. Timar J, Csuka O, Remenar E, Repassy G, Kasler M. Progression of head and neck squamous cell cancer. Cancer Metastasis Rev. 2005;24(1):107–27.

13. Swartz MA, Lund AW. Lymphatic and interstitial flow in the tumour microenvironment: linking mechanobiology with immunity. Nat Rev Cancer. 2012;12(3):210–9.

14. Maula SM, Luukkaa M, Grenman R, Jackson D, Jalkanen S, Ristamaki R. Intratumoral lymphatics are essential for the metastatic spread and prognosis in squamous cell carcinomas of the head and neck region. Cancer Res. 2003;63(8):1920–6.

15. Kaplan RN, Riba RD, Zacharoulis S, Bramley AH, Vincent L, Costa C, MacDonald DD, Jin DK, Shido K, Kerns SA, et al. VEGFR1-positive haematopoietic bone marrow progenitors initiate the pre-metastatic niche. Nature. 2005;438(7069):820–7.

16. Deng J, Liu Y, Lee H, Herrmann A, Zhang W, Zhang C, Shen S, Priceman SJ, Kujawski M, Pal SK, et al. S1PR1-STAT3 signaling is crucial for myeloid cell colonization at future metastatic sites. Cancer Cell. 2012;21(5):642–54.

17. Joyce JA, Pollard JW. Microenvironmental regulation of metastasis. Nat Rev Cancer. 2009;9(4):239–52.

18. Lorusso G, Ruegg C. New insights into the mechanisms of organ-specific breast cancer metastasis. Semin Cancer Biol. 2012;22(3):226–33.

19. Langley RR, Fidler IJ. The seed and soil hypothesis revisited--the role of tumor-stroma interactions in metastasis to different organs. Int J Cancer. 2011;128(11):2527–35.

20. Mathot L, Stenninger J. Behavior of seeds and soil in the mechanism of metastasis: a deeper understanding. Cancer Sci. 2012;103(4):626–31.

21. Genden EM, Ferlito A, Bradley PJ, Rinaldo A, Scully C. Neck disease and distant metastases. Oral Oncol. 2003;39(3):207–12.

22. Renner G. Small cell carcinoma of the head and neck: a review. Semin Oncol. 2007;34(1):3–14.

23. Witt RL. Major salivary gland cancer. Surg Oncol Clin N Am. 2004;13(1):113–27.

24. Okura M, Aikawa T, Sawai NY, Iida S, Kogo M. Decision analysis and treatment threshold in a management for the N0 neck of the oral cavity carcinoma. Oral Oncol. 2009;45(10):908–11.

25. Sobin LH, Wittekind C: TNM classification of malignant Tumours; 2002.

26. de Marqui AB, Vidotto A, Polachini GM, Bellato Cde M, Cabral H, Leopoldino AM, de Gois Filho JF, Fukuyama EE, Settanni FA, Cury PM, et al. Solubilization of proteins from human lymph node tissue and two-dimensional gel storage. J Biochem Mol Biol. 2006;39(2):216–22.

27. Bradford MM. A rapid and sensitive method for the quantitation of microgram quantities of protein utilizing the principle of protein-dye binding. Anal Biochem. 1976;72:248–54.

28. Laemmli UK. Cleavage of structural proteins during the assembly of the head of bacteriophage T4. Nature. 1970;227(5259):680–5.

29. Paes Leme AF, Sherman NE, Smalley DM, Sizukusa LO, Oliveira AK, Menezes MC, Fox JW, Serrano SM. Hemorrhagic activity of HF3, a snake venom metalloproteinase: insights from the proteomic analysis of mouse skin and blood plasma. J Proteome Res. 2012;11(1):279–91.

30. Henrique T, Jose Freitas da Silveira N, Henrique Cunha Volpato A, Mioto MM, Carolina Buzzo Stefanini A, Bachir Fares A, da Silva Castro G, Andrade J, Masson C, Veronica Mendoza Lopez R, Daumas Nunes F, et al. HNdb: an integrated database of gene and protein information on head and neck

squamous cell carcinoma. Database. 2016;2016. https://doi.org/10.1093/database/baw026.

31. Kanehisa M, Goto S. KEGG: Kyoto encyclopedia of genes and genomes. Nucleic Acids Res. 2000;28(1):27–30.

32. Ashburner M, Ball CA, Blake JA, Botstein D, Butler H, Cherry JM, Davis AP, Dolinski K, Dwight SS, Eppig JT, et al. Gene ontology: tool for the unification of biology. The gene ontology consortium. Nat Genet. 2000;25(1):25–9.

33. Edgar R, Domrachev M, Lash AE. Gene expression omnibus: NCBI gene expression and hybridization array data repository. Nucleic Acids Res. 2002; 30(1):207–10.

34. da Huang W, Sherman BT, Lempicki RA. Bioinformatics enrichment tools: paths toward the comprehensive functional analysis of large gene lists. Nucleic Acids Res. 2009;37(1):1–13.

35. da Huang W, Sherman BT, Lempicki RA. Systematic and integrative analysis of large gene lists using DAVID bioinformatics resources. Nat Protoc. 2009; 4(1):44–57.

36. Dvorakova M, Jerabkova J, Prochazkova I, Lenco J, Nenutil R, Bouchal P. Transgelin is upregulated in stromal cells of lymph node positive breast cancer. J Proteome. 2016;132:103–11.

37. Flores-Perez A, Marchat LA, Sanchez LL, Romero-Zamora D, Arechaga-Ocampo E, Ramirez-Torres N, Chavez JD, Carlos-Reyes A, Astudillo-de la Vega H, Ruiz-Garcia E, et al. Differential proteomic analysis reveals that EGCG inhibits HDGF and activates apoptosis to increase the sensitivity of non-small cells lung cancer to chemotherapy. Proteomics Clin Appl. 2016;10(2):172–82.

38. Haonon O, Rucksaken R, Pinlaor P, Pairojkul C, Chamgramol Y, Intuyod K, Onsurathum S, Khuntikeo N, Pinlaor S. Upregulation of 14-3-3 eta in chronic liver fluke infection is a potential diagnostic marker of cholangiocarcinoma. Proteomics Clin Appl. 2016;10(3):248–56.

39. Peng XC, Gong FM, Chen Y, Qiu M, Cheng K, Tang J, Ge J, Chen N, Zeng H, Liu JY. Proteomics identification of PGAM1 as a potential therapeutic target for urothelial bladder cancer. J Proteome. 2016;132:85–92.

40. Camisasca DR, da Ros GL, Soares MR, Sandim V, Nogueira FC, Garcia CH, Santana R, de Oliveira SP, Buexm LA, de Faria PA, et al. A proteomic approach to compare saliva from individuals with and without oral leukoplakia. J Proteome. 2017;151:43–52.

41. Oliveira BM, Coorssen JR, Martins-de-Souza D. 2DE: the phoenix of proteomics. J Proteome. 2014;104:140–50.

42. Fukumoto S, Yamauchi N, Moriguchi H, Hippo Y, Watanabe A, Shibahara J, Taniguchi H, Ishikawa S, Ito H, Yamamoto S, et al. Overexpression of the aldo-keto reductase family protein AKR1B10 is highly correlated with smokers' non-small cell lung carcinomas. Clin Cancer Res. 2005;11(5):1776–85.

43. Penning TM. AKR1B10: a new diagnostic marker of non-small cell lung carcinoma in smokers. Clin Cancer Res. 2005;11(5):1687–90.

44. Chen J, He QY, Yuen AP, Chiu JF. Proteomics of buccal squamous cell carcinoma: the involvement of multiple pathways in tumorigenesis. Proteomics. 2004;4(8):2465–75.

45. Wang Z, Feng X, Liu X, Jiang L, Zeng X, Ji N, Li J, Li L, Chen Q. Involvement of potential pathways in malignant transformation from oral leukoplakia to oral squamous cell carcinoma revealed by proteomic analysis. BMC Genomics. 2009;10:383.

46. He QY, Chen J, Kung HF, Yuen AP, Chiu JF. Identification of tumor-associated proteins in oral tongue squamous cell carcinoma by proteomics. Proteomics. 2004;4(1):271–8.

47. Alves VA, Nonogaki S, Cury PM, Wunsch-Filho V, de Carvalho MB, Michaluart-Junior P, Moyses RA, Curioni OA, Figueiredo DL, Scapulatempo-Neto C, et al. Annexin A1 subcellular expression in laryngeal squamous cell carcinoma. Histopathology. 2008;53(6):715–27.

48. Silistino-Souza R, Rodrigues-Lisoni FC, Cury PM, Maniglia JV, Raposo LS, Tajara EH, Christian HC, Oliani SM. Annexin 1: differential expression in tumor and mast cells in human larynx cancer. Int J Cancer. 2007;120(12):2582–9.

49. Uma RS, Naresh KN, D'Cruz AK, Mulherkar R, Borges AM. Metastasis of squamous cell carcinoma of the oral tongue is associated with down-regulation of epidermal fatty acid binding protein (E-FABP). Oral Oncol. 2007;43(1):27–32.

50. Fang LY, Wong TY, Chiang WF, Chen YL. Fatty-acid-binding protein 5 promotes cell proliferation and invasion in oral squamous cell carcinoma. J Oral Pathol Med. 2010;39(4):342–8.

51. Zhu Z, Xu X, Yu Y, Graham M, Prince ME, Carey TE, Sun D. Silencing heat shock protein 27 decreases metastatic behavior of human head and neck squamous cell cancer cells in vitro. Mol Pharm. 2010;7(4):1283–90.

52. Lee JH, Sun D, Cho KJ, Kim MS, Hong MH, Kim IK, Lee JS. Overexpression of human 27 kDa heat shock protein in laryngeal cancer cells confers chemoresistance associated with cell growth delay. J Cancer Res Clin Oncol. 2007;133(1):37–46.

53. Saussez S, Decaestecker C, Lorfevre F, Cucu DR, Mortuaire G, Chevalier D, Wacreniez A, Kaltner H, Andre S, Toubeau G, et al. High level of galectin-1 expression is a negative prognostic predictor of recurrence in laryngeal squamous cell carcinomas. Int J Oncol. 2007;30(5):1109–17.

54. Alves PM, Godoy GP, Gomes DQ, Medeiros AM, de Souza LB, da Silveira EJ, Vasconcelos MG, Queiroz LM. Significance of galectins-1, −3, −4 and −7 in the progression of squamous cell carcinoma of the tongue. Pathol Res Pract. 2011;207(4):236–40.

55. Masood N, Malik FA, Kayani MA. Expression of xenobiotic metabolizing genes in head and neck cancer tissues. Asian Pac J Cancer Prev : APJCP. 2011;12(2):377–82.

56. Masood N, Kayani MA. Expression patterns of carcinogen detoxifying genes (CYP1A1, GSTP1 & GSTT1) in HNC patients. Pathol Oncol Res : POR. 2013; 19(1):89–94.

57. Yamashina M, Sato K, Tonogi M, Tanaka Y, Yamane GY, Katakura A. Evaluation of superficial oral squamous cell malignancy based on morphometry and immunoexpression of cytokeratin 13 and cytokeratin 17. Acta Cytol. 2014;58(1):67–75.

58. Hamakawa H, Fukuzumi M, Bao Y, Sumida T, Kayahara H, Onishi A, Sogawa K. Keratin mRNA for detecting micrometastasis in cervical lymph nodes of oral cancer. Cancer Lett. 2000;160(1):115–23.

59. Takahashi M, Suzuki S, Ishikawa K. Cyclophilin A-EMMPRIN interaction induces invasion of head and neck squamous cell carcinoma. Oncol Rep. 2012;27(1):198–203.

60. Huang CF, Sun ZJ, Zhao YF, Chen XM, Jia J, Zhang WF. Increased expression of peroxiredoxin 6 and cyclophilin a in squamous cell carcinoma of the tongue. Oral Dis. 2011;17(3):328–34.

61. Kudo Y, Iizuka S, Yoshida M, Nguyen PT, Siriwardena SB, Tsunematsu T, Ohbayashi M, Ando T, Hatakeyama D, Shibata T, et al. Periostin directly and indirectly promotes tumor lymphangiogenesis of head and neck cancer. PLoS One. 2012;7(8):e44488.

62. Shen Z, Jiang Z, Ye D, Xiao B, Zhang X, Guo J. Growth inhibitory effects of DJ-1-small interfering RNA on laryngeal carcinoma Hep-2 cells. Med Oncol. 2011;28(2):601–7.

63. Zhu XL, Wang ZF, Lei WB, Zhuang HW, Hou WJ, Wen YH, Wen WP. Tumorigenesis role and clinical significance of DJ-1, a negative regulator of PTEN, in supraglottic squamous cell carcinoma. J Exp Clin Cancer Res : CR. 2012;31:94.

64. Tripathi SC, Matta A, Kaur J, Grigull J, Chauhan SS, Thakar A, Shukla NK, Duggal R, DattaGupta S, Ralhan R, et al. Nuclear S100A7 is associated with poor prognosis in head and neck cancer. PLoS One. 2010;5(8):e11939.

65. Kesting MR, Sudhoff H, Hasler RJ, Nieberler M, Pautke C, Wolff KD, Wagenpfeil S, Al-Benna S, Jacobsen F, Steinstraesser L. Psoriasin (S100A7) up-regulation in oral squamous cell carcinoma and its relation to clinicopathologic features. Oral Oncol. 2009;45(8):731–6.

66. Mitra RS, Zhang Z, Henson BS, Kurnit DM, Carey TE, D'Silva NJ. Rap1A and rap1B ras-family proteins are prominently expressed in the nucleus of squamous carcinomas: nuclear translocation of GTP-bound active form. Oncogene. 2003;22(40):6243–56.

67. Thul PJ, Lindskog C. The human protein atlas: a spatial map of the human proteome. Protein Sci. 2018;27(1):233–44.

68. Severino P, Alvares AM, Michaluart P Jr, Okamoto OK, Nunes FD, Moreira-Filho CA, Tajara EH. Global gene expression profiling of oral cavity cancers suggests molecular heterogeneity within anatomic subsites. BMC Res Notes. 2008;1:113.

69. Krop I, Marz A, Carlsson H, Li X, Bloushtain-Qimron N, Hu M, Gelman R, Sabel MS, Schnitt S, Ramaswamy S, et al. A putative role for psoriasin in breast tumor progression. Cancer Res. 2005;65(24):11326–34.

70. Le QT, Shi G, Cao H, Nelson DW, Wang Y, Chen EY, Zhao S, Kong C, Richardson D, O'Byrne KJ, et al. Galectin-1: a link between tumor hypoxia and tumor immune privilege. J Clin Oncol. 2005;23(35):8932–41.

71. Biron-Shental T, Schaiff WT, Ratajczak CK, Bildirici I, Nelson DM, Sadovsky Y. Hypoxia regulates the expression of fatty acid-binding proteins in primary term human trophoblasts. Am J Obstet Gynecol. 2007;197(5):516 e511–6.

72. Chaudary N, Hill RP. Increased expression of metastasis-related genes in hypoxic cells sorted from cervical and lymph nodal xenograft tumors. Lab Invest. 2009;89(5):587–96.

73. Chaudary N, Hill RP. Hypoxia and metastasis. Clin Cancer Res. 2007;13(7): 1947–9.

74. Gry M, Rimini R, Stromberg S, Asplund A, Ponten F, Uhlen M, Nilsson P. Correlations between RNA and protein expression profiles in 23 human cell lines. BMC Genomics. 2009;10:365.

75. Rauch J, Ahlemann M, Schaffrik M, Mack B, Ertongur S, Andratschke M, Zeidler R, Lang S, Gires O. Allogenic antibody-mediated identification of head and neck cancer antigens. Biochem Biophys Res Commun. 2004; 323(1):156–62.

76. Melle C, Ernst G, Winkler R, Schimmel B, Klussmann JP, Wittekindt C, Guntinas-Lichius O, von Eggeling F. Proteomic analysis of human papillomavirus-related oral squamous cell carcinoma: identification of thioredoxin and epidermal-fatty acid binding protein as upregulated protein markers in microdissected tumor tissue. Proteomics. 2009;9(8):2193–201.

77. Lopez RV, Levi JE, Eluf-Neto J, Koifman RJ, Koifman S, Curado MP, Michaluart-Junior P, Figueiredo DL, Saggioro FP, de Carvalho MB, et al. Human papillomavirus (HPV) 16 and the prognosis of head and neck cancer in a geographical region with a low prevalence of HPV infection. Cancer Causes Control : CCC. 2014;25(4):461–71.

78. Pang J, Liu WP, Liu XP, Li LY, Fang YQ, Sun QP, Liu SJ, Li MT, Su ZL, Gao X. Profiling protein markers associated with lymph node metastasis in prostate cancer by DIGE-based proteomics analysis. J Proteome Res. 2010;9(1):216–26.

79. Fujita K, Kume H, Matsuzaki K, Kawashima A, Ujike T, Nagahara A, Uemura M, Miyagawa Y, Tomonaga T, Nonomura N. Proteomic analysis of urinary extracellular vesicles from high Gleason score prostate cancer. Sci Rep. 2017;7:42961.

80. Wang W, Chu HJ, Liang YC, Huang JM, Shang CL, Tan H, Liu D, Zhao YH, Liu TY, Yao SZ. FABP5 correlates with poor prognosis and promotes tumor cell growth and metastasis in cervical cancer. Tumour Biol. 2016;37(11):14873–83.

81. Bao Z, Malki MI, Forootan SS, Adamson J, Forootan FS, Chen D, Foster CS, Rudland PS, Ke Y. A novel cutaneous fatty acid-binding protein-related signaling pathway leading to malignant progression in prostate cancer cells. Genes Cancer. 2013;4(7–8):297–314.

82. Ruse M, Broome AM, Eckert RL. S100A7 (psoriasin) interacts with epidermal fatty acid binding protein and localizes in focal adhesion-like structures in cultured keratinocytes. J Invest Dermatol. 2003;121(1):132–41.

83. Melle C, Ernst G, Schimmel B, Bleul A, von Eggeling F. Colon-derived liver metastasis, colorectal carcinoma, and hepatocellular carcinoma can be discriminated by the ca(2+)-binding proteins S100A6 and S100A11. PLoS One. 2008;3(12):e3767.

84. Al-Haddad S, Zhang Z, Leygue E, Snell L, Huang A, Niu Y, Hiller-Hitchcock T, Hole K, Murphy LC, Watson PH. Psoriasin (S100A7) expression and invasive breast cancer. Am J Pathol. 1999;155(6):2057–66.

85. Tachibana M, Ohkura Y, Kobayashi Y, Sakamoto H, Tanaka Y, Watanabe J, Amikura K, Nishimura Y, Akagi K. Expression of apolipoprotein A1 in colonic adenocarcinoma. Anticancer Res. 2003;23(5b):4161–7.

86. Vidotto A, Henrique T, Raposo LS, Maniglia JV, Tajara EH. Salivary and serum proteomics in head and neck carcinomas: before and after surgery and radiotherapy. Cancer Biomark. 2010;8(2):95–107.

87. Nomura H, Uzawa K, Yamano Y, Fushimi K, Ishigami T, Kato Y, Saito K, Nakashima D, Higo M, Kouzu Y, et al. Network-based analysis of calcium-binding protein genes identifies Grp94 as a target in human oral carcinogenesis. Br J Cancer. 2007;97(6):792–801.

88. Polachini GM, Sobral LM, Mercante AM, Paes-Leme AF, Xavier FC, Henrique T, Guimaraes DM, Vidotto A, Fukuyama EE, Gois-Filho JF, et al. Proteomic approaches identify members of cofilin pathway involved in oral tumorigenesis. PLoS One. 2012;7(12):e50517.

89. de Jong R, Leoni G, Drechsler M, Soehnlein O. The advantageous role of annexin A1 in cardiovascular disease. Cell Adhes Migr. 2017;11(3):261–74.

90. Zhang X, Li X, Zheng L, Lei L. ANXA1 silencing increases the sensitivity of cancer cells to low-concentration arsenic trioxide treatment by inhibiting ERK MAPK activation. Tumori. 2015;101(4):360–7.

91. Zhu DW, Yang X, Yang CZ, Ma J, Liu Y, Yan M, Wang LZ, Li J, Zhang CP, Zhang ZY, et al. Annexin A1 down-regulation in oral squamous cell carcinoma correlates to pathological differentiation grade. Oral Oncol. 2013; 49(6):542–50.

92. Han G, Lu K, Huang J, Ye J, Dai S, Ye Y, Zhang L. Effect of Annexin A1 gene on the proliferation and invasion of esophageal squamous cell carcinoma cells and its regulatory mechanisms. Int J Mol Med. 2017;39(2):357–63.

93. Pantaleao L, Rocha GHO, Reutelingsperger C, Tiago M, Maria-Engler SS,

Solito E, Farsky SP. Connections of annexin A1 and translocator protein-18kDa on toll like receptor stimulated BV-2 cells. Exp Cell Res. 2018;367:282–90.

94. Guo C, Liu S, Sun MZ. Potential role of Anxa1 in cancer. Future Oncol. 2013; 9(11):1773–93.

95. Galvao I, Vago JP, Barroso LC, Tavares LP, Queiroz-Junior CM, Costa VV, Carneiro FS, Ferreira TP, Silva PM, Amaral FA, et al. Annexin A1 promotes timely resolution of inflammation in murine gout. Eur J Immunol. 2017; 47(3):585–96.

96. Hassan MN, Belibasakis GN, Gumus P, Ozturk VO, Emingil G, Bostanci N. Annexin-1 as a salivary biomarker for gingivitis during pregnancy. J Periodontol. 2018; https://doi.org/10.1002/JPER.17-0557.

97. Wan YM, Tian J, Qi L, Liu LM, Xu N. ANXA1 affects cell proliferation, invasion and epithelial-mesenchymal transition of oral squamous cell carcinoma. Exp Ther Med. 2017;14(5):5214–8.

98. Moraes LA, Kar S, Foo SL, Gu T, Toh YQ, Ampomah PB, Sachaphibulkij K, Yap G, Zharkova O, Lukman HM, et al. Annexin-A1 enhances breast cancer growth and migration by promoting alternative macrophage polarization in the tumour microenvironment. Sci Rep. 2017;7(1):17925.

99. Biaoxue R, Xiguang C, Hua L, Tian F, Wenlong G. Increased level of annexin A1 in bronchoalveolar lavage fluid as a potential diagnostic indicator for lung cancer. Int J Biol Markers. 2017;32(1):e132–40.

100. Bizzarro V, Belvedere R, Migliaro V, Romano E, Parente L, Petrella A. Hypoxia regulates ANXA1 expression to support prostate cancer cell invasion and aggressiveness. Cell Adhes Migr. 2016:1–14. https://doi.org/10.1080/19336918.2016.1259056.

101. Tu Y, Johnstone CN, Stewart AG. Annexin A1 influences in breast cancer: controversies on contributions to tumour, host and immunoediting processes. Pharmacol Res. 2017;119:278–88.

102. Kulasinghe A, Kenny L, Perry C, Thiery JP, Jovanovic L, Vela I, Nelson C, Punyadeera C. Impact of label-free technologies in head and neck cancer circulating tumour cells. Oncotarget. 2016;7(44):71223–34.

103. Kulasinghe A, Tran TH, Blick T, O'Byrne K, Thompson EW, Warkiani ME, Nelson C, Kenny L, Punyadeera C. Enrichment of circulating head and neck tumour cells using spiral microfluidic technology. Sci Rep. 2017;7:42517.

104. Kulasinghe A, Schmidt H, Perry C, Whitfield B, Kenny L, Nelson C, Warkiani ME, Punyadeera C. A collective route to head and neck Cancer metastasis. Sci Rep. 2018;8(1):746.

14

Chromosomal microarray analysis in developmental delay and intellectual disability with comorbid conditions

Yanjie Fan[1†], Yanming Wu[1,2†], Lili Wang[1], Yu Wang[1], Zhuwen Gong[1], Wenjuan Qiu[1], Jingmin Wang[3], Huiwen Zhang[1], Xing Ji[1], Jun Ye[1], Lianshu Han[1], Xingming Jin[4], Yongnian Shen[5], Fei Li[4,6], Bing Xiao[1], Lili Liang[1], Xia Zhang[1], Xiaomin Liu[1], Xuefan Gu[1*] and Yongguo Yu[1,5*] ⓘ

Abstract

Background: Developmental delay (DD) and intellectual disability (ID) are frequently associated with a broad spectrum of additional phenotypes. Chromosomal microarray analysis (CMA) has been recommended as a first-tier test for DD/ID in general, whereas the diagnostic yield differs significantly among DD/ID patients with different comorbid conditions.

Methods: To investigate the genotype-phenotype correlation, we examined the characteristics of identified pathogenic copy number variations (pCNVs) and compared the diagnostic yields among patient subgroups with different co-occurring conditions.

Results: This study is a retrospective review of CMA results generated from a mixed cohort of 710 Chinese patients with DD/ID. A total of 247 pCNVs were identified in 201 patients (28%). A large portion of these pCNVs were copy number losses, and the size of copy number losses was generally smaller than gains. The diagnostic yields were significantly higher in subgroups with co-occurring congenital heart defects (55%), facial dysmorphism (39%), microcephaly (34%) or hypotonia (35%), whereas co-occurring conditions of skeletal malformation (26%), brain malformation (24%) or epilepsy (24%) did not alter the yield. In addition, the diagnostic yield nominally correlated with ID severity.

Conclusion: Varied yields exist in DD/ID patients with different phenotypic presentation. The presence of comorbid conditions can be among factors to consider when planning CMA.

Keywords: Chromosomal microarray, Developmental delay, Intellectual disability, Pathogenic copy number variations, Comorbid conditions

Background

Developmental delay (DD) and intellectual disability (ID) are estimated to affect ~ 1% of the children across the world [1]. Genetic factors play a major part in DD/ID (up to ~ 47.5%) [2]. Identifying the genetic cause is crucial for accurate etiological diagnosis and refined clinical management. Chromosomal microarray analysis (CMA) has been recommended as a first-tier genetic test for unexplained DD/ID and congenital malformations [3, 4]. The reported diagnostic yields of clinical CMA vary between 12 and 20%, depending on the population and methods used [3, 5]. A wide spectrum of phenotypes can be present in the DD/ID cohorts, including different degrees of ID severity [1] and co-occurrence of other conditions, like epilepsy, autism or dysmorphic features [6]. The diagnostic yields in subgroups of patients with different clinical manifestation are not clear yet. Further assessment of the diagnostic yields in DD/ID patients with different ID severity and co-occurring condition is desired, for it could offer clinicians the phenotypic clues of pathogenic copy number variations (CNVs).

* Correspondence: guxuefan@xinhuamed.com.cn; yuyongguo@shsmu.edu.cn
†Yanjie Fan and Yanming Wu contributed equally to this work.
[1]Department of Pediatric Endocrinology/Genetics, Xinhua Hospital affiliated to Shanghai Jiao Tong University School of Medicine, Shanghai Institute for Pediatric Research, 1665 Kongjiang Road, Shanghai 200092, China
Full list of author information is available at the end of the article

In this study, we reviewed CMA results generated from a Chinese cohort of 710 patients with DD/ID as the main manifestation. We characterized the property and physical distribution of pathogenic CNVs (pCNVs), and compared the yield of CMA among patients with different ID severity and comorbid conditions. Together we delineated the genotypes, diagnostic yields and phenotypes in a DD/ID cohort with heterogeneous manifestations.

Methods

Patients

This is a retrospective study conducted in Endocrine and Genetic Department, Xinhua Hospital and Shanghai Children's Medical Center, China. CMA results from 710 patients (432 males and 278 females, age range from 1 month to 29 years old, average 4.2 years old, visited the clinic during the period of March 2011 to February 2016) were reviewed. Two criteria were met for inclusion in this study: 1) individuals who presented DD/ID as the main manifestation, with or without additional features such as congenital heart defects (CHD), autism, dysmorphism et al.; 2) individuals with whole-genome microarray analysis done. The exclusion criteria were individuals who had central nervous system infection, brain injury or intracranial tumor. This study was reviewed and approved by the ethical committee of Xinhua hospital and Shanghai Children's Medical Center, China, and informed consent was obtained from the patients or parents (for patients under 18 years old).

The phenotypic information of patients were assessed routinely in the clinic, including family history, pre/peri-natal history, physical examination, standardized measure of intelligence/development, instrumental evaluations (brain MRI, EEG, ultrasound etc.). These clinical records were collected, categorized and accessed electronically in this study. Patient were classified based on ID severity: mild (IQ level 55–70), moderate (IQ level 40–55), severe (IQ level 25–40) and profound ID (IQ level below 25), when the standardized measure of intelligence was valid and available. For comparison of the diagnostic yields in Table 1.II/III, only patients with clinical record indicating negative for the specific condition is counted as "without select condition". For example, in the group of "abnormal blood biochemistry", only patients who went through tandem mass spectrometry of blood samples with a normal biochemical profile returned were counted as "without select condition". For the groups of kidney/urinary tract, gastrointestinal or respiratory tract anomalies, clinicians did not perform detailed examination of these systems in most patients, thus we did not conduct statistical analysis in these groups. For "pre–/peri-natal problems", conditions included intrauterine growth retardation, pre- or post-term birth and low APGAR score etc. "Family history" was considered positive when first- or second-degree relative with DD/ID was reported. For "karyotypical abnormalities", patients with abnormal results of karyotype were counted as "with select condition". These patients were included as they comprised a portion of DD/ID patients referred to CMA, with the main purpose to confirm the chromosomal abnormality and further delineate the spanning of gain or loss.

Chromosomal microarray analysis

500 μl peripheral venous blood was withdrawn to ethylenediamine tetra-acetic acid (EDTA) tubes. Genomic DNA was extracted with GentraPuregene Kit (Qiagen, Germany) or Lab-Aid 820 kit (ZSandx, China). Detection of genomic CNVs was performed with Affymetrix-CytoScan HD or 750 K arrays (average probe spacing 1.1 kb and 4.1 kb, respectively) following the manufacturer's instructions. Array results were visualized and analyzed by Chromosome Analysis Suite software (Affymetrix, USA). The parental origin of CNVs was examined by CMA or quantitative real-time polymerase chain reaction.

Variant filtering

Size threshold for CNV analysis was set at > 100 kb for gains, > 50 kb for losses and > 10 Mb for loss of heterozygosity. Next, analysis was restricted to rare CNVs - those with < 80% overlap of any common CNVs (< 1% frequency) in the DGV (Database of Genomic Variants) or a database of 2691 phenotypically normal controls (offered by Affymetrix). Interpretation and report of CNVs followed the ACMG guideline [7]. The CNVs deemed benign were not reported.

Statistical analysis

All statistical analyses were performed on Vassarstats (http://www.vassarstats.net/). The correlation between select condition and pCNV finding was analyzed by Fisher's exact test on a 2×3 or 2×2 contingency table (row: the number of patients with or without certain condition; column: the number of patients with or without pCNVs identified). Analysis was only done in conditions with patients number above 50. Odds ratio was calculated, and statistical differences were defined as $p < 0.01$, two-tailed test.

Results

The clinical overview and overall diagnostic yield

In this retrospective study, a total of 710 patients with DD/ID as the main manifestation were included. Among this cohort, standardized measure of intelligence was available in 345 patients. Based on the degree of ID severity, the patients can be categorized to "mild" (140),

Table 1 Diagnostic yields in patients categorized by ID severity and co-occurring conditions

I. Based on ID severity

	total	P#	Yield	P-value
Mild	140	27	19%	0.08
Moderate	105	23	22%	
Severe	85	28	33%	
Profound	15	2	13%	
Not categorized	365	121	33%	/

II. Based on co-occurring conditions present in > 50 patients, with statistical analysis performed

	With select condition			Without select condition			Odds ratio	P-value
	total	P#	Yield	total	P#	Yield		
SS[a]	201	65	32%	136	30	22%	1.69	0.048
CHD[b]	98	54	55%	110	20	18%	**5.52**	**2.66E-08**
Gonadal dysplasia	50	18	36%	103	20	19%	2.33	0.03
Skeletal malformation	62	16	26%	24	3	13%	2.44	0.251
Facial dysmorphism	201	79	39%	194	39	20%	**2.57**	**4.27E-05**
Microcephaly	128	43	34%	140	25	18%	**2.33**	**0.0033**
Brain malformation	147	36	24%	148	29	20%	1.33	0.328
Epilepsy	62	15	24%	115	23	20%	1.28	0.567
Hypotonia	54	19	35%	113	18	16%	**2.87**	**0.00613**
Pre/peri-natal problems	160	50	31%	234	50	21%	1.67	0.034
SS + dysmorphism	79	30	38%	71	9	13%	**4.22**	**6.70E-04**
SS + microcephaly	66	25	38%	74	14	19%	2.61	0.015
SS + brain malformation	56	17	30%	45	9	20%	1.74	0.261
CHD + dysmorphism	50	31	62%	61	8	13%	**10.81**	**9.10E-08**

III. Based on co-occurring conditions present in < 50 patients

	total	P#	Yield		total	P#	Yield
Family history	38	7	18%	Macrocephaly	14	2	14%
Autism	20	3	15%	Hypertonia	26	6	23%
Muscle weakness	10	4	40%	Cleft lip/palate	8	7	88%
Obesity	16	10	63%	Low weight	47	23	49%
Ocular/auditory anomalies	50	8	16%	Kidney/urinary tract anomalies	12	5	42%
Gastrointestinal anomalies	10	3	30%	Respiratory tract anomalies	6	4	67%
Abnormal blood biochemistry	33	9	27%	Karyotypical abnormalities	26	24	92%

[a]SS-short stature; [b]CHD-congenital heart defects
P# number of patients with pCNVs identified, *Odds ratio* yielding pCNVs in patients with select condition versus without select condition, based on fisher's exact; *p*-value < 0.01, two-tailed were displayed in bold

"moderate" (105), "severe" (85) and "profound" (15) (Table 1I). Only 161 patients present DD/ID as the main manifestation without other phenotype reported, and the rest of the cohort were with one or more comorbid conditions, as listed in Table 1 part II/III. The most common conditions co-occurring with DD/ID were short stature (201 patients), facial dysmorphism (201 patients), pre/peri-natal problems (160 patients), brain malformation (147), microcephaly (128) and congenital heart defects (98).

The overall diagnostic rate was 28% - 201 patients were found to harbor pathogenic CNVs. One hundred nine patients (16%) were found with variants of uncertain clinical significance (VOUS), and 400 patients (56%) received a negative result (no CNV or only benign CNVs found). A total of 406 CNVs were reported to the patients (Fig. 1b), including 247 pathogenic CNVs (pCNVs, 61%), 18 VOUS-likely pathogenic (VOUS-LP, 4%), 136 VOUS (36%) and 5 VOUS-likely benign (VOUS-LB, 1%).

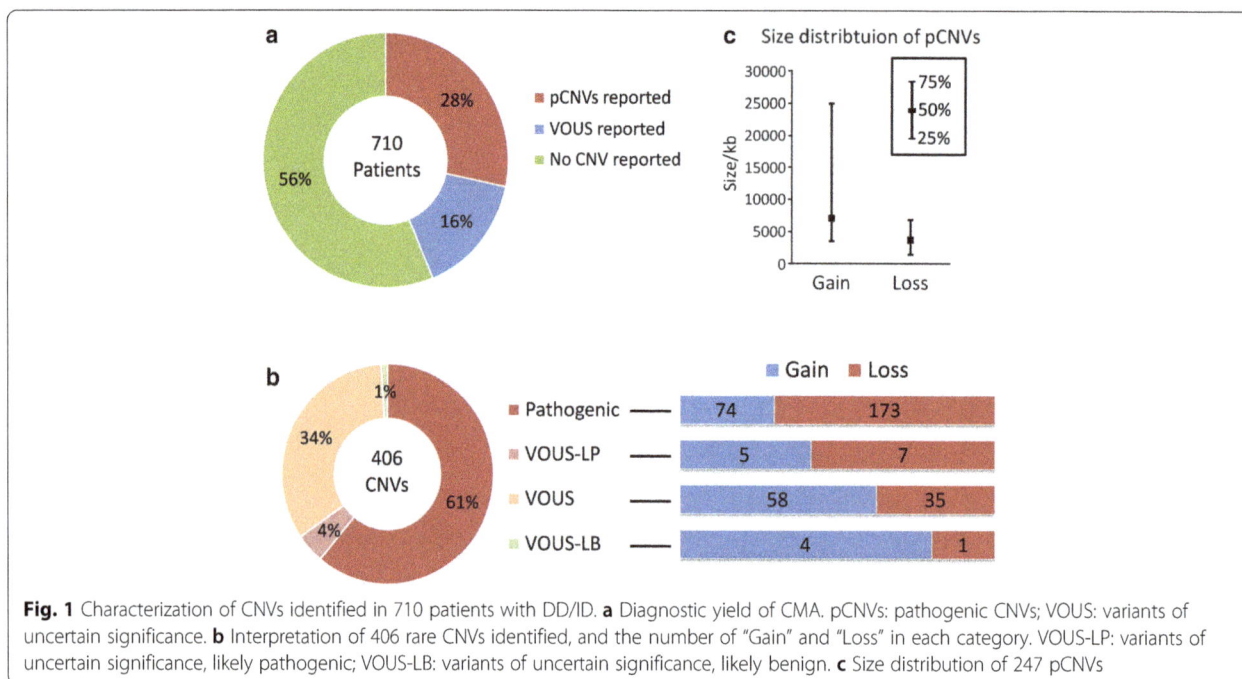

Fig. 1 Characterization of CNVs identified in 710 patients with DD/ID. **a** Diagnostic yield of CMA. pCNVs: pathogenic CNVs; VOUS: variants of uncertain significance. **b** Interpretation of 406 rare CNVs identified, and the number of "Gain" and "Loss" in each category. VOUS-LP: variants of uncertain significance, likely pathogenic; VOUS-LB: variants of uncertain significance, likely benign. **c** Size distribution of 247 pCNVs

Characterization of pCNVs

We characterized the property, size and physical distribution of pCNVs. Among 247 pCNVs identified, 173 were losses and 74 were gains (Fig. 1b). A bias towards loss was observed in pCNVs - the proportion of loss increased accordingly with the interpretation of CNV towards pathogenicity, from "VOUS-LB", "VOUS", "VOUS-LP" to pathogenic (Fig. 1b). Regarding the size of CNVs, losses were generally smaller than gains (Fig. 1c), with a median size of 3724 kb compared to 7047 kb of gains. Regarding the physical distribution, pCNVs distributed over all chromosomes, and most terminals were covered by gains or losses found in these 201 patients (Fig. 2). Enrichment of pCNVs was found in chr7, chr15 and chr22, mainly due to a few common syndromes identified in our cohorts – William Beuren syndrome (29 patients), Prader-Willi/Angelmen syndrome (21 patients), 22q11.2 deletion (5 patients) and 22q13.3 deletion (7 patients), respectively. The chromosomes with less frequent CNVs (frequency below 5) were chr6, chr9, chr14, chr16, chr19, chr20 and chrY. A full list of pCNVs analyzed was included in Additional file 1: Table S1.

Diagnostic yields in select conditions

When patients were divided to subgroups based on ID severity, the group of severe ID obtained the highest diagnostic yield of 33%, compared with 13–22% for the mild, moderate and profound group (Table 1a). The yield nominally increased with ID severity,

though not statistically significant ($p = 0.084$, fisher's exact, two-tailed).

To assess the diagnostic yields in DD/ID patients with co-occurring conditions, the cohort were divided to subgroups based on the presence of following conditions or their combination: pre/peri-natal problems, family history, short stature, congenital heart defects and twenty other conditions (Table 1, also see Methods for details). The number of patients with pCNVs identified and the diagnostic rate of each group was listed in Table 1 part II/III. Odds ratio (OR) of yielding a pathogenic finding in the presence of select condition was calculated (Table 1.II) and plotted (Fig. 3) when the number of patients with select condition was above 50. Four conditions when co-occurring with DD/ID showed a statistically higher chance of yielding pCNVs - congenital heart defects (55%, OR:5.52), facial dysmorphism (39%, OR:2.57), microcephaly (34%, OR:2.33), hypotonia (35%, OR:2.87) - markedly higher than the 28% overall diagnostic rate. In the presence of two comorbid conditions - short stature and facial dysmorphism, or congeital heart defects and facial dysmorphism, the yield was also markedly elevated (38%, OR:4.22; 62%, OR:10.81, respectively). Karyotypical abnormalities were known in 26 patients prior to CMA. Among these patients, 24 (92%) were identified with pCNVs, including 11 cases with the genomic content of marker chromosomes revealed, 3 cases with gain or loss found in "balanced rearrangement" (based on karyotype), 9 cases with gain/loss confirmed and spanning clarified, and 1 case with pCNV identified in a region

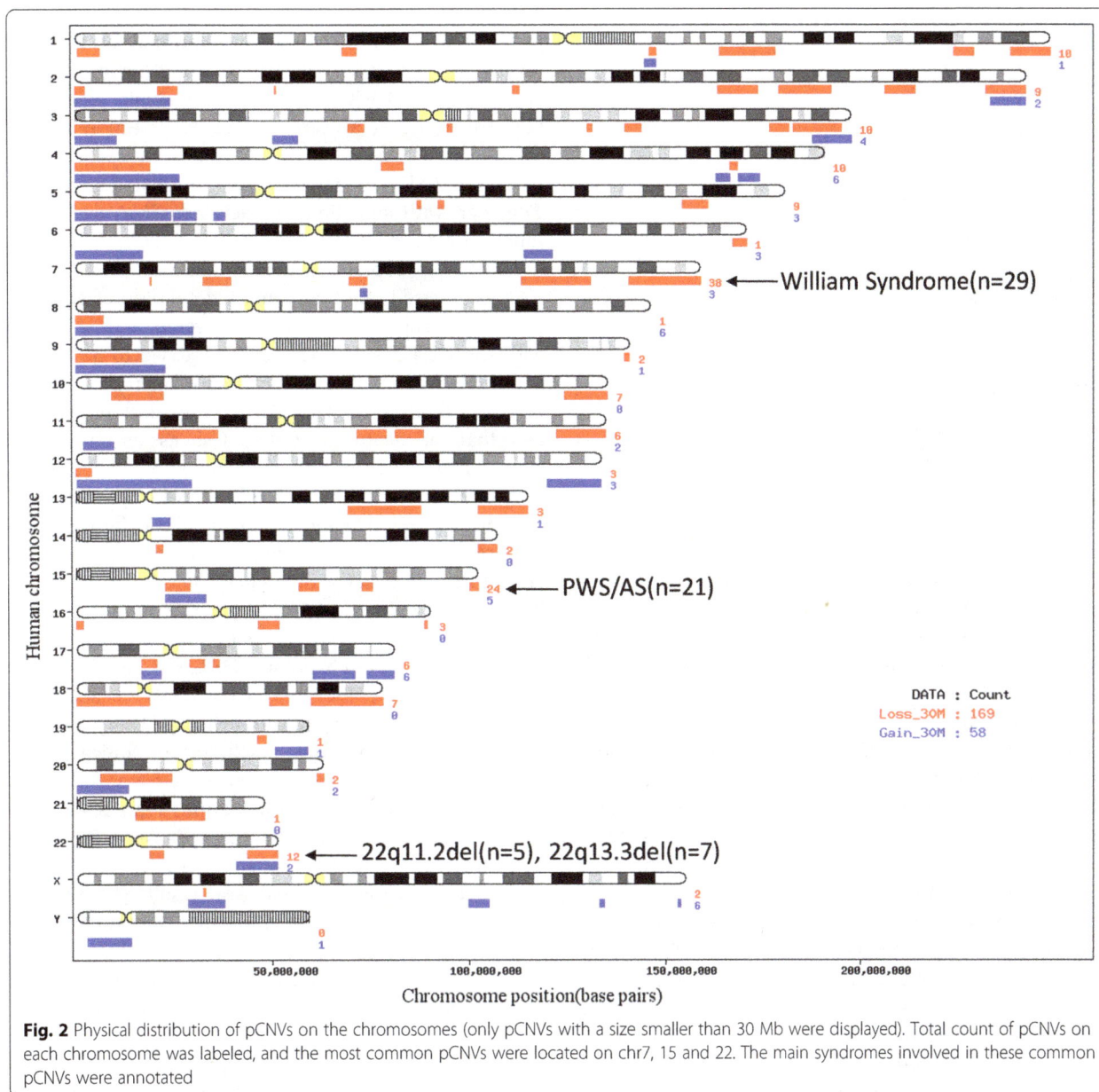

Fig. 2 Physical distribution of pCNVs on the chromosomes (only pCNVs with a size smaller than 30 Mb were displayed). Total count of pCNVs on each chromosome was labeled, and the most common pCNVs were located on chr7, 15 and 22. The main syndromes involved in these common pCNVs were annotated

other than the structural rearrangement site detected by karyotypical analysis. The rest 2 with no pCNV identified were patients with karyotypic results showing balanced rearrangement.

Discussion
More losses than gains in pCNVs
In this study, an increasing proportion of losses were observed with the pathogenic interpretation of CNVs. This is consistent with the notion that many gains present in the human genome are benign. Based on the CNV study on 59,898 exomes by Exome Aggregation Consortium, most phenotypically normal individuals possess higher number of duplications than

deletions [8]. The proportion of losses in the pCNVs can also be influenced by the interpretation, as the evidence guiding copy number losses towards pathogenic interpretation is more readily available than gains (in 1247 genes curated by ClinGen expert team, 250 genes have been rated as "sufficient evidence for haploinsufficiency", while only three genes were rated as "sufficient evidence for triplosensitivity", https://www.ncbi.nlm.nih.gov/projects/dbvar/clingen/index.shtml).

The phenotypes associated with pCNV finding
Though CMA has been recommended as the first-tier genetic test for DD/ID, it remains costly and majority of patients could not obtain a diagnosis after the test [9].

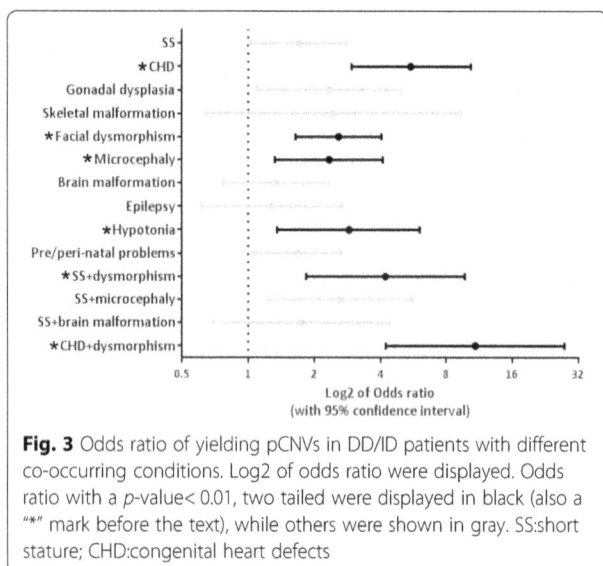

Fig. 3 Odds ratio of yielding pCNVs in DD/ID patients with different co-occurring conditions. Log2 of odds ratio were displayed. Odds ratio with a p-value< 0.01, two tailed were displayed in black (also a "*" mark before the text), while others were shown in gray. SS:short stature; CHD:congenital heart defects

Development of next-generation sequencing offers another option for genetic diagnostics of DD/ID. Based on a recent study, whole exome sequencing identified 29.3% conclusive diagnoses in a cohort of 150 patients with complex pediatric neurological conditions [10]. In the foreseeable future, the option between CMA and whole exome sequencing for DD/ID is likely to be put into discussion. Delineating the phenotypic clues of pathogenic CNVs can offer hints for the best cost-effectiveness, though a definite answer should come from the direct comparison of diagnostic yields between next-generation sequencing and CMA.

In our study, diagnostic yield of CMA appeared to correlate positively with ID severity (mild:19%, moderate:22% and severe:33%, Table 1.I), though the correlation was not statistically significant ($p = 0.08$, Fisher's exact). The number of profound ID cases in our cohort was small to generate a reliable conclusion. A study based on 349 individuals in Italy reported a higher detection rate of causative CNVs in mixed ID (21.5%, IQ < 70) than borderline ID (8.8%, IQ:70–85), but no further categorization of severity in the mixed ID cohort was assessed [11]. Larger datasets are needed to warrant the correlation between ID severity and CMA yield, ideally in a non-syndromic ID cohort.

The comorbidity of congenital heart defects (CHD) in DD/ID is the strongest single phenotype associated with pCNV finding in our study, with an odds ratio of 5.52. When additional comorbid condition is present, the effect size can be even larger - 62% yield was found in DD/ID patients with co-occurring CHD and facial dysmorphism (OR:10.81). This is consistent with a prior study by Shoukier et al., based on CMA results from 342 children with unexplained DD/ID in Europe - they

found CHD was more frequently seen in children with pCNVs compared to those with normal array CGH results [12]. There are also reports about higher yields in syndromic CHD with additional phenotypic indications [13, 14]. Geng et al. reported 22.7% detection rate of pathogenic CNVs in CHD patients with co-occurring DD/ID or ASD, compared to 4.3% in isolated cases [15]. Together with our finding, elevated CMA yield was found in comorbidity of CHD and DD/ID, and resorting to CMA is appropriate in such conditions.

Short stature is another comorbid condition frequently seen in our cohort (201/710). The overall yield of DD/ID with short stature was 32%, and increased to 38% when additional feature of dysmorphism or microcephaly was present (Table 1.II). Though the statistical power was less than adequate ($p = 0.048$, Fisher's exact) in our study, short stature has been reported to be more frequently seen in DD/ID children with pCNVs [12], thus it is a possible indication of pCNV finding. The yield of CMA reported in short stature was between 4% [16] -10% [17], and the difference could be attributed to the varied proportion of syndromic patients.

In cases of DD/ID comorbid with other neurological abnormalities, we found hypotonia (35%, OR:2.87, $p = 0.006$) and microcephaly (34%, OR:2.33, $p = 0.003$) was associated with higher CMA yield, but not epilepsy (24%, $p = 0.567$), brain malformations (24%, $p = 0.328$) or autism (15%) (Table 1, all statistical comparisons were based on fisher's exact). This is consistent with previous reports - microcephaly and hypotonia, but not epilepsy, were more frequently seen in DD/ID patients harboring pathogenic CNVs than those with normal array results [12, 18]. The documented yield of CMA in patients comorbid of DD/ID and autism varied (12.7% [19], 14% [11], 22% [20] and 26.1% [21]), and in our small subset of 20 patients, three were found to harbor pCNVs, resulting an intermediate yield of 15%.

One of the largest genotype-phenotype analysis so far - Cooper et al. investigated the rare CNV burden on 15,767 individuals in a mixed ID cohorts, and found greater enrichment of CNVs in patients with craniofacial anomalies and heart defects compared to those with epilepsy and autism [22]. Though the burden of rare CNVs cannot directly translate to clinically relevant findings, the overall trend should be informative. Our findings generally agreed that facial dysmorphism and CHD were more indicative of pCNV findings than epilepsy and autism. We additionally found gonadal dysplasia, skeletal malformation and pre/peri-natal problems were not associated with increased yield. The literature on CMA yield in DD/ID comorbid with these conditions is not sufficient, and relevant findings are subjected to further investigation.

A few other conditions, not commonly seen in DD/ID, were reviewed in this study but without statistical comparison performed (Table 1.III). Cleft lip/palate was found in 8 DD/ID patients, and CMA revealed pCNVs in 7 out of 8 patients (88%). These pCNVs were located at different regions, including 7p21 deletion (Saethre–Chotzen syndrome), partial trisomy of chromosome 9, 7q11.23 deletion, 10q26 deletion and 8q22-q24 duplication etc.. Since the reported yield of CMA in cleft lip/palate was between 11 and 14.8% based on larger cohorts [23, 24], our finding of high yield could be incidental as the number of patients was small. Another condition -abnormal biochemical profile - was not associated with elevated diagnostic yield in our DD/ID patients (yield: 27%, versus 29% in patients with normal biochemical results). Recent studies report that inborn errors of metabolism contribute to 1–5% of ID etiology [25]. American Pediatric Association also recommended considering the metabolic screening for children presenting with DD/ID [5]. In our study, patients referred to CMA after metabolic screening were mostly those without clear indication of a monogenic metabolic disorder. Our results did not support the atypical biochemical profile as a phenotypic indication of pCNV finding.

Karyotypical abnormality referred to CMA

Karyotypical abnormalities were known in some DD/ID patients prior to CMA. They were still referred mainly for further delineating the intervals of genomic aberration. Notably, in the 5 patients with karyotypically balanced rearrangement, 2 were identified to harbor micro-deletion/duplications with clinically relevant CNVs based on CMA. This highlights the possibility of genomic content loss/gain in those karyotypically balanced structural variations.

Limitations of this study

There are a number of limitations in our study: 1. the sample size is modest, especially those patients with fully accessible clinical information, which limited the statistical power in the comparison of yields based on disease severity and comorbid conditions. 2. Certain conditions can be a matter of clinical judgment like facial dysmorphism, and certain defects may be overlooked in patients without comprehensive evaluation of multiple systems. 3. The diagnostic yield in our study was overall higher than reported, which could be accounted by the patient selection. Patients with karyotypical abnormality were not excluded. In addition, metabolic screening was routinely done in our clinic, which excludes those with identifiable inborn errors of metabolism due to monogenic variants. Nonetheless, the patients in our study, with broad range of phenotypes, can be representative of DD/ID cohorts.

Conclusions

In conclusion, this study assessed the yield of CMA based on phenotypic features in a highly heterogeneous DD/ID cohort. The results suggest a disparity of gains and losses in identified pCNVs, and varied yields exist in patients with different phenotypic presentation. Congenital heart defects, microcephaly, hypotonia and facial dysmorphism co-occurring with DD/ID associate with an increased probability of pCNV finding. The presence of these comorbid conditions can be among factors to consider when planning CMA on DD/ID patients.

Abbreviations
ACMG: American College of Medical Genetics and Genomics; CHD: Congenital heart defects; CMA: Chromosomal microarray analysis; DD: Developmental delay; DGV: Database of genomic variants; ID: Intellectual disability; LB: Likely benign; LP: Likely pathogenic; pCNVs: Pathogenic copy number variations; VOUS: Variants of uncertain clinical significance

Acknowledgements
We acknowledge all the patients and families. We thank Dr.Yiping Shen (Boston children's hospital) and Dr.Yu Sun (Xinhua hospital, Shanghai) for constructive comments and discussion. We are also grateful for the expert team of Society of Medical Genetics, Chinese Medical Doctor Association in the following institutions for enrollment and referral of patients - Maternal and Child Health Hospital of Guangxi Zhuang Autonomous Region; Beijing Children's Hosptial; Shengjing Hospital; Children's Hospital of Fudan University; Guangzhou Women and Children's Medical Center; Shanghai Children's Hospital; Maternal and Child Health Hospital of Hunan Province; Nanjing Children's Hospital; Wenzhou Medical College.

Funding
Funding for this project was from the National Natural Science Foundation of China (No. 81500972, to YF; No. 81670812, to YGY), the Shanghai Municipal Education Commission (No.15CG14, to YF), the Shanghai Municipal Science and Technology Commission (No.15YF1409600, to YF), and Shanghai Jiao Tong University School of Medicine (No.15ZH3003, to YGY), Shanghai Health Bureau (20134005 to WJQ) and Precision Medical Research of National Key Research and Development Program (2016YFC0905100 to WJQ and XFG). The funding organizations played no role in the design of the study, collection, analysis and interpretation of data and in writing the manuscript.

Authors' contributions
YF and YW1 performed the analysis, prepared the figures and tables and wrote the manuscript. LW, YW2 and ZG performed the CMA experiments. WQ, JW, HZ, XJ1, JY, LH, XJ2, YS, FL, BX and LL recruited the patients and collected clinical information. XZ and XL reviewed and analyzed the clinical data. XG and YY recruited patients and supervised the study. All authors have read and approved the manuscript.

Competing interests
The authors declare that they have no competing interests.

Author details
[1]Department of Pediatric Endocrinology/Genetics, Xinhua Hospital affiliated to Shanghai Jiao Tong University School of Medicine, Shanghai Institute for Pediatric Research, 1665 Kongjiang Road, Shanghai 200092, China.

[2]Department of Pediatrics, People's Hospital of Shanghai Pudong New District, 490 South Chuanhuan Road, Shanghai 201200, China. [3]Department of Pediatrics, Peking University First Hospital, 8 Xishiku Dajie Xicheng District, Beijing 100034, China. [4]Department of Developmental and Behavioral Pediatrics, Shanghai Children's Medical Center, Shanghai Jiao Tong University School of Medicine, 1678 Dongfang Road, Shanghai 200127, China. [5]Department of Endocrinology, Shanghai Children's Medical Center, Shanghai Jiao Tong University School of Medicine, 1678 Dongfang Road, Shanghai 200127, China. [6]MOE-Shanghai Key Laboratory of Children's Environmental Health, Xinhua Hospital affiliated to Shanghai Jiao Tong University School of Medicine, 1665 Kongjiang Rd, Shanghai 200092, China.

References

1. Maulik PK, Mascarenhas MN, Mathers CD, Dua T, Saxena S. Prevalence of intellectual disability: a meta-analysis of population-based studies. Res Dev Disabil. 2011;32(2):419–36.

2. Moeschler JB, Shevell M. Clinical genetic evaluation of the child with mental retardation or developmental delays. Pediatrics. 2006;117(6):2304–16.

3. Miller DT, Adam MP, Aradhya S, Biesecker LG, Brothman AR, Carter NP, Church DM, Crolla JA, Eichler EE, Epstein CJ, et al. Consensus statement: chromosomal microarray is a first-tier clinical diagnostic test for individuals with developmental disabilities or congenital anomalies. Am J Hum Genet. 2010;86(5):749–64.

4. [Expert consensus on the clinical application of chromosomal microarray analysis in pediatric genetic diseases]. Zhonghua er ke za zhi = Chinese J Pediatr. 2016;54(6):410–3.

5. Moeschler JB, Shevell M. Comprehensive evaluation of the child with intellectual disability or global developmental delays. Pediatrics. 2014;134(3):e903–18.

6. Arvio M, Sillanpaa M. Prevalence, aetiology and comorbidity of severe and profound intellectual disability in Finland. J Intellect Disabil Res. 2003;47(Pt 2):108–12.

7. Kearney HM, Thorland EC, Brown KK, Quintero-Rivera F, South ST. American College of Medical Genetics standards and guidelines for interpretation and reporting of postnatal constitutional copy number variants. Genet Med. 2011;13(7):680–5.

8. Ruderfer DM, Hamamsy T, Lek M, Karczewski KJ, Kavanagh D, Samocha KE, Daly MJ, MacArthur DG, Fromer M, Purcell SM. Patterns of genic intolerance of rare copy number variation in 59,898 human exomes. Nat Genet. 2016;48(10):1107–11.

9. Vissers LE, Gilissen C, Veltman JA. Genetic studies in intellectual disability and related disorders. Nat Rev Genet. 2016;17(1):9–18.

10. Vissers LE, van Nimwegen KJ, Schieving JH, Kamsteeg EJ, Kleefstra T, Yntema HG, Pfundt R, van der Wilt GJ, Krabbenborg L, Brunner HG, et al. A clinical utility study of exome sequencing versus conventional genetic testing in pediatric neurology. Genet Med. 2017;

11. Battaglia A, Doccini V, Bernardini L, Novelli A, Loddo S, Capalbo A, Filippi T, Carey JC. Confirmation of chromosomal microarray as a first-tier clinical diagnostic test for individuals with developmental delay, intellectual disability, autism spectrum disorders and dysmorphic features. Eur J Paediatr Neurol. 2013;17(6):589–99.

12. Shoukier M, Klein N, Auber B, Wickert J, Schroder J, Zoll B, Burfeind P, Bartels I, Alsat EA, Lingen M, et al. Array CGH in patients with developmental delay or intellectual disability: are there phenotypic clues to pathogenic copy number variants? Clin Genet. 2013;83(1):53–65.

13. Richards AA, Santos LJ, Nichols HA, Crider BP, Elder FF, Hauser NS, Zinn AR, Garg V. Cryptic chromosomal abnormalities identified in children with congenital heart disease. Pediatr Res. 2008;64(4):358–63.

14. Syrmou A, Tzetis M, Fryssira H, Kosma K, Oikonomakis V, Giannikou K, Makrythanasis P, Kitsiou-Tzeli S, Kanavakis E. Array comparative genomic hybridization as a clinical diagnostic tool in syndromic and nonsyndromic congenital heart disease. Pediatr Res. 2013;73(6):772–6.

15. Geng J, Picker J, Zheng Z, Zhang X, Wang J, Hisama F, Brown DW, Mullen MP, Harris D, Stoler J, et al. Chromosome microarray testing for patients with congenital heart defects reveals novel disease causing loci and high diagnostic yield. BMC Genomics. 2014;15:1127.

16. van Duyvenvoorde HA, Lui JC, Kant SG, Oostdijk W, Gijsbers AC, Hoffer MJ, Karperien M, Walenkamp MJ, Noordam C, Voorhoeve PG, et al. Copy number variants in patients with short stature. Eur J Hum Genet. 2014;22(5):602–9.

17. Zahnleiter D, Uebe S, Ekici AB, Hoyer J, Wiesener A, Wieczorek D, Kunstmann E, Reis A, Doerr HG, Rauch A, et al. Rare copy number variants are a common cause of short stature. PLoS Genet. 2013;9(3):e1003365.

18. Caballero Perez V, Lopez Pison FJ, Miramar Gallart MD, Gonzalez Alvarez A, Garcia Jimenez MC, Garcia Iniguez JP, Orden Rueda C, Gil Hernandez I, Fuertes Rodrigo C, Fernando Martinez R, et al. Phenotype in patients with intellectual disability and pathological results in array CGH. Neurologia. 2017;32(9):568–78.

19. Nicholl J, Waters W, Mulley JC, Suwalski S, Brown S, Hull Y, Barnett C, Haan E, Thompson EM, Liebelt J, et al. Cognitive deficit and autism spectrum disorders: prospective diagnosis by array CGH. Pathology. 2014;46(1):41–5.

20. Shen Y, Dies KA, Holm IA, Bridgemohan C, Sobeih MM, Caronna EB, Miller KJ, Frazier JA, Silverstein I, Picker J, et al. Clinical genetic testing for patients with autism spectrum disorders. Pediatrics. 2010;125(4):e727–35.

21. Oikonomakis V, Kosma K, Mitrakos A, Sofocleous C, Pervanidou P, Syrmou A, Pampanos A, Psoni S, Fryssira H, Kanavakis E, et al. Recurrent copy number variations as risk factors for autism spectrum disorders: analysis of the clinical implications. Clin Genet. 2016;89(6):708–18.

22. Cooper GM, Coe BP, Girirajan S, Rosenfeld JA, Vu TH, Baker C, Williams C, Stalker H, Hamid R, Hannig V, et al. A copy number variation morbidity map of developmental delay. Nat Genet. 2011;43(9):838–46.

23. Emy Dorfman L, Leite JC, Giugliani R, Riegel M. Microarray-based comparative genomic hybridization analysis in neonates with congenital anomalies: detection of chromosomal imbalances. J Pediatr. 2015;91(1):59–67.

24. Cao Y, Li Z, Rosenfeld JA, Pursley AN, Patel A, Huang J, Wang H, Chen M, Sun X, Leung TY, et al. Contribution of genomic copy-number variations in prenatal oral clefts: a multicenter cohort study. Genet Med. 2016;18(10):1052–5.

25. Michelson DJ, Shevell MI, Sherr EH, Moeschler JB, Gropman AL, Ashwal S. Evidence report: genetic and metabolic testing on children with global developmental delay: report of the quality standards Subcommittee of the American Academy of neurology and the practice Committee of the Child Neurology Society. Neurology. 2011;77(17):1629–35.

Integrative pathway-based survival prediction utilizing the interaction between gene expression and DNA methylation in breast cancer

So Yeon Kim[1], Tae Rim Kim[1], Hyun-Hwan Jeong[2,3] and Kyung-Ah Sohn[1*]

Abstract

Background: Integrative analysis on multi-omics data has gained much attention recently. To investigate the interactive effect of gene expression and DNA methylation on cancer, we propose a directed random walk-based approach on an integrated gene-gene graph that is guided by pathway information.

Methods: Our approach first extracts a single pathway profile matrix out of the gene expression and DNA methylation data by performing the random walk over the integrated graph. We then apply a denoising autoencoder to the pathway profile to further identify important pathway features and genes. The extracted features are validated in the survival prediction task for breast cancer patients.

Results: The results show that the proposed method substantially improves the survival prediction performance compared to that of other pathway-based prediction methods, revealing that the combined effect of gene expression and methylation data is well reflected in the integrated gene-gene graph combined with pathway information. Furthermore, we show that our joint analysis on the methylation features and gene expression profile identifies cancer-specific pathways with genes related to breast cancer.

Conclusions: In this study, we proposed a DRW-based method on an integrated gene-gene graph with expression and methylation profiles in order to utilize the interactions between them. The results showed that the constructed integrated gene-gene graph can successfully reflect the combined effect of methylation features on gene expression profiles. We also found that the selected features by DA can effectively extract topologically important pathways and genes specifically related to breast cancer.

Keywords: Multi-omics, Integrative analysis, Random walk, Denoising autoencoder, Pathway, Breast cancer, Gene expression, DNA methylation

* Correspondence: kasohn@ajou.ac.kr
[1]Department of Computer Engineering, Ajou University, Suwon 16499, South Korea
Full list of author information is available at the end of the article

Background

Integrative analysis on multi-omics data to find bio-markers or pathway features highly associated with cancer has received considerable attention [1–6]. Considering the rich information contained in multi-omics data, many studies have investigated the interrelationships among multiple meta-dimensional data for improved biological interpretation and analysis [7–12]. To understand the interaction between different types of genomic features requires more sophisticated modeling and analysis. In particular, the causal relationships between gene expression data and DNA methylation have been extensively studied [13–16]. For joint analysis of gene expression and methylation data in cancer, pathway and subtype information have proven especially useful [17–19]. In this study, we address the problem of pathway-driven integrated analysis of gene expression and methylation data in cancer.

To combine pathway information into genomic analysis and cancer prediction, several methods of inferring pathway activity have been proposed [20–24]. For example, the mean and median of the expression values of pathway member genes can be used for precise cancer classification [24]. In [20], pathway activity inference method of condition-responsive genes (the pathway member genes whose combined expression show optimal discriminative power for the disease phenotype) have been proposed to incorporate pathway information into the precise disease classification. Pathway activity inference approaches using probabilistic inference have been used for combining multiple types of omics data and a better cancer classification [21–23]. However, those existing pathway-based methods simply take pathways as the set of genes and have ignored the topological importance of the hub genes in the pathway network that can be highly associated with diseases. In this respect, Liu, et al. proposed a directed random walk (DRW)-based pathway inference method to identify the topologically important genes and pathways by weighting the genes in the pathway network [25]. Because this original DRW method targeted a single profile of gene expression data, recent approaches have focused on integrating multiple types of data, for example, gene expression and metabolite data [26]. Directed random walk on a gene-metabolite graph (DRW-GM) was performed guided by pathway information, and identified important differential genes and risk pathways in prostate cancer.

In this study, we propose a DRW-based approach on an integrated gene-gene graph especially redefined for gene expression and methylation data in order to extract important pathway and gene features for survival prediction. We first construct an integrated gene-gene graph by adding edges between gene expression and methylation features as well as edges within each profile. In constructing the integrated gene-gene graph, we consider two approaches: one that adds bi-directional edges between expression and methylation features of the same gene that has both profiles, and another that considers only the anti-correlated interactions between the expression and methylation data. For the edges within each single profile, we adopt the pathway-based interaction graph from the previous study [25]. DRW is then performed, which produces the weight values of both expression and methylation features. The initial weights of the gene expression nodes are measured by DESeq2 [27], which is a method for differential gene expression analysis in count data from high-throughput sequencing assays. The methylation feature nodes are initially weighted by using a two-tailed t-test between two phenotypes. By using the output from the DRW, a pathway activity profile is computed. In summary, integrative DRW (iDRW) on a graph defined over gene expression and methylation features transforms the combined profile of gene expression and methylation data into a single pathway profile. To further extract important pathway features, we apply a denoising autoencoder (DA) [28] to the pathway profile matrix. DA has proven to be effective in selecting robust features against input noise and extracting more specific cancer-related pathways or genes [29–31]. The resulting features are validated on a survival prediction task of breast cancer patients. The topologically significant pathways and pathway member genes are identified and analyzed as well. The overall process of the proposed approach is illustrated in Fig. 1.

The pathway features selected with our scheme are based on gene expression and methylation features as well as interactions between the two. These extracted pathway features are effective at improving the prediction performance when compared to the gene-based profile or other pathway-driven methods. We also reveal that the iDRW method with a denoising autoencoder selects a more cancer-specific pathways or genes as compared to that directly selected by the iDRW method.

Methods

Dataset

Gene expression and DNA methylation data of 868 breast cancer patients were obtained from the TCGA dataset of the Broad Institute GDAC Firehose [32]. Gene expression data from RNA sequencing consisted of 17,673 genes, which are upper-quartile normalized RSEM count estimates in the Broad Institute GDAC Firehose [33]. DNA methylation data were obtained as a gene-level feature of 17,037 genes by selecting the probe having a minimum correlation with expression data for each gene [34]. We removed genes in which more than half had gene expression values of 0. In contrast to gene expression data, 5134 missing values were present in the methylation data. To impute missing values, we replaced them with a

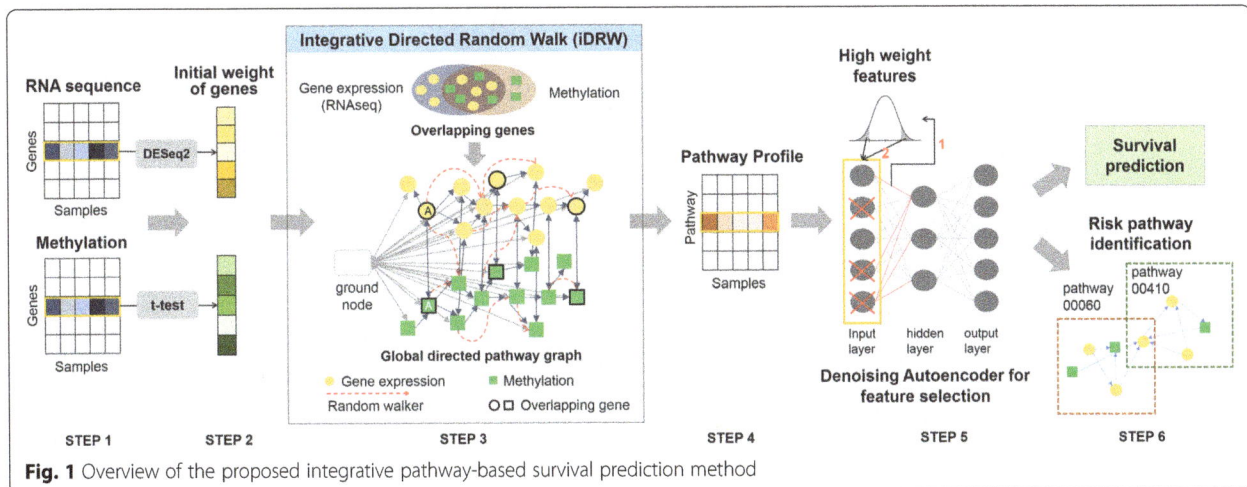

Fig. 1 Overview of the proposed integrative pathway-based survival prediction method

median of the corresponding patient's data. For each breast cancer patient, the vital status and survival days were recorded. Among 868 patients, we extracted 568 samples that had both RNA sequencing and methylation data. We removed patients whose survival days were not recorded or wrongly so as negative values. In this study, we split the patients into good (> 3 years) and poor (≤ 3 years) groups with respect to their survival days [35]. Patients who were living (vital status reported as 1) but whose survival days were less than 3 years were removed. In total, 465 samples were divided into two groups of 218 good and 247 poor. Finally, the gene expression and methylation data were normalized for the mean to be 0 and standard deviation to be 1 over all samples.

Pathway-based global directed integrated gene-gene graph

To transform each gene profile into a pathway profile, a DRW-based method was performed on a global directed gene-gene graph, which was constructed based on both 150 metabolic and 150 non-metabolic KEGG pathways [25]. Interactions between genes in the global directed graph were manually drawn from the KEGG database [36] by researchers in [25]. The global directed graph contained 4113 genes and 40,875 directed edges. Details regarding the construction method of the global directed graph are provided in [25].

To define the directed graph across gene expression and methylation data, we first included all edges in the global directed graph from [25] within each profile. In addition, the interactions between 16,454 overlapping genes in the two profiles were defined in the global directed graph. As most of the methylation profiles inhibited the genes in the gene expression data [37], we experimented with two cases. First, we assigned bi-directional edges to all overlapping genes between gene expression and methylation data. Second, we only assigned the edge when the expression and methylation values of

the same gene were anti-correlated. Correlation was measured by the Pearson correlation and significance test of a correlation coefficient was performed. The correlation coefficient with a negative value and p-value of a significant test < 0.05 meant that the methylation profile might inhibit the corresponding gene expression. The final integrated gene-gene graph contained 4113 genes as nodes, which were either from the gene expression data or methylation profiles. The number of directed edges in the graph was 88,440 when all overlapping edges were added and 81,750 (the removal of edges is about 7.6% of all overlapping edges) when only the anti-correlated edges were added.

DRW-based method on an integrated gene-gene graph

We utilized the recently proposed DRW method (DRW-GM) [26] to integrate information in a graph constructed from multiple profiles. To perform random walk, the initial weights of the genes should be assigned. As the DRW-GM method is specifically designed to integrate gene expression profiles and metabolomic profiles, the weights of the genes were modified for the graph from the gene expression and methylation profiles. For each gene profile, W_0 is constructed as:

$$W_0 = - \log\left(w_g + \epsilon\right)$$

where w_g is the weight of the gene g in the directed integrated gene-gene graph G, and $\epsilon = 2.2e^{-16}$. The weight of the gene is the p-value from either a two-tailed t-test for the methylation profiles or a DESeq2, which is a method for differential gene expression analysis based on negative binomial distribution for RNA sequence genes [27]. Each gene weight vector is normalized to scale the range between 0 and 1. Finally, W_0 is L_1-normalized to a unit vector. A random walker starts on a source node s and transits to a randomly selected neighbor or returns to the source node s with a restart probability r at each time step t. The DRW method is formally defined as:

$$W_{t+1} = (1-r)M^T W_t + r W_0$$

where W_t is the weight vector in which the i-th element represents the probability of being at node i at time step t; M is a row-normalized adjacency matrix of the directed integrated gene-gene graph G; r is the restart probability, which is set to 0.7 (as it was previously shown that the performance of the DRW method is not sensitive to the varying r [25]), and W_0 is the initial weight vector of genes in the graph G. At each time step, W_t is updated and guaranteed to converge to a steady state W_∞ [38] when $|W_{t+1} - W_t| < 10^{-10}$.

Pathway activity inference

For a j-th pathway P_j containing n_j differential genes $(g_1, g_2, ..., g_{n_j})$ whose p-value (w_g) is < 0.05, the pathway activity is defined as:

$$a(P_j) = \frac{\sum_{i=1}^{n_j} W_\infty(g_i) * score(g_i) * z(g_i)}{\sqrt{\sum_{i=1}^{n_j}(W_\infty(g_i))^2}}$$

where $W_\infty(g_i)$ is the weight of gene g_i from the DRW method, $z(g_i)$ is the normalized expression vector of g_i across overall samples, and $score(g_i)$ is either a log_2 fold change from the DESeq2 [27] analysis if g_i is a gene from the gene expression data, or a $sign(tscore(g_i))$ from two-tailed t-test statistics if g_i is a gene with the methylation feature. For DESeq2 in the gene expression data, log_2 fold change indicates the extent to which gene expression values have changed between groups of samples. For each pathway, the pathway activity is computed from the normalized gene expression values for each sample, which corresponds to a pathway profile. As a result, the pathway profile is used as an input to a classification model.

Feature selection and ranking strategy

To select pathway features, the pathways are first scored by the weight matrix from DA [28]. Given an input $x \in \mathbb{R}^d$ that is a feature vector and corrupted input $\tilde{x} \in \mathbb{R}^d$ that is perturbed by a random binomial error, $\tilde{x}$ is mapped to a hidden representation $y \in \mathbb{R}^p$ as follows:

$$y = s(W\tilde{x} + b)$$

where s is a sigmoid activation function, W is a weight matrix that is randomly initialized depending on its input and hidden layer size, b is a bias, and y is a latent representation of the encoded $\tilde{x}$ by the encoder. y is then used as an input into a decoder to reconstruct z as follows:

$$z = s(W^T y + b^T)$$

Here, z C input of x given y. To calculate the reconstruction error, we used a mean squared error, not the cross-entropy as the scale of our data was not in [0, 1]. $L(xz)$, which is the loss on the reconstruction of the original input x from z, is defined as:

$$L(xz) = \frac{\|x-z\|^2}{2}$$

For feature importance scoring purposes, we used a single hidden layer because the input features are scored by the weight matrix between input and hidden layers, and the more abstract features are selected when using the more number of hidden layers which can lead to lose pathway information. Note that the purpose of using DA in this study was primarily for feature selection than for accurate reconstruction of the original input. To rank the pathway features, we first trained the DA to obtain the weight matrix between input and hidden layers. The weight of each input feature was then defined as the mean value of the weight vector of the input node to all hidden nodes. We experimented with a varying number of hidden nodes (50, 100, 150, 200). As the number of hidden nodes did not greatly affect the list of selected pathway features and the final classification performance, the number of hidden nodes was set to 200. In the experiments, the selected pathway features from DA combined with the iDRW method (iDRW+DA) were compared with those obtained using the iDRW method. The pathway features were ranked by their p-values from the t-test of pathway activities across samples with the iDRW method. Therefore, the ranked features by the iDRW+DA method were selected to best fit the classification model using a greedy search as performed in [25].

Classification performance evaluation

We performed a logistic regression analysis using the extracted features. A 5-fold cross validation was conducted to evaluate the classification performance. We first divided the entire samples into five folds. We then trained the regression model using four folds and validated the performance using the remaining fold. For each fold, the top-N pathway features that yielded the best classification performance were selected; this was measured by area under the curve (AUC) and the accuracy. AUC is the area under the Receiving operating characteristic (ROC) curve evaluating the trade-off between true positive rate (sensitivity) and false positive rate (1- specificity) and the accuracy measures the proportion of true positives and true negatives; the more AUC and the accuracy is, the better the trained regression model classifies the test samples into good and poor group. To select the best pathway features, we repeated the entire cross validation process 10 times and assessed the pathway features that appeared more than three times in a union of 50 feature sets. Finally, the average AUC and accuracy after 10 repeats of the process using five folds was used as a final classification performance.

Results

Performance comparison on a single type of feature data

To check the utility of the pathway profiles obtained using the DRW method, we first experimented with each single-layered feature data. The performances were evaluated using four types of data: RNA-seq gene expression profile, methylation profile, RNA-seq pathway profile, and methylation pathway profile. The pathway profiles were obtained by the original DRW method. The classification performance was evaluated using the selected top-N pathway features ranked by their t-test scores. For a fair comparison, top-N genes of the gene profiles were also ranked by their DESeq2 or t-test scores. Note that the genes and pathways are weighted via two-group (good and poor groups) comparison that is considered as a supervised learning task. Figure 2 shows the average AUC and the accuracy from a 5-fold cross validation measured using a logistic regression model. As shown in Fig. 2, the overall performance using the pathway

profiles from the DRW method was better than that when using the gene profiles. These findings reveal that the pathway features extracted using the DRW method can improve the prediction performance when compared to the gene features. We also determined that the performance difference between RNA-seq data and the methylation profile was considerable when using pathway profiles. This means that gene expression plays a more critical role in survival prediction in a breast cancer patient group than does a methylation profile. Moreover, this difference was particularly remarkable when raw feature values were transformed into pathway features.

Performance comparison of the pathway-based prediction methods on combined feature data

To show the utility of the proposed method on the combined feature data, we compared different pathway-based prediction methods on the combined RNA-seq and DNA methylation data (Fig. 3). First, we simply employed means (Mean) and medians (Median) of the expression values of the significant pathway member genes to construct a pathway profile matrix. To show the utility of the integrated gene-gene graph, we also assessed the performance when the pathway profiles obtained from the RNA-seq and methylation data were concatenated (DRW-concat).

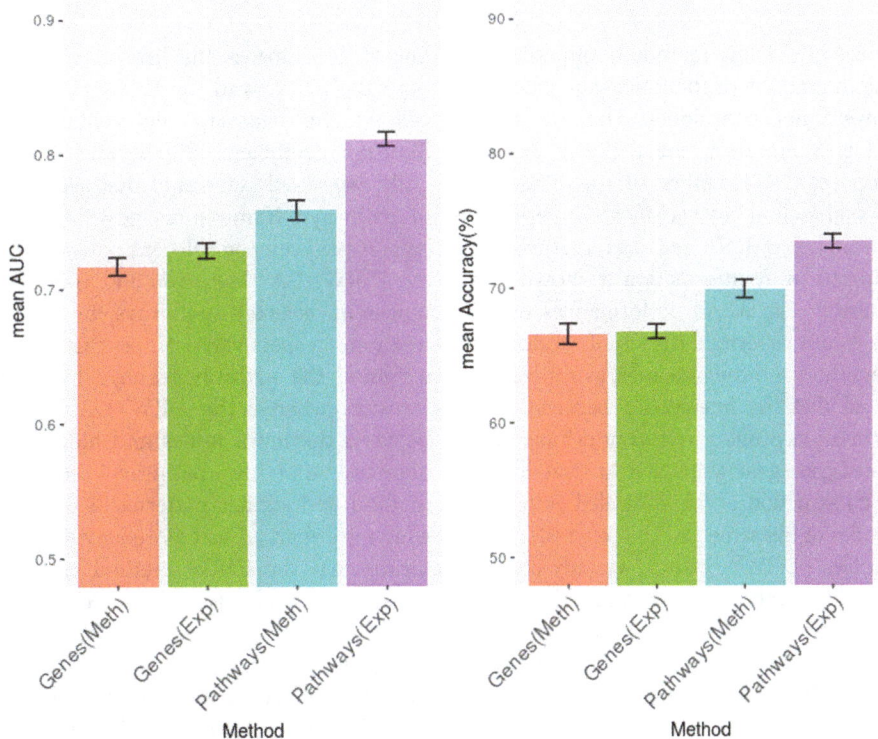

Fig. 2 Classification performance comparison between a single type of feature data and converted pathway profiles by DRW in terms of mean AUC (left) and mean accuracy (right) after 10 repeats of 5-fold cross validation process. Gene and pathway profiles with gene expression and methylation profiles were evaluated. The pathway profiles were obtained by the original DRW method. Error bars represent the standard error of the mean values

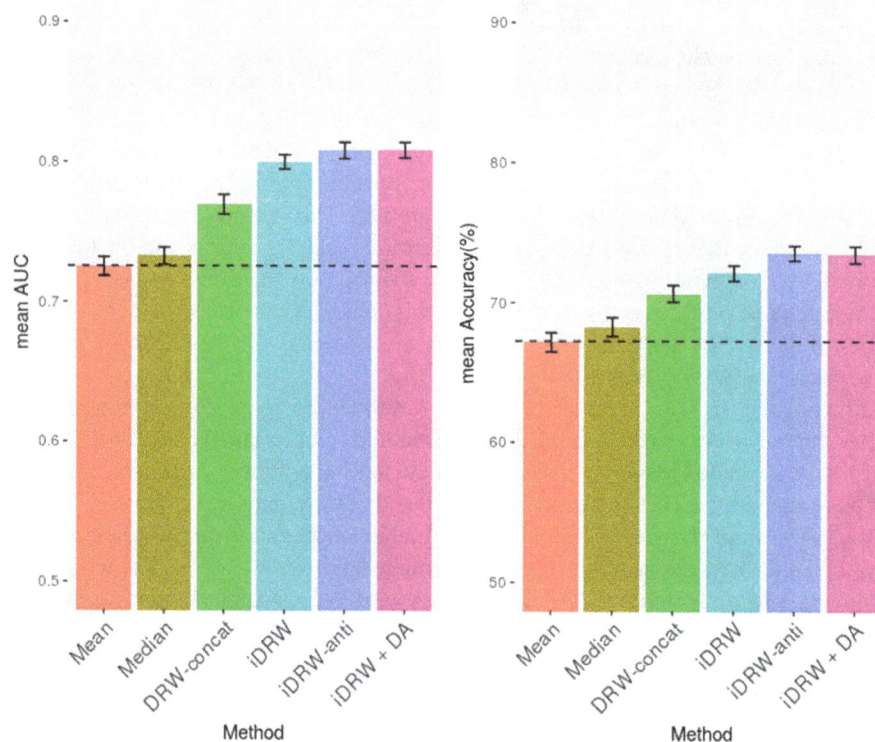

Fig. 3 Classification performance comparison of the pathway-based prediction methods on the combined feature data. Mean AUC (left) and mean accuracy (right) after 10 repeats of 5-fold cross validation process are shown. Error bars represent the standard error of the mean values

In this method, we used the DRW method to obtain pathway profiles but the interaction of the RNA sequence and methylation data were not considered. The last three results shown in Fig. 3 are from the pathway profiles obtained by the proposed DRW method on the integrated gene-gene graph. As a baseline, the classification performance over the concatenated RNA-seq and methylation profile without using pathway information is shown as a dotted horizontal line in Fig. 3. All performances of the iDRW-based methods outperformed the simple concatenation of the DRW method and the baselines, as expected.

These results reveal that the interactions between gene expression and methylation profiles have considerable joint effect on the integrated gene-gene graph and survival prediction. Regarding the construction of the integrated graph, we first linked all the nodes of the same gene between RNA-seq and methylation profiles (iDRW). Second, we only considered the anti-correlated interactions (iDRW-anti). The classification performance of iDRW combined with the DA (iDRW+DA) was the best, whereas the performance difference between the three iDRW methods was marginal.

Identification of significant pathways and genes in breast cancer

In our study, we could extract significant pathway features from both the iDRW outputs and the iDRW+ DA.

Figure 4 compares the lists of selected pathways from both the iDRW and the iDRW+DA as a heatmap. Each cell in the heatmap represents similarity using the Simpson coefficient [39] between two lists of differentially expressed genes and methylation sites from a pair of pathways. It measures how many genes were overlapped between the selected pathways by the iDRW and the iDRW+DA. The rows and columns in the heatmap represent selected pathways by DA and the iDRW method, respectively. Note that the iDRW method weighted the pathway features by the two-tailed t-test statistics, whereas the iDRW+DA used the weight matrix between the input nodes and hidden nodes in DA. We observed that the pathways selected by the iDRW method had similar patterns to those from iDRW+DA, which are marked as colored rows in the heatmap. This means that the iDRW method can detect general and non-specific pathways such as MAPK signaling pathway (86 genes), pathways in cancer (86 genes), and endocytosis (47 genes). However, iDRW+DA identified dorso-ventral axis formation as a top-scoring pathway which is an extremely specific pathway and contains four differentially expressed genes: ETS proto-oncogene 1, transcription factor (ETS1); notch 2 (NOTCH); mitogen-activated protein kinase 3 (MAPK3); and SOS Ras/Rac guanine nucleotide exchange factor 1 (SOS1). The dorso-ventral axis formation

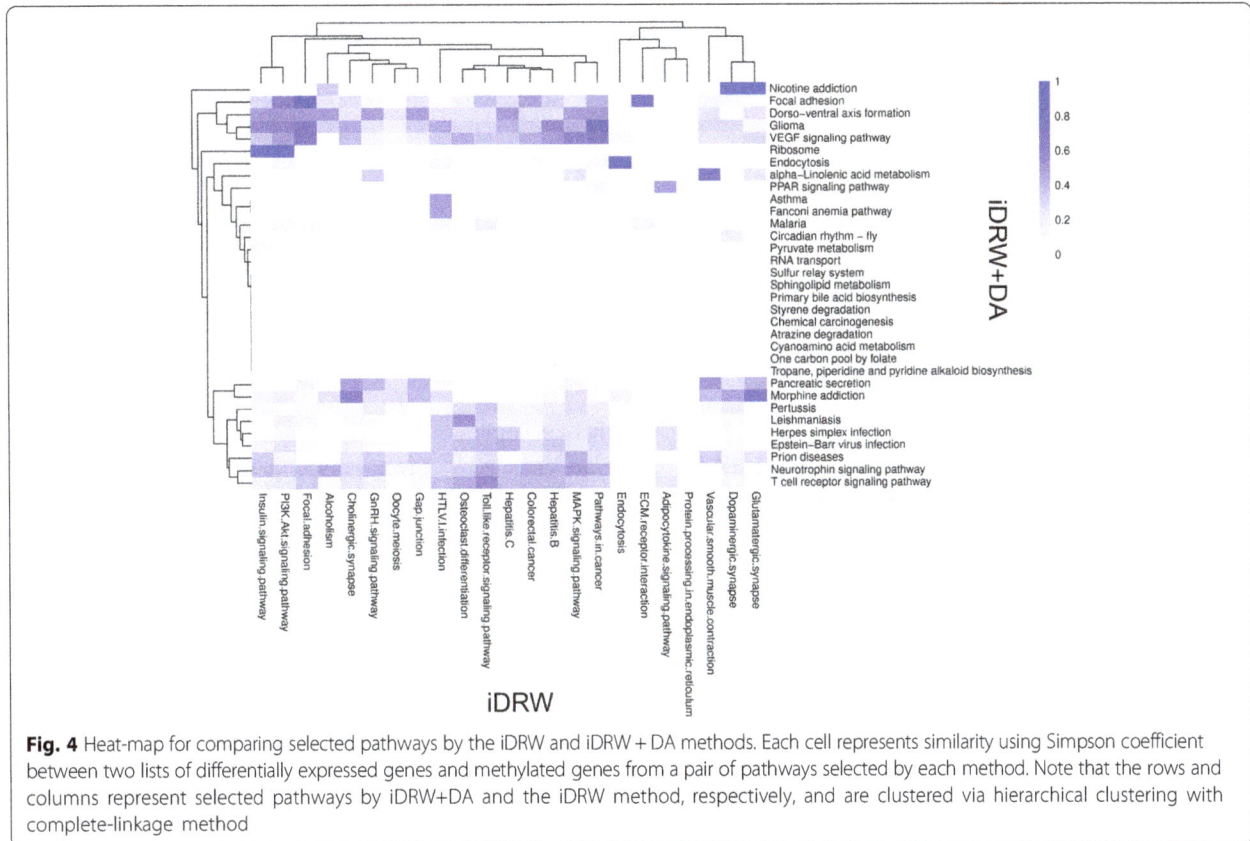

Fig. 4 Heat-map for comparing selected pathways by the iDRW and iDRW + DA methods. Each cell represents similarity using Simpson coefficient between two lists of differentially expressed genes and methylated genes from a pair of pathways selected by each method. Note that the rows and columns represent selected pathways by iDRW+DA and the iDRW method, respectively, and are clustered via hierarchical clustering with complete-linkage method

is related to the Wnt signaling pathway [40]. Wnt signaling pathway is one of the closely associated pathways with cancer [41]. We also found that approximately 40% of patients (439 of 1098) showed genetic alterations for the four genes in the pathway from the Breast Invasive Carcinoma dataset in the cBioPortal (http://www.cbioportal.org/), as shown in Fig. 5. Moreover, the DisGeNET database (http://www.disgenet.org), which shows relations between genes and diseases, indicates that those genes are associated with cancer-related diseases or disorders such as precancerous conditions (umls: C0032927), follicular thyroid carcinoma (umls: C0206682), and tumor initiation (umls: C0598935). We did not identify any strong evidence of association with pancreatic secretion (KEGG ID: hsa04972). However, we found that 13 genes in the pancreatic secretion pathway may regulate blood circulation as a means of releasing nucleic acids [42]. The circulating nucleic acids by the biological process can be a biomarker of breast cancer. Based on our findings, we can hypothesize that the top-ranked pathways can be directly associated with the survivability of breast cancer patients given additional biological experiments.

One of the advantages of our method is that it can obtain both differentially expressed genes from gene expression data as well as differentially methylated genes in each pathway. Thus, we can perform a joint analysis

of the gene expression and methylation data. Table 1 shows the risk-active pathways selected by the proposed iDRW+DA method. The pathways that appear more than five times during 50 iterations are shown, and the number of significant pathway member genes from the gene expression and methylation data are also reported. The top-ranked pathways (i.e., dorso-ventral axis formation, pancreatic secretion, and neurotrophin signaling pathway) are reported as breast-cancer-related pathways as shown above. The genes in the top-10 pathways in Table 1 are also visualized in the gene-gene network shown in Fig. 6. The hub genes in the network play a crucial role in pathways selected by both the iDRW+DA method and the iDRW method. For example, MAPK3, transforming protein p21 (HRAS), and v-akt murine thymoma viral oncogene homolog 1 (AKT1) were all reported as highly related to the MAPK signaling pathway (KEGG ID: map 04010) known to be associated broadly with many cancers [43, 44]. In addition, PTK2 protein tyrosine kinase 2 (PTK2), phosphatidylinositol 3-kinase regulatory subunit gamma (PIK3R3), and phosphatidylinositol-4,5-bisphosphate 3-kinase catalytic subunit delta (PIK3CD) are shown to be related to pathways in cancer (KEGG ID: map 05200) [9]. Additionally, we investigated the association between the genes in the network and breast cancer using a gene-disease association (GDA) score from DisGeNET

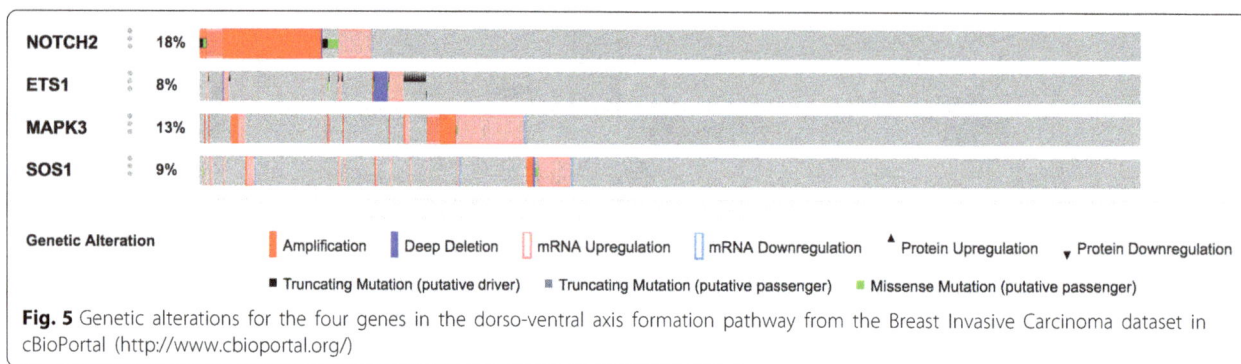

Fig. 5 Genetic alterations for the four genes in the dorso-ventral axis formation pathway from the Breast Invasive Carcinoma dataset in cBioPortal (http://www.cbioportal.org/)

database. Note that the hub genes whose degrees in the network are greater than 4 and those genes detected in differential methylation regions are selected (which are colored in Fig. 6). Based on these criteria, 38 genes are used as input to the DisGeNET database. The GDA score above 0.2 for a gene can be interpreted to mean that it is strongly related to the disease, and the GDA score of a gene above 0 reveals that an association between that gene and the disease may be found in public databases and publications. Moreover, if the GDA score for a gene is 0, then no reports exist in any database or literature showing evidence of association between the gene and the disease. According to the GDA scores, 73.69% of hub genes (28 of 38) have GDA scores above 0 for breast cancer-related diseases, and we can claim that among hub-genes in the network, these genes are highly related to the breast cancer-related diseases. Table 2 summarizes the top-5 genes (as ranked by GDA scores from the DisGeNET database) that are associated with each disease. Based on

these results, we can conclude that the genes and pathways detected by the proposed iDRW+DA method are related to breast cancer.

Discussion

The selected pathways by iDRW+DA showed different patterns in comparison with the iDRW method. As the heatmap in Fig. 4 shows, only two pathways of Focal adhesion (KEGG ID: map 04510) and Endocytosis (KEGG ID: map 04144) were identified by both the iDRW+DA method and the iDRW method. In the iDRW+DA method, the genes in the pathways of sphingolipid metabolism (KEGG ID: map 00600), one carbon pool by folate (KEGG ID: map 00670), and chemical carcinogenesis (KEGG ID: map 05204) were detected and previous studies reported that these pathways are associated with breast cancer. The pathway of sphingolipid metabolism is activated by the steroid hormone estrogen. Estrogen includes a variety of cytoplasmic second messengers

Table 1 Risk-active pathways identified by the proposed method (iDRW+DA)

Pathway ID	Pathway name	Frequency[a]	Total genes[b]	DE genes	DM genes
map 04320	Dorso-ventral axis formation	10/50	27	4	0
map 04972	Pancreatic secretion	8/50	65	26	3
map 04722	Neurotrophin signaling pathway	7/50	90	47	3
map 05020	Prion diseases	7/50	30	12	0
map 00670	One carbon pool by folate	5/50	33	6	1
map 00592	alpha-Linolenic acid metabolism	5/50	23	8	1
map 00620	Pyruvate metabolism	5/50	96	7	1
map 03320	PPAR signaling pathway	5/50	61	13	1
map 04660	T cell receptor signaling pathway	5/50	85	52	8
map 04510	Focal adhesion	5/50	148	83	11
map 03010	Ribosome	5/50	143	1	0
map 05214	Glioma	5/50	52	27	0
map 04711	Circadian rhythm - fly	5/50	8	4	1
map 00960	Tropane, piperidine, and pyridine alkaloid biosynthesis	5/50	26	1	0

[a]Frequency: the number of times the pathway has been selected over 10 times of 5-fold cross validation process (50 iterations)
[b]Total genes: the number of genes mapped to the pathway in the KEGG database
Note that the number of differentially expressed genes (DE genes) and differentially methylated genes (DM genes) are also shown (p-value of DESeq2 or t-test < 0.05)

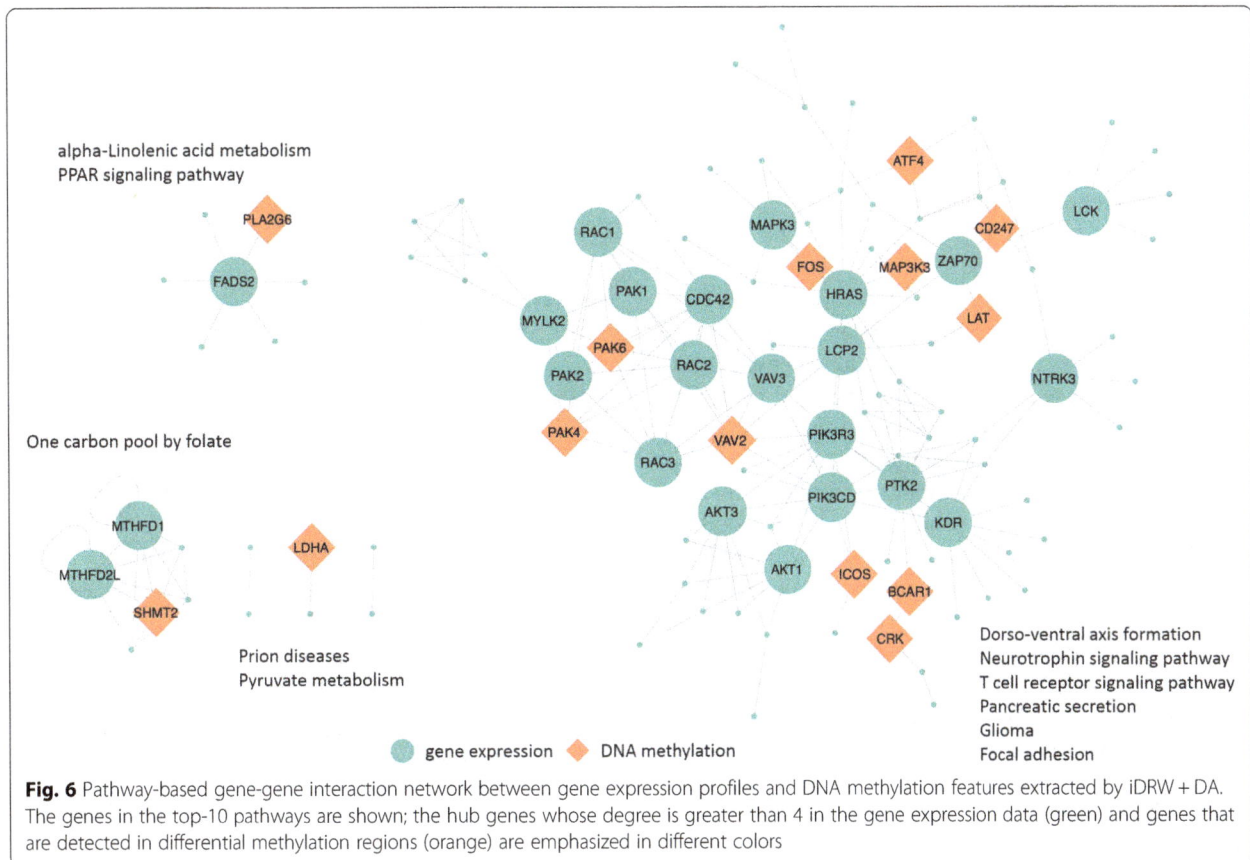

Fig. 6 Pathway-based gene-gene interaction network between gene expression profiles and DNA methylation features extracted by iDRW + DA. The genes in the top-10 pathways are shown; the hub genes whose degree is greater than 4 in the gene expression data (green) and genes that are detected in differential methylation regions (orange) are emphasized in different colors

Table 2 Top-5 genes ranked by GDA scores from the DisGeNET database (http://www.disgenet.org/) that are associated with breast-cancer-related diseases

Disease ID	Disease	Gene	GDA score
C0678222	Breast Carcinoma	AKT1	0.2418
		PIK3CD	0.0448
		MAPK3	0.0118
		HRAS	0.0077
		BCAR1	0.0074
C0006142	Malignant neoplasm of breast	AKT1	0.2420
		PIK3CD	0.0475
		KDR	0.0119
		MAPK3	0.0110
		PAK1	0.0095
C3539878	Triple Negative Breast Neoplasms	PIK3CD	0.0047
		AKT1	0.0022
		AKT3	0.0011
		MAPK3	0.0011
		KDR	0.0008

linked to a multitude of tissue-specific effects, and Sukocheva et al. reported that this hormone triggers the sphingolipid signaling cascade in various tissues, including breast cancer [45]. We also identified chemical carcinogenesis (KEGG ID: map 05204) using our method. In many cases, chemical and physical agents play a critical role in cancer induction, and one study shows that diethylstilbestrol (DES) and bisphenol A (BPA) are estrogen-like endocrine disruption chemicals that induce continual epigenetic changes affecting emerging breast cancer [46]. Moreover, many studies revealed that one carbon pool by folate (KEGG ID: map 00670) is related to cancer. Experiments revealed that one carbon pool by folate is upregulated in a cancer cell line [47]. Furthermore, Shuvalov et al. reported cancer-related metabolism is a hallmark of cancesr. In particular, one-carbon metabolism is reported as the keystone of them all [48]. Thus, we can conclude that the proposed iDRW+DA method contributes to identifying more specific cancer-related pathways, whereas the iDRW method tends to find generally important pathways for cancers. The main difference between the iDRW and iDRW+DA methods is the pathway features ranking strategy. Taken pathway profiles as an input, the pathways are ranked by the t-test statistics (iDRW) or the weight matrix of DA (iDRW+DA). Denoising process of DA can differentiate the features more and discover interesting structure in the input [28]. As it is shown that DA is effective at capturing more distinctive features by learning latent representations of the input [28], we can observe that the iDRW +DA method detects more cancer-specific pathways despite that the performance difference between iDRW and iDRW+DA methods was marginal.

Conclusions

In this study, we proposed a DRW-based method on an integrated gene-gene graph with expression and methylation profiles in order to utilize the interactions between them. DA-based feature selection was also employed to discover more cancer-specific genes and pathways. The results showed that the constructed integrated gene-gene graph can successfully reflect the combined effect of methylation features on gene expression profiles. The classification performance of the methods showed that pathway-based prediction outperforms gene-based methods. We also found that the selected features by DA can effectively extract topologically important pathways and genes specifically related to breast cancer. Although the classification performance improvement by DA was found to be marginal in our study, DA can extract specific cancer-related biomarkers and facilitate the analysis of biologically meaningful features. The proposed method also identified known breast-cancer-related genes and risk-active pathways successfully. As the integrated gene-gene graph utilized the pathway information using multi-omics data, our study showed that an effective joint analysis on gene expression and methylation data is possible under our framework.

Abbreviations
AUC: Area under the curve; DA: Denoising autoencoder; DRW: Directed random walk; GDA: Gene-disease association

Acknowledgements
We gratefully acknowledge the TCGA Consortium and all its members for the TCGA Project initiative, for providing sample, tissues, data processing and making data and results available. The results published here are in whole or part based upon data generated by The Cancer Genome Atlas pilot project established by the NCI and NHGRI. Information about TCGA and the investigators and institutions that constitute the TCGA research network can be found at http://cancergenome.nih.gov.

Funding
This research was supported by Basic Science Research Program through the National Research Foundation of Korea (NRF) funded by the Ministry of Education [NRF- 2016R1D1A1B03933875]. The publication cost of this article was funded by NRF of Korea [2016R1D1A1B03933875] and Ajou university.

Authors' contributions
SK, TK, HJ, and KS designed the study. SK, TK, and HJ implemented the idea and performed the experiments. SK, TK, HJ, and KS developed the idea and performed the analysis. SK, TK, HJ, and KS wrote the paper. All authors read and approved the final manuscript.

Competing interests
The authors declare that they have no competing interests.

Author details
[1]Department of Computer Engineering, Ajou University, Suwon 16499, South Korea. [2]Department of Molecular and Human Genetics, Baylor College of Medicine, Houston, TX 77030, USA. [3]Jan and Dan Duncan Neurological Research Institute, Texas Children's Hospital, Houston, TX 77030, USA.

References
1. H-h J, Leem S, Wee K, Sohn K-A. Integrative network analysis for survival-associated gene-gene interactions across multiple genomic profiles in ovarian cancer. J Ovarian Res. 2015;8(1):42.
2. Kim D, Joung J-G, Sohn K-A, Shin H, Park YR, Ritchie MD, Kim JH. Knowledge boosting: a graph-based integration approach with multi-omics data and genomic knowledge for cancer clinical outcome prediction. J Am Med Inform Assoc. 2014;22(1):109–20.
3. Kim D, Li R, Lucas A, Verma SS, Dudek SM, Ritchie MD. Using knowledge-driven genomic interactions for multi-omics data analysis: metadimensional models for predicting clinical outcomes in ovarian carcinoma. J Am Med Inform Assoc. 2017;24(3):577–87.
4. Kim D, Shin H, Sohn K-A, Verma A, Ritchie MD, Kim JH. Incorporating inter-relationships between different levels of genomic data into cancer clinical outcome prediction. Methods. 2014;67(3):344–53.
5. Zhang W, Li F, Nie L. Integrating multiple 'omics' analysis for microbial biology: application and methodologies. Microbiology. 2010;156(2):287–301.
6. Gevaert O, Villalobos V, Sikic BI, Plevritis SK. Identification of ovarian cancer driver genes by using module network integration of multi-omics data. Interface Focus. 2013;3(4):20130013.
7. Higdon R, Earl RK, Stanberry L, Hudac CM, Montague E, Stewart E, Janko I, Choiniere J, Broomall W, Kolker N. The promise of multi-omics and clinical data integration to identify and target personalized healthcare approaches in autism spectrum disorders. Omics. 2015;19(4):197–208.
8. Meng C, Kuster B, Culhane AC, Gholami AM. A multivariate approach to the integration of multi-omics datasets. BMC Bioinformatics. 2014;15(1):162.
9. Kristensen VN, Lingjærde OC, Russnes HG, Vollan HKM, Frigessi A, Børresen-Dale A-L. Principles and methods of integrative genomic analyses in cancer. Nat Rev Cancer. 2014;14(5):299–313.
10. Sanchez-Garcia F, Villagrasa P, Matsui J, Kotliar D, Castro V, Akavia U-D, Chen B-J, Saucedo-Cuevas L, Barrueco RR, Llobet-Navas D. Integration of genomic data enables selective discovery of breast cancer drivers. Cell. 2014;159(6): 1461–75.
11. Ritchie MD, Holzinger ER, Li R, Pendergrass SA, Kim D. Methods of integrating data to uncover genotype-phenotype interactions. Nat Rev Genet. 2015;16(2):85–97.
12. Gonzalez-Reymundez A, de los Campos G, Gutierrez L, Lunt SY, Vazquez AI. Prediction of years of life after diagnosis of breast cancer using omics and omic-by-treatment interactions. Eur J Hum Genet. 2017;25(5):538–44.
13. Yang X, Han H, De Carvalho DD, Lay FD, Jones PA, Liang G. Gene body methylation can alter gene expression and is a therapeutic target in cancer. Cancer Cell. 2014;26(4):577–90.
14. Jiao Y, Widschwendter M, Teschendorff AE. A systems-level integrative framework for genome-wide DNA methylation and gene expression data identifies differential gene expression modules under epigenetic control. Bioinformatics. 2014;30(16):2360–6.
15. Network CGA. Comprehensive molecular portraits of human breast tumors. Nature. 2012;490(7418):61.
16. Anjum S, Fourkala E-O, Zikan M, Wong A, Gentry-Maharaj A, Jones A, Hardy R, Cibula D, Kuh D, Jacobs IJ. A BRCA1-mutation associated DNA methylation signature in blood cells predicts sporadic breast cancer incidence and survival. Genome Med. 2014;6(6):47.
17. Creixell P, Reimand J, Haider S, Wu G, Shibata T, Vazquez M, Mustonen V, Gonzalez-Perez A, Pearson J, Sander C. Pathway and network analysis of cancer genomes. Nat Methods. 2015;12(7):615.
18. Michaut M, Chin S-F, Majewski I, Severson TM, Bismeijer T, de Koning L, Peeters JK, Schouten PC, Rueda OM, Bosma AJ. Integration of genomic, transcriptomic and proteomic data identifies two biologically distinct

Integrative pathway-based survival prediction utilizing the interaction between gene expression and DNA...

165

subtypes of invasive lobular breast cancer. Sci Rep. 2016;6:18517.

19. Lee G, Bang L, Kim SY, Kim D, Sohn K-A. Identifying subtype-specific associations between gene expression and DNA methylation profiles in breast cancer. BMC Med Genet. 2017;10(1):28.

20. Lee E, Chuang H-Y, Kim J-W, Ideker T, Lee D. Inferring pathway activity toward precise disease classification. PLoS Comput Biol. 2008;4(11):e1000217.

21. Vaske CJ, Benz SC, Sanborn JZ, Earl D, Szeto C, Zhu J, Haussler D, Stuart JM. Inference of patient-specific pathway activities from multi-dimensional cancer genomics data using PARADIGM. Bioinformatics. 2010;26(12):i237–45.

22. Su J, Yoon B-J, Dougherty ER. Accurate and reliable cancer classification based on probabilistic inference of pathway activity. PLoS One. 2009;4(12):e8161.

23. Khunlertgit N, Yoon B-J. Identification of Robust Pathway Markers for Cancer through Rank-Based Pathway Activity Inference. Adv Bioinformatics. 2013;2013:8.

24. Guo Z, Zhang T, Li X, Wang Q, Xu J, Yu H, Zhu J, Wang H, Wang C, Topol EJ. Towards precise classification of cancers based on robust gene functional expression profiles. BMC Bioinformatics. 2005;6(1):58.

25. Liu W, Li C, Xu Y, Yang H, Yao Q, Han J, Shang D, Zhang C, Su F, Li X, et al. Topologically inferring risk-active pathways toward precise cancer classification by directed random walk. Bioinformatics. 2013;29(17):2169–77.

26. Liu W, Bai X, Liu Y, Wang W, Han J, Wang Q, Xu Y, Zhang C, Zhang S, Li X, et al. Topologically inferring pathway activity toward precise cancer classification via integrating genomic and metabolomic data: prostate cancer as a case. Sci Rep. 2015;5:13192.

27. Love MI, Huber W, Anders S. Moderated estimation of fold change and dispersion for RNA-seq data with DESeq2. Genome Biol. 2014;15(12):550.

28. Vincent P, Larochelle H, Bengio Y, Manzagol P-A: Extracting and composing robust features with denoising autoencoders. In: Proceedings of the 25th international conference on Machine learning: 2008. ACM: 1096–1103.

29. Tan J, Ung M, Cheng C, Greene CS: Unsupervised feature construction and knowledge extraction from genome-wide assays of breast cancer with denoising autoencoders. In: Pacific Symposium on Biocomputing Pacific Symposium on Biocomputing: 2015. NIH Public Access: 132.

30. Tan J, Hammond JH, Hogan DA, Greene CS. Adage-based integration of publicly available pseudomonas aeruginosa gene expression data with denoising autoencoders illuminates microbe-host interactions. mSystems. 2016;1(1):e00025–15.

31. Hira ZM, Gillies DF. A review of feature selection and feature extraction methods applied on microarray data. Adv Bioinformatics. 2015;2015:13.

32. Center BITGDA: Analysis-ready standardized TCGA data from Broad GDAC Firehose 2016_01_28 run. In.: Broad Institute of MIT and Harvard; 2016.

33. Li B, Ruotti V, Stewart RM, Thomson JA, Dewey CN. RNA-Seq gene expression estimation with read mapping uncertainty. Bioinformatics. 2009;26(4):493–500.

34. Kim D, Li R, Dudek SM, Ritchie MD. Predicting censored survival data based on the interactions between meta-dimensional omics data in breast cancer. J Biomed Inform. 2015;56:220–8.

35. Liedtke C, Mazouni C, Hess KR, André F, Tordai A, Mejia JA, Symmans WF, Gonzalez-Angulo AM, Hennessy B, Green M, et al. Response to Neoadjuvant therapy and long-term survival in patients with triple-negative breast Cancer. J Clin Oncol. 2008;26(8):1275–81.

36. Kanehisa M, Goto S. KEGG: Kyoto encyclopedia of genes and genomes. Nucleic Acids Res. 2000;28(1):27–30.

37. Yoo S, Takikawa S, Geraghty P, Argmann C, Campbell J, Lin L, Huang T, Tu Z, Foronjy RF, Spira A, et al. Integrative analysis of DNA methylation and gene expression data identifies EPAS1 as a key regulator of COPD. PLoS Genet. 2015;11(1):e1004898.

38. Lü L, Zhang Y-C, Yeung CH, Zhou T. Leaders in social networks, the delicious case. PLoS One. 2011;6(6):e21202.

39. Bass JIF, Diallo A, Nelson J, Soto JM, Myers CL, Walhout AJM. Using networks to measure similarity between genes: association index selection. Nat Meth. 2013;10(12):1169–76.

40. Navarro-Garberi M, Bueno C, Martinez S. Wnt1 signal determines the patterning of the diencephalic dorso-ventral axis. Brain Struct Funct. 2016;221(7):3693–708.

41. Zhan T, Rindtorff N, Boutros M. Wnt signaling in cancer. Oncogene. 2017; 36(11):1461–73.

42. Schwarzenbach H. Circulating nucleic acids as biomarkers in breast cancer. Breast Cancer Res. 2013;15(5):211.

43. Monlish DA, Cavanaugh JE. Abstract 2242: the MAPK and PI3K signaling pathways in breast cancer: crosstalk mechanisms and the effect on cell proliferation. Cancer Res. 2012;72(8 Supplement):2242.

44. Wagner EF, Nebreda AR. Signal integration by JNK and p38 MAPK pathways in cancer development. Nat Rev Cancer. 2009;9(8):537–49.

45. Sukocheva O, Wadham C. Role of sphingolipids in oestrogen signalling in breast cancer cells: an update. J Endocrinol. 2014;220(3):R25–35.

46. Roberts SM, James RC, Williams PL: Principles of toxicology: environmental and industrial applications: John Wiley & Sons; 2014.

47. Ertel A, Verghese A, Byers SW, Ochs M, Tozeren A. Pathway-specific differences between tumor cell lines and normal and tumor tissue cells. Mol Cancer. 2006; 5(1):55.

48. Shuvalov O, Petukhov A, Daks A, Fedorova O, Vasileva E, Barlev NA. One-carbon metabolism and nucleotide biosynthesis as attractive targets for anticancer therapy. Oncotarget. 2017;8(14):23955.

16

Blood pressure signature genes and blood pressure response to thiazide diuretics: results from the PEAR and PEAR-2 studies

Ana Caroline C. Sá[1,2], Amy Webb[3], Yan Gong[1], Caitrin W. McDonough[1], Mohamed H. Shahin[1], Somnath Datta[4], Taimour Y. Langaee[1], Stephen T. Turner[5], Amber L. Beitelshees[6], Arlene B. Chapman[7], Eric Boerwinkle[8], John G. Gums[9,10], Steven E. Scherer[11], Rhonda M. Cooper-DeHoff[1,12], Wolfgang Sadee[13] and Julie A. Johnson[1,2,12]*

Abstract

Background: Recently, 34 genes had been associated with differential expression relative to blood pressure (BP)/ hypertension (HTN). We hypothesize that some of the genes associated with BP/HTN are also associated with BP response to antihypertensive treatment with thiazide diuretics.

Methods: We assessed these 34 genes for association with differential expression to BP response to thiazide diuretics with RNA sequencing in whole blood samples from 150 hypertensive participants from the Pharmacogenomic Evaluation of Antihypertensive Responses (PEAR) and PEAR-2 studies. PEAR white and PEAR-2 white and black participants ($n = 50$ for each group) were selected based on the upper and lower quartile of BP response to hydrochlorothiazide (HCTZ) and to chlorthalidone.

Results: FOS, DUSP1 and PPP1R15A were differentially expressed across all cohorts (meta-analysis p-value $< 2.0 \times 10^{-6}$), and responders to HCTZ or chlorthalidone presented up-regulated transcripts. Rs11065987 in chromosome 12, a trans-eQTL for expression of FOS, PPP1R15A and other genes, is also associated with BP response to HCTZ in PEAR whites (SBP: $\beta = -2.1$; $p = 1.7 \times 10^{-3}$; DBP: $\beta = -1.4$; $p = 2.9 \times 10^{-3}$).

Conclusions: These findings suggest FOS, DUSP1 and PPP1R15A as potential molecular determinants of antihypertensive response to thiazide diuretics.

Keywords: Pharmacogenomics, Hypertension, Thiazide diuretics, Personalized medicine, RNA-Seq, eQTL

Background

Hypertension (HTN) is the most important modifiable risk factor for cardiovascular diseases- coronary artery disease, myocardial infarction, heart failure, stroke and peripheral vascular diseases; controlling blood pressure (BP) is critical for reducing long-term mortality and morbidity rates [1]. Despite the plethora of therapeutic options, selection of the initial anti-HTN treatment remains empirical. Worldwide, 1 billion people suffer from HTN [2] but only about 50% of those under drug therapy achieve the treatment goal, which highlights that anti-HTN drug selection for a specific patient likely impacts therapy success [3, 4].

Thiazide diuretics (TD) are a centerpiece of anti-HTN therapy due to their effectiveness, and safety profile in the management of HTN. Among the available anti-HTN medications, HCTZ, chlorthalidone and other TD are considered first line options for most patients with un-complicated essential HTN, and are highly recommended for patients requiring more than one anti-HTN therapy for control of BP [5]. However, TD have variable efficacy, and less than 50% of HCTZ-treated patients achieve BP

* Correspondence: johnson@cop.ufl.edu
[1]Center for Pharmacogenomics, Department of Pharmacotherapy and Translational Research, College of Pharmacy, University of Florida, P.O.Box 100484, Gainesville, FL 32610-0486, USA
[2]Graduate Program in Genetics and Genomics, University of Florida, Gainesville, FL, USA
Full list of author information is available at the end of the article

control [3]. The inter-individual variability in BP response to TD is likely to contribute to suboptimal BP control.

Using a genome-wide association (GWAS) approach, two replicated regions, one in PRKCA (protein kinase C, alpha) and the other one near GNAS (G protein alpha subunit), were identified with clinically relevant effects on BP response to HCTZ [6]. Despite the successes, the GWAS approach provides only one dimension of molecular information about BP response to anti-HTN treatment. While it is a critical dimension, analyzing DNA variation alone is insufficient for achieving an understanding of the multidimensional complexity of BP response to TD. In this context, transcriptomics (gene expression profiling) has been described as an innovative approach that enables biomarker discovery associated with different diseases and traits [7–10].

Recently, Huan et al. [9] identified 34 genes associated with differential expression relative to BP/HTN, which in aggregate explain ~ 9% of inter-individual variability in BP. In addition, previous findings suggest that some signals from HTN GWAS may predict anti-HTN drug response [11]. This study tests the hypothesis that some of the differentially expressed genes associated with BP/HTN are also associated with BP response to antihypertensive treatment with TD. We assessed the association of these 34 genes with differential expression to BP response to TD by applying RNA sequencing data from the Pharmacogenomic Evaluation of Antihypertensive Responses (PEAR) and PEAR-2 studies.

Methods

Study population and ethics statement
This study includes data from PEAR and PEAR-2 (NCT00246519, NCT01203852 www.clinicaltrials.gov), which were previously described in details [12]. Briefly, PEAR was a multicenter, randomized clinical trial with the primary aim of evaluating the role of genetic variability on BP response of HCTZ and/or atenolol treated patients. Study participants ($n = 768$) with uncomplicated HTN were randomized to receive monotherapy of either the thiazide diuretic HCTZ, or the beta-blocker atenolol for a period of 9 weeks. Fasting blood and urine samples were collected at baseline (untreated), after 9 weeks of monotherapy, and after 9 weeks of combination therapy. BP responses were assessed using office, home, and 24-h ambulatory BP and then a composite BP response was constructed [13].

The PEAR-2 clinical trial included a hypertensive population similar to the one in PEAR, and for which metoprolol, a beta-blocker, and chlorthalidone, a thiazide-like diuretic, were tested. Details of this prospective, clinical trial were previously published [14]. Briefly, 417 hypertensive participants were treated in a sequential monotherapy design with metoprolol and then chlorthalidone with at least 4 week washout periods prior to each active treatment. Data collected included home and clinic BP measurements, adverse metabolic effects, fasting whole blood, and urine samples.

Gene expression profile with RNA-Seq
PEAR whites and PEAR-2 white and black participants were selected for gene expression profiling with RNA-Seq based on the differences in their BP response to HCTZ and chlorthalidone treatment, respectively. A total of 150 patients with BP responses to either HCTZ or chlorthalidone in the top and bottom quartiles from each of the three cohorts were selected and classified as poor BP responders (non-responders) and good BP responders (responders). Sample size was selected based on the theoretical statistical calculations [15], which revealed that with 32 million reads per sample (average number of RNA-Seq reads generated), coefficient of variation (σ) = 0.8, two-sided α level = 0.05, and 25 samples per group (25 responders and 25 non-responders to thiazide diuretics) we have greater than 80% power to detect two-fold differences in expression.

We determined the mean changes of serum potassium concentrations and uric acid levels in non-responders before and after treatment with HCTZ and chlorthalidone with the premise that if the cause of the nonresponse for BP lowering was nonadherence, then these individuals would also not have any adverse metabolic responses that are typically seen with thiazide. We also compared changes from baseline to after treatment serum potassium and uric acid using paired t-tests. Potassium depletion and uric acid elevation are commonly observed secondary to treatment with TD [16–18], and were lab parameters with statistically significant change in the overall clinical study from PEAR participants [19, 20].

Using whole blood samples collected before HCTZ or chlorthalidone monotherapy, RNA was extracted using the PAXgene Blood RNA kit IVD (Qiagen, Valenica, CA). The selection of poly(A) mRNA from total RNA was performed using Sera-Mag Magnetic Oligo(dT) Beads (Illumina, San Diego,CA) according to the manufacturer's protocol. 100 ng of RNA was then used as a template for cDNA synthesis. Libraries were prepared following the strand-specific protocol [21]. DNA clusters were generated using the Illumina cluster station, followed by 100 cycles of paired-end sequencing on the Illumina HiSeq 2000, performed at Baylor Human Genome Sequencing Center in Texas. For data quality control purposes, read duplicates removal was implemented using Picard (http://broadinstitute.github.io/picard/) MarkDuplicates option.

The 100 bp reads generated in the paired-end RNA sequencing were uniquely mapped to the human reference genome (hg19) using TopHat v2.0.10 [22] allowing for four reads mismatches, read edit distance of six, one mismatch in the anchor region of a spliced read, and a maximum of five multi-hits. Transcript assembly was performed using Cufflinks v2.2.1. Statistical analysis were carried out with Cuffdiff and gene expression levels are reported in fragments per kilobase per million reads (FPKM), considering reads mapped to exonic regions of the 34 genes previously associated with BP/HTN [9].

Additionally, we performed differential expression analysis using alternative tools in order to adjust the expression levels for age, sex and baseline diastolic BP because we observed, for these variables, statistically significant differences between participants classified as responders and non-responders to thiazide diuretics (Table 1). Other common covariates in association studies of hypertension, such as Body Mass Index (BMI) and smoking were not included as covariates because previous analysis of BP response in PEAR [23] established that these variables were not associated with BP response. By using BAM files from TopHat 2 alignments, we were able to count the number of reads for each known human genes (Gencode gene annotation release 18) applying the htseq-count function from the HTSeq bioconductor package [24]. Counts were modeled to a Negative Binomial distribution using a generalized linear model in edgeR [25].

Statistical methods

Based on the fact that the BP signature genes, selected for this analysis, were discovered in whites, the primary data analysis was also performed in whites treated with HCTZ or chlorthalidone. Associations of differences in expression levels of these genes in responders compared to non-responders to TD was evaluated using a t-test to quantify the statistical significance in the differences observed among the gene expression measurements

(FPKM). Bonferroni corrected P values < 0.0015 (0.05/34) were considered statistically significant. In addition, we assessed the statistical significance (hypergeometric test) of the overlap between the 34 BP signature genes and the 29 genes associated with thiazide diuretics blood pressure response at the whole transcriptome level (FDR p-value < 0.05) [29].

For each differentially expressed gene in PEAR or in PEAR-2 whites (6 in total), we attempted replication in PEAR-2 blacks and the alternate group of whites in order to validate the association of the genes with BP response to TD. A strict approach was established for validation with Bonferroni corrected P value ($< 0.05/6 = 0.008$) and the same fold change direction (either up or down regulation) as the primary analysis in whites treated with HCTZ or chlorthalidone.

For those genes that passed the validation criteria, the differential expression results from each study cohort were combined in a meta-analysis, using standardized p-values to follow the assumption of the Fisher p-value combination method implemented by the R package MetaRNASeq [26]. We considered that genes with meta-analysis p values $< 2.0 \times 10^{-6}$ (0.05/25,000) achieved transcriptome-wide association with BP response to TD.

To evaluate whether *FOS*, *DUSP1* and *PPP1R15A* robustly predict BP response to TD, PEAR participants were assigned into the derivation cohort for logistic regression model building. PEAR-2 whites constituted the validation cohort, in which area under the receiver operator curve was calculated in the R ROCR package [27], for model evaluation. The TD prediction model was compared to logistic regression model including randomly selected genes from whole transcriptome analysis. Twenty randomly selected genes were sampled (R function "sample", 20 rounds), and each random signature was fitted to a logistic regression model to assess the probability of random

Table 1 Characteristics of PEAR and PEAR-2 participants classified as responder and non-responders for the RNA-Seq analysis

| Characteristics | Whites (n = 99) | | | | Blacks (n = 50) | |
| | HCTZ | | Chlorthalidone | | Chlorthalidone | |
	Responders (n = 24)	Non-responders (n = 25)	Responders (n = 25)	Non-responders (n = 25)	Responders (n = 25)	Non-responders (n = 25)
Age	48 ± 12	48 ± 8	53 ± 8	48 ± 10	52 ± 8	50 ± 10
Female, n (%)	11 (44%)	10 (40%)	15 (75%)[a]	5 (25%)[a]	12 (48%)	12 (48%)
BMI, kg^{a}m^{-2}	29 ± 5	32 ± 6	32 ± 5	30.5 ± 5	30 ± 6	31 ± 5
Baseline DBP	93 ± 5	94 ± 4	97 ± 6[a]	93 ± 5[a]	98 ± 6[a]	93 ± 4[a]
Baseline SBP	146 ± 10	144 ± 10	152 ± 11[a]	144 ± 9[a]	152 ± 10[a]	146 ± 10[a]
DBP response to TD	−9 ± 6[b]	0.06 ± 4[b]	−14 ± 4[b]	−0.2 ± 2[b]	−17 ± 4[b]	−1.4 ± 3[b]
SBP response to TD	−12 ± 6[b]	−0.9 ± 6[b]	−22 ± 7[b]	−1.5 ± 5[b]	−27 ± 7[b]	−4.4 ± 5[b]

Mean and Standard Deviation values for the continuous variables were presented
BMI body mass index, *SBP* systolic blood pressure, *DBP* diastolic blood pressure, *TD* thiazide diuretics
[a]Significant at the 0.05 probability level
[b]Significant at the 0.001 probability level

gene signature performing better than the TD genes. Gene expression measures in FPKM were used for this analysis.

Genomics analysis

Previous studies have explored the genome-wide genotyping results for the PEAR and PEAR-2 studies in much more detail [6, 11]. GWAS data for chlorthalidone in PEAR-2 will be reported separately. Briefly, DNA samples were genotyped using Illumina Human Omni-1Million Quad BeadChip and 2.5 M-8 BeadChip (Illumina, San Diego CA) for PEAR and PEAR-2, respectively. Genotypes were called using GenTrain2 clustering algorithm (GenomeStudio, Illumina, San Diego CA). MaCH software (version 1.0.16) was used to impute SNPs based on HapMapIII haplotypes.

In order to identify SNPs potentially regulating the expression of the genes differentially expressed in the RNA-Seq data, we consulted the Blood eQTL browser [28]. The SNPs identified as eQTL for the differentially expressed genes were then evaluated in the PEAR and PEAR2 GWAS data, to test for a genetic association with BP response to TD. SNP associations with BP response were evaluated using previously conducted GWAS analyses [6] that included data on systolic and diastolic BP responses to HCTZ in 228 whites participants from PEAR, and responses to chlorthalidone in 185 white and 142 black participants from PEAR-2. PLINK software was used to run the analysis with adjustment for age, sex, pre-HCTZ/chlorthalidone BP and population substructure by considering the first and second principal components (PC1 and PC2) in all our analysis.

Results

Table 1 summarizes baseline and demographic characteristics from PEAR white participants treated with HCTZ and PEAR-2 white and black participants treated with chlorthalidone who were selected for RNA-Sequencing. For PEAR, age, body mass index (BMI), sex and baseline BP were not statistically different between participants classified as responders and non-responders to HCTZ. However, in PEAR-2 white participants, differences in sex and baseline BP were statistically significant between responders and non-responders to chlorthalidone. Differences in baseline BP were also observed in PEAR-2 blacks between responders and non-responders to chlorthalidone.

After treatment with HCTZ and chlorthalidone, there were significant reductions on serum potassium concentrations and significant increases serum uric acid levels in participants classified as non-responders (Additional file 1: Table S1). These changes are consistent with previously reported metabolic effects after treatment with

TD [19, 20], and suggest high treatment adherence in the group of BP non-responders to TD.

In order to identify genes with differential expression involved in BP response to TD, whole transcriptome sequences were generated from 149 participants treated with HCTZ or chlorthalidone. One of the samples from HCTZ responders did not achieve enough library yield for adequate performance in sequencing. On average, 32 million reads per sample were mapped to the human reference genome (hg 19) and about 93% were uniquely mapped (Additional file 1: Figure S1). Whole transcriptome analyses from the PEAR and PEAR2 studies were previously published [29].

At a Bonferroni corrected alpha (0.0015), six genes were differentially expressed in whites treated with HCTZ or chlorthalidone (Additional file 1: Table S2). Of those GPR56, FOS and FGFBP2 were common between the gene lists as significant for BP response to TD at the whole transcriptome level (FDR p-value < 0.05 in PEAR or PEAR-2 whites) [29] and the BP signature genes (Additional file 1: Table S2). A hypergeometric test ($p = 9.0 \times 10^{-7}$) showed that this overlap between the 29 genes associated to TD BP response at the whole transcriptome level [29] and the 34 BP signature genes is statistically significant. For each gene differentially expressed ($P < 0.0015$) in PEAR or PEAR-2 white participants, we attempted replication in the other group of white study participants and in black participants from PEAR-2 (Additional file 1: Table S2). Of the six genes identified, FOS and DUSP1 were differentially expressed and showed consistent fold change direction in all 3 cohorts (Table 2), passing the stringent Bonferroni corrected alpha at 0.008 for validation. PPP1R15A showed consistent directional fold change in all three cohorts, and met the Bonferroni threshold p value in PEAR whites given HCTZ (Fold Change (Responders/non-responders): 1.27, $p = 1.15 \times 10^{-3}$) and PEAR-2 blacks given chlorthalidone (Fold Change: 1.29, $p = 1.75 \times 10^{-3}$), while only achieving nominal significance in PEAR-2 whites (Fold Change: 1.19, $p = 3.61 \times 10^{-2}$) (Table 2). The meta-analysis of all participants with RNA-Seq data included FOS, DUSP1 and PPP1R15A, and confirmed transcriptome-wide associations that far exceeded transcriptome wide (and genome wide) significance for FOS ($p = 2 \times 10^{-12}$), DUSP1 ($p = 9.5 \times 10^{-12}$) and PPP1R15A ($p = 3.6 \times 10^{-8}$) expression and BP response to TD (Table 2). Even though the statistical strength of the association lessened after the adjustment for age, sex and baseline BP, the fold change direction remains consistent across PEAR whites and PEAR-2 whites and blacks regardless of the statistical methods used (Additional file 1: Table S3).

The combination of FOS, DUSP1 or PPP1R15A gene expression in a logistic regression model was statistically significant ($P = 0.02$), and explained 23.3% of the variability in drug response to TD in the derivation cohort

Table 2 Genes differentially expressed between responders and non-responders to HCTZ and chlorthalidone in all 3 cohorts, with consistent direction and transcriptome-wide statistical significance when meta-analyzed

Genes	HCTZ Whites				Chlorthalidone Whites				Chlorthalidone Blacks				Meta-analysis
	Non-resp.	Resp.	Fold Change	P value	Non-resp.	Resp.	Fold Change	P value	Non-resp.	Resp.	Fold Change	P value	P value
FOS	39.2	49.5	1.26	2.90E-03	29.4	38.0	1.29	1.15E-03	24.6	35.9	1.46	5.00E-05	2.08E-12
DUSP1	76.0	105.2	1.38	1.50E-04	71.5	92.8	1.30	1.35E-03	63.3	81.7	1.29	3.55E-03	9.50E-12
PPP1R15A	38.3	48.7	1.27	1.15E-03	29.9	35.5	1.19	3.61E-02	27.6	35.6	1.29	1.75E-03	3.64E-08

Fold change corresponds to gene expression levels in responders divided by levels in non-responders, in fragments per kilobase per million reads (FPKM)

(PEAR). For independent assessment of this model in PEAR-2, the area under the curve was 0.71, indicative of the model's good prediction for BP response to TD (Fig. 1). Additionally, this model performed better than randomly selected signature genes of identical size, re-sampled 20 times (P range: = 0.045–0.96) (Additional file 1: Figure S2).

Based on data in the Blood eQTL browser [28], we identified 4 trans-eQTLs (rs11065987, rs653178, rs10774625 and rs11066301) associated with reduced expression of both *FOS* and *PPP1R15A* (Additional file 1: Table S4). Because of the high linkage disequilibrium between these SNPs (Additional file 1: Figure S3), we selected a representative SNP (rs11065987) to test for an association with BP response with TD. Rs11065987 was associated with SBP and DBP response to HCTZ in PEAR whites (SBP: $\beta = -2.1$; $p = 1.7 \times 10^{-3}$; DBP: $\beta = -1.4$; $p = 2.9 \times 10^{-3}$) (Fig. 2) and showed consistent directional association in PEAR-2 whites that did not reach statistical significance in PEAR-2 whites or blacks treated with chlorthalidone (Additional file 1: Table S4).

In order to investigate *FOS* and *PPP1R15A* co-expression, we calculated the Pearson correlation coefficient between the log transformation of expression levels of these genes. *FOS* and *PPP1R15A* showed strong positive correlation with $r^2 = 0.9$ in PEAR whites treated with HCTZ and $r^2 = 0.8$ in PEAR-2 whites treated with chlorthalidone. This indicates

potential common co-regulatory mechanism involving the expression of these genes and driven by rs11065987 or its proxy SNPs.

Discussion

Despite the widespread use of TD, there is large inter-individual variability in BP or drug response, which has motivated the identification of genetic markers with the potential to optimize antihypertensive treatment selection. GWAS results have definitely contributed to enlarge the current knowledge on the potential role of genetics in inter-individual variability in drug response in general and also to thiazide BP response [6, 11]. However, this approach provides only one dimension of molecular information in thiazide BP response, which may not be sufficient to understand the complexity of this phenotype. Gene expression has been shown to have predictive and prognostic value in disease genomics studies, applying transcriptomics tools for the characterization of novel cancer subtypes [30–32] or the identification of signature genes for hypertension [9, 33], heart failure [34–36] and other diseases. Recent studies presented a remarkable effect of whole transcriptome gene expression data in enriching for drug responders to docetaxel and cisplatin treatment of breast cancer [37], and to erlotinib in non-small cell lung cancer [38]. Each

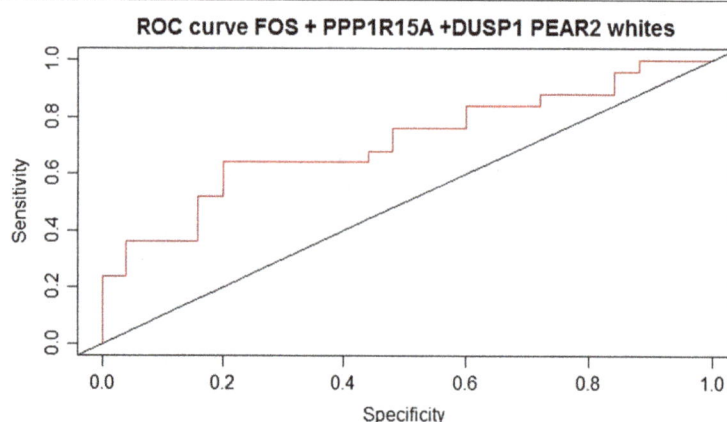

Fig. 1 Receiver operator curve for assessment of logistic regression model prediction in PEAR-2. Statistical model including thiazide diuretic (TD) genes FOS, DUSP1 and PPP1R15A showed area under the curve was 0.71, indicative of the model's good prediction for blood pressure response to TD. Gene expression measures reported in Fragments per Kilobase of Exon per Million mapped (FPKM)

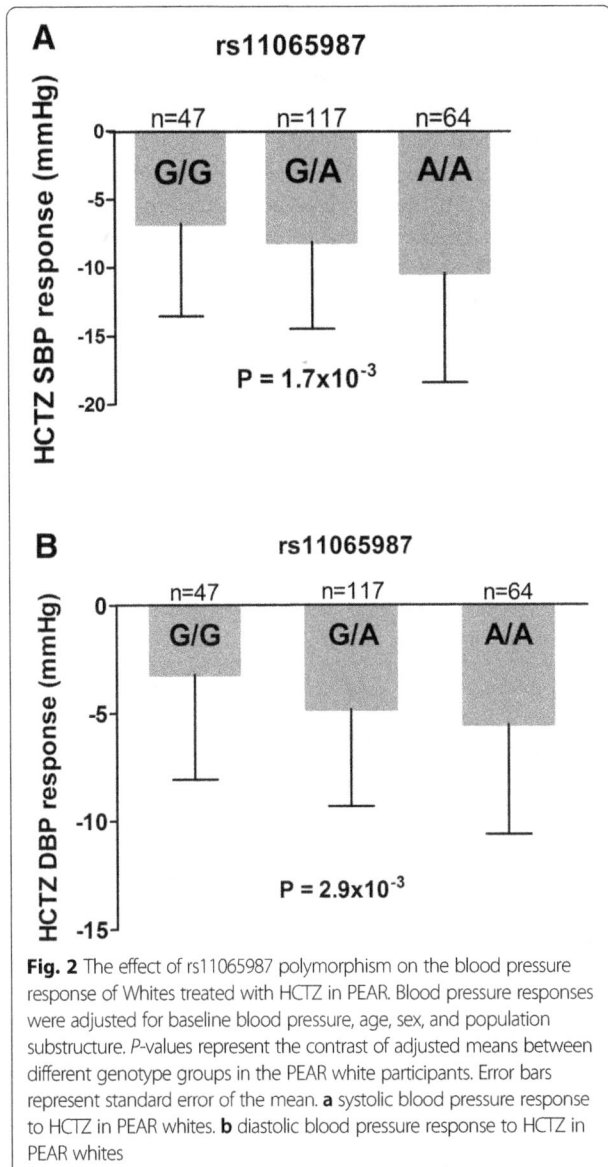

Fig. 2 The effect of rs11065987 polymorphism on the blood pressure response of Whites treated with HCTZ in PEAR. Blood pressure responses were adjusted for baseline blood pressure, age, sex, and population substructure. *P*-values represent the contrast of adjusted means between different genotype groups in the PEAR white participants. Error bars represent standard error of the mean. **a** systolic blood pressure response to HCTZ in PEAR whites. **b** diastolic blood pressure response to HCTZ in PEAR whites

three different cohorts treated with TD, with consistent directional fold change in whites treated with HCTZ and whites and blacks treated with chlorthalidone.

Among these three genes, only *FOS* has been associated previously with the pathophysiology of HTN. Expression of FOS (FBJ murine osteosarcoma viral oncogene homolog, also known as AP-1 transcription factor subunit), a leucine zipper protein that when dimerized with JUN forms a transcription factor complex, is linked to neuronal activation of vasomotor areas in mice [39]. Also, the blockade of *FOS* expression with oligonucleotides attenuates high BP in HTN-induced and spontaneously HTN mice [40].

We did not find any direct evidence in the literature of the involvement of DUSP1 and PPP1R15A that could account mechanistically for a potential susceptibility for HTN and/or BP response to thiazides. However, we found that these genes are involved in biological processes related to BP regulatory mechanisms. For instance, DUSP1 has shown consistent inhibition of ERK 1/2 (Extracellular Regulated Kinases) signaling in vitro and in vivo [41], with potential attenuation on the effects of angiotensin II-mediated vascular smooth muscle cell (VSMC) proliferation and vasoconstriction [42].

PPP1R15A is a regulatory subunit for phosphatase protein (PP) 1 [43]. PP1 is the catalytic subunit for myosin phosphatases, a key convergence point on contractility pathways in VSMC, that dephosphorylates the myosin light chain and initiates the relaxation process for vasodilation [44]. Of relevance, PP1 has a highly specific inhibitor 1 (I-1) which, when activated by protein kinase A, forms a heterotrimeric complex with PP1 and PPP1R15A [43]. This specific interaction of PPP1R15A with the C-terminal region of I-1 engenders strong PP1 inhibition [43] and a potential amplification of contractile response in VSMC [45]. In addition, recent research shows that I-1 regulates thiazide-sensitive NaCl cotransporter (NCC) activity and phosphorylation in the distal convoluted tube (DCT), and loss of I-1 expression in mice lowers arterial BP [46]. Since there is no concrete evidence of the consequences of I-1/PPP1R15A interaction in the regulation of contractile signaling, in VSMC, or in the regulation of NCC activity in DCT, we can only speculate that PPP1R15A may be important for BP regulatory mechanisms. Further experimental validation will be crucial to close the link between PPP1R15A interactions with I-1 for the regulation of PP1 and NCC activity in VSMC and DCT.

In addition, we found rs11065987 associated with both systolic and diastolic BP responses to HCTZ in PEAR whites, and it is also associated in *trans* with decreased expression of two genes in our top list of BP signature genes: *FOS* and *PPP1R15A*, which are co-expressed in the whole blood samples tested in this study.

of these studies highlights the potential scientific insights that can be gained through experimental approaches that apply gene expression data. In this study, we investigated differences in gene expression underlying extreme BP response to thiazides in white and black participants from PEAR and PEAR-2. Such approaches have the potential to provide methods for precision medicine, but additionally may provide previously unrecognized insights into BP regulation and responses to antihypertensive drugs.

Herein, we have shown that applying transcriptome sequencing data helped us to identify molecular markers potentially implicated in BP response to TD. Among the 34 genes previously documented to influence BP/HTN, *FOS*, *DUSP1* and *PPP1R15A* mRNAs were differentially expressed between responders and non-responders in

rs11065987, the leading SNP in a small haplotype block, is an intergenic SNP in chromosome 12, where the closest gene is BRCA1 associated protein and previous cardiovascular disease GWA studies identified 12q4 as a risk locus for coronary artery disease and HTN [47]. Further experiments will be valuable to understand the mechanisms involved in gene expression regulation in the chromosome 12q4 region that could potentially affect BP regulation as well.

Although it is not clear how FOS, DUSP1 and PPP1R15A are involved in BP regulation, the differences in gene expression documented in this study taken together with evidence of gene expression regulatory mechanism with *trans*-eQTLs associated with BP response to HCTZ suggest that these genes may be markers of response to TD. Further functional studies may provide additional insights to the field.

This study presents some limitations. First, the number of samples with RNA-Seq data may have limited the power to identify additional genes differentially expressed as well as to validate some of the transcriptomics signals; however, we enhanced the power of the number of samples tested by taking an extreme phenotype approach. Second, using RNA from whole blood for RNA-Seq data analysis may have limited the detection of the expression of some genes/regulatory mechanisms that might be cell type-specific. However, it may be challenging to select only one tissue in order to investigate gene expression as a marker of BP regulation since drug response to anti-HTN might arise from a variety of target tissues such as heart, brain, kidney or vasculature. Not only are these tissues difficult to access in relatively healthy patients, as hypertensive patients are, but it is also not obvious which tissue should be used. Thus we are using whole blood as a surrogate for multiple tissues. Moreover, the original study that served as the basis for selection of BP signature genes also used whole blood samples for that transcriptome-wide gene expression study due to the convenience to identify biomarkers using easily accessible body fluids [9].

Conclusions

For over half century, thiazide diuretics have been a centerpiece of antihypertensive therapy with more than 100 million prescriptions annually in the US alone. Its large inter-individual variability in BP response emphasizes the need for molecular predictors of drug response that hold potential for improving the antihypertensive therapy. Results of the present study suggest that whole transcriptome data can provide insights into genes potentially involved in the pharmacogenetic phenotype of antihypertensive drug response. We were able to demonstrate that genes previously identified through BP/HTN transcriptome profiling that are also relevant determinants of BP response to TD. Specifically, *FOS, DUSP1*

and *PPP1R15A*, through their differential expression, may be involved in the response to TD. To strengthen the finding, through use of a publicly available eQTL database, we found an eQTL (SNP) of *FOS* and *PPP1R15A* that associated with BP response to TD and other SNPs with evidence of gene expression regulatory mechanisms. Further work is needed to understand the mechanistic basis by which differential expression of *FOS, DUSP1* and *PPP1R15A* may influence BP regulation and response to TD.

Abbreviation

BP: Blood Pressure; DBP: Diastolic Blood Pressure; eQTL: Expression Quantitative Trait Loci; ERK: Extracellular Regulated Kinases; FDR: False Discovery Rate; GWAS: Genome-wide Association Studies; HCTZ: Hydrochlorothiazide; HTN: Hypertension; PEAR: Pharmacogenomics Evaluation of Antihypertensives Response; PP: Phosphatase Protein; RNA-Seq: RNA Sequencing; SBP: Systolic Blood Pressure; SNP: Single Nucleotide Polymorphis; VSMC: Vascular Smooth Muscle Cell

Acknowledgements

We thank the valuable contributions of the Pharmacogenomics Evaluation of Antihypertensive Responses (PEAR) study participants, support staff, and study physicians. We also thank University of Florida Research Computing (http://www.rc.ufl.edu/) for providing computational resources and support as well as BCM-HGSC personnel including Viktoriya Korchina, HarshaVardhan Doddapaneni, Donna Muzny and Richard Gibbs that have contributed to the research results reported in this publication.

Funding

The Pharmacogenomics Evaluation of Antihypertensive Responses (PEAR) study was supported by the National Institute of Health Pharmacogenetics Research Network grant U01-GM074492 and the National Center for Advancing Translational Sciences under the award number UL1 TR000064 (University of Florida), UL1 TR000454 (Emory University), and UL1 TR000135 (Mayo Clinic). The PEAR study was also supported by funds from the Mayo Foundation. RNA-Seq data production was supported by the National Institutes of Health Pharmacogenetics Research Network grants U19-GM061388 and U19-GM061390.

Authors' contributions

ACCS drafted the manuscript and prepared the figures and tables. ACCS and AW performed the RNA-Seq data analyses. SD, MHS, YG and CWM developed the analysis plan for analysis and quality control of the RNA-Seq data and the statistical analysis of the data, and assisted in interpretation of the data. TYL and SES performed the laboratory work for sequencing, and assisted in the analysis and interpretation of the data. JAJ, STT, EB, RMC, WS, ABC, SES, JGG and ALB conceptualized the study and study design and secured funding. JAJ, RMC, STT, ABC, JGG conducted the clinical trial. All authors provided critical review of manuscript. All authors read and approved the final manuscript.

Competing interests

The authors declare that they have no competing interests.

Author details

[1]Center for Pharmacogenomics, Department of Pharmacotherapy and Translational Research, College of Pharmacy, University of Florida, P.O.Box 100484, Gainesville, FL 32610-0486, USA. [2]Graduate Program in Genetics and Genomics, University of Florida, Gainesville, FL, USA. [3]Department of Biomedical Informatics, College of Medicine, The Ohio State University, Columbus, OH, USA. [4]Department of Biostatistics, University of Florida,

Blood pressure signature genes and blood pressure response to thiazide diuretics: results from the PEAR...

173

Gainesville, FL, USA. [5]Division of Nephrology and Hypertension, Mayo Clinic, Rochester, MN, USA. [6]Division of Endocrinology, Diabetes and Nutrition, University of Maryland, Baltimore, MD, USA. [7]Department of Medicine, University of Chicago, Chicago, IL, USA. [8]Division of Epidemiology, University of Texas at Houston, Houston, TX, USA. [9]Department of Pharmacotherapy and Translational Research, College of Pharmacy, University of Florida, Gainesville, USA. [10]Department of Community Health and Family Medicine, College of Medicine, University of Florida, Gainesville, FL, USA. [11]Human Genome Sequencing Center, Baylor College of Medicine, Houston, TX, USA. [12]Department of Medicine, Division of Cardiovascular Medicine, University of Florida, Gainesville, FL, USA. [13]Department of Cancer Biology and Genetic, College of Medicine, Center for Pharmacogenomics, Ohio State University, Columbus, OH, USA.

References

1. Oparil S, Schmieder RE. New approaches in the treatment of hypertension. Circ Res. 2015;116(6):1074–95.
2. Mozaffarian D, Benjamin EJ, Go AS, Arnett DK, Blaha MJ, Cushman M, et al. Executive summary: heart disease and stroke Statistics-2016 update a report from the American Heart Association. Circulation. 2016;133(4):447–54.
3. Materson BJ. Variability in response to antihypertensive drugs. Am J Med. 2007;120(4):10–20.
4. Materson BJ, Reda DJ, Cushman WC, Massie BM, Freis ED, Kochar MS, et al. Single-drug therapy for hypertension in men. A comparison of six antihypertensive agents with placebo. The Department of Veterans Affairs Cooperative Study Group on antihypertensive agents. N Engl J Med. 1993; 328(13):914–21.
5. James PA. 2014 Evidence-based guideline for the Management of High Blood Pressure in adults: report from the panel members appointed to the eighth joint National Committee (JNC 8) (vol 311, pg 507, 2014). Jama-J Am Med Assoc. 2014;311(17):1809.
6. Turner ST, Boerwinkle E, O'Connell JR, Bailey KR, Gong Y, Chapman AB, et al. Genomic association analysis of common variants influencing antihypertensive response to hydrochlorothiazide. Hypertension. 2013;62(2): 391–7.
7. Chepelev I, Wei G, Tang QS, Zhao KJ. Detection of single nucleotide variations in expressed exons of the human genome using RNA-Seq. Nucleic Acids Res. 2009;37(16):e106.
8. Himes BE, Jiang XF, Wagner P, Hu RX, Wang QY, Klanderman B, et al. RNA-Seq transcriptome profiling identifies CRISPLD2 as a glucocorticoid responsive gene that modulates cytokine function in airway smooth muscle cells. PLoS One. 2014;9(6)
9. Huan T, Esko T, Peters MJ, Pilling LC, Schramm K, Schurmann C, et al. A meta-analysis of gene expression signatures of blood pressure and hypertension. PLoS Genet. 2015;11(3):e1005035.
10. Peng ZY, Cheng YB, Tan BCM, Kang L, Tian ZJ, Zhu YK, et al. Comprehensive analysis of RNA-Seq data reveals extensive RNA editing in a human transcriptome. Nat Biotechnol. 2012;30(3):253.
11. Gong Y, McDonough CW, Wang Z, Hou W, Cooper-DeHoff RM, Langaee TY, et al. Hypertension susceptibility loci and blood pressure response to antihypertensives: results from the pharmacogenomic evaluation of antihypertensive responses study. Circ Cardiovasc Genet. 2012;5(6):686–91.
12. Johnson JA, Boerwinkle E, Zineh I, Chapman AB, Bailey K, Cooper-DeHoff RM, et al. Pharmacogenomics of antihypertensive drugs: rationale and design of the Pharmacogenomic evaluation of antihypertensive responses (PEAR) study. Am Heart J. 2009;157(3):442–9.
13. Turner ST, Schwartz GL, Chapman AB, Beitelshees AL, Gums JG, Cooper-DeHoff RM, et al. Power to identify a genetic predictor of antihypertensive drug response using different methods to measure blood pressure response. J Transl Med. 2012;10:47.
14. Hamadeh IS, Langaee TY, Dwivedi R, Garcia S, Burkley BM, Skaar TC, et al. Impact of CYP2D6 polymorphisms on clinical efficacy and tolerability of metoprolol tartrate. Clin Pharmacol Ther. 2014;96(2):175–81.
15. Hart SN, Therneau TM, Zhang Y, Poland GA, Kocher JP. Calculating sample size estimates for RNA sequencing data. J Comput Biol. 2013;20(12):970–8.
16. Shafi T, Appel LJ, Miller ER 3rd, Klag MJ, Parekh RS. Changes in serum potassium mediate thiazide-induced diabetes. Hypertension. 2008;52(6): 1022–9.
17. Gosfield E Jr. Thiazide-induced hyperuricemia. N Engl J Med. 1963;268:562.
18. Duarte JD, Cooper-DeHoff RM. Mechanisms for blood pressure lowering and metabolic effects of thiazide and thiazide-like diuretics. Expert Rev Cardiovasc Ther. 2010;8(6):793–802.
19. Smith SM, Anderson SD, Wen S, Gong Y, Turner ST, Cooper-Dehoff RM, et al. Lack of correlation between thiazide-induced hyperglycemia and hypokalemia: subgroup analysis of results from the pharmacogenomic evaluation of antihypertensive responses (PEAR) study. Pharmacotherapy. 2009;29(10):1157–65.
20. Smith SM, Gong Y, Turner ST, Cooper-DeHoff RM, Beitelshees AL, Chapman AB, et al. Blood pressure responses and metabolic effects of hydrochlorothiazide and atenolol. Am J Hypertens. 2012;25(3):359–65.
21. Levin JZ, Yassour M, Adiconis X, Nusbaum C, Thompson DA, Friedman N, et al. Comprehensive comparative analysis of strand-specific RNA sequencing methods. Nat Methods. 2010;7(9):709–15.
22. Trapnell C, Hendrickson DG, Sauvageau M, Goff L, Rinn JL, Pachter L. Differential analysis of gene regulation at transcript resolution with RNA-seq. Nat Biotechnol. 2013;31(1):46.
23. Turner ST, Schwartz GL, Chapman AB, Beitelshees AL, Gums JG, Cooper-DeHoff RM, et al. Plasma renin activity predicts blood pressure responses to beta-blocker and thiazide diuretic as monotherapy and add-on therapy for hypertension. Am J Hypertens. 2010;23(9):1014–22.
24. Anders S, Pyl PT, Huber W. HTSeq-a Python framework to work with high-throughput sequencing data. Bioinformatics. 2015;31(2):166–9.
25. Robinson MD, McCarthy DJ, Smyth GK. edgeR: a Bioconductor package for differential expression analysis of digital gene expression data. Bioinformatics. 2010;26(1):139–40.
26. Rau A, Marot G, Jaffrezic F. Differential meta-analysis of RNA-seq data from multiple studies. BMC Bioinformatics. 2014;15:91.
27. Sing T, Sander O, Beerenwinkel N, Lengauer T. ROCR: visualizing classifier performance in R. Bioinformatics. 2005;21(20):3940–1.
28. Westra HJ, Peters MJ, Esko T, Yaghootkar H, Schurmann C, Kettunen J, et al. Systematic identification of trans eQTLs as putative drivers of known disease associations. Nat Genet. 2013;45(10):1238–43.
29. Sa ACC, Webb A, Gong Y, McDonough CW, Datta S, Langaee TY, et al. Whole transcriptome sequencing analyses reveal molecular markers of blood pressure response to thiazide diuretics. Sci Rep. 2017;7(1):16068.
30. Zhan F, Huang Y, Colla S, Stewart JP, Hanamura I, Gupta S, et al. The molecular classification of multiple myeloma. Blood. 2006;108(6):2020–8.
31. Agnelli L, Bicciato S, Mattioli M, Fabris S, Intini D, Verdelli D, et al. Molecular classification of multiple myeloma: a distinct transcriptional profile characterizes patients expressing CCND1 and negative for 14q32 translocations. J Clin Oncol. 2005;23(29):7296–306.
32. Tan IB, Ivanova T, Lim KH, Ong CW, Deng N, Lee J, et al. Intrinsic subtypes of gastric cancer, based on gene Expr pattern, predict survival and respond differently to chemotherapy. Gastroenterology. 2011;141(2):476–85, 85 e1–11.
33. Glastonbury CA, Vinuela A, Buil A, Halldorsson GH, Thorleifsson G, Helgason H, et al. Adiposity-dependent regulatory effects on multi-tissue transcriptomes. Am J Hum Genet. 2016;99(3):567–79.
34. di Salvo TG, Yang KC, Brittain E, Absi T, Maltais S, Hemnes A. Right ventricular myocardial biomarkers in human heart failure. J Card Fail. 2015;21(5):398–411.
35. Di Salvo TG, Guo Y, Su YR, Clark T, Brittain E, Absi T, et al. Right ventricular long noncoding RNA expression in human heart failure. Pulm Circ. 2015; 5(1):135–61.
36. Liu Y, Morley M, Brandimarto J, Hannenhalli S, Hu Y, Ashley EA, et al. RNA-Seq identifies novel myocardial gene expression signatures of heart failure. Genomics. 2015;105(2):83–9.
37. Geeleher P, Cox NJ, Huang RS. Clinical drug response can be predicted using baseline gene expression levels and in vitro drug sensitivity in cell lines. Genome Biol. 2014;15(3):R47.
38. Wheeler HE, Aquino-Michaels K, Gamazon ER, Trubetskoy VV, Dolan ME, Huang RS, et al. Poly-omic prediction of complex traits: OmicKriging. Genet Epidemiol. 2014;38(5):402–15.
39. Minson J, Arnolda L, LlewellynSmith I, Pilowsky P, Chalmers J. Altered c-fos in rostral medulla and spinal cord of spontaneously hypertensive rats. Hypertension. 1996;27(3):433–41.
40. Rao F, Zhang L, Wessel J, Zhang K, Wen G, Kennedy BP, et al. Tyrosine hydroxylase, the rate-limiting enzyme in catecholamine biosynthesis - discovery of common human genetic variants governing transcription, autonomic activity, and blood pressure in vivo. Circulation. 2007;116(9): 993–1006.

41. Duff JL, Monia BP, Berk BC. Mitogen-activated protein (map) kinase is regulated by the map kinase phosphatase (Mkp-1) in vascular smooth-muscle cells. J Biol Chem. 1995;270(13):7161–6.

42. Touyz RM, Deschepper C, Park JB, He G, Chen X, Neves MF, et al. Inhibition of mitogen-activated protein/extracellular signal-regulated kinase improves endothelial function and attenuates Ang II-induced contractility of mesenteric resistance arteries from spontaneously hypertensive rats. J Hypertens. 2002;20(6):1127–34.

43. Connor JH, Weiser DC, Li S, Hallenbeck JM, Shenolikar S. Growth arrest and DNA damage-inducible protein GADD34 assembles a novel signaling complex containing protein phosphatase 1 and inhibitor 1. Mol Cell Biol. 2001;21(20):6841–50.

44. Terrak M, Kerff F, Langsetmo K, Tao T, Dominguez R. Structural basis of protein phosphatase 1 regulation. Nature. 2004;429(6993):780–4.

45. Lipskaia L, Bobe R, Chen J, Turnbull IC, Lopez JJ, Merlet E, et al. Synergistic role of protein phosphatase inhibitor 1 and sarco/endoplasmic reticulum Ca2+ -ATPase in the acquisition of the contractile phenotype of arterial smooth muscle cells. Circulation. 2014;129(7):773–85.

46. Picard N, Trompf K, Yang CL, Miller RL, Carrel M, Loffing-Cueni D, et al. Protein phosphatase 1 inhibitor-1 deficiency reduces phosphorylation of renal NaCl cotransporter and causes arterial hypotension. J Am Soc Nephrol. 2014;25(3):511–22.

47. Ikram MK, Sim X, Jensen RA, Cotch MF, Hewitt AW, Ikram MA, et al. Four novel loci (19q13, 6q24, 12q24, and 5q14) influence the microcirculation in vivo. PLoS Genet. 2010;6(10):e1001184.

17

Distributed gene clinical decision support system based on cloud computing

Bo Xu, Changlong Li, Hang Zhuang, Jiali Wang, Qingfeng Wang, Chao Wang* and Xuehai Zhou

Abstract

Background: The clinical decision support system can effectively break the limitations of doctors' knowledge and reduce the possibility of misdiagnosis to enhance health care. The traditional genetic data storage and analysis methods based on stand-alone environment are hard to meet the computational requirements with the rapid genetic data growth for the limited scalability.

Methods: In this paper, we propose a distributed gene clinical decision support system, which is named GCDSS. And a prototype is implemented based on cloud computing technology. At the same time, we present CloudBWA which is a novel distributed read mapping algorithm leveraging batch processing strategy to map reads on Apache Spark.

Results: Experiments show that the distributed gene clinical decision support system GCDSS and the distributed read mapping algorithm CloudBWA have outstanding performance and excellent scalability. Compared with state-of-the-art distributed algorithms, CloudBWA achieves up to 2.63 times speedup over SparkBWA. Compared with stand-alone algorithms, CloudBWA with 16 cores achieves up to 11.59 times speedup over BWA-MEM with 1 core.

Conclusions: GCDSS is a distributed gene clinical decision support system based on cloud computing techniques. In particular, we incorporated a distributed genetic data analysis pipeline framework in the proposed GCDSS system. To boost the data processing of GCDSS, we propose CloudBWA, which is a novel distributed read mapping algorithm to leverage batch processing technique in mapping stage using Apache Spark platform.

Keywords: Clinical decision support system, Cloud computing, Spark, Alluxio, Genetic data analysis, Read mapping

Background

Clinical decision support system (CDSS) provides clinicians, staff, patients, and other individuals with knowledge and person-specific information to enhance health and health care [1]. CDSS can effectively break the limitations of doctors' knowledge and reduce the possibility of misdiagnosis to guarantee the quality of medical care with a lower medical expenses. Genetic diagnosis have

the advantages of early detection, early discovery, early prevention and early treatment [2].

With the development of next-generation sequencing (NGS) technology, the number of newly sequenced data increase exponentially in recent years [3]. How to store and analyze the large amount of genetic data has become a huge challenge. Therefore, faster genetic data storage and analysis technologies are urgently needed. The current best practice genomic variant calling pipeline [4] is that use the Burrows-Wheeler Alignment tool (BWA) [5] to map genetic sequencing data to a reference and use the Genome Analysis Toolkit (GATK) [6] to produce

* Correspondence: cswang@ustc.edu.cn
School of Computer Science and Technology, University of Science and Technology of China, Hefei 230027, China

high-quality variant calls, which takes approximately 120 h to process a single, high-quality human genome using a single, beefy node [7]. It need more time to compute when the sequencing depth is deeper or the length of reads is longer. What's more, time is equal to life in the medical field, especially in emergency. Therefore, it is significant to accelerate the processing of genetic data for CDSS [8]. However, the traditional genetic data storage and analysis technology based on stand-alone environment are hard to meet the computational requirements with the rapid data growth for the limited scalability [2].

In order to solve the problems mentioned above, we propose GCDSS, a distributed gene clinical decision support system based on cloud computing technology. There are two main challenges in implementing GCDSS and improving its performance.

The first one is to design and implement a distributed genetic data analysis pipeline framework. The genetic data analysis usually involves a large amount of data, varied data formats and complicate analysis process. It is difficult to design and implement such framework. The second challenge is the limited scalability of traditional read mapping algorithms. Read mapping is the first and time-consuming step in the whole genetic data analysis pipeline. The lengths of the read are generally range from several to thousands of bases. A sample can typically produce billions of reads. It is critical and difficult for subsequent analysis to map these reads to the reference genome quickly and accurately.

In order to meet the challenges, we considered distributed storage, distributed computing framework and distributed algorithms. Also, we exploit cloud computing technology to parallelize genetic data analysis pipeline. We claim the following contributions and highlights:

1) In this paper, we design a distributed genetic data analysis pipeline framework for GCDSS and implements its prototype based on cloud computing technology. The unified pipeline framework effectively integrates read mapping and calibration, the variant discovery and genotyping, disease identification and analysis into the framework.

2) A novel distributed read mapping algorithm CloudBWA is presented in this paper. It enable traditional BWA-MEM [9] algorithms run in a horizontally scalable distributed environment based on Apache Spark. CloudBWA supports different genomics data formats, which facilitates the distributed storage of the large amount of genetic data. Also, we design and implement batch processing strategy to improve the performance of read mapping algorithm.

Our experimental result shows that GCDSS has an excellent scalability and an outstanding performance.

We first summarize the related work in following aspects:

A. *Genetic data analysis pipeline*

Over the past few years, a large number of distributed genetic data analysis pipeline frameworks have emerged in research institutions, such as Illumina [10], UCLA [11, 12], AMPLab [7, 13–15] and Broad Institute of MIT and Harvard [4, 12]. CS-BWAMEM [11], a fast and scalable read aligner at the cloud scale for genome sequencing, is developed by UCLA, which is for distributed read mapping, and implemented distributed sort and mark duplicates. Adam [7, 14], the distributed genomics data formats, and Avocado [13], the distributed variant discovery and genotyping algorithms, are presented by AMPLab. Moreover, Avocado has not implemented distributed read mapping. Distributed local sequence alignment algorithms DSW [16] and CloudSW [16] both achieve outstanding performance.

B. *Read mapping*

At present, BWA [5, 9, 17] is one of the best popular read mapping tool, which consists of BWA-SW [17], BWA-MEM [9] and BWA-backtrack [5]. SNAP, BWA and other traditional read mapping algorithms have a shortcoming of limited scalability. CS-BWAMEM is a fast and scalable read aligner at the cloud scale for genome sequencing, but it only support paired-end read mapping. SparkBWA is a tool that integrates the BWA [5, 9, 17] on a Apache Spark framework running on the top of Hadoop. Nevertheless, the I/O overhead of SparkBWA is extremely large because it has to read and wirte disk too many times [2]. SparkBWA can be error when numPartitions size is too large to run on Spark, such as the size of numPartitions is larger than the number of Spark workers. Moreover, if numPartitions size is relative small, it may result in uneven distribution of data and calculations, which ultimately reduce the performance of the system.

C. *Cloud computing*

Over the past decade or so, Hadoop [18], HDFS [19], Spark [20] and Alluxio [21] have been implemented and released as open source, which have greatly promoted the academic research and industrial applications. Especially in recent years, cloud computing technology has developed rapidly and become more mature, its performance has also been greatly improved [22–24]. Cloud computing has the characteristics of good fault tolerance, easy to expand, large scale, low cost and distributed, which has been widely used in academia and industry [25, 26]. However, the absorption of those technologies in the scientific field is slow [27].

Methods

The GCDSS architecture includes the general overview, the workflow, the specific implementation and corresponding API respectively. This section especially put concentration on the design method and implementation for building the data analysis framework in distribution pipeline.

System architecture

GCDSS uses genetic data for clinicians, patients, employees, and others to provide intelligent knowledge and personalized information to assist in clinical decision-making and help enhance health. The difference between GCDSS and traditional CDSS is that GCDSS mainly uses the genetic data to analyze and process, instead of using the data of traditional Chinese medicine or modern medicine to build the system. With the development of NGS technology, the number of newly sequenced data has exhibited an exponential increase in recent years. The traditional genetic data storage and analysis technology based on stand-alone environment have limited scalability, which has been difficult to meet the computational requirements of rapid data growth. This paper aims to design and implement a distributed gene clinical decision support system by using cloud computing technology.

As shown in Fig. 1, the GCDSS system workflow is composed of three stages: NGS data processing, variant discovery and genotyping, disease identification, and

discovery. In this section, we will describe these stages respectively.

1) The NGS processing

The NGS data processing mainly consists of read mapping and calibration.

After achieving sequencing data from high-throughput sequencer like HiSeq X Ten of Illumina, GCDSS system needs to map billions of the raw reads to the reference genome. In the next step, it obtains the most probable location of every read, which is normally referred to read mapping. The Read mapping stage is generally complicated and critical for subsequent analysis, as it needs to accurately and efficiently map billions of reads to the reference genome. To address the scalability problem of traditional read mapping algorithms, we employ a distributed read mapping algorithm, named CloudBWA based on the cloud computing techniques. The CloudBWA will be described in detail in the next Section.

During the process of genetic sequencing by sequencer, errors during sample preparation and sequencing can lead to the duplication of some reads. To improve the accuracy of subsequent analysis, we detect duplicates by reads' alignment position and orientation after read mapping, and the reads that have identical position and orientation in RDD [28] are assumed to be duplicates. All duplicate reads but the highest quality read are marked as duplicates. We can remove duplicate reads easily by filter function of Spark.

Since a lot of read mapping algorithms have adopted greedy strategy, which leads to inaccurate local alignment, it is necessary to LR for the inaccurate alignment after read mapping. The LR algorithm first identify regions as targets from reads, and then compute the convex hull of overlapping targets, and next classify reads and realignment reads of RDD.

During the process of genetic sequencing, systemic errors produced by the sequencer can lead to the incorrect assignment of base quality scores. BQSR is quite necessary for improving subsequent analysis accuracy. The correction is applied by estimating the error probability for each set of covariates under a beta-binomial model [7].

2) Genotyping and variant discovery

The second phase of the GCDSS workflow includes variant discovery and genotyping, both of which are intended to discover the possible variant in analysis-ready reads, as well as the genotyping procedure. Due to that the majority of variants is named single nucleotide polymorphism (SNP), and SNPs normally

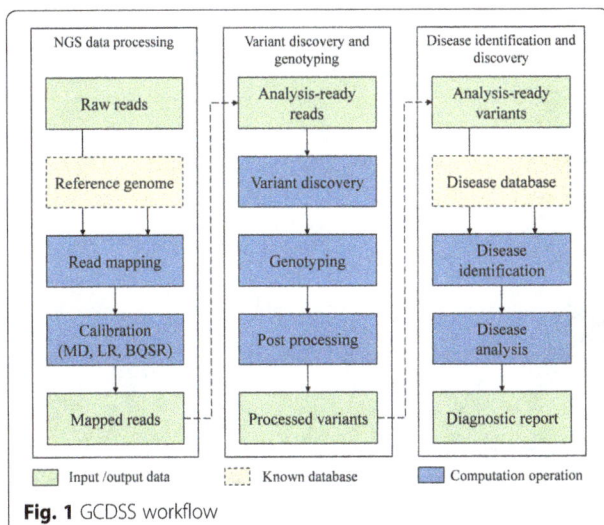

Fig. 1 GCDSS workflow

have stable heredity, wide distribution, and easy detection, therefore in this paper we mainly focus on the variant discovery and genotyping of SNP, and employ the insertion-deletion polymorphism (Indel) accordingly.

In this paper, we use Genotyping, which employs the biallelic genotyper [10] to obtain the sample genotype. Especially, it first marks the variants in the relevant variant RDD and gets the observations, and then for the next step, it turns the single variant observation into the genotype call, and finally creates a genotype RDD.

3) Disease identification

Finally, the last stage is the disease identification and discovery. As illustrated in Fig. 2, this disease identification phase is composed of two steps: the associated database construction and data analysis for the association.

The associated database construction stage mainly uses public database to build an associated database especially for the discovered variations with known diseases. It is acknowledged that NCBI has a public variation database whose size is as large as about 26 gigabytes with around 150 million variations [29]. In the databased, each variation contains the information with following items: the chromosome, position, variant id, reference base, alternate base. NCBI also provides a mapping database of disease and variation. The number of information in the mapping database is about 19,000. Each item contains the OMIM id, the locus id, the SNP, locus symbol, SNP id and so on. Meanwhile, the Online mendelian inheritance in man (OMIM) also provides a comprehensive and timely research support of human genes descriptions and phenotypes, as well as the relationships between them [30]. In this paper, we employ OMIM as disease database at present, due to that OMIM describes a wide variety of disease-related medical features, diagnosis measures, treatment measures, state-of-the-art research progress and other materials.

Also, the main steps to build an association database are listed as below:

(1) Preprocessing and mapping the variation and disease database.
(2) Analyzing the variation database comprehensively, then mapping the variation and disease database, filtering out the variations which are not related to disease.
(3) Obtaining the association database by integrating the processed disease database, which should include the variation and corresponding disease information.

We provide two modes for association database. The simple mode only focuses on the disease id, position, chromosome name, reference base, variant id, and the alternate base. In addition to information of simple mode, the complex mode also includes the locus symbol, method, title, and the link to the corresponding description on the OMIM website. The link can be accessed to the latest OMIM website page with the latest information.

System implementation
In this paper, GCDSS employs a hierarchical structure with cloud computing techniques. The system architecture of GCDSS consists of four layers: storage layer, computing layer, service layer and application layer.

Distributed storage
The first layer is the storage layer, which mainly in charges of storing the related data, including original genetic data, variant data, and disease data.

HDFS is designed to store and manage very large data sets. HDFS has the characteristics of high reliability, excellent scalability and high performance, which has been widely used in various fields. In GCDSS, HDFS is used

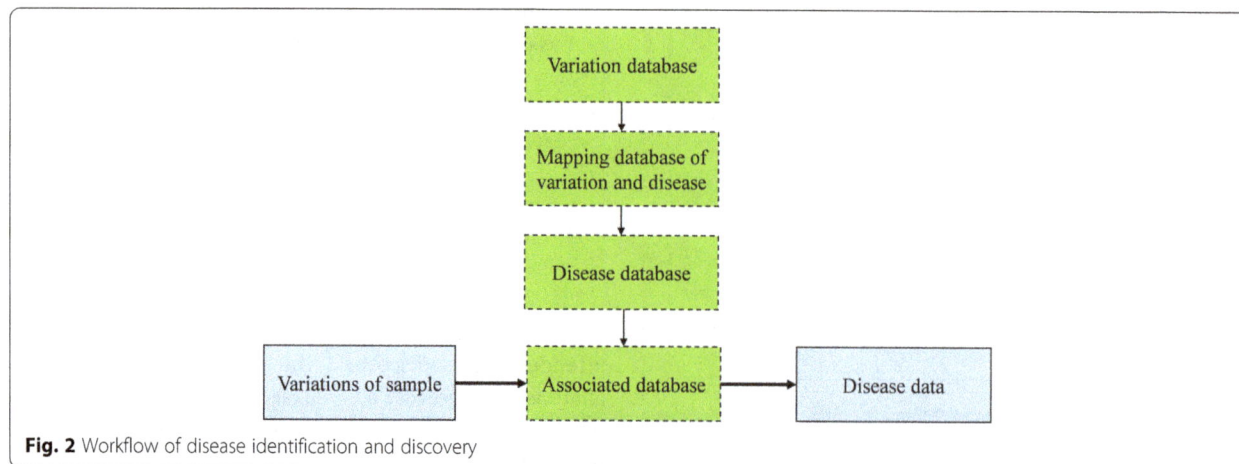

Fig. 2 Workflow of disease identification and discovery

as persistence in storage layer, which is mainly used to store large files or important data, including original sequencing data in FASTQ, result data in Adam format and so on.

However, the data in HDFS is stored in disk, which has limited I/O performance. To improve the read and write performance, we employ Alluxio as primary storage in the process of computing, which speeds up I/O performance by serving data from memory in local node rather than disks, and reduces network traffic between nodes by caching hot files in memory. Between different operations or Spark applications, GCDSS store intermediate data into Alluxio, which avoids storing intermediate data into disk and saves time.

In order to facilitate the calculation of Spark, we need to create several new RDDs by reading data from Alluxio or HDFS. To reduce repeat calculation in Spark application, we cache the RDD in memory by invoking persist or cache functions of Spark in different scenario. For example, we cache the data in memory while there are a series of transformations before an action.

After analyzing genetic data, we obtain result data and need show it to users. We employ NoSQL database Neo4j to show the result. Neo4j is a robust (fully ACID) transactional property graph database. It can vividly display the attributes of different things and their relationship and has high distributed query performance. We leverage Neo4j to store the result data, including information of the sample and its disease data, and provide query function for users.

To address the above problems, we leverage Adam system to convert traditional genetic data formats to Parquet format [31]. To be specific, the Columnar parquet formats can provide storage to minimize the I/O bandwidth and space [7].

Distributed computing framework

The computing layer is mainly responsible for analyzing genetic data and obtaining related results. Computing layer is based on Apache Spark, a memory-based distributed computing framework. Spark has the characteristics of excellent scalability and high performance. Spark is far more efficient than MapReduce [32] in memory, or 10x faster on disk. Spark provides different APIs in Java, Scala, and Python, which makes it easier to be used and compatible with other software like SAMtools [33].

BWA [5] is one of the most widely used read mapping algorithms. It has great accuracy and high performance in single node. BWA-MEM [9] is the newest algorithm in BWA tool. Therefore, we select BWA-MEM to read mapping. In this paper, we present CloudBWA, a distributed read mapping algorithm based on cloud computing technology. CloudBWA integrates BWA into Spark, which is based on Adam system for the genetic data formats, such as FASTA, FASTQ, SAM, and VCF, etc. [11]. Meanwhile We employ Avocado [10] Avocado to accomplish the variant discovery and genotyping.

Distributed algorithms

In order to facilitate the genetic data analysis in distribution, we implement several distributed algorithms, including the extract-transform-load library (ETLlib), the base algorithm library (BAlib), the conversion library (Clib) and the upload/download library (UPlib).

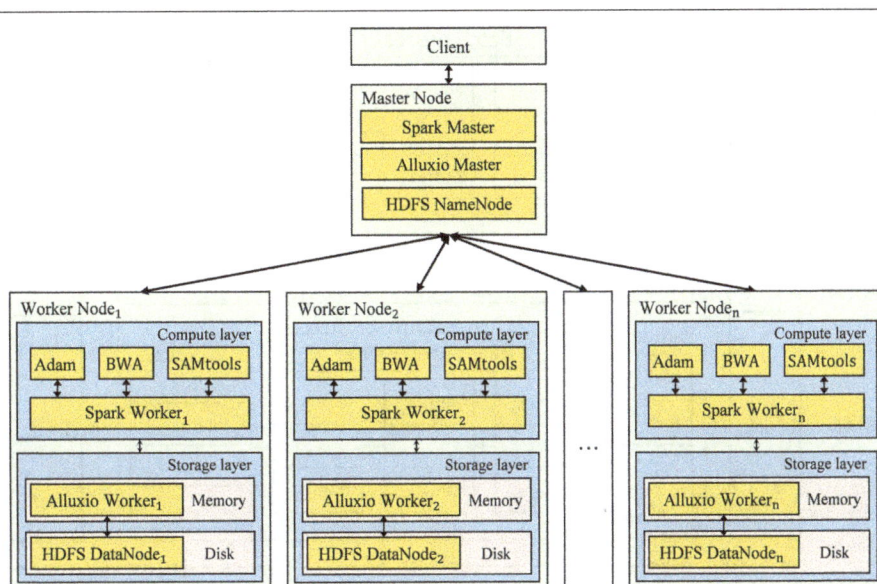

Fig. 3 Framework of the CloudBWA algorithm

BAlib is a general algorithm library to distributed process and analyze the genetic data processing and analysis, including read mapping algorithm, Indel realignment algorithm, base quality score recalibration algorithm, mark duplicates algorithm, sorting algorithm, variants discovery algorithm, genotyping algorithm, disease identification and analysis algorithm and so on.

ETLlib is a library which is responsible for the extraction, cleaning, conversion and loading of genetic data, which is used to process the raw data and facilitates subsequent operations.

UPlib is a library dedicated to the uploading and downloading genetic data. As the usual FASTA, FASTQ and SAM data formats are not suitable for distributed environments at present, uploading files from the local file system requires related operations to process them. Moreover, it also requires related operations to process for downloading data from DFS to local file system.

Clib is a library designed for converting different data formats. It provides mutual conversion functions between standalone data formats FASTA, FASTQ, SAM, VCF and distributed data formats Adam [2].

Distributed read mapping algorithm

In order to solve the scalability problems of the conventional read mapping algorithms, in this paper we propose a distributed read mapping algorithm CloudBWA, which is based on cloud computing techniques. This section describes the CloudBWA framework and the CloudBWA workflow respectively.

First, the CloudBWA framework is shown in Fig. 3, CloudBWA usually employs a Master-slave framework. In general, the Master node is primarily responsible for manage the metadata and the cluster, which combines Spark Master, Alluxio Master and HDFS NameNode. In comparison, the Slave node consists of two layers: a storage layer and a compute layer. The specifications of both layers are presented in Distributed read mapping algorithm section.

The CloudBWA workflow mainly utilizes Spark and the BWA tools to a distributed read mapping framework, including data storage and conversion. As presented in Fig. 4, the CloudBWA algorithm is composed of three stages: the data preprocessing stage, the Map stage, and the post-processing stage.

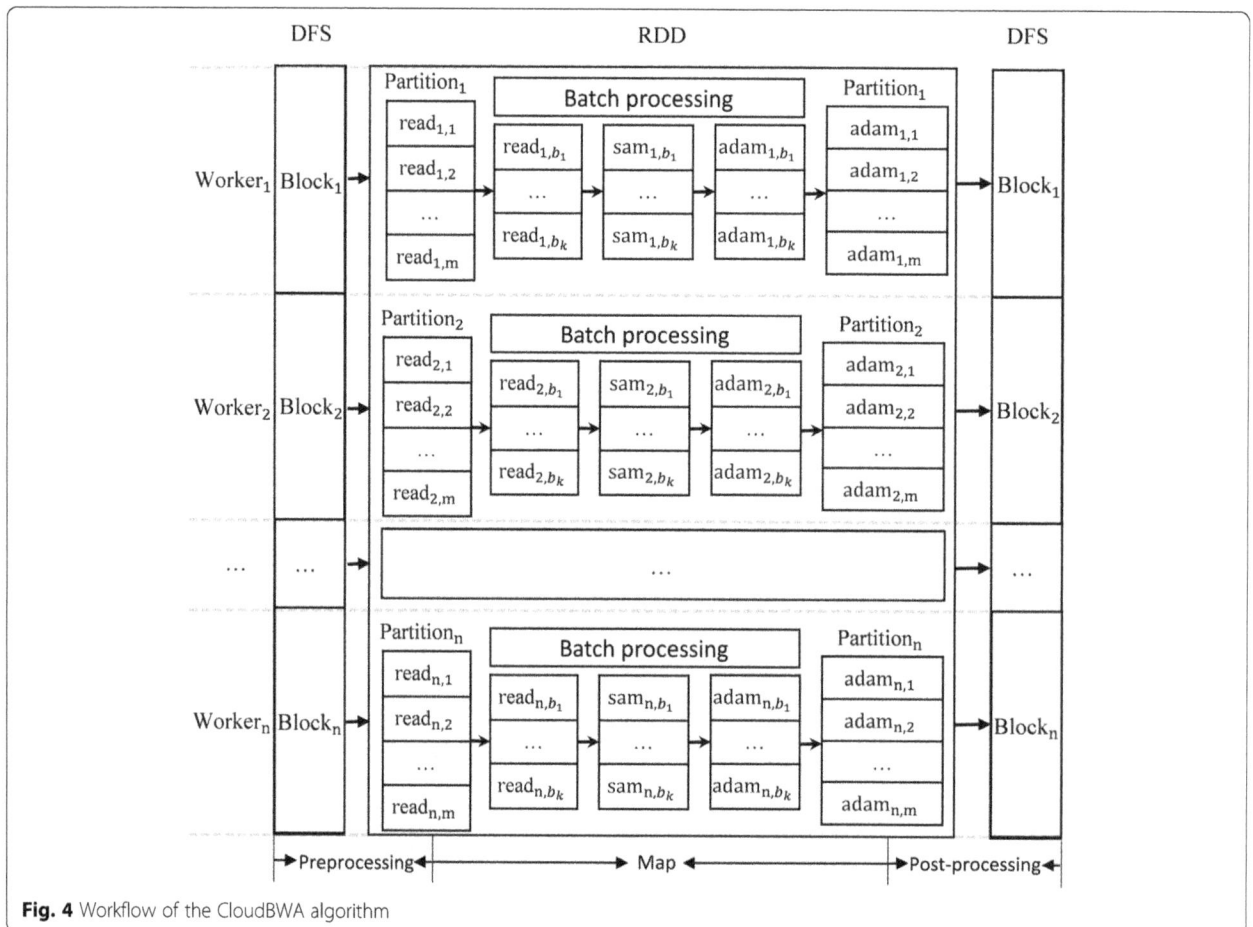

Fig. 4 Workflow of the CloudBWA algorithm

1) Preprocessing

The preprocessing stage mainly reads data from the distributed file system (DFS) and works on the pre-process procedure. The DFS supported by CloudBWA has Alluxio and HDFS. Alluxio is small capacity and fast speed, and HDFS is more stable and larger capacity, but the read and write speed is relatively slower.

Data preprocessing contains following steps:

(1) Inputting data. CloudBWA supports input genetic data in forms of the traditional FASTA, FASTQ and VCF formats, and then uses Adam to convert them into distributed data formats. CloudBWA also supports input genetic data in forms of Parquet data format.
(2) Converting data. Since the Map phase requires information such as the sequence and name of the read, it is necessary to extract and convert.
(3) Filtering data. Filtering out the data which is not in accordance with the requirements.
(4) Pairing reads. It is necessary to pairing paired-end reads in preprocessing phase. Otherwise, it will increase the overhead of subsequent computation if paired-end reads are distributed in different nodes. CloudBWA pairs reads by invoking the Spark's groupBy function and using the name of reads as key. Users can also specify the size of numPartitions, which can be used to adjust the number of partitions in each node and weaken the effect of stragglers.
(5) Caching data. To reduce repeat computation, caching processed data into memory.

2) Map

Table 1 Real datasets

Public datasets	Description	Number
GRCh38	Reference genome	About 3.2 billion base
ERR000589	Paired-end reads	23,928,016 reads
SRR062634	Paired-end reads	48,297,986 reads

This Map phase employs batch processing techniques to speed up the data processing procedure. When the batch is too small, the utilization rate of computing resources is not high. When the batch is too large, it will increase the system memory and CPU load and result in lower performance. So it is critical for the performance of CloudBWA to select the size of the batch.

As illustrated in Fig. 4, a new RDD of reads is generated after the preprocessing stage. Each RDD has several or a number of partitions. To facilitate the description comprehensively, each node in the Fig. 4 has only one partition, which can actually be adjusted by numPartitions in preprocessing phase. Considering that the data distribution is sufficiently uniform, each partition has m pairs of reads. Paired-end reads of $Partition_1$ are named as $read_{1, 1}$ to $read_{1, m}$. The paired-end reads in different partitions are generally different. CloudBWA provides two output mode: SAM and Adam mode. Assuming the size of batch is k. The Map phase are composed of following steps:

(1) Loading the reference genome. The mapPartitions function of Spark is used to process each partition. The jBWA [34] is called to launch the reference genome that has already been built BWA index.
(2) Read mapping stage. When the size of batch reaches k, the CloudBWA architecture will call the jBWA to do the read mapping process. If the remaining batch size of the partition is less than k,

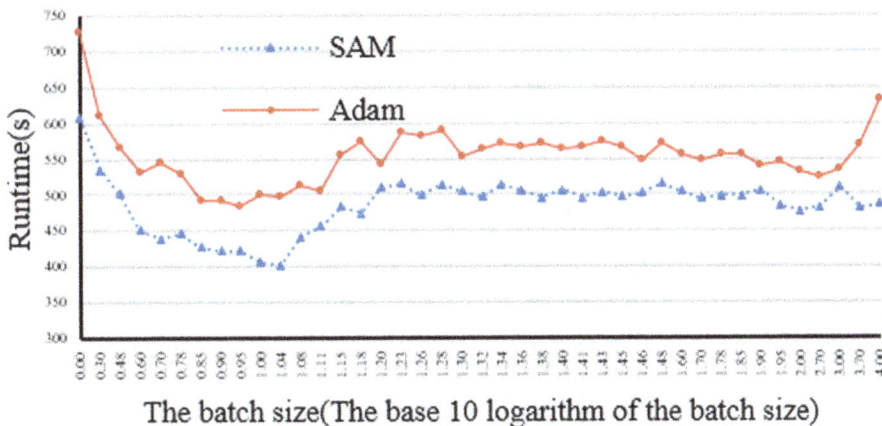

Fig. 5 Impact evaluation of different batch size and output mode

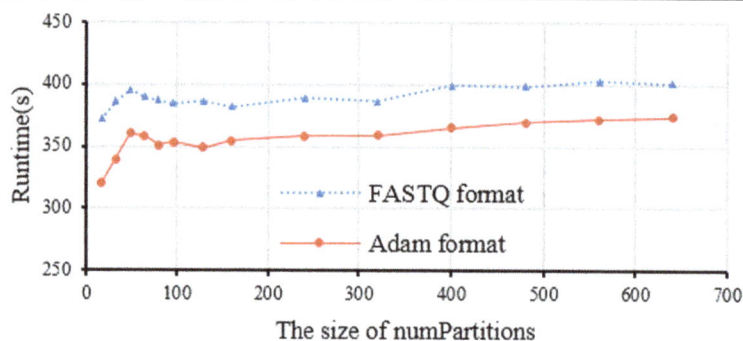

Fig. 6 Impact evaluation of different input data format

they will be mapped. For example, $read_{1,b_1}$ will be processed and return to sam_{1,b_1} by read mapping. The sam_{1,b_1} is SAM format string.

(3) Unifying the expression stage. Due to that jBWA may return multiple results after mapping, they need to be filtered and transformed. CloudBWA designs and implement a processing mechanism to unify the expression.

(4) Processing in Adam mode. If the output is formatted as Adam mode, CloudBWA will invoke SAM tools to convert SAM format string into SAM Record format, and obtains or generates the reference sequence dictionary SQ, read group RG and program information PG, and then convert them into Adam format.

(5) After processing an entire batch, the next batch of reads in the partition will be processed from (2) until the genetic data of the partition is processed.

(6) When the whole partition is finished, CloudBWA will release the related data and operations of jBWA. When all the partitions are processed, CloudBWA will start the next phase automatically.

3) *Post processing*

CloudBWA needs to do a post processing after the map phase. The main steps are shown as follows:

(1) Generating RDD. CloudBWA needs to obtain the reference sequence dictionary SQ, read group RG and program information PG, and then combines them with mapped reads in map phase to generate a new SAM or Adam RDD.

(2) If the output mode is SAM mode, CloudBWA will save SAM RDD into DFS or return SAM RDD.

(3) If the output mode is Adam mode, CloudBWA will return Adam RDD or save Adam RDD into DFS with specified storage block size and compression method.

Using Adam format output and storage increases computational overhead, but reduces storage space because Adam uses Parquet column storage, which can compress easily and has smaller storage space [2]. When the three phases are completed, CloudBWA completes the distributed read mapping.

Results

The main goal of this paper is to solve the scalability problems of traditional genetic data analysis pipeline. In this section, we evaluate GCDSS in two major aspects: performance and scalability. CloudBWA is a distributed read mapping algorithm in GCDSS. The major aim of CloudBWA is address the second challenge: the scalability of traditional read mapping algorithms is limited. Read mapping is rather time-consuming in the whole genetic data analysis pipeline. Therefore, we focused on the evaluation of CloudBWA. We also evaluate the feasibility of the GCDSS prototype.

All our experiments are performed on an 8-node local cluster. The operation system of each node is Ubuntu-14.04.1. Each node has a dual core Intel Xeon W3505 CPU with 22GB of RAM, and it is connected via Gigabit Ethernet. The version of Apache Spark is 1.5.2. The Alluxio version is 1.3.0. The version of HDFS is 2.6.0. The version of Java JDK is 1.8.0_121. The version

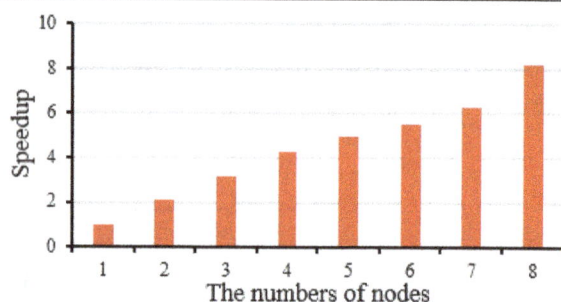

Fig. 7 The speedup improvement by increasing the number of nodes

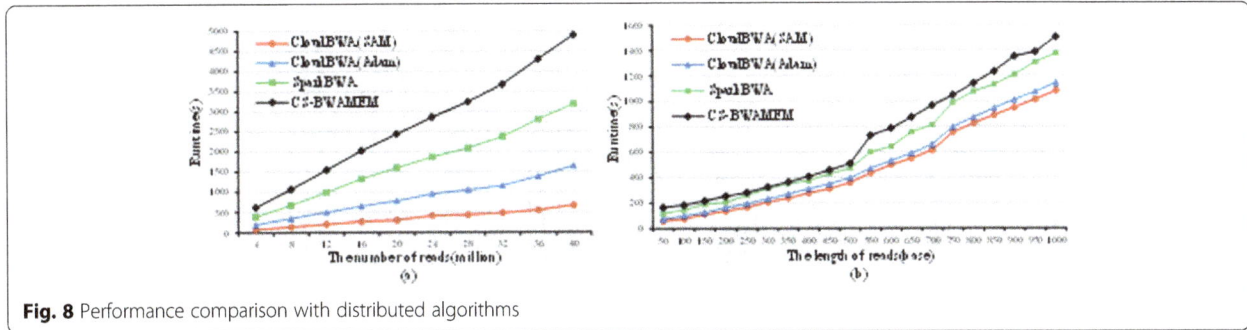

Fig. 8 Performance comparison with distributed algorithms

of Scala is 2.10.5. We employ wgsim [35] to generate simulation data. The version of wgsim is 0.3.2. The parameters of wgsim are set as default besides description. In order to validate algorithm or system in real environment, we use real datasets ERR000589 and SRR062634 (see Table 1) that are the same as SparkBWA [20]. ERR000589 has 23,928,016 reads and the length of each read is 51 base. SRR062634 has 48,297,986 reads and the length of each read is 100 base. Their sequencing platform is Illumina.

CloudBWA is measured with different metrics, including the impact of different parameters on CloudBWA, the scalability evaluation, the performance comparison.

Performance evaluation

We evaluated the impact of different parameters on CloudBWA, including the batch size and number of the Partitions.

(1) Impact of the batch sizes and output mode

The experimental raw data reads are generated by wgsim with 20 million of reads at 50 base length. The memory of the Spark node is configured as 20G. The size of numPartitions is set to 32. Adam uses GZIP software to compress the data. Reference is chromosome 1 of GRCh38. We use HDFS as the distributed file system with FASTQ as the input format of reads.

Figure 5 illustrates impact evaluation of batch size and output mode on CloudBWA framework. The experimental result proposes that SAM mode is more efficient than the Adam mode for all possible batch sizes. This is due to that Adam format needs more computation resources, including the conversion and compression process. When batch size is only 1 read, the runtime of SAM and Adam mode is remarkable. When the batch size increases, the runtime of SAM mode will decrease at first and then increase accordingly, and finally become stable. The run time of Adam mode will rise when batch size is considerable. The runtime is the least when batch size is about 10 reads.

Impact of different data format and numPartitions

CloudBWA supports both FASTQ and Adam input format. We use the same experimental data as the first experiment. The output mode is SAM mode with 10 reads for the batch size. We use Alluxio as the distributed file system with FASTQ as the input format of reads. The CloudBWA is evaluated with different numPartitions sizes.

Figure 6 demonstrates the impact of different input data formats on the CloudBWA. The experimental result illustrates that Adam input format is more efficient than FASTQ format. Adam format achieves 9.6% performance improvement over SAM format on average. When inputting data with Adam format in DFS, CloudBWA

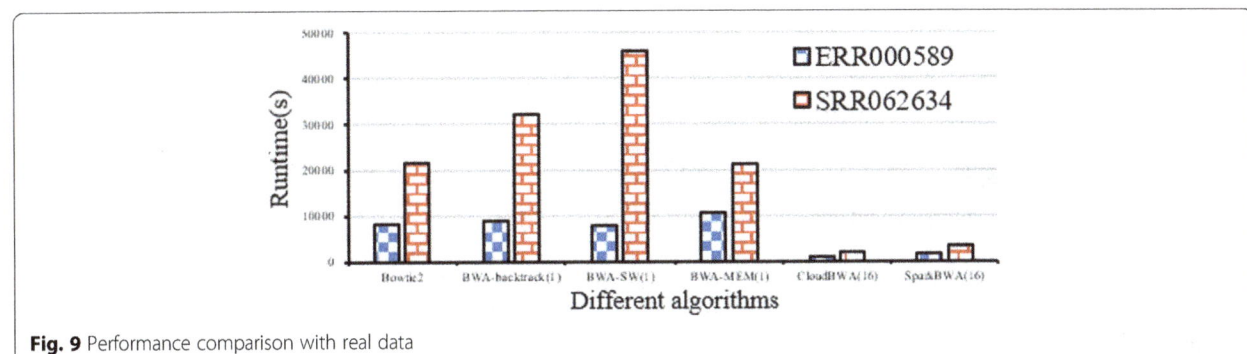

Fig. 9 Performance comparison with real data

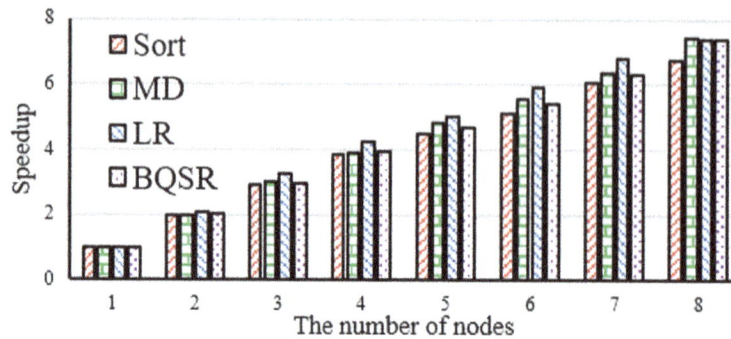

Fig. 10 Performance evaluation of calibration

can directly process the data, which avoids extra transformation overhead like FASTQ format. The experimental result shows that with the growth in numPartitions, the running time of CloudBWA will grow quickly, and then becomes flat with minor increments. When the size of numPartitions is 16, the runtime of CloudBWA is the least. At present, CloudBWA employs BWA to read mapping in each partition, including loading index file and releasing related data.

Scalability evaluation

In order to measure the scalability of CloudBWA, we run the algorithm with different number of nodes. The data are the same as the first experiment. Every node uses one core. The numPartitions size is 16 with Adam input data format. The output mode is SAM with 10 reads for the batch size.

Figure 7 illustrates the speedup improvement of CloudBWA architecture in line with the number of nodes growth. The experimental result shows that CloudBWA achieves approximately linear speedup when the number of nodes grows from 1 to 8.

Comparison

We use different experiments to compare the performance of CloudBWA and other related algorithms, including stand-alone algorithms and distributed algorithms.

Comparison with distributed algorithms

We compare CloudBWA with different distributed algorithms, including SparkBWA [20] and CS-BWAMEM [13], both of which are the state-of-the-art read mapping algorithms in distribution. The version of CS-BWAMEM is 0.2.2, with output format is Adam and 100 reads batch size. The version of SparkBWA is 0.2 with SAM output format and numPartitions size is 8 The SparkBWA uses two threads in each node. The version of CloudBWA is 1.0.1, with numPartitions size at 16 and batch size at 10 reads. The three algorithms use 8 nodes and 16 cores in cluster.

Figure 8 illustrates the performance comparison with both distributed algorithms. In particular, Fig. 8a uses different number of reads, which is from 4 million to 40 million, and their length is 50 base. The experimental results demonstrate that CloudBWA is more efficient than the SparkBWA and CS-BWAMEM algorithm in different number of reads. The Adam mode of CloudBWA achieves average 1.84 times speedup over CS-BWAMEM. The SAM mode of CloudBWA gains up to 2.63 times speedup over SparkBWA. Figure 8b evaluates the results for different length of reads, which is from 50 to 1000 base. The numbers illustrate that CloudBWA is more efficient than SparkBWA and CS-BWAMEM in various length of reads. The Adam mode of CloudBWA gains up to 2.22 times speedup over CS-BWAMEM. The SAM mode of

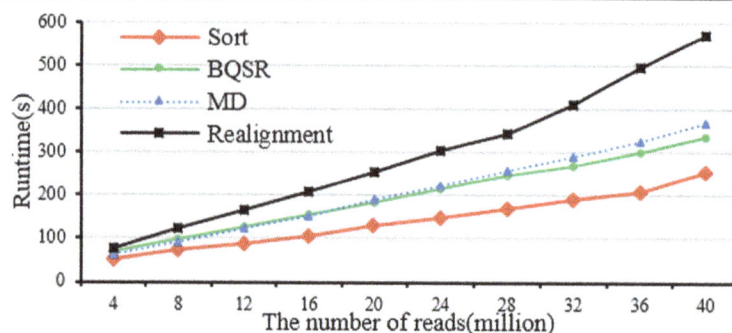

Fig. 11 Scalability evaluation of calibration

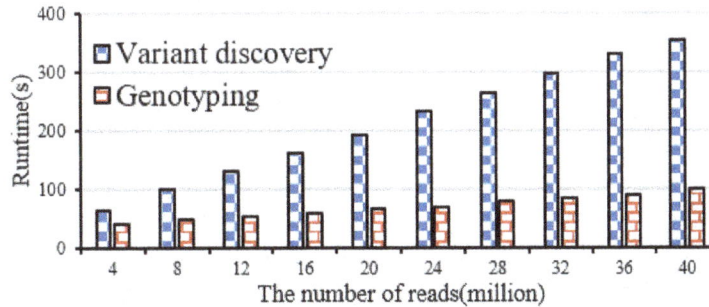

Fig. 12 Performance evaluation of variant discovery and genotyping

CloudBWA achieves 1.44 times speedup over SparkBWA on average.

Comparison with real data

In order to more fully validate CloudBWA, we design two different experiments with real data (see Table 1).

The stand-alone algorithms use one node and one core. The distributed algorithms use 8 nodes with 16 cores. The version of CloudBWA is 1.2.0. CloudBWA uses 160 as NumPartitions size and 11 as batch size for ERR000589. CloudBWA uses 128 as NumPartitions size and 10 reads as batch size for SRR062634. We cannot obtain experiment result of CS-BWAMEM because of it has out of memory error in real data.

Figure 9 illustrates the performance comparison with real data. The parameter of parentheses is the number of processor cores. The experimental result illustrates that CloudBWA has outstanding performance. For ERR000589, CloudBWA (16) achieves 11.59, 8.39, 1.66 times speedup over BWA-MEM (1), BWA-SW (1), SparkBWA (16), respectively. For SRR0062634, CloudBWA (16) achieves 11.02, 23.86, 1.68 times speedup over BWA-MEM (1), BWA-SW (1), SparkBWA (16), respectively.

Discussion

After evaluating the CloudBWA, which is the key component algorithm in GCDSS, we also measure the other GCDSS's components. We especially focus on the performance and scalability analysis.

Calibration evaluation

The experimental benchmarks and configurations are the same as the experiment of A 3) (1). The length of reads is set to 50.

Performance of calibration

Figure 10 illustrates the performance of calibration. The experimental results demonstrate that sort is the fastest process and LR is the slowest process in the calibration procedure. MD is actually slower than BQSR at the beginning, but MD is far more efficient when the number of reads is more than 20 million. With the growth in the population of reads, the four operations' runtime of calibration are also approximately linear increasing.

Scalability of calibration

Figure 11 demonstrates the scalability of calibration. The experimental result reveals that the four operations of calibration achieve about linear speedup when the number of nodes increases from 1 to 8 in cluster.

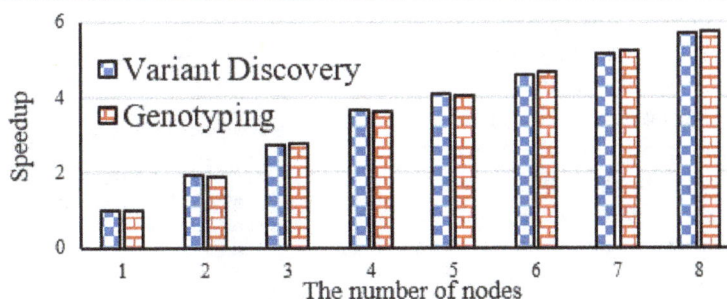

Fig. 13 Scalability evaluation of variant discovery and genotyping

Table 2 Evaluation of disease identification and discovery

Number of raw reads	4,000,000	20,000,000	40,000,000
Number of mapped reads	3,911,329	19,553,895	39,107,115
Number of mate mapped reads	3,824,558	19,117,950	38,234,922
Reads number after variant discovery	3,655,139	17,772,692	37,313,251
Reads number after genotyping	5071	13,797	15,571
Reads number after disease analysis	3	14	34

Variant discovery and genotyping evaluation

The experimental benchmarks and configurations are the same as the experiment of A 3) (1). The length of reads is set to 50.

Performance evaluation

Figure 12 illustrates performance of variant discovery and genotyping. The experimental result shows that with the growth of the number of reads, the runtime of variant discovery and genotyping both are around near linear.

Scalability evaluation

Figure 13 tells scalability of variant discovery and genotyping. The experimental result shows that variant discovery and genotyping both achieve near linear speedup in line with the growth the number of nodes from 1 to 8.

Disease identification and discovery evaluation

Disease identification and discovery also plays a vital role of the GCDSS. We also accomplish several experiments to measure the disease identification and discovery. In order to analyze the GCDSS system comprehensively, this paper also incorporates the benchmarks same as the previous read mapping and variant analysis.

Table 2 tells the evaluation results of disease identification and discovery. We select 4 million, 20 million, and 40 million respectively. The experiment result shows that the corresponding number of data are 3, 14, and 34 after the data are analyzed by disease identification and discovery of GCDSS.

Conclusions

In this paper, we have presented GCDSS, which is a distributed gene clinical decision support system based on cloud computing techniques. In particular, we incorporated a distributed genetic data analysis pipeline framework in the proposed GCDSS system. To boost the data processing of GCDSS, we propose CloudBWA, which is a novel distributed read mapping algorithm to leverage batch processing technique in mapping stage using Apache Spark platform. The experimental results show that CloudBWA is able to achieve outstanding performance with excellent scalability. Compared to state-of-the-art distributed read mapping algorithms, CloudBWA

achieves up to 2.63 times speedup over SparkBWA. Compared with unicore read mapping algorithms, CloudBWA with 16 cores achieves up to 11.59 times speedup over BWA-MEM with uniprocessor. We also evaluated other GCDSS's key components, including calibration, variant discovery, genotyping, disease identification, and discovery. The experimental results illustrate that GCDSS also achieves remarkable speedup with satisfying scalability.

In the future, we plan to exploit numerous technologies to further improve performance and increase the variety of disease analysis.

Acknowledgements
The authors would like to thank all the reviewers from BIBM conferences and BMC journal for their valuable feedbacks and suggestions.

Funding
Publication costs were funded by the National Key Research and Development Program of China (under Grant 2017YFA0700900), Suzhou Research Foundation (No.SYG201625). This research was also supported by the NSFC (No.61772482), Anhui Provincial NSF (No.1608085QF12), and Youth Innovation Promotion Association CAS (No. 2017497), Fundamental Research Funds for the Central Universities (WK2150110003), and the State Key Laboratory of Computer Architecture, Institute of Computing Technology, CAS (CARCH201709).

Authors' contributions
BX and CL analyzed and interpreted the data, and they are major contributors in writing the manuscript. HZ, JW and QW performed the algorithms analysis and evaluated experimental results. CW and XZ designed and implemented the GCDSS. All authors read and approved the final manuscript. CW is the corresponding author.

Competing interests
The authors declare that they have no competing interests.

References
1. Osheroff JA, et al. A roadmap for national action on clinical decision support. J Am Med Inform Assoc. 2007;14(2):141–5.
2. Xu B, et al. Distributed gene clinical decision support system based on cloud computing. In: Bioinformatics and Biomedicine (BIBM), 2017 IEEE International Conference on: IEEE; 2017.
3. Muir P, et al. The real cost of sequencing: scaling computation to keep pace with data generation. Genome Biol. 2016;17(1):1.
4. Auwera GA, et al. From FastQ data to high-confidence variant calls: the genome analysis toolkit best practices pipeline. Curr Protoc Bioinformatics. 2013;43:11.10.1-33.
5. Li H, Durbin R. Fast and accurate short read alignment with burrows-wheeler transform. Bioinformatics. 2009;25(14):1754–60.
6. McKenna A, et al. The genome analysis toolkit: a MapReduce framework for analyzing next-generation DNA sequencing data. Genome Res. 2010; 20(9):1297–303.
7. Nothaft FA, et al. Rethinking data-intensive science using scalable analytics systems. In: Proceedings of the 2015 ACM SIGMOD International Conference on Management of Data: ACM; 2015.
8. Wang C, et al. Heterogeneous cloud framework for big data genome sequencing. IEEE/ACM Trans Comput Biol Bioinform (TCBB). 2015;12(1): 166–78.
9. Li, H., Aligning sequence reads, clone sequences and assembly contigs with BWA-MEM. arXiv preprint arXiv:1303.3997; 2013.

10. Nothaft, F., Scalable genome resequencing with ADAM and avocado. 2015.

11. Massie, M., et al., Adam: Genomics formats and processing patterns for cloud scale computing. EECS Department, University of California, Berkeley, Tech. Rep. UCB/EECS-2013-207; 2013.

12. Zaharia, M., et al., Faster and more accurate sequence alignment with SNAP. arXiv preprint arXiv:1111.5572; 2011.

13. Chen, Y.-T., et al., CS-BWAMEM: a fast and scalable read aligner at the cloud scale for whole genome sequencing. High Throughput Sequencing Algorithms and Applications (HITSEQ); 2015.

14. Chen, Y.-T., Memory system optimizations for customized computing--from single-Chip to datacenter; 2016.

15. Spark meets Genomics: Helping Fight the Big C with the Big D. Available from: https://spark-summit.org/2014/david-patterson/.

16. Parsian M. Data Algorithms: Recipes for Scaling Up with Hadoop and Spark: O'Reilly Media, Inc.; 2015.

17. Xu, B., et al., DSA: Scalable Distributed Sequence Alignment System Using SIMD Instructions. arXiv preprint arXiv:1701.01575, 2017.

18. Xu, B., et al., Efficient Distributed Smith-Waterman Algorithm Based on Apache Spark. 2017 IEEE 10th International Conference on Cloud Computing; 2017.

19. Li H, Durbin R. Fast and accurate long-read alignment with burrows–wheeler transform. Bioinformatics. 2010;26(5):589–95.

20. Abuín JM, et al. SparkBWA: speeding up the alignment of high-throughput DNA sequencing data. PLoS One. 2016;11(5):e0155461.

21. White T. Hadoop: The definitive guide: O'Reilly Media, Inc.; 2012.

22. Shvachko K, et al. The hadoop distributed file system. In: 2010 IEEE 26th symposium on mass storage systems and technologies (MSST): IEEE; 2010.

23. Zaharia M, et al. Spark: cluster computing with working sets. HotCloud. 2010;10:10.

24. Li H, et al. Tachyon: reliable, memory speed storage for cluster computing frameworks. In: Proceedings of the ACM symposium on cloud computing: ACM; 2014.

25. Wang C, et al. GenServ: genome sequencing services on scalable energy efficient accelerators. In: Web Services (ICWS), 2017 IEEE International Conference on: IEEE; 2017.

26. Wang C, et al. Big data genome sequencing on zynq based clusters. In: Proceedings of the 2014 ACM/SIGDA international symposium on field-programmable gate arrays: ACM; 2014.

27. Wang C, et al. Genome sequencing using mapreduce on FPGA with multiple hardware accelerators. In: Proceedings of the ACM/SIGDA international symposium on field programmable gate arrays: ACM; 2013.

28. Zaharia M, et al. Resilient distributed datasets: a fault-tolerant abstraction for in-memory cluster computing. In: Proceedings of the 9th USENIX conference on networked systems design and implementation: USENIX Association; 2012.

29. Rodrigues Pereira, R., Identifying potential cis-regulatory variants associated with allele-specific expression. 2016.

30. Amberger JS, et al. OMIM. Org: online Mendelian inheritance in man (OMIM®), an online catalog of human genes and genetic disorders. Nucleic Acids Res. 2015;43(D1):D789–98.

31. Parquet, A. Apache Parquet. http://parquet.incubator.apache.org; Available from: http://parquet.apache.org/.

32. Dean J, Ghemawat S. MapReduce: simplified data processing on large clusters. Commun ACM. 2008;51(1):107–13.

33. Li H, et al. The sequence alignment/map format and SAMtools. Bioinformatics. 2009;25(16):2078–9.

34. Forer L, et al. Cloudflow-a framework for mapreduce pipeline development in biomedical research. In: Information and Communication Technology, Electronics and Microelectronics (MIPRO), 2015 38th International Convention on: IEEE; 2015.

35. Li H. wgsim-Read simulator for next generation sequencing. http://github.com/lh3/wgsim; 2013.

18

Transposase mapping identifies the genomic targets of BAP1 in uveal melanoma

Matthew Yen[1], Zongtai Qi[2], Xuhua Chen[2], John A. Cooper[1], Robi D. Mitra[2] and Michael D. Onken[1]*

Abstract

Background: BAP1 is a histone deubiquitinase that acts as a tumor and metastasis suppressor associated with disease progression in human cancer. We have used the "Calling Card System" of transposase-directed transposon insertion mapping to identify the genomic targets of BAP1 in uveal melanoma (UM). This system was developed to identify the genomic loci visited by transcription factors that bind directly to DNA; our study is the first use of the system with a chromatin-remodeling factor that binds to histones but does not interact directly with DNA.

Methods: The transposase *piggyBac* (PBase) was fused to BAP1 and expressed in OCM-1A UM cells. The insertion of transposons near BAP1 binding sites in UM cells were identified by genomic sequencing. We also examined RNA expression in the same OCM-1A UM cells after BAP1 depletion to identify BAP1 binding sites associated with BAP1-responsive genes. Sets of significant genes were analyzed for common pathways, transcription factor binding sites, and ability to identify molecular tumor classes.

Results: We found a strong correlation between multiple calling-card transposon insertions targeted by BAP1-PBase and BAP1-responsive expression of adjacent genes. BAP1-bound genomic loci showed narrow distributions of insertions and were near transcription start sites, consistent with recruitment of BAP1 to these sites by specific DNA-binding proteins. Sequence consensus analysis of BAP1-bound sites showed enrichment of motifs specific for YY1, NRF1 and Ets transcription factors, which have been shown to interact with BAP1 in other cell types. Further, a subset of the BAP1 genomic target genes was able to discriminate aggressive tumors in published gene expression data from primary UM tumors.

Conclusions: The calling card methodology works equally well for chromatin regulatory factors that do not interact directly with DNA as for transcription factors. This technique has generated a new and expanded list of BAP1 targets in UM that provides important insight into metastasis pathways and identifies novel potential therapeutic targets.

Keywords: Genomic mapping, Transcription, BAP1, Uveal melanoma

Background

BAP1 is a histone deubiquitinase that remodels chromatin to regulate gene expression. The BAP1 polypeptide is the catalytic subunit of the polycomb-repressive deubiquitinase complex, which requires either ASXL1 or ASXL2 [1], and which can include HCFC1, OGT and other factors [2]. This complex, a component of the polycomb pathway, removes mono-ubiquitin from histone H2A [1]. The HCFC1 subunit is a transcriptional co-activator that can bind transcription factors such as E2F, YY1, and Ets-related transcription factors [3, 4]; however, its role in targeting BAP1 to chromatin has not been fully elucidated.

Melanomas arising from the pigmented layers (uvea) of the eye are highly aggressive cancers: almost half of patients with uveal melanoma (UM) die from metastatic disease, even after the primary tumor is completely removed by surgical excision of the eye [5], because we are unable to prevent or treat metastatic spread of the cancer [5]. UMs can be divided into two

* Correspondence: mdonken@wustl.edu
[1]Department of Biochemistry and Molecular Biophysics, Washington University School of Medicine, 660 S. Euclid Ave., St. Louis, MO 63110, USA
Full list of author information is available at the end of the article

classes by molecular and genetic analysis of the tumor. Class 1 UMs have a favorable prognosis; the cancers are low-grade, indolent, and rarely metastasize. Class 2 UMs have a dismal prognosis; they are high-grade, aggressive and nearly always metastasize [6]. Over 95% of class 2 UMs show complete loss of expression of BAP1 protein [7], with inactivating somatic mutations in the *BAP1* gene in 80% of these tumors [8]. Loss of BAP1 causes UM cells to assume a rounded, epithelioid morphology, to deposit distinctive extracellular matrix materials, and to grow well under clonogenic conditions [9, 10], and BAP1-depleted UM cells display increased diapedesis through endothelial monolayers in a cell-culture model of transendothelial migration [11], which may reflect their ability to metastasize. BAP1 mutations have been found in other aggressive cancers, including skin-derived melanomas, mesotheliomas, and renal cell carcinomas [12–17], suggesting a general role for BAP1 as a suppressor of metastasis in cancer.

Transposon integration by targeted transposases has been used to identify genomic regions in several contexts [18]. The coordinates and numbers of insertions of transposons reflect the locations where the factor binds and the proportion of time the factor is bound to the locus. The "calling card" methodology fuses a piggyBac transposase to a protein of interest [19], and uses multiple bar-coded transposon donor plasmids to improve the spatial and temporal demarcation of integration sites [20]. Here, we modified the technique, originally developed for DNA-binding transcription factors, to detect the interactions of chromatin with BAP1 complex, which does not bind directly to DNA. Our results provide novel insights into the biology of BAP1 in cancer tumor suppression and metastasis.

Methods

Cell culture and reagents

The coding region of human BAP1 cDNA (NM_004656.2) from pReceiver-M12 BAP1 (GeneCopoeia, Rockville, MD) was fused to cDNA encoding the hyperactive piggyBac transposase derived from a pCMV-hyPBase plasmid, generously provided by Dr. Allan Bradley [21]. Both N-terminal and C-terminal fusions were prepared, using Gibson assembly [22]. For BAP1-PBase, BAP1 was placed at the 5′ end of hyPBase with an 18-aa linker, KLGGGAPAVGGGPKAADK. For PBase-BAP1, BAP1 was placed at the 3′ end of hyPBase, with the same linker. Plasmid clones were maintained and expanded in DH5-α cells in carbenicillin, and the identities of plasmids were confirmed by DNA sequencing of all regions that underwent PCR amplification (Genewiz; South Plainfield, NJ). Forty uniquely bar-coded piggyBac transposon plasmids [20] were used as donors

for the calling card protocol. The 40 plasmids were divided into four sets of 10 donors per experiment.

OCM-1A cells were originally derived by Dr. June Kan-Mitchell [23]. Cells were cultured in growth medium: RPMI 1640 with 10% FBS and penicillin/streptomycin (Gibco; Carlsbad, CA) at 37 °C in 5% CO_2. Cells were transfected using TransIT-LT1 transfection reagent (Mirus; Madison, WI) according to manufacturer's instructions. After 24 h, the medium was replaced with growth medium containing 1.4 µg/mL puromycin. Cells were maintained under selection for 2 weeks, at which point large visible colonies were formed. Colonies were harvested by trypsinization and centrifugation, and cell pellets were stored at − 80 °C.

Preparation of genomic DNA

The following procedure was adapted and modified from [19]. Genomic DNA was isolated from cell pellets using a High MW Cell DNA Isolation Kit (EZ Bioresearch, St. Louis, MO) according to manufacturer instructions. For each sample, three independent digests were performed with Taq1, Msp1, and CviQ (New England Biolabs, Ipswich, MA) using 20 µg of genomic DNA and following manufacturer protocols. Each separate digested genomic DNA sample was purified using a Qiaquick PCR Purification Kit (Qiagen), self-ligated with T4 Ligase (New England Biolabs) at 15 °C for 18–24 h, and purified with Amicon Ultra-0.5 mL Centrifugal 30 k filters (Millipore; Billerica, MA) with 5-min spins (instead of the standard protocol of 10–30 min). The circularized genomic material from the three independent digests were pooled for each experimental sample and inverse PCR was performed using piggyBac transposon-specific primers. DNA fragments from 200 to 1000 bp were isolated and yields were quantified by UV absorbance. Next-gen sequencing was performed on the MiSeq 2×250 (Illumina) by the Center for Genomic Sciences and Systems Biology at Washington University in St. Louis, using the transposon-specific sequencing primer.

Calling card data analysis

Raw reads were mapped back to the human genome (hg19) with Bowtie2. Significant Calling Cards peaks were called with a modified version of the previously described algorithm [19]. Briefly, transposon insertions were clustered into peaks with a maximum distance of 5 kb between insertions. Significant peaks were identified using the Poisson distribution to test for enrichment over the background (unfused transposase) Calling Card data. The expected number of hops per TTAA was locally estimated from the background Calling Card data by considering regions centered directly under the Calling Card peak, 1 kb from the Calling Card peak, or 5 kb from the Calling Card peak, and taking the maximum of the three estimated parameters. Peaks were annotated with nearby gene information using bedtools.

Lentiviral shRNA knockdown of BAP1

The following was modified from Mooren et al. [24]. Lentiviral pLKO.1 shRNA plasmid targeting *BAP1* (NM_004656.2-2658s1c1) was designed by the RNAi consortium (TRC) and obtained from the Children's Discovery Institute / Genome Sequencing Center at Washington University. Lentiviral shRNA expression plasmids were cotransfected into HEK293T cells with the plasmids pCMV-dR8.2 dvpr and pCMV-VSV-G. After 72 h, viral particles were harvested. OCM-1A cells were infected with lentivirus in growth medium with 8 μg/mL protamine sulfate. After 24 h, medium was changed to fresh growth medium containing 1.4 μg/mL puromycin. OCM-1A cells were harvested for analysis of protein and RNA 6 days post infection.

RNA sequencing and analysis

RNA was isolated using the Qiagen RNeasy Mini Kit according to manufacturer instructions, including the optional DNase I step. Second-strand cDNA synthesis was performed using SuperScript IV (ThermoFisher Scientific; Waltham, MA) according to manufacturer instructions. Next-gen RNA sequencing was performed on the Illumina HiSeq2500 1×50 by the Genome Technology Access Center (Washington University). Three biological replicates for *BAP1* and control (GFP) knockdowns were sequenced. RNA-Seq analysis was performed by the Genomic Technology Access Center at Washington University. Reads were aligned to the Ensembl release 76 top-level assembly with STAR version 2.0.4b. Gene counts were derived from the number of uniquely aligned unambiguous reads by Subread:featureCount version 1.4.5. Transcript counts were produced by Sailfish version 0.6.3. Sequencing performance was assessed for total number of aligned reads, total number of uniquely aligned reads, genes and transcripts detected, ribosomal fraction known junction saturation and read distribution over known gene models with RSeQC version 2.3.

Gene-level and transcript counts were imported into the R/Bioconductor package. EdgeR and TMM normalization size factors were calculated to adjust for samples with differences in library size. Genes or transcripts not expressed in any sample were excluded from further analysis. The TMM size factors and the matrix of counts were imported into R/Bioconductor package Limma. Weighted likelihoods based on the observed mean-variance relationship of every gene/

transcript and sample were calculated for all samples with the voomWithQualityWeights function. Generalized linear models were then created to test for gene/ transcript level differential expression. Differentially expressed genes and transcripts were then filtered for FDR adjusted *p*-values less than or equal to 0.01. Gene ontology (GO) and pathway analyses was performed using Gene Set Enrichment Analysis (GSEA) [25]. GO groups were assembled by merging the lists of genes from related GO terms that were significantly enriched in the signature gene set. GSEA was also used to identify published molecular signatures (curated by the Broad Institute: http://broadinstitute.org/ GSEA) that showed significant overlap ($p < 0.001$) with response to BAP1 depletion.

DNA motif analysis

BAP1-PBase calling card peaks with five or more insertions were used for Hypergeometric Optimization of Motif EnRichment (HOMER) analysis (available at: http://homer.ucsd.edu). Peaks were analyzed separately depending on whether they were associated with genes showing significant change ($p < 0.01$) in expression after *BAP1* depletion, and whether the associated gene increased or decreased expression upon Bap1 depletion. HOMER was used to identify enriched motifs in genomic regions (findMotifsGenome.pl) using the given size of each peak.

Results

The calling card system identifies genomic regions bound by BAP1

We fused the piggyBac transposase (PBase) to BAP1 with a flexible 18-aa linker at either end of BAP1 (Fig. 1). Each fusion construct was cotransfected with PB donor plasmids into OCM-1A UM cells; unfused PBase served as a negative control. Next-gen sequencing of genomic DNA revealed specific clusters of genomic reads associated with BAP1-PBase fusion constructs and not present in control samples. The BAP1-PBase and PBase-BAP1 fusion constructs produced 199,209 and 179,244 genomic transposon insertions, respectively, and these insertion sites clustered into 7,810 (see Additional file 1) and 7,634 (see Additional file 2) genomic peaks. Peaks were called by accounting for background hops (i.e. a call required enrichment of BAP1 hops over background). Only a small subset of genomic peaks showed directly overlapping insertion peaks with both fusion constructs (Fig. 2a). For each construct, many genes were found to contained multiple, non-overlapping peaks. We clustered the genomic peaks based on closest gene (5,883 for BAP1-PBase and 5,542 for PBase-BAP1), and the targeted genes showed substantial overlap (47% for BAP1-PBase and 50% for PBase-BAP1; Fig. 2b). The

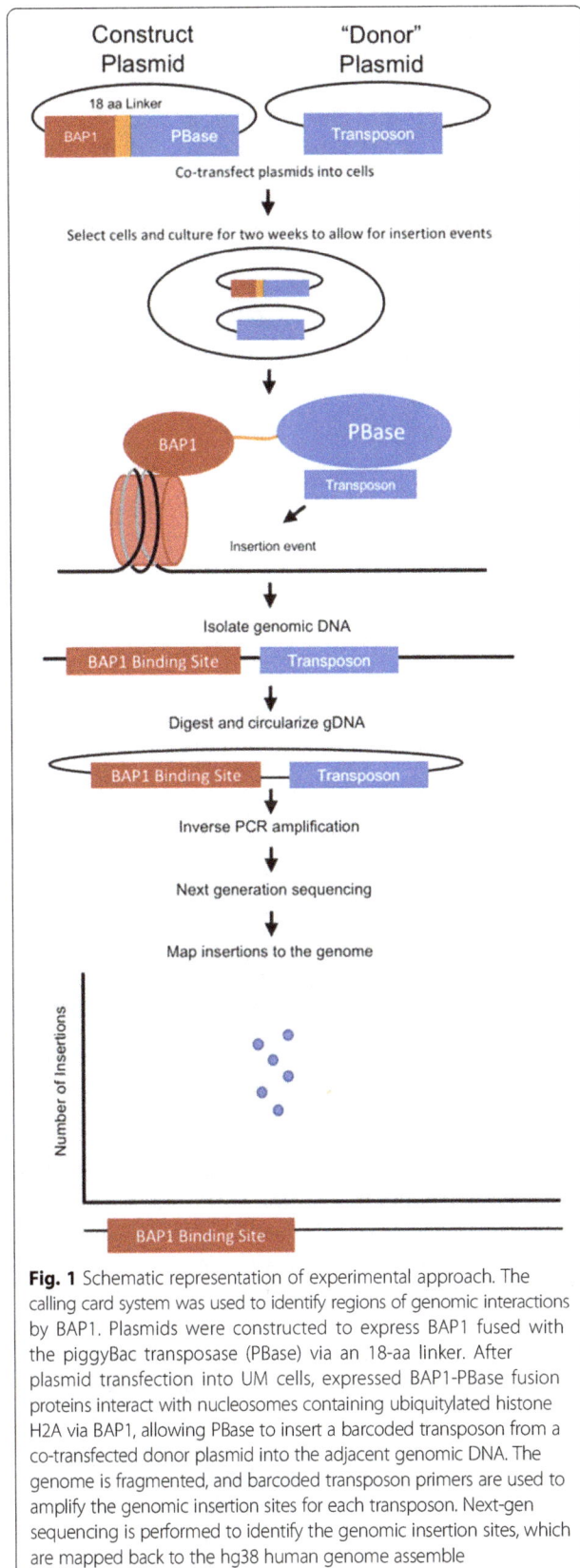

Fig. 1 Schematic representation of experimental approach. The calling card system was used to identify regions of genomic interactions by BAP1. Plasmids were constructed to express BAP1 fused with the piggyBac transposase (PBase) via an 18-aa linker. After plasmid transfection into UM cells, expressed BAP1-PBase fusion proteins interact with nucleosomes containing ubiquitylated histone H2A via BAP1, allowing PBase to insert a barcoded transposon from a co-transfected donor plasmid into the adjacent genomic DNA. The genome is fragmented, and barcoded transposon primers are used to amplify the genomic insertion sites for each transposon. Next-gen sequencing is performed to identify the genomic insertion sites, which are mapped back to the hg38 human genome assemble

BAP1-PBase fusion generated more high-number insertion sites than did the PBase-BAP1 fusion, with higher maximum numbers of transposons per locus (86 for BAP1-PBase vs. 58 for PBase-BAP1).

BAP1 interacts with chromatin near transcription start sites

Many genomic peaks with high numbers of insertions were narrow and centered close to transcription start sites. The distances of each BAP1-PBase or PBase-BAP1 genomic peak to the nearest transcription start site were determined and plotted as histograms (Fig. 3). As a control, we analyzed distances from transcription start sites for randomly selected regions of the genome (Fig. 3). Mann-Whitney U tests revealed that BAP1-PBase and PBase-BAP1 peaks were both significantly closer to transcription start sites ($p < 0.0001$ for both). One concern was that PBase alone might be predisposed to target transposons to open chromatin and thus near active transcription start sites. Comparing BAP1-fusion insertions with all background insertions, we found distances to transcription start sites as highly enriched for both fusions ($p < 0.0001$, Mann-Whitney U tests). Thus, BAP1 binds specifically near transcription start sites.

BAP1 genomic targets show BAP1-dependent gene expression

To ascertain whether genes targeted by BAP1 in the calling card analysis were functionally regulated by BAP1, we performed RNA-Seq on OCM-1A cells depleted of BAP1 by lentiviral shRNAs targeting BAP1. GFP-targeting shRNAs served as a negative control [10]. BAP1 protein levels decreased by 68–74%, compared to GFP controls, by immunoblot (see Additional file 3). BAP1 transcript levels decreased similarly, to 75%, compared to controls based on RNA-seq (see Additional file 4). RNA-Seq results revealed a significant response for 70% (3,565 / 5,033) of BAP1-targeted genes with > 5 insertions. Among the significant gene targets, 22% (784 / 3,565) exhibited greater than two-fold changes in expression in response to BAP1 depletion (Fig. 4a-b and (Additional file 5)). Genes with five or fewer insertions did not show a significant association with expression changes (Fisher's exact test, $p > 0.01$; Fig. 4a). This level of concordance between genomic insertion and expression change is remarkable. By comparison, a study of multiple transcription factors found that less than 15% of transcription factor-bound target genes were perturbed upon knockdown of the transcription factor [26].

We performed pathway and gene ontology analyses on the 784 genes identified by the combination of > 2-fold BAP1-sensitive RNA expression changes and calling-card transposon targeting. The top three pathways enriched for the 244 up-regulated targets were the

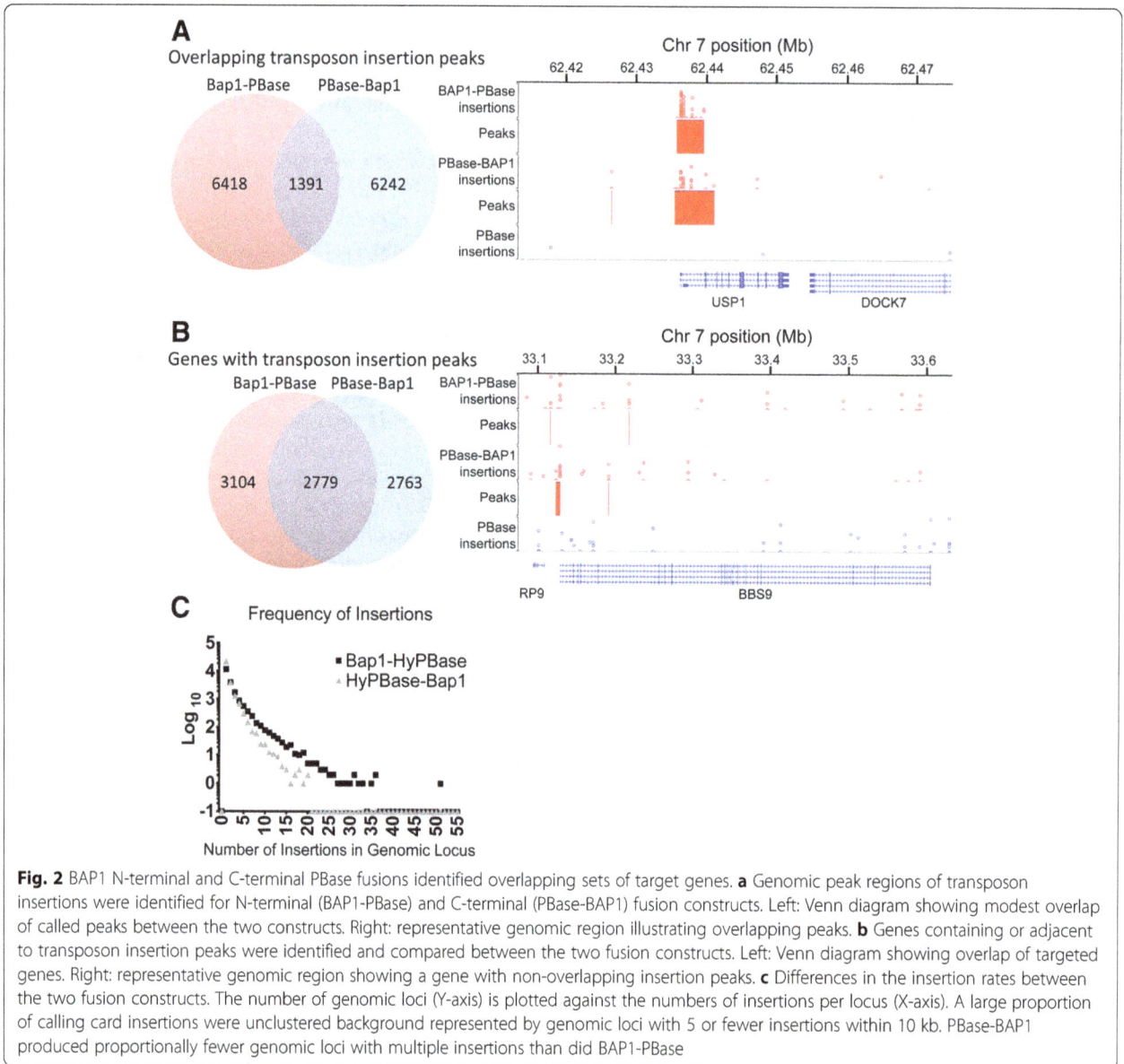

Fig. 2 BAP1 N-terminal and C-terminal PBase fusions identified overlapping sets of target genes. **a** Genomic peak regions of transposon insertions were identified for N-terminal (BAP1-PBase) and C-terminal (PBase-BAP1) fusion constructs. Left: Venn diagram showing modest overlap of called peaks between the two constructs. Right: representative genomic region illustrating overlapping peaks. **b** Genes containing or adjacent to transposon insertion peaks were identified and compared between the two fusion constructs. Left: Venn diagram showing overlap of targeted genes. Right: representative genomic region showing a gene with non-overlapping insertion peaks. **c** Differences in the insertion rates between the two fusion constructs. The number of genomic loci (Y-axis) is plotted against the numbers of insertions per locus (X-axis). A large proportion of calling card insertions were unclustered background represented by genomic loci with 5 or fewer insertions within 10 kb. PBase-BAP1 produced proportionally fewer genomic loci with multiple insertions than did BAP1-PBase

HIF1α, β3-integrin signaling, and p53 signaling pathways (see Additional file 6). The top three pathways enriched for the 540 down-regulated targets were the Gαi (G-protein), PDGF-Rβ signaling, and the EGFR signaling pathways (see Additional file 6). Gene ontology analysis identified significant differential regulation of ontologies associated with development and differentiation, and with the cytoskeleton (Fig. 4c). BAP1-depletion was associated with up-regulation of genes involved in transcription, translation, and protein regulation (Fig. 4c), and down-regulation of genes involved in vesicular transport, membrane formation, and cell projections (Fig. 4c). Two highly significant ($p < 0.001$) molecular signatures were identified by Gene Set Enrichment Analysis of BAP1 calling-card target genes associated with gene expression response to BAP1 depletion (see Additional file 7):

an Epithelial-to-Mesenchymal Transition (EMT) signature was associated with up-regulated genes; and a polycomb-mediated lysine27-trimethylation of histone H3 in Embryonic Stem Cells was associated with down-regulated genes (Fig. 4d). These analyses suggest that, in UM cells, BAP1 coordinates several downstream pathways through its genomic targets that are important to metastatic spread and survival by regulating differentiation, lineage specificity and stemness.

BAP1 is recruited to specific DNA-binding motifs

Our data suggested recruitment of BAP1 to specific genes by DNA-binding proteins, as opposed to random scanning for monoubiquitylated histones. Genomic loci associated with genes that were up-regulated versus down-regulated in response to BAP1 depletion were

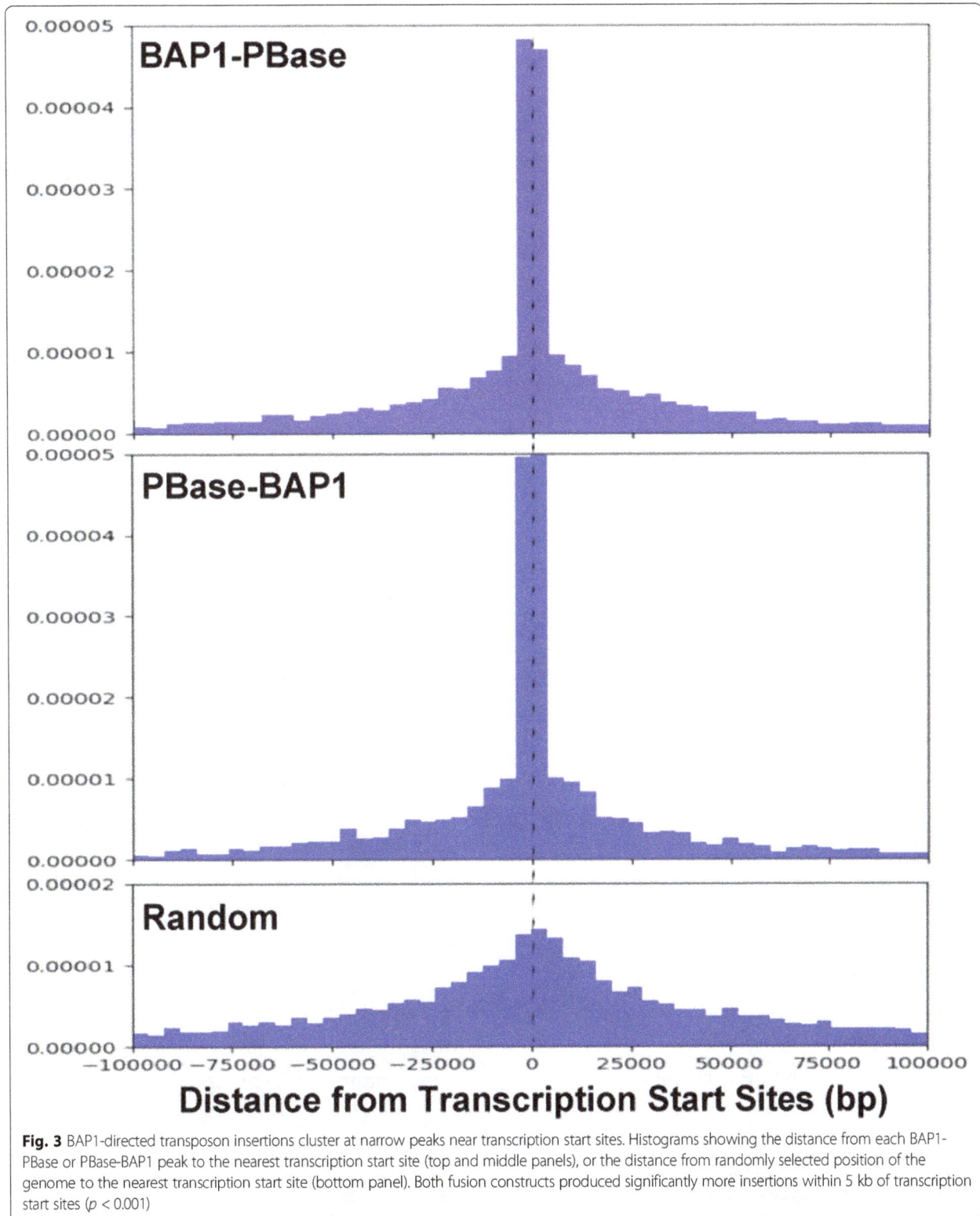

Fig. 3 BAP1-directed transposon insertions cluster at narrow peaks near transcription start sites. Histograms showing the distance from each BAP1-PBase or PBase-BAP1 peak to the nearest transcription start site (top and middle panels), or the distance from randomly selected position of the genome to the nearest transcription start site (bottom panel). Both fusion constructs produced significantly more insertions within 5 kb of transcription start sites ($p < 0.001$)

analyzed separately (see Additional file 8). HOMER analysis is designed for use with large data sets ($\sim 10,000$ peaks), so de novo motif analysis could not be performed due to the small number of peaks in each data set

(approximately 500–600) being analyzed. Enrichment was found for a number of motifs bound by transcription factors that have been previously identified to form complexes with BAP1 [4], including NRF1, Ets factors, and

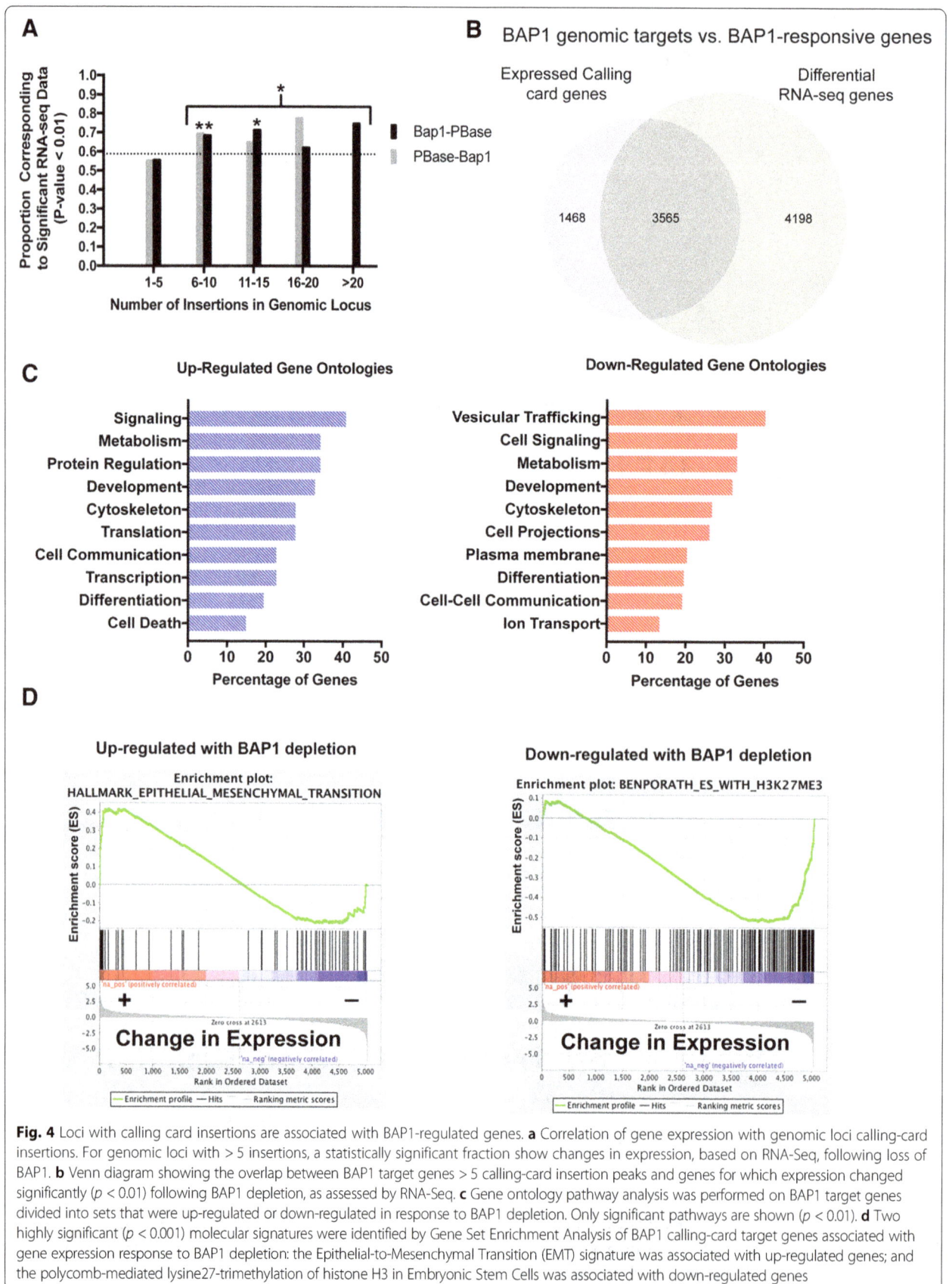

Fig. 4 Loci with calling card insertions are associated with BAP1-regulated genes. **a** Correlation of gene expression with genomic loci calling-card insertions. For genomic loci with > 5 insertions, a statistically significant fraction show changes in expression, based on RNA-Seq, following loss of BAP1. **b** Venn diagram showing the overlap between BAP1 target genes > 5 calling-card insertion peaks and genes for which expression changed significantly ($p < 0.01$) following BAP1 depletion, as assessed by RNA-Seq. **c** Gene ontology pathway analysis was performed on BAP1 target genes divided into sets that were up-regulated or down-regulated in response to BAP1 depletion. Only significant pathways are shown ($p < 0.01$). **d** Two highly significant ($p < 0.001$) molecular signatures were identified by Gene Set Enrichment Analysis of BAP1 calling-card target genes associated with gene expression response to BAP1 depletion: the Epithelial-to-Mesenchymal Transition (EMT) signature was associated with up-regulated genes; and the polycomb-mediated lysine27-trimethylation of histone H3 in Embryonic Stem Cells was associated with down-regulated genes

YY1. Surprisingly, the up- and down-regulated gene sets were both enriched for NRF1 and YY1 suggesting that other transcription factors on the same promoters are determining direction and magnitude of change in gene expression. On the other hand, only up-regulated genes were enriched for Ets factor binding sites, suggesting the existence of a BAP1-containing co-activator complex specifically associated with Ets-factors.

BAP1 calling card targets are linked to the metastatic signature

UM tumors are classified clinically by gene expression profiling of primary tumor samples [6, 27, 28]. We cross-referenced our list of 784 highly significant BAP1 genomic target genes to the list of genes from primary tumor expression analysis [6]. We used comparative marker selection to cluster the genes based on tumor class to determine whether BAP1-responsive genomic target genes correlated with the phenotypic distinction between class 1 and class 2 tumors, (Fig. 5a) (see Additional file 9). We found that a subset of BAP1 targets were able to discriminate molecular class in primary tumors, so we performed unsupervised principal component analysis on the patient sample gene expression data using only genes identified by our analysis as BAP1 genomic targets. This identified a subset of 79 genes able to differentiate class 1

from class 2 tumors with clear discrimination of the tumors into two distinct groups (Fig. 5b). Enrichment analysis of these genes identified targets of ETS2, NF1, E2F4, and ELK1 in the discriminators that were upregulated in Class 2 tumors, and targets of FOXO4, CHX10, and SOX9 in the downregulated discriminators (see Additional file 10). These genes represent a direct link between the genomic function of BAP1 and the metastatic gene expression signature associated with BAP1 loss in UM tumors.

Discussion
Calling card methodology and chromatin modifying factors

The calling card methodology identifies genomic localizations of transcription factors that bind DNA directly [19]. We show that this novel approach can also identify genomic loci occupied by a chromatin-remodeling factor, BAP1, which does not bind to DNA directly. We found that fusions of BAP1 with transposase at either the N-terminus and C-terminus did not impair transposase function, and that while a substantial number (32%) of the genes were identified by both the N-terminal and C-terminal fusion constructs, the majority were identified by only one (Fig. 2b). By combining the lists of

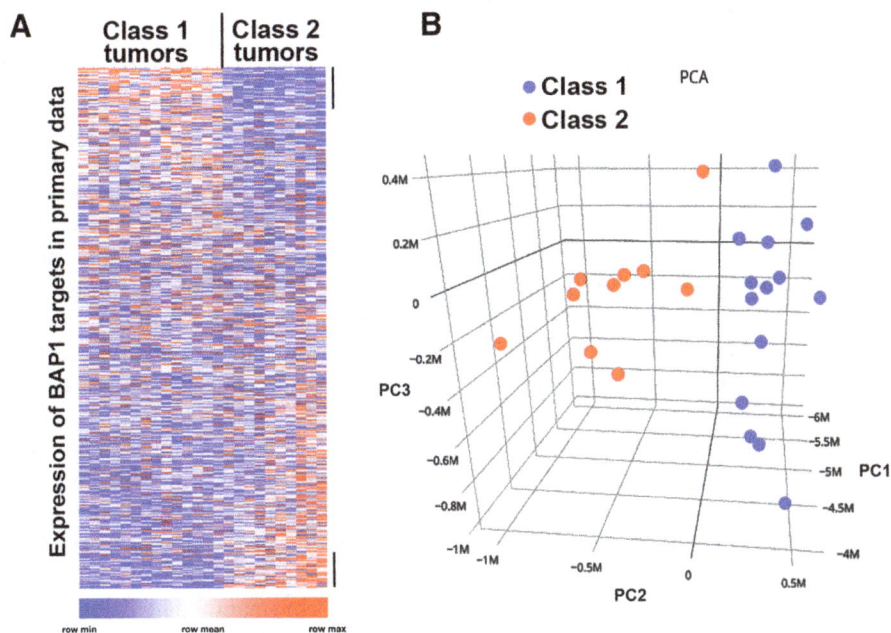

Fig. 5 BAP1 calling-card target genes distinguish molecular class in primary UM tumors. Gene expression values from published microarray data of primary UM tumors [6] were analyzed for genes identified in this study as having BAP1-targeted insertions and significant gene expression response to BAP1 depletion. a Heatmap showing relative gene expression (blue to red) of BAP1 targets in primary UM tumors. Each column is one human tumor. Each row is one gene. Genes were clustered by comparative marker selection based on tumor class (see Additional file 9). Maximum and minimum values were normalized for each row and do not represent global maxima or minima. Black bars indicate genes with significant differential expression (p < 0.01). b Unsupervised principal component analysis of published tumor data using only BAP1 calling card targets shows a portion of genes (principal component 2: PC2) that distinguish class 1 (blue circles) from class 2 (red circles) tumors

results from the two fusions, we generated a substantially larger number of statistically significant genomic loci, which may provide an important insight for future calling card studies of chromatin-remodeling factors.

Genomic recruitment of BAP1 to regulate metastasis and differentiation

Upregulated BAP1-sensitive genes were associated with motif enrichment for Ets factors including ELF1, which has been shown previously in other cell types to co-precipitates with BAP1 [4]. Motifs found in both up-regulated and down-regulated data sets included NRF1 (nuclear respiratory factor 1) and YY1 (yin yang factor 1). NRF1 regulates metabolism, proteasome degradation, and mitochondrial biogenesis [29], and like ELF1, NRF1 has been shown previously in other cell types to co-precipitates with BAP1 [4], YY1 also co-precipitates with BAP1 [4], and YY1 regulates development, cell cycling, tumorigenesis, cell death, and a number of other pathways [30]. We suggest that recruitment of BAP1 by NRF1 and YY1 to specific genes requires the co-recruitment of tissue and lineage specific transcription factors to drive the aggressive nature of class 2 UM tumors.

We found pathways related to Epithelial-to-Mesenchymal Transition (EMT) and embryonic stem cell differentiation affected by depletion of BAP1 in UM cells. Prior studies of gene expression in response to loss of BAP1 have been performed in two other cell types, which showed substantial differences from each other, suggesting that the targets of BAP1 vary depending on cell lineage. In melanocytic cells, BAP1 is important for expression of genes involved in melanoblast and neural crest differentiation [10]. In contrast, in hematopoietic cells, loss of BAP1 affected pathways related to hematopoietic differentiation [31]. Although 45% of these genes were also targets of BAP1 binding in UM cells (35% of calling card genes were in the ChIP-Seq list), none of the hematopoietic differentiation genes responded to BAP1 depletion in our UM cells. In human non-small cell lung carcinoma cells (H1299 cells) [32], BAP1 depletion negatively regulated the FoxK2-target genes *MCM3*, *CDC14a*, and *CDKN1B*. Although two of these (*MCM3* and *CDC14a*) were targets of BAP1 binding in UM cells, we found no significant response in gene expression to BAP1 depletion. Taken together, these observations suggest that BAP1's role in differentiation depends on specific changes in gene expression defined by other lineage-specific regulators. This agrees with our observation that BAP1 is recruited by NRF1 and YY1 to both up- and down-regulated genes. Thus, the pathways regulated by BAP1 that link its loss to metastasis – as it is in UM tumors – also depend on the tissue and lineage contexts of the tumor.

Novel BAP1 targets are sufficient to identify aggressive tumors

The genomic loci identified by the calling card analysis represent bona fide, biologically valid, physiologically relevant targets of BAP1. First, genes adjacent to genomic loci targeted by BAP1 show differential expression when BAP1 is depleted: 70% of genes identified by calling-card analysis showed BAP1-sensitive expression; and conversely, 45% of all BAP1-sensitive genes were adjacent to genomic loci targeted in the calling-card analysis. Second, the genomic insertions identified by calling-card analysis clustered as narrow peaks near gene promoters with motifs known to bind transcription factors that interact with BAP1. Third, and most important, the subset of BAP1-responsive, Calling Card genes identified here are able to discriminate aggressive, class 2 primary tumor samples from human patients.

Identification of class 2 tumors is vital for clinical prognosis of the individual patient [27], and loss of BAP1 expression is seen in > 90% of metastasizing, class 2 tumors [7]. Comparing our BAP1-responsive, calling card target genes with the published expression data from primary UM patient samples [6], we identified several BAP1 genomic targets that were able to discriminate between class 1 and class 2 UM tumors.

Conclusions

We used the calling card methodology to identify the genomic regions occupied by the chromatin-remodeling factor, BAP1, despite its inability to bind directly to DNA. This both expands the possible uses of the calling card technique to other chromatin-remodeling factors – as well as transcriptional co-activators and co-repressors – and identifies for the first time the genomic targets of BAP1 in UM cells. Far from targeting broad regions of modified histones, we found that BAP1 interacts with the genome at narrow regions around transcription start sites and is targeted to these sites by a specific set of DNA motifs. We suggest that BAP1 is recruited by NRF1, YY1, and Ets factors to specific sets of genes that are co-regulated by other tissue and lineage determinants. Importantly, several BAP1 genomic targets were able to discriminate aggressive class 2 UM tumors, demonstrating the first functional link between the role of BAP1 in chromatin remodeling and the phenotypic switch to metastasizing tumors. Moreover, this link suggests that the class 2 gene expression profile may serve as a functional readout for loss of BAP1 activity in UM tumors. Understanding the roles of these class-discriminating BAP1 genomic targets in the broader context of tumor progression will provide new insights into the cellular mechanisms of UM metastasis.

Additional files

Additional file 1: BAP1-PBase genomic peaks. List of genomic regions of transposon insertion from the BAP1-PBase construct giving location, number of insertion events (hops), significance, and nearest gene (Feature).

Additional file 2: PBase-BAP1 genomic peaks. List of genomic regions of transposon insertion from the PBase-BAP1 construct giving location, number of insertion events (hops), significance, and nearest gene (Feature).

Additional file 3: Immunoblot to confirm knockdown of BAP1. Immunoblot of protein collected from the three independent experiments that were used for RNA-seq expressing control or BAP1-specific shRNAs in OCM-1A cells. Specific bands for BAP1 and GAPDH are indicated.

Additional file 4: Table summarizing the RNA-seq results. Differential gene expression results in BAP1-knockdown compared to control OCM-1A cells are shown from the RNA-seq data. Each row gives the unique Ensembl identifier, gene name, and description for each gene, as well as the log of the fold change (logFC), average expression, adjusted *p*-value, and linear fold change.

Additional file 5: BAP1-sensitive calling-card target genes. List of the 784 genes identified by the combination of > 2-fold BAP1-sensitive RNA expression changes and calling-card transposon targeting. Each row gives the gene name, unique Ensembl identifier, and description for each gene. Linear fold change and adjusted p-value in gene expression are from RNA-seq data. Experimental hops, p-value, and fusion construct data are from the calling card experiments.

Additional file 6: Pathways associated with BAP1 target genes. The ten most significant pathways associated with BAP1 calling-card target genes that were up-regulated (positive response) or down-regulated (negative response) in response to BAP1 depletion. Pathways were identified by GSEA.

Additional file 7: GSEA terms associated with BAP1 target genes. Gene set enrichment analysis based on gene expression values for the 784 genes identified by the combination of > 2-fold BAP1-sensitive RNA expression changes and calling-card transposon targeting. Each row gives the name of the curated GSEA term, and the nominal enrichment score, *p*-value, false discovery rate (FDR), family-wise error rate (FWER), and rank-at-max value calculated by the GSEA software.

Additional file 8: DNA motifs associated with BAP1 binding. HOMER was used to identify DNA motifs that were significantly enriched in genomic regions containing BAP1 calling card insertions. Calling card loci were divided into three categories based on response of associated genes to BAP1 depletion, and analyzed separately.

Additional file 9: Heatmap data. Gene expression values from published microarray data of primary UM tumors depicted in heatmap in Fig. 5a. Each row gives the gene rank assigned by comparative marker selection, which molecular class shows upregulation, and the name of each gene. Signal-to-noise ratio (SNR), p-values, false discovery rate (FDR), Bonferroni correction, family-wise error rate (FWER), fold change, means and standard deviations were all calculated by the comparative marker selection software. The original expression values from the published data [6] used to assemble the heatmap are included.

Additional file 10: GSEA terms associated with top BAP1 target genes. Gene set enrichment analysis on the subset of 79 BAP1 targets that were able to discriminate molecular class in primary tumors. Each row gives the name of the curated GSEA term, the number of overlapping genes (size), enrichment score (ES), nominal enrichment score (NES), nominal p-value, false discovery rate (FDR), family-wise error rate (FWER), and rank-at-max value calculated by the GSEA software.

Abbreviations
GO: Gene ontology; GSEA: Gene set enrichment analysis; HOMER: Hypergeometric optimization of motif enrichment; PBase: *piggyBac* transposase; UM: Uveal melanoma

Acknowledgements
The authors are grateful to Dr. Jerry Y. Niederkorn for the OCM-1A UM cell line. The authors are grateful to Jessica Hoisington-Lopez for her expert assistance with the use of the Illumina Genome Analyzer.

Funding
This work was supported by an institutional research grant from the American Cancer Society [to MDO] and grants from the National Institutes of Health [GM118171, GM38542 to JAC]. Funding for open access charge: National Institutes of Health.

Authors' contributions
MY, JAC, RDM and MDO planned the experiments. MY, ZQ, XC, and MDO performed experiments. MY, ZQ, JAC, RDM and MDO analyzed data and provided comments. MY, JAC, RDM and MDO wrote the paper. All authors have read and approved the manuscript.

Competing interests
The authors declare that they have no competing interests.

Author details
[1]Department of Biochemistry and Molecular Biophysics, Washington University School of Medicine, 660 S. Euclid Ave., St. Louis, MO 63110, USA. [2]Department of Genetics and Center for Genome Sciences and Systems Biology, Washington University School of Medicine, 660 S. Euclid Ave., St. Louis, MO 63110, USA.

References
1. Scheuermann JC, de Ayala Alonso AG, Oktaba K, Ly-Hartig N, McGinty RK, Fraterman S, Wilm M, Muir TW, Muller J. Histone H2A deubiquitinase activity of the Polycomb repressive complex PR-DUB. Nature. 2010;465:243–7.
2. Sowa ME, Bennett EJ, Gygi SP, Harper JW. Defining the human deubiquitinating enzyme interaction landscape. Cell. 2009;138:389–403.
3. Tyagi S, Chabes AL, Wysocka J, Herr W. E2F activation of S phase promoters via association with HCF-1 and the MLL family of histone H3K4 methyltransferases. Mol Cell. 2007;27:107–19.
4. Yu H, Mashtalir N, Daou S, Hammond-Martel I, Ross J, Sui G, Hart GW, Rauscher FJ 3rd, Drobetsky E, Milot E, Shi Y, Affar el B. The ubiquitin carboxyl hydrolase BAP1 forms a ternary complex with YY1 and HCF-1 and is a critical regulator of gene expression. Mol Cell Biol. 2010;30:5071–85.
5. Balch CM, Gershenwald JE, Soong SJ, Thompson JF, Atkins MB, Byrd DR, Buzaid AC, Cochran AJ, Coit DG, Ding S, Eggermont AM, Flaherty KT, Gimotty PA, Kirkwood JM, McMasters KM, Mihm MCJ, Morton DL, Ross MI, Sober AJ, Sondak VK. Final version of 2009 AJCC melanoma staging and classification. J Clin Oncol. 2009;27:6199–206.
6. Onken MD, Worley LA, Ehlers JP, Harbour JW. Gene expression profiling in uveal melanoma reveals two molecular classes and predicts metastatic death. Cancer Res. 2004;64:7205–9.
7. van de Nes JA, Nelles J, Kreis S, Metz CH, Hager T, Lohmann DR, Zeschnigk M. Comparing the prognostic value of BAP1 mutation pattern, chromosome 3 status, and BAP1 immunohistochemistry in uveal melanoma. Am J Surg Pathol. 2016;40:796–805.
8. Harbour JW, Onken MD, Roberson ED, Duan S, Cao L, Worley LA, Council ML, Matatall KA, Helms C, Bowcock AM. Frequent mutation of BAP1 in metastasizing uveal melanomas. Science. 2010;330:1410–3.
9. Onken MD, Ehlers JP, Worley LA, Makita J, Yokota Y, Harbour JW. Functional gene expression analysis uncovers phenotypic switch in aggressive uveal melanomas. Cancer Res. 2006;66:4602–9.

10. Matatall KA, Agapova OA, Onken MD, Worley LA, Bowcock AM, Harbour JW. BAP1 deficiency causes loss of melanocytic cell identity in uveal melanoma. BMC Cancer. 2013;13:371.

11. Onken MD, Li J, Cooper JA. Uveal melanoma cells utilize a novel route for Transendothelial migration. PLoS One. 2014;9:e115472.

12. Bott M, Brevet M, Taylor BS, Shimizu S, Ito T, Wang L, Creaney J, Lake RA, Zakowski MF, Reva B, Sander C, Delsite R, Powell S, Zhou Q, Shen R, Olshen A, Rusch V, Ladanyi M. The nuclear deubiquitinase BAP1 is commonly inactivated by somatic mutations and 3p21.1 losses in malignant pleural mesothelioma. Nat Genet. 2011;43:668–72.

13. Pena-Llopis S, Vega-Rubin-de-Celis S, Liao A, Leng N, Pavia-Jimenez A, Wang S, Yamasaki T, Zhrebker L, Sivanand S, Spence P, Kinch L, Hambuch T, Jain S, Lotan Y, Margulis V, Sagalowsky AI, Summerour PB, Kabbani W, Wong SW, Grishin N, Laurent M, Xie XJ, Haudenschild CD, Ross MT, Bentley DR, Kapur P, Brugarolas J. BAP1 loss defines a new class of renal cell carcinoma. Nat Genet. 2012;44:751–9.

14. Wiesner T, Obenauf AC, Murali R, Fried I, Griewank KG, Ulz P, Windpassinger C, Wackernagel W, Loy S, Wolf I, Viale A, Lash AE, Pirun M, Socci ND, Rutten A, Palmedo G, Abramson D, Offit K, Ott A, Becker JC, Cerroni L, Kutzner H, Bastian BC, Speicher MR. Germline mutations in BAP1 predispose to melanocytic tumors. Nat Genet. 2011;43:1018–21.

15. Testa JR, Cheung M, Pei J, Below JE, Tan Y, Sementino E, Cox NJ, Dogan AU, Pass HI, Trusa S, Hesdorffer M, Nasu M, Powers A, Rivera Z, Comertpay S, Tanji M, Gaudino G, Yang H, Carbone M. Germline BAP1 mutations predispose to malignant mesothelioma. Nat Genet. 2011;43:1022–5.

16. Abdel-Rahman MH, Pilarski R, Cebulla CM, Massengill JB, Christopher BN, Boru G, Hovland P, Davidorf FH. Germline BAP1 mutation predisposes to uveal melanoma, lung adenocarcinoma, meningioma, and other cancers. J Med Genet. 2011;48:856–9.

17. Je EM, Lee SH, Yoo NJ. Somatic mutation of a tumor suppressor gene BAP1 is rare in breast, prostate, gastric and colorectal cancers. APMIS. 2012;120:855–6.

18. Dirks RA, Stunnenberg HG, Marks H. Genome-wide epigenomic profiling for biomarker discovery. Clin Epigenetics. 2016;8:122.

19. Wang H, Mayhew D, Chen X, Johnston M, Mitra RD. "Calling cards" for DNA-binding proteins in mammalian cells. Genetics. 2012;190:941–9.

20. Qi Z, Wilkinson MN, Chen X, Sankararaman S, Mayhew D, Mitra RD. An optimized, broadly applicable piggyBac transposon induction system. Nucleic Acids Res. 2017;45:e55. https://doi.org/10.1093/nar/gkw1290.

21. Yusa K, Zhou L, Li MA, Bradley A, Craig NL. A hyperactive piggyBac transposase for mammalian applications. Proc Natl Acad Sci U S A. 2011;108:1531–6.

22. Gibson DG. Enzymatic assembly of overlapping DNA fragments. Methods Enzymol. 2011;498:349–61.

23. Kan-Mitchell J, Mitchell MS, Rao N, Liggett PE. Characterization of uveal melanoma cell lines that grow as xenografts in rabbit eyes. Invest Ophthalmol Vis Sci. 1989;30:829–34 PMID: 2722439.

24. Mooren OL, Li J, Nawas J, Cooper JA. Endothelial cells use dynamic actin to facilitate lymphocyte Transendothelial migration and maintain the monolayer barrier. Mol Biol Cell. 2014;25:4115–29.

25. Subramanian A, Tamayo P, Mootha VK, Mukherjee S, Ebert BL, Gillette MA, Paulovich A, Pomeroy SL, Golub TR, Lander ES, Mesirov JP. Gene set enrichment analysis: a knowledge-based approach for interpreting genome-wide expression profiles. Proc Natl Acad Sci U S A. 2005;102:15545–50.

26. Cusanovich DA, Pavlovic B, Pritchard JK, Gilad Y. The functional consequences of variation in transcription factor binding. PLoS Genet. 2014; 10:e1004226.

27. Onken MD, Worley LA, Tuscan MD, Harbour JW. An accurate, clinically feasible multi-gene expression assay for predicting metastasis in uveal melanoma. J Mol Diagn. 2010;12:461–8.

28. Onken MD, Worley LA, Char DH, Augsburger JJ, Correa ZM, Nudleman E, Aaberg TMJ, Altaweel MM, Bardenstein DS, Finger PT, Gallie BL, Harocopos GJ, Hovland PG, McGowan HD, Milman T, Mruthyunjaya P, Simpson ER, Smith ME, Wilson DJ, Wirostko WJ, Harbour JW. Collaborative ocular oncology group report number 1: prospective validation of a multi-gene prognostic assay in uveal melanoma. Ophthalmology. 2012;119:1596–603.

29. Bugno M, Daniel M, Chepelev NL, Willmore WG. Changing gears in Nrf1 research, from mechanisms of regulation to its role in disease and prevention. Biochim Biophys Acta. 2015;1849:1260–76.

30. Gordon S, Akopyan G, Garban H, Bonavida B. Transcription factor YY1: structure, function, and therapeutic implications in cancer biology. Oncogene. 2006;25:1125–42.

31. Dey A, Seshasayee D, Noubade R, French DM, Liu J, Chaurushiya MS, Kirkpatrick DS, Pham VC, Lill JR, Bakalarski CE, Wu J, Phu L, Katavolos P, LaFave LM, Abdel-Wahab O, Modrusan Z, Seshagiri S, Dong K, Lin Z, Balazs M, Suriben R, Newton K, Hymowitz S, Garcia-Manero G, Martin F, Levine RL, Dixit VM. Loss of the tumor suppressor BAP1 causes myeloid transformation. Science. 2012;337:1541–6.

32. Okino Y, Machida Y, Frankland-Searby S, Machida YJ. BRCA1-associated protein 1 (BAP1) deubiquitinase antagonizes the ubiquitin-mediated activation of FoxK2 target genes. J Biol Chem. 2015;290:1580–91.

19

Current landscape of personalized medicine adoption and implementation in Southeast Asia

Huey Yi Chong[1], Pascale A. Allotey[2] and Nathorn Chaiyakunapruk[1,3,4,5*]

Abstract

Background: The emergence of personalized medicine (PM) has raised some tensions in healthcare systems. PM is expensive and health budgets are constrained - efficient healthcare delivery is therefore critical. Notwithstanding the cost, many countries have started to adopt this novel technology, including resource-limited Southeast Asia (SEA) countries. This study aimed to describe the status of PM adoption in SEA, highlight the challenges and to propose strategies for future development.

Methods: The study included scoping review and key stakeholder interviews in four focus countries – Indonesia, Malaysia, Singapore, and Thailand. The current landscape of PM adoption was evaluated based on an assessment framework of six key themes – healthcare system, governance, access, awareness, implementation, and data. Six PM programs were evaluated for their financing and implementation mechanisms.

Results: The findings revealed SEA has progressed in adopting PM especially Singapore and Thailand. A regional pharmacogenomics research network has been established. However, PM policies and programs vary significantly. As most PM programs are champion-driven and the available funding is limited, the current PM distribution has the potential to widen existing health disparities. Low PM awareness in the society and the absence of political support with financial investment are fundamental barriers. There is a clear need to broaden opportunities for critical discourse about PM especially for policymakers. Multi-stakeholder, multi-country strategies need to be prioritized in order to leverage resources and expertise.

Conclusions: Adopting PM remains in its infancy in SEA. To achieve an effective PM adoption, it is imperative to balance equity issues across diverse populations while improving efficiency in healthcare.

Keywords: Personalized medicine, Pharmacogenomics, Implementation, Southeast Asia

Background

Driven by a spectrum of genomic breakthroughs, personalized medicine (PM) is the central theme across healthcare systems, mainly in the United Kingdom (UK), the United States (US), and the European Union (EU). Commonly, it is known as an emerging field in which the application of specific biological markers, often genetic [1, 2], enables diagnosis and disease management to

be more accurately targeted at the individual patient [3]. By providing "the right treatment to the right patient at the right time", a paradigm shift in healthcare from the current "one-size-fits-all" to a more personalized approach can be realized.

Despite its high cost, many countries have started to adopt this novel PM technology including Southeast Asia (SEA). At the same time, these healthcare systems are striving towards universal health coverage (UHC) to ensure everyone has access to needed health services, without undue financial hardship, financial constraint remains as one of the main challenges in attaining and maintaining UHC [4, 5]. Adopting expensive PM would place increasing strain on the already constrained

---

* Correspondence: nathorn.chaiyakunapruk@monash.edu
[1]School of Pharmacy, Monash University Malaysia, Subang Jaya, Selangor, Malaysia
[3]Center of Pharmaceutical Outcomes Research (CPOR), Department of Pharmacy Practice, Faculty of Pharmaceutical Sciences, Naresuan University, Phitsanulok, Thailand
Full list of author information is available at the end of the article

healthcare budget, further raises concerns on equitable, affordable and sustainable of such healthcare delivery to populations in the context of UHC. Thus, the need of an efficient healthcare delivery is highly critical.

Based on valuable experience from "early adopters", several pressing issues were highlighted: limited availability of evidence for clinical utility; lack of awareness among providers, patients and families; limited access to genetic testing; lack of reimbursement for genetic testing; the need for real-time, point-of-care integration of test results with the electronic health record (EHR) and clinical decision support (CDS) tools; and ethical, legal, and social concerns [6–9]. Primarily, both economic challenges and operational issues present the most significant obstacles to the development of PM adoption and implementation [10, 11]. To harness PM in SEA, changes at multilevel in the healthcare systems are essential to improve the quality of patient care and health system productivity.

Given the complexities of PM adoption and implementation, this study aimed to describe the current policy and program approaches by different stakeholders in SEA to promote PM adoption and implementation, highlight the challenges and to propose strategies for future development.

Methods

The overall methodology of the study was adapted from Shafie et al. [12] and Lim et al [13]. The human research ethics approval was granted by Monash University Human Research Ethics Committee (reference number: 2017–8622).

Study settings

Southeast Asia, a region of 11 countries with 2.2 billion people [13]. Based on the World Bank income categories, this region consists of high-, upper middle-, lower middle-income countries [14]. A total of 4 focus countries were selected and reviewed in this study – Indonesia, Malaysia, Singapore, and Thailand. This was mainly due to the capacity for regional cooperation and openness, and fairly developed national health programs in these countries.

Assessment framework

In this study, the current landscape of PM adoption and implementation in SEA was evaluated using an assessment framework. This framework focused on six major key themes – (i) healthcare system, (ii) governance, (iii) access, (iv) awareness, (v) implementation, and (vi) data (Additional file 1). These were identified through multiple sources from reference countries (the UK, the US, the EU, Australia, and Canada). Sources included PM initiative/strategic plan, published government report, and published literature. The framework was further

supplemented using the World Health Organization (WHO) framework for action in strengthening health systems [15] and the WHO action framework for the Western Pacific region towards UHC [4].

Personalized medicine is not a rigid concept, but rather encompasses different types of technology. Given the diversity and heterogeneity of PM programs available in SEA, six PM programs – targeted oncology therapy/ companion diagnostic, pharmacogenomics (PGx) testing, newborn screening, prenatal diagnosis, cancer risk screening, and advanced multigene sequencing were selected to further evaluate the current financing and integration mechanisms in SEA's healthcare system.

Data sources

A scoping review was undertaken using electronic databases – PubMed, EMBASE, CINAHL, Cochrane Library, and Web of Science, as well as appropriate grey literature, e.g. Ministry of Health websites, published policy documents, and national guidelines, as well as Google Scholar. The search strategy used is presented in Additional file 2. Considering that the completion of human genome sequencing in April 2003 [16], searches were restricted by date from 1 January 2004 to 31 January 2017, further limited to the focus countries. Any literature that reported on the PM adoption was included. Multiple sources of evidence with no restriction on type of study design were included in this review. Data related to the key themes were extracted.

A semi-structured interview with key opinion leaders (KOLs) in four focus SEAs was conducted. These KOLs were researchers and clinicians, identified and contacted through government channels and expert connections. A snowball sampling technique was used in which other potential participants were nominated by initial through connections in the field. An interview guide was developed with open questions surrounding the key themes and any obvious gap collected from the literature review. This guide was validated to address any ambiguity or duplicate. The interviews were conducted from May to July 2017. Interviewees were briefed about the objectives of the research and gave their informed consent to participate and for the interview to be audio-recorded. Country-specific information related to the key themes was extracted from the interview transcript to supplement the findings derived from the review.

In this study, we focused on the current status of PM adoption and implementation in the public healthcare settings. Findings in SEA from literature and interview were then benchmarked with that of any reference countries.

Results

The literature search yielded 9537 articles across 5 electronic databases. After removal of duplicates, there were

9503 unique articles. A total of 698 articles were selected for further screening and 30 articles were included in this study. Furthermore, a number of relevant articles, government guidelines/reports and websites were found from other sources and included in the review - eight journal articles, six government guidelines/reports, and three websites. The list of included articles is presented in Additional file 3. As for the KOL interviews, 11 KOLs from four focus countries participated in the interview. They were researchers ($n = 6$, 55%) and clinicians ($n = 5$, 45%) involved in the provision of PM service in their country. At least 2 KOLs were interviewed from each country. The sociodemographic characteristics of the KOLs interviewed are presented in Table 1.

In general, the four focus SEA countries have made progress towards PM adoption. However, significant heterogeneity of the PM adoption and implementation in terms of the key themes was noted (Table 2). Among them, Singapore and Thailand have made remarkable efforts in PM adoption – an upcoming national PM initiative in Singapore aiming for a nationwide PM adoption, while Thailand has progressed ahead with the introduction of PGx card for patients. On the other hand, PM-related activities remain largely in the research stage and/or as special clinical services in selected national hospitals and university hospitals in Malaysia and Indonesia. A regional research group – South East Asian Pharmacogenomics Research Network (SEAPharm) has been established with six Asian countries (Japan, Korea, Indonesia, Malaysia, Taiwan, and Thailand), and the latest additions of Singapore and Vietnam. This was initiated by Thailand and Japan – Thailand Centre of Excellence for Life Sciences (TCELS), Department of Medical Sciences in Ministry of Public Health (MOPH), Ramathibodi Hospital in Mahidol University, and Riken Centre for Integrative Medical Sciences.

Table 1 Sociodemographic characteristics of key opinion leaders participated ($n = 11$) in the interview

Sociodemographic variables	N	%
Gender ($n = 11$)		
Male	6	55
Female	5	45
Country ($n = 11$)		
Indonesia	2	18
Malaysia	4	36
Singapore	2	18
Thailand	3	28
Professional role ($n = 11$)		
Clinician	5	45
Researcher	6	55

Healthcare systems

The healthcare delivery capabilities and financing among these focus countries vary. Majority of the countries have relatively high healthcare coverage, 98–100%. However, an alarmingly high out-of-pocket (OOP) expenditure of more than 40% was noted in Indonesia (46.9%) and Singapore (54.8%). To date, a national PM initiative is yet to be implemented except Singapore, a high-income country (HIC) is in the drafting process. Furthermore, Thailand, a developing low- and middle-income country (LMIC), has been engaging in PGx research since 2004 through the Thai PGx Project with investments from TCELS.

Besides targeted oncology therapy/companion diagnostics and newborn screening are delivered as routine practice in four focus countries, the availability of other PM programs is limited, either in a few major tertiary/university hospitals or in the research stage. Interestingly, PGx testing of *HLA-B*15:02* prior to carbamazepine (CBZ) initiation has been incorporated as the standard of care in Singapore and Thailand.

In terms of PM-specific healthcare providers, the workforce remains insufficient – 2 cancer clinical geneticist in Singapore, 6 (Singapore) to 22 (Thailand) clinical/medical geneticists, and approximately 2–20 genetic counsellors in Malaysia and Singapore. At present, genetic counsellor is not commonly available as there is no official position within Malaysia's Ministry of Health (MOH), while no formal training of genetic counsellor in Thailand as well.

Governance

The absence of governance and legislation in the provision of PM and genetic data, neither specific guideline nor regulation is formalized among all focus countries. Nevertheless, there are a few frameworks related to genomics/genetics already in place. As early as 2004, Thailand promulgated the National Biotechnology Policy Framework 2004–2009, where genomics and bioinformatics were identified as key strategy areas for improving the health of the Thai people, developing new bio-businesses as well as creating a self-sufficient economy. In Malaysia and Singapore, a national guideline on medical genetics service and/or genetic testing provides some degree of ethical oversights on the use of genetic in healthcare.

Since genetic data is categorized as medical data, thus its confidentiality is governed under the existing legislation in each country. In addition, recommendations on issues – the protection of privacy and confidentiality of genetic information in biomedical research, and access to genetic information by employers and insurers are governed under the national guideline aforementioned in Malaysia and Singapore. Only Singapore is drafting a PM-specific provision standard that incorporates the

Table 2 Current PM adoption in four focus SEA countries based on six key themes

Key themes	Indicators	Indonesia	Malaysia	Singapore	Thailand
Healthcare system	General				
	GDP per capita (Current USD)	3500	11,306	56,007	5970
	Healthcare financing system	Social health insurance	Tax-funded	Mixture from tax revenue, insurer and patient	Social health insurance
	Healthcare expenditure per capita (USD)	99	456	2752	360
	THE (% of GDP, 2014)	2.8	4.2	4.9	6.5
	Health coverage (%)	48	100	100	98
	OOP health expenditure (% of THE, 2014)	46.9	35.3	54.8	7.9
	PM-specific				
	Presence of PM-related healthcare service delivery				
	1. Targeted oncology therapy	Yes	Yes	Yes	Yes
	2. PGx testing	No[a]	No[a]	Yes[b]	Yes[c]
	3. Newborn screening	Yes (congenital hypothyroidism)	Yes (congenital hypothyroidism, G6PD)	Yes (congenital hypothyroidism, G6PD, inherited metabolic disorders)	Yes (congenital hypothyroidism, thalassemia, phenylketonuria)
	4. Cancer risk screening	No[a]	Yes[d]	Yes[d]	No[a]
	5. Advance genome sequencing	No	No	Yes[e]	Yes[e]
	Presence of PM-related healthcare workforce				
	1. Medical geneticist	Yes (NR)	Yes (9)	Yes (6 + 2 cancer geneticist)	Yes (11)
	2. Genetic counsellors	Yes (NR)	Yes (2)	Yes (≈10)	No
	Financing mechanism				
	1. Capacity-building	NR	NR	NR	NR
	2. Infrastructure	NR	NR	NR	NR
	3. Research	Cyclic grants from government, university, international collaborators	Cyclic, one-off grant from government, university	Funding from A*STAR	Cyclic, one-off grant from government, university
Governance	National strategy/plan	No	No	National PM initiative (in progress)	No
	Comprehensive PM legislation/guideline	No	No[f]	No[f]	No
	Ethical, social, legal framework on PM provision	No	No	PM-specific provision standard is in progress	No
	Ethical, social, legal framework for genetic data	No	Yes, but no laws related to genetic discrimination by insurance companies	PM-specific standard is in progress[g]	Yes, but no laws related to genetic discrimination by insurance companies
	National PM research centre or large-scale research initiative	No	No	GIS; POLARIS; SAPhIRE; PRISM	PGx projects by TCELS
	Direct to consumer test legislation or code of conduct	No	No	Bioethics Advisory Committee recommendations	Existing consumer law
	PM working group with multiple stakeholders	No	No	Yes	Yes

Table 2 Current PM adoption in four focus SEA countries based on six key themes *(Continued)*

Key themes	Indicators	Indonesia	Malaysia	Singapore	Thailand
Access	HTA body	Yes Major hospitals	Yes National	Yes National	Yes National
	PM-specific HTA framework	No	No	No[h]	No
	Multi-stakeholder decision-making group	Yes	Yes	Yes	Yes
Awareness	Patient support/advocacy groups	No	Yes	Yes, but not specific	Yes, but not specific
	Efforts to increase public awareness	Yes	Yes	Yes	Yes
	Patient involvement in healthcare and/or research	Low in research	Low in research	Moderate in research	High in research
Implementation	Centre of excellence/leading institute in PM service	Dr Cipto Mangunkusumo Hospital; Center for Biomedical Research in Diponegoro University	Institute of Medical Research	PRISM	Ramathibodi Hospital; Khon Kaen University Hospital; Siriraj Hospital
	Education and training for PM and non-PM specialized healthcare workforce including medical school	Yes	Yes	Yes	Yes
Data	EHR	No	No	Yes	Yes
	Biobank	Hospital-level biobanks	Malaysian Cohort Biobank; UKMMC-UMBI Biobank	SingHealth Tissue Repository; National University Health System Tissue Repository	Hospital-level biobanks
	Database	Indonesian National Genetic Database	Malaysian Human Variome Project	Singapore Genome Variation Project database; Singapore Human Mutation/ Polymorphism Database; Singapore PGx Portal	Thailand Mutation and Variation database
	Patient registry with genetic/genomic data	No	Thalassemia Registry	Singapore Polyposis Registry; Thalassemia Registry; National Birth Defect Registry	No

Notes
[a] Available through special request
[b] HLA-B*15:02 screening is mandatory in Singapore. UGT1A*6 and UGT1A1*28 testing are available in National Cancer Centre
[c] HLA-B*15:02 screening is routinely practised in major hospitals. A variety of other PGx testings are available as service in several university hospitals
[d] BRCA screening is available in a few national/university/ specialised hospitals: University Malaya Medical Centre, Hospital Kuala Lumpur in Malaysia; National Cancer Centre Singapore, National University Hospital in Singapore
[e] Next-generation sequencing is available in leading hospital: SingHealth-POLARIS in Singapore; Ramathibodi Hospital in Thailand
[f] Some degree of ethical oversights are governed under the existing national medical genetics service and/or genetic testing guideline
[g] Includes informed consent, security and confidentiality of information, and disclosure of test results to third parties outside direct healthcare providers
[h] Genetic test is evaluated as medical device

Abbreviations
*A*STAR* Agency for Science and Technology Research, *EHR* electronic health record, *GDP* gross domestic product, *GIS* Genome Institute of Singapore, *HTA* health technology assessment, *NR* not reported or insufficient information, *OOP* out-of-pocket, *PGx* pharmacogenomics, *PM* personalized medicine, *POLARIS* Personalized OMIC Lattice for Advanced Research and Improving Stratification, *PRISM* SingHealth Duke-NUS Institute of Precision Medicine, *SAPhIRE* Surveillance and Pharmacogenomics Initiative for Adverse Drug Reactions, *TCELS* Thailand Centre of Excellence Life Sciences, *THE* total health expenditure, *UKMMC* University Kebangsaan Malaysia Medical Centre, *UMBI* UKM Medical Biology Institute, *USD* United States dollar

ethical, social, legal framework of this provision in healthcare and genetic data.

Local PM research plays an integral role in improving the ability to respond to local disease threats by translating locally discovered genomic biomarkers into clinical applications. In all focus countries, research is mostly conducted at the institutional level, with the support of cyclic grants from government, university, or international collaborators. Furthermore, insufficient funding remains one of the main challenges to sustain PM research. Only a few large-scale research initiatives in Singapore and Thailand have been funded with considerable governmental financial supports such as Singapore's Agency for Science and Technology Research (A*STAR) and Thailand's TCELS, a public organization under the Thai Ministry of Science and Technology.

In Singapore, there are several major players – government agency, clinician, and researcher/academia driving the development of PM adoption. Since 2000, a cascade of major development strategies ranging from research to clinical application marks an important milestone in the roadmap of Singapore's PM adoption (Table 3). Notably, the SingHealth Duke-National University Singapore Institute of Precision Medicine (PRISM) is one of key drivers underpinning the upcoming national PM initiative. Under PRISM's initiative, a multi-dimensional database, "SPECTRA" will be developed from 5000 healthy Asian volunteers that incorporates genomic, clinical, lifestyle, and imaging data, subsequently to serve as reference database for disease-oriented studies by specialty centers and across the nation.

While in Thailand, a genotyping initiative was launched in consistence with the Thai biotechnology policy framework. Catalyzed by an initial investment of THB 120 million by TCELS, six PGx projects were initiated on diseases common among Thai – human immunodeficiency virus, CBZ- and allopurinol-induced severe cutaneous adverse reactions (SCARs), acute childhood lymphoblastic leukemia, oncology chemotherapy, aspirin responsiveness, and thalassemia-hemoglobin E.

As part of the SEAPharm's collaborative effort, "100 Pharmacogene Project" has been recently announced. This will involve genomes sequencing from 1000 patients from 10 SEA participating members. A pharmacogene database will be produced consisting of genetic variations of 100 pharmacogenes associated with drug efficacy and safety among SEA populations. At the same time, a research guideline will be proposed to support this regional, large-scale research work.

In the UK, PM adoption in the National Health Service (NHS) has been long supported by high-level political endorsement [17]. A national strategic vision has been set out by the Human Genomics Strategy Group through specific recommendations on steps needed for the NHS to benefit from PM adoption. These recommendations include (i) translating genomic innovation into quality-assured care pathways; (ii) developing an equitable, affordable, and high-quality service delivery; (iii) setting up the bioinformatics platform; (iv) preparing the workforce; (v) developing the legal and ethical framework; and (vi) engaging the public and building awareness [18]. Furthermore, specific funding has been allocated for development of policies on genomics in healthcare, approximately €200,000 per year in the UK [19]. At present, PM research continues to receive substantial investment from the federal government in the UK, the US, and Canada [18, 20, 21]. Similarly, in Australia, the recognition of strong leadership and governance in PM adoption will be substantiated, in consistence with the call in the upcoming National Health Genomics Policy Framework as the most critical priority area to be addressed. Consequently, improvements in all other priority areas of the Framework would be achieved accordingly. With the joint national leadership and strong governance arrangements at the state, national, international levels, nationally unified directions will be provided to promote consistent and coordinated implementation of activities across Australia in the integration of genomics into the Australian health system [22].

Access

Despite the upsurge of health technology assessments (HTAs) and the corresponding bodies in four focus countries at the national or hospital level, current

Table 3 Major milestones in the development of PM adoption in Singapore

Year	Organisation/ Initiative	Funder/Collaboration	Aim
2000	GIS[i]	A*STAR	To use genomic sciences to achieve improvements in human health and public prosperity
2013	POLARIS	GIS, SingHealth	To deliver better patient outcomes through research within SingHealth institutions[j]
2014	SAPhIRE	BMRC and the HSA, GIS, and the Translational Laboratory for Genetic Medicine	To develop an active surveillance network for ADR monitoring and discovery of genomic biomarkers that are predictive of specific ADRs
2015	PRISM	SingHealth and Duke-NUS Medical School	To drive, promote and standardize the use of PM and Precision Health for improving patient care, focusing on diseases relevant to Asian populations

Notes

[i] National flagship program for the genomic sciences

[j] This includes Singapore General Hospital, National Cancer Centre Singapore, Singapore National Eye Centre, and NUS Health System

Abbreviations

A*STAR Agency for Science and Technology Research, ADR adverse drug reaction, BMRC Biomedical Research Council, GIS Genome Institute of Singapore, HSA Health Sciences Authority, NUS National University of Singapore, POLARIS Personalised OMIC Lattice for Advanced Research and Improving Stratification, PRISM SingHealth Duke-National University Singapore Institute of Precision Medicine, SAPhIRE Surveillance and Pharmacogenomics Initiative for Adverse Drug Reactions

approaches to economic evaluation to support decision making are largely focused on reimbursement of drug. Given the absence of specific HTA framework for PM interventions, the current HTA state to comprehensively guide decisions on the reimbursement and coverage of PM is limited. Among the four focus countries, only Singapore's Agency of Care Effectiveness is currently evaluating genetic testing as medical device.

In addition, many jurisdictions have adopted a cost-effective threshold to guide the decision-making process [23]. It is revealed that the application of a general threshold of THB 160,000 per quality-adjusted life year gained for oncology PM in Thailand [24].

The Pharmaceutical Benefits Advisory Committee in Australia has introduced a guideline for HTA submission of hybrid technologies and co-dependent technologies. This includes clinical evaluation on evidence related to prognostic effect of the biomarker, performance and accuracy of the proposed test, change in clinical management, and clinical evaluation of the co-dependent technologies, as well as economic evaluation that captures both accurate and inaccurate test results among eligible population [25, 26]. While the UK Genetic Testing Network Steering Group has endorsed and adapted the analytic validity, clinical validity, clinical utility, and ethical, legal and social issues as core principles to produce a "Gene Dossier" for evaluating genetic tests in the NHS [27]. Furthermore, the UK National Institute for Health and Care Excellence evaluates companion diagnostics using either the Diagnostics Assessment Program or the Technology Appraisal process with the focus of incorporating clinical evidence in terms of the test's predictive value and ability to identify the eligible patient population [28, 29].

Awareness

A lack of specific information on genetic/genomic available to the public and patients, corresponding to the poor awareness of PM, except for oncology-related information from various sources – digital media, the existing patient advocacy and support groups such as information dissemination on *BRCA1* and *BRCA2* genetic screening by the Breast Cancer Singapore, awareness campaigns on cancer and related research by Cancer Research Malaysia including *BRCA* genetic screening, as well as the Hereditary Breast and Ovarian Cancer Campaign by Cancer Advocacy Society of Malaysia. Through online education, information related to targeted oncology therapy for the treatment of breast cancer and *HER2* in breast cancer is made available by the National University Hospital Singapore and the "Yayasan Kanser Payudara Indonesia" (Indonesia Breast Cancer Association). Beyond oncology, there is a general trend that education efforts are uncommon and clinicians are often the main source of information at the point-of-care.

In Thailand, education programs on PGx testings have been actively carried out by the TCELS and Ramathibodi Hospital. As a result, several PGx books and reports were released for decision makers, clinicians, scientists, and layman. Notably, an educational PGx mobile application is developed to raise the awareness on PGx among patients and public.

As part of the EU's International Consortium for PM (ICPerMed) Action Plan, a European Knowledge Platform will be developed to improve both health and digital literacy using web-based and social media instruments over short and medium term. Best practices of patient engagement approaches will be developed to enhance patients' experience and their need to participate and make informed decision on their healthcare, as well as their involvement in all phases of PM's research and development [30]. Several important European organizations are aiming to promote the ideas of PM. Among them, the European Alliance for Personalized Medicine collaborates with health experts and patient advocates through developing case studies, organizing workshops, education, training, and communication [31].

Implementation

Overall, a few major healthcare institutes have been leading in the provision of PM programs as their service in four focus countries. Unlike targeted oncology therapy/companion diagnostics with supports from manufacturers, the availability and integration of other PM programs are mainly driven by successful research projects previously conducted by local champions. This corresponds to the availability of these services are mainly in the national capital or university hospitals.

The availability of clinical expertise varies widely across the region with an overall significant lack of genetic expertise. Although genetics/genomics are integrated into the medical school curricula, continuing education and training for healthcare providers remains to be insufficient in all focus countries as there is neither formal training program nor capacity building program in place.

In Thailand, the launching of PGx card by Ramathibodi Hospital represents an important progress in PM adoption. It aims to summarize patients' *HLA* gene variant information predicting risk of developing SCARs from specific drugs.

In the UK, NHS England specialized services has progressed in setting up a network consisting of genomic technology centers, biomedical diagnostic hubs and regional genetics centers. This enables NHS to advance the use of genomic information into mainstream clinical medicine. New education and training programs have been developed and implemented across the UK as part of the Department of Health Modernizing Scientific

Careers program. The programs aim to ensure training for whole NHS workforce on genomics and PM [18].

Data

Genetic/genomic data is complex and its significance to the individual patient changes throughout the patient's life. The EHR implementation is an important tool in PM adoption especially the support using a CDS enables clinicians in making informed decisions at the point-of-care. However, a nationwide EHR system is available in Singapore and Thailand.

Furthermore, patient registry is critical in the management of genetic diseases. Although there are patient registries with genetic data in Malaysia and Singapore, only Singapore Polyposis Registry and Singapore Thalassemia Registry are utilized to facilitate identification, surveillance and management of families and individuals at high risk of colorectal cancer and thalassemia. For research purposes, several genetic databases and/or biobanks have been established, either at the national or hospital level in all focus countries.

In the UK, work is underway in consistence with the NHS Paperless 2020 program through NHS digital. This aims to create a fully interoperable EHR (incorporating genomic, clinical and diagnostic, medicines, and lifestyle data), supported by information sharing and data linkage [32]. In the early 2000s, the Electronic Medical Records and Genomics Network, a US National Human Genome Research Institute–funded consortium that combines genomic with EHR for large scale, high-throughput genetic research in support of implementing genomic medicine [33]. It has demonstrated that data captured through routine clinical care are sufficient to generate findings for large-scale genetic research. Data harmonization, an important issue needs to be addressed when dealing with a spectrum of big data generated from PM research. As part of the EU's ICPerMed Action Plan, research will be undertaken to ensure the appropriate alignment of existing and future datasets with important information for PM, thus promoting the development and implementation of existing as well as innovative PM strategies along the value chain [30].

Comparison of the financing and implementation of PM programs

Among six PM programs investigated, information gathered related to 3 of these programs was sufficient to make a meaningful comparison of their financing and integration mechanisms (Table 4). Thus, this comparison included (i) trastuzumab/HER2 testing for targeted oncology therapy, (ii) HLA-B*15:02 screening for PGx testing, and (iii) congenital hypothyroidism screening for newborn screening. Unlike trastuzumab/HER2 testing and congenital hypothyroidism screening are provided

routinely in all focus countries, HLA-B*15:02 screening is available as the standard care in Singapore and Thailand, but not in Malaysia and Indonesia despite the high allele frequency in SEA (> 15%) [34].

Trastuzumab was introduced into the market with enormous manufacturer support including, but not limited to the sponsorship of HER2 testing and the readily available clinical and economic evidence. The remaining two PM programs are champion-driven, predominantly by clinicians. The HLA-B*15:02 screening was initiated by the Health Sciences Authority (HSA)'s pharmacovigilance unit in Singapore, while in Thailand by clinicians and MOPH. The congenital hypothyroidism screening was introduced since 1990s in all focus countries except Indonesia in 2008 by the association of pediatricians. Both involved a lengthy process to advocate their adoption. Apart from HTA studies, locally-conducted observational pilot studies were employed to demonstrate the value of this screening to policymakers.

Limited funding remains a major hurdle for a widespread PM service. This is most evident in Indonesia, up to today, the financial allocation has never been adequate for all newborns to be screened for congenital hypothyroidism after 9 years of its nationwide introduction in 2008. Even though the coverage of trastuzumab/HER2 testing by national health programs, these are publicly reimbursed with the existing, tight budget allocation in Malaysia or partially subsidized under the "Medication Assistance Fund" in Singapore. However, in Indonesia, HER2 testing is not covered under the national health insurance scheme. As for HLA-B*15:02 screening, its reimbursement policy is highly dependent on the cost of genetic testing in Thailand (<THB 1000). While in Singapore, multi-stakeholder discussions with clinicians, HSA were held to address pertinent issues to further reduce the genotyping cost and turnaround time prior to its mandatory implementation [35]. Today, it is partially subsidized up to 75%.

The integration of the PM programs into healthcare varies significantly. For trastuzumab/HER2 testing, its integration as a package has been largely supported by the relevant manufacturers. This usually follows with consistent, timely changes in both international and local clinical practice guidelines. This has led to a more successful PM oncology application due to the adequate level of awareness and education on PM among oncologists. On the other hand, various efforts were introduced for HLA-B*15:02 screening by MOH and clinicians, including the issuance of a "Dear Healthcare Professional Letter" on HLA-B*15:02 screening prior to CBZ as the standard of care, and its recommendation in product insert in Singapore; a warning inserted on the association of HLA-B*15:02 and SCARs with CBZ use in the Thai clinical practice guideline for epilepsy. Furthermore, to better

Table 4 Comparison of the financing and integration mechanisms of three most common PM programs in SEA

Indicators		Targeted oncology therapy and companion diagnostic	Pharmacogenomics testing	Newborn screening
		Trastuzumab	HLA-B*15:02	Congenital hypothyroidism
Availability as routine practice	Yes	Indonesia Malaysia Singapore Thailand	Singapore (nationwide) Thailand (major hospitals)	Indonesia (10 provinces in 2017) Malaysia Singapore Thailand
	No	–	Malaysia (special request) Indonesia (research)	–
Stakeholder that initiated the PM program	Pharmaceutical company	Indonesia Malaysia Singapore Thailand	–	–
	Clinicians	–	Singapore Thailand	Indonesia Malaysia Singapore Thailand
Financing mechanism	Covered in national health program	Indonesia (HER2 testing as OOP expenses) Malaysia Thailand	Thailand (Cap at THB1000)	Indonesia (Limited budget) Malaysia Thailand
	Partial subsidy by the national health programs	Singapore (under Medical Assistance Fund scheme)	Singapore (Up to 75% subsidy)	Singapore (60% subsidy)
Monitoring framework	Clinical outcome	Malaysia (in future plan) Thailand	Singapore	–
Integration in healthcare	Change in local clinical practice guideline	Indonesia Malaysia Singapore Thailand	Thailand Singapore	Indonesia Malaysia Singapore Thailand
	Availability of CDS in EHR	NR	Singapore Thailand (some hospitals)	NA
Presence of healthcare information	Physician	Indonesia Malaysia Singapore Thailand	Singapore Thailand	Indonesia Malaysia Singapore Thailand
	Patient	Singapore	Thailand	Indonesia Malaysia Singapore Thailand

Abbreviations
CDS clinical decision support, *EHR* electronic health record, *NA* not applicable, *NR* not reported or insufficient information, *OOP* out-of-pocket, *THB* Thai Baht

integrate *HLA-B*15:02* screening into the clinical practice, CDS within the EHR system has been deployed in Singapore and Thailand. But for congenital hypothyroidism screening, the information is made available through routine educational programs or at point-of-care by physician during an antenatal care.

To date, outcomes of all PM programs have not been monitored in a standardized framework, with clinical audits for trastuzumab in the future planning. For *HLA-B*15:02* screening in Singapore, the clinical outcome monitoring was based on the number of CBZ-related SCARs reported. Since the initiation of testing in 2013, no cases have been reported to the HSA's pharmacovigilance unit.

Discussion

In general, there is increasing interest among clinicians and researchers in PM in SEA. However, due to functional silo of each stakeholder especially clinicians, the PM output and effort are fragmented at the institutional level. At the same time, majority of healthcare systems in SEA are still facing fundamental issues in providing basic healthcare services to all citizens. As a result, the current PM adoption is slow and haphazard across SEA. To adopt PM as a national health agenda, ensuring sustainable funding and consistent political support are central for the capacity building of expertise and infrastructure at both research and clinical settings.

From the broad overview of PM initiatives across the focus countries in SEA, we have developed the following observations and recommendations:

(1) Wide variations of PM adoption and implementation across the region.
   The increasing efforts in adopting and implementing various PM programs are driven by local champions. These services are predominantly located at the more affluent parts of the country. In addition, the limited funding remains a challenge to sustain PM delivery. For the example, despite the coverage of trastuzumab under the national health program in all focus countries, HER2 testing remains as an OOP expense in Indonesia. An equitable patient access to trastuzumab is limited as HER2 testing is more readily affordable among the rich. It is also worth noting that there is a potential risk of financial burden among trastuzumab patients in Malaysia as its provision is highly dependent on the existing limited budget allocation. Thus, the current implementation and distribution of PM programs has the potential to widen the existing health disparities, and realization of its potential can be uneven.
   The problem with inequitable patient access may be further aggravated by the low awareness on genetics/genomics and PM among patients and public. In consistence with evidence of increasing disparities in the uptake of PM in the US, these low levels of awareness will reduce patient requests for testing, in turn decreasing the testing rate among eligible minority patients [36]. This is further supported by the lack of familiarity with PM, even in the US, 73% of individuals not having heard the term [37]. Clearly, there is a need to increase health literacy on PM's value proposition among patients, leading to an improved in the access to PM services, as well as achieving equity in PM. Moreover, with patient empowerment in their healthcare, this helps accelerate strategies to overcome other barriers in PM adoption [38].

(2) The situation across SEA countries offers substantial improvement opportunities for all aspects.
   Despite some countries have more policies and support structures in place than others, significant gaps are present for all aspects, particularly the absence of governance in PM. Effective governance at the system level is the cornerstone in shaping a robust PM policy framework. Essentially, high-level commitment from a wide range of stakeholders is critical in this interactive, multi-centric process. Thus, key stakeholders are coordinated and jointly working towards an agreed institutional goal and expectation in PM adoption.

Another notable bottleneck to PM adoption is the lack of information and communication technology platform in this region, including the need for improved CDS capabilities in an EHR. As genomic information is complex in nature, the primary role of CDS should focus on collect, disseminate, process complex health information at the point-of-care. However, this complexity increases with the latest update from additional guidelines and the discovery of clinically important gene-drug relationships [39]. Clearly, EHR represents an essential component to be integrated, and a significant need to develop a CDS framework capable of leveraging complex information on a widespread scale. Furthermore, the genetics/genomics competency among the healthcare workforce is a fundamental building block in this PM transformation. Due to the current shortage of PM specialist, it is particularly important for non-PM specialized health professionals such as primary care providers to provide PM services [40]. Since 2007, the US National Coalition for Health Professional Education in Genetics has outlined a minimum set of core competencies – knowledge, skills, and attitude for all health professionals from all disciplines [41]. In the primary care settings, essential skills among non-PM health professionals include taking family histories, conducting family-history assessments, interpret results of genetic tests, provide genetics/genomics education to patients, and make appropriate referrals for genetic evaluation [41, 42]. Despite the availability of many education programs for non-PM health professionals [40], recent surveys reveal they remain unprepared at large [43–46], demonstrating knowledge gaps [47]. To address this, strengthening the existing educational/training programs is at prime time [40] to more robust, rigorous pre- and post-graduate programs integrated with genomics curriculum. It is worth highlighting that developing additional educational programs for other disciplines of nongenetic health professionals is desirable. For example, the availability of an in-house pharmacists increases the utilization of PGx testing in a primary care setting [48]. The potential leading role of pharmacist in PGx adoption is further emphasized by a KOL in our interview. Therefore, by leveraging the strengths of each healthcare discipline through a competent multidisciplinary clinical team, patient care can be improved significantly with PM advancement.

The access of PM requires immediate attention. Several related aspects represent major challenges for PM adoption in SEA – the lack of cost-effectiveness evidence for PM, the inadequacy of

HTA approach for PM, and the use of a fixed cost-effectiveness threshold. Apart from Thailand, the HTA bodies in other SEA countries are in an early stage. With substantial limited human capacity, this impedes the synthesis of local cost-effectiveness data. Nevertheless, such data is especially critical to make a nuanced decision involving the uptake of high-cost PM in resource-limited SEA countries. Moreover, the current approach used to evaluate PM have been criticized as it falls short in demonstrating the multidimensional value of PM. Due to the high cost of PM and the emerging evidence base derived from a small subgroup of patients, imprecise, unfavorable cost-effectiveness findings of PM are often resulted against a fixed cost-effective threshold [49]. As a result, the delay in patient access to PM is more pronounced with further deterioration of health outcomes in SEA. To better allocate scarce resources and allow timely patient access, several strategies are essential to improve the decision-making framework – (i) investment on capacity building on HTA [50]; (ii) refinement of the current assessment approach and tool to address the greater complexity exerts by PM [51]; and (iii) the use of multicriteria decision analysis may assist in guiding the proper valuation of PM in a consistency and transparent manner [49, 52].

(3) PM adoption poses tremendous challenge across the region, as the upfront costs remain high and resources are limited.

At present, most of the SEA region are not only prioritizing chronic and communicable diseases [12], but also facing financing challenges due to the rapid demographic transition [53]. This current situation renders a strong skepticism around costly PM adoption. An augmented concern in which the financial sustainability of current basic UHC might be undermined due to PM. Despite the plummeting cost of genome sequencing with time, the high start-up costs arising from setting up infrastructure, human development, and education and research are seen as significant obstacles [54]. Although financial stability appears to be a prerequisite for PM adoption, other LMICs such as India, Mexico, and Brazil have made remarkable strides in utilizing genomic technologies [54–57].

In common, the foremost effort in PM adoption in these LMICs is to build research capacity. This is because the research findings from HICs may be difficult to be extrapolated due to the differences in genomic/genetic profile. In SEA, multidisciplinary collaborative works between institutions should be encouraged to avoid competition and wasteful duplicates. In addition, to facilitate the sustainable future improvement in PM research, several potential solutions are suggested. These include increasing research funding, establishing centers of excellence, encouraging international collaborations, and organizing specialized training programs [54].

(4) Value recognition of PM among policymakers across SEA to drive a PM era.

Engaging policymakers is the most salient step in this PM transformation. Political will and institutional leadership are highlighted as the key factors in developing a vision and a plan, and in the implementation of population-based genotyping initiatives in "early adopters" from HICs and LMICs [55]. With consistent and vocal high-level political support, it helps in initiating, driving, and maintaining a successful PM adoption and implementation [58]. The interest among policymakers to adopt PM across SEA remains low due to the lack of value recognition. This can be explained by the inadequate, yet emerging evidence base of PM to convince policymakers and clinicians to change policies and practices. To reduce uncertainty among stakeholder, it begins with evidence base generation to demonstrate that PM use can improve population health outcomes in a safe, effective, and cost-effective manner. As demonstrated the extensive process of acquiring and processing new local clinical and economic evidence of three aforementioned PM programs has led to their adoption decision. Potentially, an early dialogue between policymakers and manufacturers to discuss the evidentiary requirements necessary for coverage, as well as collaborations to share research data to resolve uncertainty in genomics can be a solution [38].

Apart from policymakers, public and patients are chief actors in increasing the momentum of PM adoption. It is worth noting that enormous pressure from general public on the government to provide safer and more effective treatments has accelerated PM adoption in the US [59, 60]. Similarly, in SEA, strengthening education efforts to public and the role of patient advocacy groups is warranted in driving the PM agenda forward.

(5) There are useful lessons to be learned from global experiences to enable a more effective PM adoption and implementation into the healthcare system. Notwithstanding various attempts supported by high-level political endorsement, PM has yet to move into the mainstream healthcare practice, even in "early adopters". Owing to the staggering challenges to facilitate a PM adoption [17, 61], its development as a national health agenda has been dynamic and iterative. Based on global experiences,

reforms at multiple levels of the healthcare system are clearly required. Evidence shows that addressing eight interdependent components – resources, governance, clinical practice, education, testing, knowledge translation, CDS and maintenance has generated positive outcomes in the implementation of a PM service [58]. SEA countries can adopt and adapt the strategies from reference countries to roll out PM adoption, while ensuring the social, ethical, equity and economic implications are fully recognized and addressed. Most importantly, PM awareness barrier needs to be lifted at all levels of society, especially patients, healthcare providers, and policymakers.

(6) There is potential to organize a multi-stakeholder and multi-country approach from research to clinical implementation of PM.

Translating discovery into routine use in healthcare is complex. As PM is an emerging concept, varying awareness and views are reported among a plethora of key players and stakeholders [62, 63]. It is suggested that partnerships between scientific research bodies, regulatory agencies, politics, clinicians, pharmaceutical and diagnostic companies, and patients/public will be the key success factor [64]. No single stakeholder can set all the essential requirements to further drive the PM adoption and implementation in healthcare. In HICs, a multi-stakeholder working group or public-private partnership has been engaged to level up key efforts for an effective PM adoption and implementation [65–67].

Likewise, collaborations among SEA countries are highly recommended to leverage the regional expertise and resources. Notably, SEAPharm has made several efforts to foster collaborative research in SEA especially the upcoming large-scale population genotyping presents an exciting opportunity to catalyze PM development in this region. Useful next steps include bringing together health research funders, policy-making organizations, and patient advocacy groups to coordinate the research and health policy in SEA, akin to the EU's ICPerMed.

The study is subject to a few important limitations. First, the literature search may not have identified all articles related to PM adoption and implementation, as some of these are likely to be in the local language. Given the diversity of fragmented PM-related efforts from different stakeholders, the sample of KOLs in this study may be insufficient to capture all relevant information. Furthermore, the overall methodology undertaken in this study including the snowballing approach employed may introduce bias in the information

gathered from literature and KOLs. Nevertheless, we believe an overview of major developments related to PM adoption and implementation across SEA has been presented. Despite our attempts to recruit policymakers, none participated in our interview. However, majority of KOLs participated were clinicians and researchers with some influence in the national health policy making. This is likely because we are at the early stage of PM development, thus the lack of success stories to stimulate interest and attention on PM among policymakers in SEA. Despite four SEA countries were studied, the findings especially from Indonesia could be extrapolated to other lower middle-income countries in SEA where sparse progress in PM adoption and majority of the activities are in the research stage can be expected. Although key findings and recommendations between our study with Shafie et al. [12] and Lim et al [13] are subtle, we undertook a broader scope of PM adoption in our study.

Conclusions

Notwithstanding the increasing interest, we are still only at the beginning of PM adoption not only in SEA, but also worldwide. Harnessing the full potential of PM to improve health is likely a decades-long endeavor. To achieve an effective PM adoption, it is imperative to balance equity issues across diverse populations, while improving efficiency in healthcare. A number of hurdles present on the road to an optimal evidence-based PM adoption in healthcare systems. In this study, we highlight the more salient issues in SEA to be addressed as a matter of priority.

In short term, there is a clear need for value recognition at all levels of society especially policymakers with more awareness and education programs. Starting with SEAPharm, better efficiency in the evidence generation activity can be achieved through regional collaborative research efforts and international partnerships. This enables not only better leverage of resources and expertise in this region, but also triggers political interest and support towards PM. Subsequently, critical discourse about PM among policymakers should be initiated to explore opportunities and priorities.

In medium and long term, it is important to move forward with a national PM strategic plan and legislation, with sustainable public and private funding. The national agreed transparent evidentiary requirement of PM's efficacy, safety, cost-effectiveness, analytical validity, clinical validity, and clinical utility should be introduced to support PM access with appropriate on-going research to resolve uncertainty. At the country and regional level, a multi-stakeholder working group consisting of policymakers, clinicians, researchers, and patient advocacy groups is essential to step up coordination efforts to allow synergies in the preparation of PM adoption. Among the many initiatives needed to integrate PM into person-centered healthcare, setting up centers of excellence, EHR infrastructure, as well as capacity-building among healthcare providers are critical starting points. Finally, SEA should address the ethical, legal, social, and equity concerns following PM adoption and genetic data. Periodic monitoring and evaluating the clinical, ethical, social, and equity outcomes should be included to indicate the performance of PM delivery. With themes emphasized above, the perspective to formulate robust recommendations for SEA is provided to guide future public health practice in an era of PM.

Abbreviations

A*STAR: Agency for sciences and technology research; CBZ: Carbamazepine; CDS: Clinical decision support; EHR: Electronic health record; EU: European Union; HER2: Human epidermal growth factor receptor 2; HIC: High-income country; HLA: Human leukocyte antigen; HSA: Health sciences authority; HTA: Health technology assessment; ICPerMed: International consortium for personalized medicine; KOL: Key opinion leader; LMIC: Low- and middle-income country; MOH: Ministry of Health; MOPH: Ministry of Public Health; NHS: National Health Service; OOP: Out-of-pocket; PGx: Pharmacogenomics; PM: Personalized medicine; PRISM: SingHealth Duke-National University Singapore Institute of Precision Medicine; SCAR: Severe cutaneous adverse reaction; SEA: Southeast Asia; SEAPharm: South East Asian Pharmacogenomics Research Network; TCELS: Thailand Center of Excellence for Life Sciences; THB: Thai Baht; UHC: Universal health coverage; UK: United Kingdom; US: United States; WHO: World Health Organization

Acknowledgements

We acknowledge the contribution from all participants from four focus countries. We thank Dr. Mukdarut Bangpan for her inputs and comments.

Funding

None

Authors' contributions

HYC and NC participated in the design on the study. HYC drafted the manuscript. PAA and NC were responsible for critical revision of the manuscript for important intellectual content. All authors read and approved the manuscript.

Competing interests

The authors declare that they have no competing interests.

Author details

[1]School of Pharmacy, Monash University Malaysia, Subang Jaya, Selangor, Malaysia. [2]United Nations University International Institute for Global Health, Kuala Lumpur, Malaysia. [3]Center of Pharmaceutical Outcomes Research (CPOR), Department of Pharmacy Practice, Faculty of Pharmaceutical Sciences, Naresuan University, Phitsanulok, Thailand. [4]School of Pharmacy, University of Wisconsin, Madison, USA. [5]Asian Centre for Evidence Synthesis in Population, Implementation and Clinical Outcomes (PICO), Global Asia in the 21st Century (GA21) Platform, Monash University Malaysia, Subang Jaya, Malaysia.

References

1. Personalized Medicine Coalition (PMC). The case for personalized medicine. Washington DC: PMC; 2014.
2. Talking glossary of genetic terms: personalized medicine [https://www.genome.gov/glossary/index.cfm?id=150].
3. Pokorska-Bocci A, Stewart A, Sagoo GS, Hall A, Kroese M, Burton H. 'Personalized medicine': what's in a name? Personalized Med. 2014;11(2): 197–210.
4. World Health Organization (WHO). Universal health coverage: moving towards better health – action framework for the Western Pacific region. Geneva: WHO; 2016.
5. Van Minh H, Pocock NS, Chaiyakunapruk N, Chhorvann C, Duc HA, Hanvoravongchai P, Lim J, Lucero-Prisno DE, Ng N, Phaholyothin N, et al. Progress toward universal health coverage in ASEAN. Glob Health Action. 2014;7. https://doi.org/10.3402/gha.v3407.25856.
6. Manolio TA, Chisholm RL, Ozenberger B, Roden DM, Williams MS, Wilson R, Bick D, Bottinger EP, Brilliant MH, Eng C, et al. Implementing genomic medicine in the clinic: the future is here. Genet Med. 2013;15(4):258–67.
7. Weitzel KW, Alexander M, Bernhardt BA, Calman N, Carey DJ, Cavallari LH, Field JR, Hauser D, Junkins HA, Levin PA, et al. The IGNITE network: a model for genomic medicine implementation and research. BMC Med Genet. 2016;9(1).
8. Farrugia G, Weinshilboum RM. Challenges in implementing genomic medicine: the Mayo Clinic Center for individualized medicine. Clin Pharmacol Ther. 2013;94(2):204–6.
9. Scott SA. Clinical pharmacogenomics: opportunities and challenges at point of care. Clin Pharmacol Ther. 2013;93(1):33–5.
10. Davis J, Furstenthal L, Desai A, Norris T, Sutaria S, Fleming E, Ma P. The microeconomics of personalized medicine: today's challenge and tomorrow's promise. Nat Rev Drug Discov. 2009;8:279–86.
11. Jakka S, Rossbach M. An economic perspective on personalized medicine. HUGO J. 2013;7(1):1.
12. Shafie AA, Chaiyakunapruk N, Supian A, Lim J, Zafra M, Hassali MAA. State of rare disease management in Southeast Asia. Orphanet J Rare Dis. 2016;11:107.
13. Lim JFY, Zafra M, Mocanu JD, Umareddy I, de Lima Lopes G, Foo R, Jha A, Hickinbotham L. Preparing health systems in Southeast and East Asia for new paradigms of care/personalized medicine in cancers: are health systems ready for evolving cancer management? J Asian Public Policy. 2017; 10(3):268–86.
14. World bank country and lending groups [https://datahelpdesk.worldbank.org/knowledgebase/articles/906519-world-bank-country-and-lending-groups].
15. World Health Organization (WHO). Monitoring the building blocks of health systems: a handbook of indicators and their measurement strategies. Geneva: WHO; 2010.
16. International consortium completes human genome project [https://www.genome.gov/11006929/].
17. Pokorska-Bocci A, Kroese M, Sagoo GS, Hall A, Burton H. Personalised medicine in the UK: challenges of implementation and impact on healthcare system. Genome Med. 2014;6(4):28.
18. Human Genomics Strategy Group. Building on our inheritance: genomic technology in healthcare. London: Department of Health; 2012.
19. Mazzucco W, Pastorino R, Lagerberg T, Colotto M, d'Andrea E, Marotta C, Marzuillo C, Villari P, Federici A, Ricciardi W, et al. Current state of genomic policies in healthcare among EU member states: results of a survey of chief medical officers. Eur J Pub Health. 2017;27(5):931–7.
20. Ashley EA. The precision medicine initiative: a new national effort. J Am Med Assoc. 2015;313(21):2119–20.
21. CIHR Institute of Health Services and Policy Research Strategic Plan 2015–19 [http://www.cihr-irsc.gc.ca/e/49711.html].
22. Australian Government Department of Health. In: Health Do, editor. National Health Genomics Policy Framework, 2017–2020. Canberra: Department of Health; 2017.
23. Choosing interventions that are cost-effective (WHO-CHOICE) [http://www.who.int/choice/cost-effectiveness/en/].
24. Schwarzer R, Rochau U, Saverno K, Jahn B, Bornschein B, Muehlberger N, Flatscher-Thoeni M, Schnell-Inderst P, Sroczynski G, Lackner M, et al. Systematic overview of cost-effectiveness thresholds in ten countries across four continents. J Comp Effectiveness Res. 2015;4(5):485–504.
25. The Pharmaceutical Benefits Advisory Committee guidelines: Product type 4 - Hybrid technologies and co-dependent technologies [https://pbac.pbs.gov.au/product-type-4-codependent-technologies.html].

26. Merlin T, Farah C, Schubert C, Mitchell A, Hiller JE, Ryan P. Assessing personalized medicines in Australia: a national framework for reviewing codependent technologies. Med Decis Mak. 2013;33(3):333–42.

27. Sanderson S, Zimmern R, Kroese M, Higgins J, Patch C, Emery J. How can the evaluation of genetic tests be enhanced? Lessons learned from the ACCE framework and evaluating genetic tests in the United Kingdom. Genet Med. 2005;7(7):495–500.

28. Precision medicine & CDx market access: A NICE perspective [http://worldcdx-europe.com/wp-content/uploads/sites/92/2017/04/Day-2-Stream-B-1200-Fay-McCracken-YES.pdf].

29. Payne K, Thompson J. A: economics of pharmacogenomics: rethinking beyond QALYs? Curr Pharmacogenomics Personalized Med. 2013;11(3):187–95.

30. International Consortium for Personalised Medicine (ICPerMed). Action plan: actionable research and support activities. Cologne: ICPerMed; 2017.

31. International Consortium for Personalised Medicine (ICPerMed). Shaping Europe's vision for personalised medicine: strategic research and innovation agenda. Cologne: PerMed; 2015.

32. Graham E. In: NHS England M, Diagnostics and Personalised Medicine Unit, editor. Improving outcomes through personalised medicine. Leeds: NHS; 2016.

33. Gottesman O, Kuivaniemi H, Tromp G, Faucett WA, Li R, Manolio TA, Sanderson SC, Kannry J, Zinberg R, Basford MA, et al. The electronic medical records and genomics (eMERGE) network: past, present, and future. Genet Med. 2013;15(10):761–71.

34. Leckband SG, Kelsoe JR, Dunnenberger HM, George AL, Tran E, Berger R, Müller DJ, Whirl-Carrillo M, Caudle KE, Pirmohamed M. Clinical pharmacogenetics implementation consortium guidelines for HLA-B genotype and carbamazepine dosing. Clin Pharmacol Ther. 2013;94(3):324–8.

35. National Human Genome Research Institute (NHGRI). International experience part 2: Singapore - Cynthia Sung. Bethesda: NHGRI; 2015.

36. Armstrong K. Equity in precision medicine: is it within our reach? J Natl Compr Cancer Netw. 2017;15(3):421–3.

37. Garfeld S, Douglas MP, MacDonald KV, Marshall DA, Phillips KA. Consumer familiarity, perspectives and expected value of personalized medicine with a focus on applications in oncology. Personalized Med. 2015;12(1):13–22.

38. Pritchard DE, Moeckel F, Villa MS, Housman LT, McCarty CA, McLeod HL. Strategies for integrating personalized medicine into healthcare practice. Personalized Med. 2017;14(2):141–52.

39. Hicks JK, Dunnenberger HM, Gumpper KF, Haidar CE, Hoffman JM. Integrating pharmacogenomics into electronic health records with clinical decision support. Am J Health Syst Pharm. 2016;73(23):1967–76.

40. Talwar D, Tseng TS, Foster M, Xu L, Chen LS. Genetics/genomics education for nongenetic health professionals: a systematic literature review. Genet Med. 2017;19(7):725–32.

41. Jenkins J, Blitzer M, Boehm K, Feetham S, Gettig E, Johnson A, Lapham EV, Patenaude AF, Reynolds PP, Guttmacher AE. Recommendations of core competencies in genetics essential for all health professionals. Genet Med. 2001;3:155.

42. Skirton H, Lewis C, Kent A, Farndon P, Bloch-Zupan A, Coviello D: Core competencies for all health professionals in Europe. Vienna: European Society of Human Genetics; 2007.

43. Christensen KD, Vassy JL, Jamal L, Lehmann LS, Slashinski MJ, Perry DL, Robinson JO, Blumenthal-Barby J, Feuerman LZ, Murray MF, et al. Are physicians prepared for whole genome sequencing? A qualitative analysis. Clin Genet. 2016;89(2):228–34.

44. Marzuillo C, Vito CD, D'Addario M, Santini P, D'Andrea E, Boccia A, Villari P. Are public health professionals prepared for public health genomics? A cross-sectional survey in Italy. BMC Health Serv Res. 2014;14:239.

45. Chow-White P, Ha D, Laskin J. Knowledge, attitudes, and values among physicians working with clinical genomics: a survey of medical oncologists. Hum Resour Health. 2017;15:42.

46. Melo DG, de Paula PK, de Araujo Rodrigues S, da Silva de Avó LR, Germano CMR, Demarzo MMP. Genetics in primary health care and the National Policy on Comprehensive Care for People with rare diseases in Brazil: opportunities and challenges for professional education. J Community Genet. 2015;6(3):231–40.

47. Johansen Taber KA, Dickinson BD. Pharmacogenomic knowledge gaps and educational resource needs among physicians in selected specialties. Pharmacogenomics Personalized Med. 2014;7:145–62.

48. Haga SB, Mills R, Moaddeb J, Allen LaPointe N, Cho A, Ginsburg GS. Primary care providers' use of pharmacist support for delivery of pharmacogenetic testing. Pharmacogenomics. 2017;18(4):359 67.

49. Carrera P, MJ IJ. Are current ICER thresholds outdated? Valuing medicines in the era of personalized healthcare. Expert Rev Pharmacoecon Outcomes Res. 2016;16(4):435–7.

50. Chootipongchaivat S, Tritasavit N, Luz A, Teerawattananon Y, Tantivess S. Factors conducive to the development of health technology assessment in Asia: impacts and policy options. Geneva: WHO; 2015.

51. Husereau D, Marshall DA, Levy AR, Peacock S, Hoch JS. Health technology assessment and personalized medicine: are economic evaluation guidelines sufficient to support decision making? Int J Technol Assess Health Care. 2014;30(2):179–87.

52. Marsh K, M IJ, Thokala P, Baltussen R, Boysen M, Kalo Z, Lonngren T, Mussen F, Peacock S, Watkins J, et al. Multiple criteria decision analysis for health care decision making--emerging good practices: report 2 of the ISPOR MCDA emerging good practices task force. Value Health. 2016;19(2):125–37.

53. Chongsuvivatwong V, Phua KH, Yap MT, Pocock NS, Hashim JH, Chhem R, Wilopo SA, Lopez AD. Health and health-care systems in Southeast Asia: diversity and transitions. Lancet. 2011;377(9763):429–37.

54. Helmy M, Awad M, Mosa KA. Limited resources of genome sequencing in developing countries: challenges and solutions. Appl Transl Genomics. 2016;9:15–9.

55. Seguin B, Hardy B-J, Singer PA, Daar AS. Genomic medicine and developing countries: creating a room of their own. Nat Rev Genet. 2008;9(6):487–93.

56. Passos-Bueno MR, Bertola D, Horovitz DDG, de Faria Ferraz VE, Brito LA. Genetics and genomics in Brazil: a promising future. Mol Genet Genomic Med. 2014;2(4):280–91.

57. Jauhari S, Rizvi SAM. An Indian eye to personalized medicine. Comput Biol Med. 2015;59:211–20.

58. Caraballo PJ, Hodge LS, Bielinski SJ, Stewart AK, Farrugia G, Schultz CG, Rohrer-Vitek CR, Olson JE, St. Sauver JL, Roger VL, et al. Multidisciplinary model to implement pharmacogenomics at the point of care. Genet Med. 2017;19(4):421–9.

59. Agyeman AA, Ofori-Asenso R. Perspective: does personalized medicine hold the future for medicine? J Pharm Bioallied Sci. 2015;7(3):239–44.

60. Jain KK. Textbook of personalized medicine. New York: Springer; 2015.

61. Horgan D, Jansen M, Leyens L, Lal JA, Sudbrak R, Hackenitz E, Busshoff U, Ballensiefen W, Brand A. An index of barriers for the implementation of personalised medicine and pharmacogenomics in Europe. Public Health Genomics. 2014;17(5–6):287–98.

62. Paci D, Ibarreta D. Economic and cost-effectiveness considerations for pharmacogenetics tests: an integral part of translational research and innovation uptake in personalized medicine. Curr Pharmacogenomics Personalized Med. 2009;7:284–96.

63. Mitropoulos K, Al Jaibeji H, Forero DA, Laissue P, Wonkam A, Lopez-Correa C, Mohamed Z, Chantratita W, Lee MTM, Llerena A, et al. Success stories in genomic medicine from resource-limited countries. Hum Genomics. 2015;9(1):11.

64. Steffen JA, Steffen JS. Driving forces behind the past and future emergence of personalized medicine. J Personalized Med. 2013;3(1):14–22.

65. Canadian Institutes of Health Research. Personalized medicine signature initiative 2010-2013. Ottawa: Canadian Institutes of Health Research; 2013.

66. Fact sheet: President Obama's Precision Medicine Initiative [https://obamawhitehouse.archives.gov/the-press-office/2015/01/30/fact-sheet-president-obama-s-precision-medicine-initiative].

67. Keogh B. Personalised medicine strategy. London: National Health Service England; 2015.

20

Role of *PUF60* gene in Verheij syndrome: a case report of the first Chinese Han patient with a de novo pathogenic variant

Qiong Xu[1], Chun-yang Li[1], Yi Wang[1], Hui-ping Li[1], Bing-bing Wu[1], Yong-hui Jiang[2,3,4,5] and Xiu Xu[1*]

Abstract

Background: Verheij syndrome is a rare microdeletion syndrome of chromosome 8q24.3 that harbors *PUF60*, *SCRIB*, and *NRBP2* genes. Subsequently, loss of function mutations in *PUF60* have been found in children with clinical features significantly overlapping with Verheij.

Case presentation: Here we present the first Chinese Han patient with a de novo nonsense variant (c.1357C > T, p.Gln453*) in *PUF60* by clinical whole exome sequencing. The 5-year-old boy presents with dysmorphic facial features, intellectual disability, and growth retardation but without apparent cardiac, renal, ocular, and spinal anomalies.

Conclusions: Our finding contributes to the understanding of the genotype and phenotype in *PUF60* related disorder.

Keywords: *PUF60*, Verheij syndrome, Intellectual disability, Chinese Han patient

Background

Verheij syndrome (VRJS) (MIM 615583) is characterized by intellectual disability, growth retardation, dysmorphic facial features, and vertebral skeletal abnormalities. Additional features include coloboma and renal and cardiac defects [1–5]. Verheij syndrome is caused by a deletion in chromosome 8q24.3. The commonly deleted intervals include two genes, poly(U)-binding-splicing factor (*PUF60*) and scribbled planar cell polarity protein (*SCRIB*). Point mutations in *PUF60* have been reported in individuals with clinical features overlapping with those associated with a 8q24.3 deletion or VRJS [2]. The *PUF60* gene encodes a protein that directly interacts with splicing factor 3B, subunit 4 (SF3B4) and plays a role in the recognition of the 3′ splice site and the recruitment of U2 and U5 small nucleolar ribonucleoprotein to the intron for splicing [2]. Mutations of the *PUF60* gene including nonsense, frameshifting, splicing site, or missense have been identified in 24 individuals [1, 2, 4–9]. Here, we report a Chinese Han

patient who carries a heterozygous de novo and novel nonsense mutation (c.1357C > T, p.Gln453*) in *PUF60* identified by clinical whole exome sequencing. This individual shares some characteristic features with previously described individuals including intellectual disability, growth retardation, and dysmorphic facial features but not other features such as cardiac, renal, ocular, and spine abnormalities [1, 2, 4–9]. This is the first report and characterization of a Chinese Han child harboring a *PUF60* variant.

Clinical summary

A 5-year-old boy was born prematurely at 36 weeks of gestation without a known cause. The birthweight was 2650 g and appropriate for gestational age. He had a significant history of poor feeding and failure of thrive as an infant. At the age of 4 years and 7 months, his weight was 13.5 kg (< 2 SD) and his height was 98 cm (< 2 SD). His head circumference was 49.5 cm (< 1 SD). He showed global developmental delay and started to walk at the age of 20 months. At the age of 4 years, his vocabulary was limited to just a few words. At present, he is able to speak simple phrases but not complex sentences. In

* Correspondence: xuxiu@fudan.edu.cn
[1]Developmental and Behavioral Pediatric Department & Child Health Care Department, Children's Hospital of Fudan University, 399 Wanyuan Road, Shanghai 201102, China
Full list of author information is available at the end of the article

addition, he has significant history of chronic diarrhea from birth to 2.5 years of age without an identifiable cause. He had an average of 5–7 loose stools per day while being breastfed during the first year. Between the ages of 1–2.5 years, he was formula-fed and had an average of 6–8 loose stools per day. The chronic diarrhea resolved after 2.5 years of age without any clinical intervention. He was also diagnosed with febrile seizures and had significant sleep disturbance. Upon the physical examination at AGE, a distinct facial dimorphism was noted and these include a short neck, thin upper lip, long philtrum, wide nasal bridge, micrognathia, and almond-shaped eyes and short palpebral fissures (Fig. 1). There was no ocular coloboma and no shoulder subluxation or generalized joint laxity. Both parents were healthy and non-consanguineous. Family history was negative for any neurodevelopmental disorder or known genetic disease. Endocrine work-up, brain magnetic resonance imaging, abdominal and renal ultrasonography, and skeletal bone survey were normal. His hearing was normal. The detail clinical description of this patient and comparison with other previously reported cases carrying *PUF60* mutations are listed in Table 1.

Genetic evaluation

Standard karyotyping was normal (46, XY). A clinical trio whole exome sequencing (WES) was performed by WuXi NextCODE Genomics, Shanghai, China (CLIA Lab ID: 99D2064856) using a previous described protocol [10]. Briefly, exome capture was performed using the Agilent SureSelect Human All Exon V5, Illumina TruSeq Rapid PE Cluster, and SBS kits (Agilent Technologies, Santa Clara, CA, USA). WES was performed on the Illumina HiSeq 2000/2500 platform. Reads were aligned to the human genome reference sequence (GRCh37/hg19 build of UCSC Genome Browser; http://genome.ucsc.edu)

with the Burrows-Wheeler Aligner v.0.6.2. Duplicate paired-end reads were marked with Picard v.1.55 (https://broadinstitute.github.io/picard/). The Genome Analysis Toolkit v.2.3–9 was used for base quality score recalibration, indel realignment, and variant discovery. Variants were annotated using a pipeline developed in-house [10] and filtered in the Exome Variant Server, gnomAD, Exome Aggregation Consortium, or the dbSNP databases. The candidate variants were confirmed by Sanger sequencing.

In this proband, a heterozygous de novo and nonsense c.1357C > T variant in exon 11 (NM_078480.2) was identified from the WES analysis and confirmed by Sanger sequencing. This variant is predicted to result in a premature stop codon (p.Gln453*) of PUF60 protein (Fig. 1). Other previously reported pathogenic variants are also diagramed in Fig. 2 for a comparison.

Discussion and conclusion

In this report, we presented the finding of a novel pathogenic variant in *PUF60* gene in a Chinese child. To our knowledge, this is the first case of a Chinese child with *PUF60* mutation. The proband's clinical presentations of intellectual disability, short stature, and dysmorphic facial features were similar with those previously reported cases with mutations in *PUF60* variants or with a deletion of 8q24.3 containing the *PUF60* or VRJS [1, 2, 4–9]. However, the vertebral anomaly, coloboma, renal defects, and cardiac defects reported in other cases were not found in our patient. In individuals with 8q24.3 deletion or VRJS, both *PUF60* and *SCRIB* genes are deleted. In an early study in zebrafish, morpholino-mediated knockdown of either *PUF60* or *Scribble* (*Scrib*) in zebrafish recapitulates some of the phenotypes of 8q24.3 deletion in humans [2]. Knockdown of either gene cause a short stature, microcephaly, and reduced jaw size.

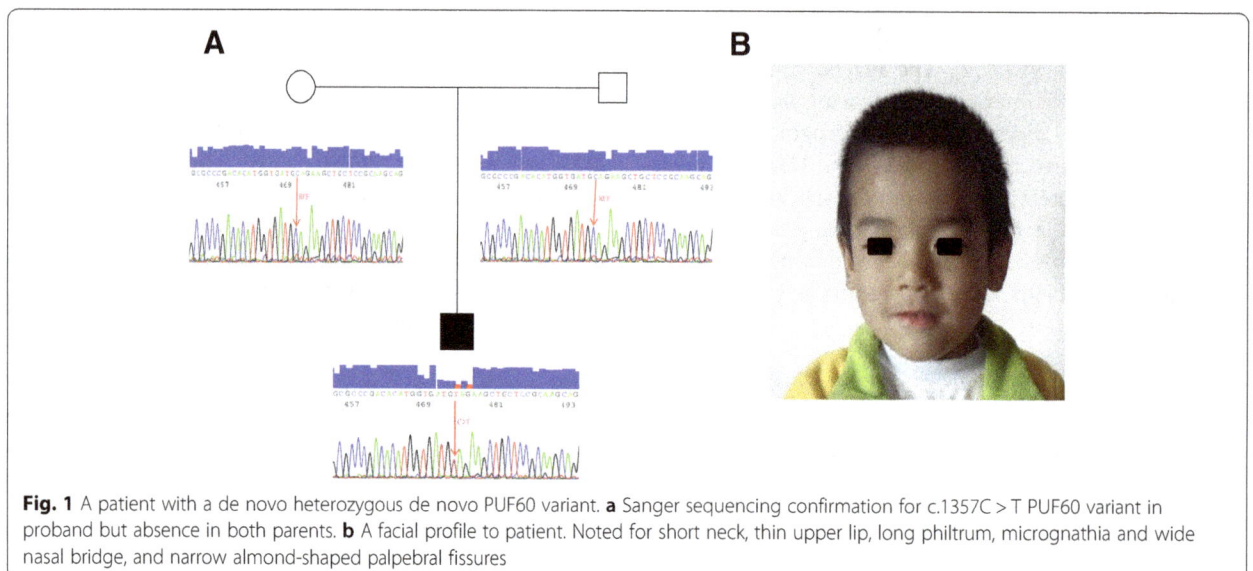

Fig. 1 A patient with a de novo heterozygous de novo PUF60 variant. **a** Sanger sequencing confirmation for c.1357C > T PUF60 variant in proband but absence in both parents. **b** A facial profile to patient. Noted for short neck, thin upper lip, long philtrum, micrognathia and wide nasal bridge, and narrow almond-shaped palpebral fissures

Table 1 Comparison of clinical features in our patient and others previously reported with the *PUF60* mutation

Clinical phenotypes	Patient 1	Previous reported with *PUF60* variants (n = 24)[2, 4–9]	Previous reported with 8q24.3 deletion (n = 7)[1, 2]
Gestation			
Pre-term	+	3/18	NA
Full-term		15/18	1/1
Height (z score < 2 SD)	+	16/23	7/7
Renal	−	6/22	4/7
Coloboma	−	8/23	4/7
Cardiac	−	13/21	5/7
Skeletal	−	15/23	5/7
Hand anomalies	−	11/20	4/7
Joint laxity	−	11/19	5/7
Feeding	+	10/17	5/7
ID (intellectual disability)	+	24/24	5/6
Auditory	−	8/14	1/5
Hypertrichosis	−	5/12	NA
Facial feature			
Long philtrum	+	16/23	7/7
Thin upper lip	+	15/23	7/7
Micro-retrognathism	+	13/22	4/7
Short neck	+	14/22	5/7
Wide nasal bridge	+	9/22	6/7

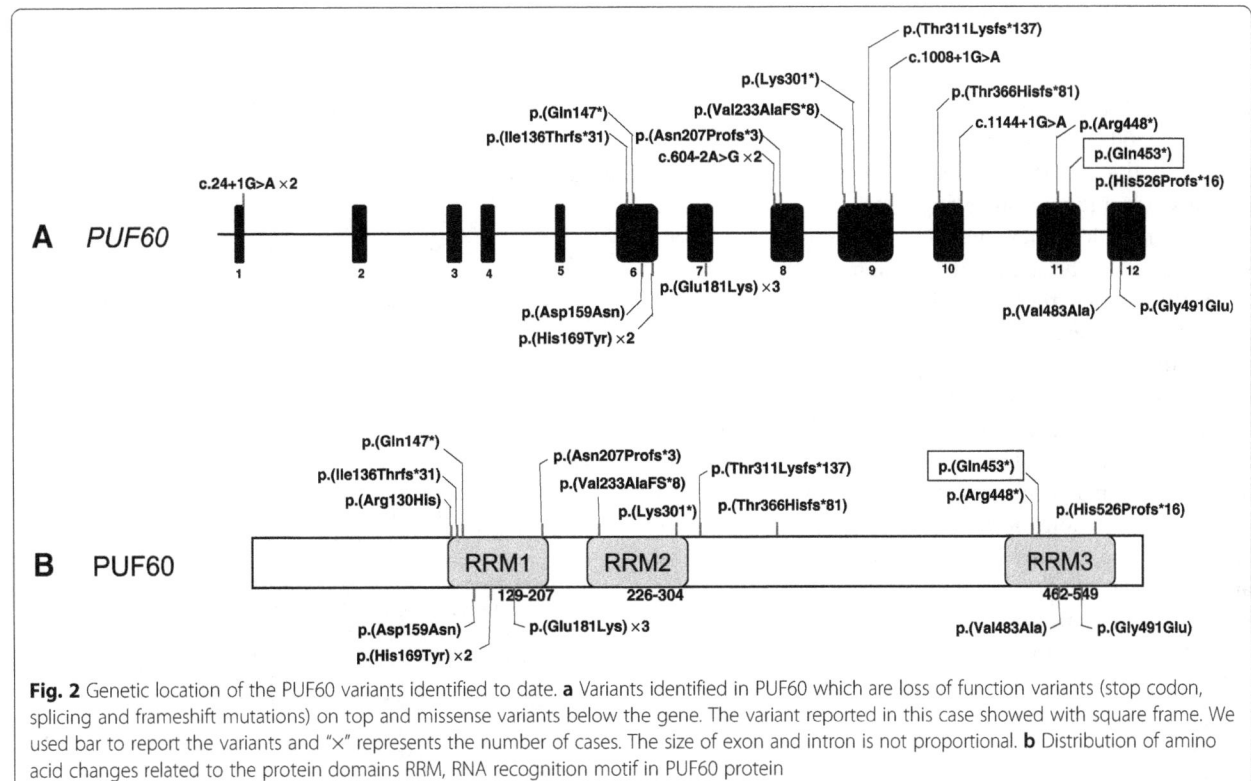

Fig. 2 Genetic location of the PUF60 variants identified to date. **a** Variants identified in PUF60 which are loss of function variants (stop codon, splicing and frameshift mutations) on top and missense variants below the gene. The variant reported in this case showed with square frame. We used bar to report the variants and "×" represents the number of cases. The size of exon and intron is not proportional. **b** Distribution of amino acid changes related to the protein domains RRM, RNA recognition motif in PUF60 protein

Knockdown of *Scrib* alone resulted in coloboma and renal abnormalities, whereas knockdown of *PUF60* alone resulted in cardiac structural defects. Knockdown of both genes result in more severe short stature phenotype. It was concluded that *PUF60* or *SCRIB* haploinsufficiency drives the majority of syndromic phenotypes found in patients with the copy number deletion of 8q24.3 or VRJS. However, several patients harboring *PUF60* point mutations have been recently described, and these individuals have clinical phenotypes that overlap significantly with patients carrying 8q24.3 deletions. These findings support a major role for *PUF60* in the phenotype of VRJS in human [1, 2, 4–9]. It remains to be seen whether mutations in *SCRIB* alone in humans may also cause the clinical problem similar to mutations of PUF60. The presentation of chronic diarrhea in our patient has not been previously reported [1, 2, 4–9]. It will be interesting to see if diarrhea is a feature of other patients harboring a *PUF60* defect.

The findings of a heterozygous de novo nonsense change of *PUF60* in our study further supports haploinsufficiency as the underlying mechanism [6]. Loss-of-function variants are predicted to result in altered dosages of different PUF60 isoforms and, consequently, abnormal splicing of targeted genes [2]. Both VRSJ syndrome and *PUF60*-related disorder encompass diverse phenotypes, suggesting that dysregulated targeted genes due to the *PUF60* deficiency may account for diverse phenotypes in humans.

Interesting to note, two reports have suggested the overlapping clinical features between *PUF60* related disorder with CHARGE syndrome. In these cases, the clinical and genetic evaluation of CHARGE syndrome is considered but the mutation study of *CHD7* is negative (PMID 29300383 and PMID: 28471317). Other have also suggested the overlapping feature between Cornelia de Lange syndrome and other craniofacial disorders caused by mutations in genes encoding the spliceosomal proteins [11, 12]. The apparent question for the future investigation is whether there is a convergent molecular mechanism among these disorders.

The majority of genetic variants in *PUF60* are predicted to be loss of function mutations, However, missense variants are also reported. Clinically, there is no significant difference between individuals carrying clear loss of function and missense variants. These may support the loss of function mechanism underlying the missense variants in these cases. However, additional phenotypical and molecular studies are warranted to clarify the genotype and phenotype correlation and whether the missense variants may result in loss of function at protein level.

This study is the first report of a Chinese Han patient carrying de novo *PUF60* heterozygous mutation. The proband exhibited many of the characteristics previously reported in PUF60 variant or VRSJ patients such as intellectual disability, growth retardation, and dysmorphic facial features [1, 2, 4–9]. However, the patient did not present with especially vertebral skeletal abnormalities, coloboma, renal defects, or cardiac defects. Clinical and molecular characterization of patients with diverse background will help us better understand the genetic diversity and prevalence of *PUF60* related disorder.

Abbreviations

PUF60: Poly(U)-binding-splicing factor; SCRIB: Scribbled planar cell polarity protein; SF3B4: Splicing factor 3B, subunit 4

Acknowledgements

We would like to thank the child and his parents whose participation made this study possible.

Funding

This study was funded by Shanghai Municipal Science and Technology Commission (grant number 15411967900) and by the National Science Foundation of China (grant number 81701496).

Authors' contributions

QX, CY, YH, XX conceived and conducted the study; QX, HP, XX identified the patients and carried out the clinical characterizations; CY, YW, BB carried out the molecular genetics studies; HP, YW, BB contributed WES analysis; QX, YH, XX wrote the manuscript; all authors read and approved the final manuscript.

Competing interests

The authors declare that they have no competing interest.

Author details

Developmental and Behavioral Pediatric Department & Child Health Care Department, Children's Hospital of Fudan University, 399 Wanyuan Road, Shanghai 201102, China. 2Department of Pediatrics, Duke University School of Medicine, Durham, NC 27710, USA. 3Department of Neurobiology, Duke University School of Medicine, Durham, NC 27710, USA. 4Program in Genetics and Genomics, Duke University School of Medicine, Durham, NC 27710, USA. Cellular Molecular Biology, Duke University School of Medicine, Durham, NC 27710, USA.

References

1. Verheij JB, de Munnik SA, Dijkhuizen T, de Leeuw N, Olde Weghuis D, van den Hoek GJ, Rijlaarsdam RS, Thomasse YE, Dikkers FG, Marcelis CL, et al. An 8.35 Mb overlapping interstitial deletion of 8q24 in two patients with coloboma, congenital heart defect, limb abnormalities, psychomotor retardation and convulsions. Eur J Med Genet. 2009;52(5):353–7.
2. Dauber A, Golzio C, Guenot C, Jodelka FM, Kibaek M, Kjaergaard S, Leheup B, Martinet D, Nowaczyk MJ, Rosenfeld JA, et al. SCRIB and PUF60 are primary drivers of the multisystemic phenotypes of the 8q24.3 copy-number variant. Am J Hum Genet. 2013;93(5):798–811.
3. Fiorentino DF, Presby M, Baer AN, Petri M, Rieger KE, Soloski M, Rosen A, Mammen AL, Christopher-Stine L, Casciola-Rosen L. PUF60: a prominent new target of the autoimmune response in dermatomyositis and Sjogren's syndrome. Ann Rheum Dis. 2016;75(6):1145–51.

Role of PUF60 gene in Verheij syndrome: a case report of the first Chinese Han patient with a de novo...

217

4. Low KJ, Ansari M, Abou Jamra R, Clarke A, El Chehadeh S, FitzPatrick DR, Greenslade M, Henderson A, Hurst J, Keller K, et al. PUF60 variants cause a syndrome of ID, short stature, microcephaly, coloboma, craniofacial, cardiac, renal and spinal features. Eur J Hum Genet. 2017;25(5):552–9.

5. Santos-Simarro F, Vallespin E, Del Pozo A, Ibanez K, Silla JC, Fernandez L, Nevado J, Gonzalez-Pecellin H, Montano VEF, Martin R, et al. Eye coloboma and complex cardiac malformations belong to the clinical spectrum of PUF60 variants. Clin Genet. 2017;92(3):350-1.

6. El Chehadeh S, Kerstjens-Frederikse WS, Thevenon J, Kuentz P, Bruel AL, Thauvin-Robinet C, Bensignor C, Dollfus H, Laugel V, Riviere JB, et al. Dominant variants in the splicing factor PUF60 cause a recognizable syndrome with intellectual disability, heart defects and short stature. Eur J Hum Genet. 2016;25(1):43–51.

7. Graziano C, Gusson E, Severi G, Isidori F, Wischmeijer A, Brugnara M, Seri M, Rossi C. A de novo PUF60 mutation in a child with a syndromic form of coloboma and persistent fetal vasculature. Ophthalmic Genet. 2017;38(6): 590–2.

8. Zhao JJ, Halvardson J, Zander CS, Zaghlool A, Georgii-Hemming P, Mansson E, Brandberg G, Savmarker HE, Frykholm C, Kuchinskaya E, et al. *Exome sequencing reveals NAA15 and PUF60 as candidate genes associated with intellectual disability.* Am J Med Genet B Neuropsychiatr Genet. 2018;177(1): 10–20.9.

9. Moccia A, Srivastava A, Skidmore JM, Bernat JA, Wheeler M, Chong JX, Nickerson D, Bamshad M, Hefner MA, Martin DM, et al. Genetic analysis of CHARGE syndrome identifies overlapping molecular biology. Genet Med. 2018. https://doi.org/10.1038/gim.2017.233. [Epub ahead of print].

10. Yang L, Kong Y, Dong X, Hu L, Lin Y, Chen X, Ni Q, Lu Y, Wu B, Wang H, et al. Clinical and genetic spectrum of a large cohort of children with epilepsy in China. Genet Med. 2018. https://doi.org/10.1038/s41436-018-0091-8. [Epub ahead of print].

11. Lehalle D, Wieczorek D, Zechi-Ceide RM, Passos-Bueno MR, Lyonnet S, Amiel J, Gordon CT. A review of craniofacial disorders caused by spliceosomal defects. Clin Genet. 2015;88(5):405–15.

12. Hastings ML, Allemand E, Duelli DM, Myers MP, Krainer AR. Control of pre-mRNA splicing by the general splicing factors PUF60 and U2AF(65). PLoS One. 2007;2(6):e538.

Permissions

The contributors of this book come from diverse backgrounds, making this book a truly international effort. This book will bring forth new frontiers with its revolutionizing research information and detailed analysis of the nascent developments around the world.

We would like to thank all the contributing authors for lending their expertise to make the book truly unique. They have played a crucial role in the development of this book. Without their invaluable contributions this book wouldn't have been possible. They have made vital efforts to compile up to date information on the varied aspects of this subject to make this book a valuable addition to the collection of many professionals and students.

This book was conceptualized with the vision of imparting up-to-date information and advanced data in this field. To ensure the same, a matchless editorial board was set up. Every individual on the board went through rigorous rounds of assessment to prove their worth. After which they invested a large part of their time researching and compiling the most relevant data for our readers.

The editorial board has been involved in producing this book since its inception. They have spent rigorous hours researching and exploring the diverse topics which have resulted in the successful publishing of this book. They have passed on their knowledge of decades through this book. To expedite this challenging task, the publisher supported the team at every step. A small team of assistant editors was also appointed to further simplify the editing procedure and attain best results for the readers.

Apart from the editorial board, the designing team has also invested a significant amount of their time in understanding the subject and creating the most relevant covers. They scrutinized every image to scout for the most suitable representation of the subject and create an appropriate cover for the book.

The publishing team has been an ardent support to the editorial, designing and production team. Their endless efforts to recruit the best for this project, has resulted in the accomplishment of this book. They are a veteran in the field of academics and their pool of knowledge is as vast as their experience in printing. Their expertise and guidance has proved useful at every step. Their uncompromising quality standards have made this book an exceptional effort. Their encouragement from time to time has been an inspiration for everyone.

The publisher and the editorial board hope that this book will prove to be a valuable piece of knowledge for researchers, students, practitioners and scholars across the globe.

Contributors

Hyun Jin Kim and So Yeon Park
Laboratory of Medical Genetics, Medical Research Institute, Cheil General Hospital and Women's Healthcare Center, Seoul, South Korea

Ji Hyae Lim
Laboratory of Medical Genetics, Medical Research Institute, Cheil General Hospital and Women's Healthcare Center, Seoul, South Korea
Department of Medical Genetics, College of Medicine, Hanyang University, 222, Wangsimni-ro, Seongdong-gu, Seoul 04763, South Korea

Hyun Mee Ryu
Laboratory of Medical Genetics, Medical Research Institute, Cheil General Hospital and Women's Healthcare Center, Seoul, South Korea
Department of Obstetrics and Gynecology, Cheil General Hospital and Women's Healthcare Center, Dankook University College of Medicine, 1-19, Mookjung-dong, Chung-gu, Seoul 100-380, South Korea

Youl-Hee Cho
Department of Medical Genetics, College of Medicine, Hanyang University, 222, Wangsimni-ro, Seongdong-gu, Seoul 04763, South Korea

You Jung Han and Moon Young Kim
Department of Obstetrics and Gynecology, Cheil General Hospital and Women's Healthcare Center, Dankook University College of Medicine, 1-19, Mookjung-dong, Chung-gu, Seoul 100-380, South Korea

Manu K. Shivakumar
Biomedical and Translational Informatics Institute, Geisinger Health System, Danville, PA, USA

Dokyoon Kim
Biomedical and Translational Informatics Institute, Geisinger Health System, Danville, PA, USA
Huck Institute of the Life Sciences, Pennsylvania State University, University Park, PA, USA

Jason E. Miller
Biomedical and Translational Informatics Institute, Geisinger Health System, Danville, PA, USA
Present Address: Department of Genetics, Institute for Biomedical Informatics, Perelman School of Medicine, University of Pennsylvania, Philadelphia, PA, USA

Younghee Lee and Seonggyun Han
Department of Biomedical Informatics, University of Utah School of Medicine, Salt Lake City, UT 84106, USA

Emrin Horgousluoglu, Shannon L. Risacher, Andrew J. Saykin and Kwangsik Nho
Department of Radiology and Imaging Sciences, Indiana University School of Medicine, Indianapolis, IN, USA

Rubén Cabanillas, Marta Diñeiro, Guadalupe A. Cifuentes, Rebeca Álvarez, Noelia Sánchez-Durán, Raquel Capín and Juan Cadiñanos
Instituto de Medicina Oncológica y Molecular de Asturias (IMOMA) S. A, Avda. Richard Grandío s/n, 33193 Oviedo, Spain

David Castillo, Patricia C. Pruneda and Gonzalo R. Ordóñez
Disease Research And Medicine (DREAMgenics) S. L., Oviedo, Spain

Ana Plasencia, Mónica Viejo-Díaz, Noelia García-González, Inés Hernando, José L. Llorente, Justo Ramón Gómez-Martínez and Faustino Núñez-Batalla
Hospital Universitario Central de Asturias, Oviedo, Spain

María Costales
Hospital Universitario Central de Asturias, Oviedo, Spain
Hospital Universitario Marqués de Valdecilla, Santander, Spain

Alfredo Repáraz-Andrade and Cristina Torreira-Banzas
Hospital Álvaro Cunqueiro, Vigo, Spain

Jordi Rosell and Nancy Govea
Hospital Universitario Son Espases, Palma de Mallorca, Spain

José A. Garrote
Hospital Universitario Río Hortega, Valladolid, Spain

Ángel Mazón-Gutiérrez
Hospital Universitario Marqués de Valdecilla, Santander, Spain

María Isidoro-García and Belén García-Berrocal
Instituto de Investigación Biomédica de Salamanca, Salamanca, Spain

Neda Stjepanovic, Natasha B. Leighl, Raymond Jang, Monika K. Krzyzanowska, Amit M. Oza, Abha Gupta and Christine Elser
Division of Medical Oncology and Hematology, Princess Margaret Cancer Centre, 610 University Ave, Toronto, ON M5G 2M9, Canada

Philippe L. Bedard, Lailah Ahmed and Lillian L. Siu
Division of Medical Oncology and Hematology, Princess Margaret Cancer Centre, 610 University Ave, Toronto, ON M5G 2M9, Canada

Cancer Genomics Program, Princess Margaret Cancer Centre, 610 University Ave, Toronto, ON M5G 2M9, Canada

Raymond H. Kim
Division of Medical Oncology and Hematology, Princess Margaret Cancer Centre, 610 University Ave, Toronto, ON M5G 2M9, Canada
Cancer Genomics Program, Princess Margaret Cancer Centre, 610 University Ave, Toronto, ON M5G 2M9, Canada
Zane Cohen Centre for Digestive Diseases, Mount Sinai Hospital, 60 Murray St, Toronto, ON M5T 3L9, Canada

Tracy L. Stockley and Suzanne Kamel-Reid
Cancer Genomics Program, Princess Margaret Cancer Centre, 610 University Ave, Toronto, ON M5G 2M9, Canada
Department of Clinical Laboratory Genetics and Department of Laboratory Medicine and Pathobiology, University of Toronto, 610 University Ave, Toronto, ON M5G 2M9, Canada

Jeanna M. McCuaig
Department of Molecular Genetics, University of Toronto, 610 University Ave, Toronto, ON M5G 2M9, Canada

Melyssa Aronson, Spring Holter and Kara Semotiuk
Zane Cohen Centre for Digestive Diseases, Mount Sinai Hospital, 60 Murray St, Toronto, ON M5T 3L9, Canada

Lisa Wang
Department of Biostatistics, Princess Margaret Cancer Centre, 610 University Ave, Toronto, ON M5G 2M9, Canada

Tsung-Yu Hsieh
Artificial Intelligence Research Laboratory, College of Information Sciences and Technology, Pennsylvania State University, University Park, PA 16802, USA

School of Electrical Engineering and Computer Science, Pennsylvania State University, University Park, PA 16802, USA
The Center for Big Data Analytics and Discovery Informatics, Pennsylvania State University, University Park, PA 16802, USA

Yasser EL-Manzalawy
Artificial Intelligence Research Laboratory, College of Information Sciences and Technology, Pennsylvania State University, University Park, PA 16802, USA
The Center for Big Data Analytics and Discovery Informatics, Pennsylvania State University, University Park, PA 16802, USA
The Clinical and Translational Sciences Institute, Pennsylvania State University, University Park, PA 16802, USA

Vasant Honavar
Artificial Intelligence Research Laboratory, College of Information Sciences and Technology, Pennsylvania State University, University Park, PA 16802, USA
The Huck Institutes of the Life Sciences, Pennsylvania State University, University Park, PA 16802, USA
School of Electrical Engineering and Computer Science, Pennsylvania State University, University Park, PA 16802, USA
The Center for Big Data Analytics and Discovery Informatics, Pennsylvania State University, University Park, PA 16802, USA
The Clinical and Translational Sciences Institute, Pennsylvania State University, University Park, PA 16802, USA

Manu Shivakumar
Biomedical and Translational Informatics Institute, Geisinger Health System, Danville, PA, USA

Dokyoon Kim
Biomedical and Translational Informatics Institute, Geisinger Health System, Danville, PA, USA

The Huck Institutes of the Life Sciences, Pennsylvania State University, University Park, PA 16802, USA

Jie-Qiong Li and Xiang-Zhen Yuan
Department of Neurology, Qingdao Municipal Hospital, Qingdao University, No.5 Donghai Middle Road, Qingdao 266071, Shandong Province, China

Jin-Tai Yu and Lan Tan
Department of Neurology, Qingdao Municipal Hospital, Qingdao University, No.5 Donghai Middle Road, Qingdao 266071, Shandong Province, China
Clinical Research Center, Qingdao Municipal Hospital, Qingdao University, Qingdao, China

Hai-Yan Li
Department of Neurology, Weihaiwei People's Hospital, Weihai, China

Xi-Peng Cao
Clinical Research Center, Qingdao Municipal Hospital, Qingdao University, Qingdao, China

Wei-An Chen
Department of Neurology, The First Affiliated Hospital of Wenzhou Medical University, Nanbaixiang Road, Wenzhou 325000, Zhejiang Province, China

Fang Li, Xiao Xiao, Raj Putatunda, Jun Yu, Xiao-Feng Yang and Hong Wang
Center for Metabolic Disease Research, Temple University Lewis Katz School of Medicine, 3500 N Broad Street, Philadelphia, PA 19140, USA

Yonggang Zhang
Center for Metabolic Disease Research, Temple University Lewis Katz School of Medicine, 3500 N Broad Street, Philadelphia, PA 19140, USA
Center for Stem Cell Research and Application, Institute of Blood Transfusion, Chinese Academy of Medical Sciences and Peking Union Medical College (CAMS and PUMC), Chengdu 610052, China

Wenhui Hu
Center for Metabolic Disease Research, Temple University Lewis Katz School of Medicine, 3500 N Broad Street, Philadelphia, PA 19140, USA
Department of Pathology and Laboratory Medicine, Temple University Lewis Katz School of Medicine, 3500 N Broad Street, Philadelphia, PA 19140, USA

Gustavo Arango and Liqing Zhang
Department of Computer Science, Virginia Tech, Blacksburg, VA 24060, USA

Layne T. Watson
Department of Computer Science, Virginia Tech, Blacksburg, VA 24060, USA
Department of Mathematics, Department of Aerospace and Ocean Engineering, Virginia Tech, Blacksburg, VA 24060, USA

Haruto Uchino, Masaki Ito, Ken Kazumata, Shuji Hamauchi, Shunsuke Terasaka and Kiyohiro Houkin
Department of Neurosurgery, Hokkaido University Graduate School of Medicine, North 15 West 7, Sapporo 0608638, Japan

Yuka Hama and Hidenao Sasaki
Department of Neurology, Hokkaido University Graduate School of Medicine, Sapporo, Japan

Morag A. Lewis and Karen P. Steel
Wolfson Centre for Age-Related Diseases, King's College London, WC2R 2LS, London, UK
Wellcome Trust Sanger Institute, Hinxton, Cambridge CB10 1SA, UK

Lisa S. Nolan, Barbara A. Cadge and Sally J. Dawson
UCL Ear Institute, University College London, WC1X 8EE, London, UK

Lois J. Matthews, Bradley A. Schulte and Judy R. Dubno
Medical University of South Carolina, Charleston, SC 29425, USA

Richa G. Thaman
Deep Hospital, Ludhiana, Punjab, India

Geeti P. Arora
Deep Hospital, Ludhiana, Punjab, India
Department of Clinical Sciences, Clinical Research Centre, Lund University, Malmö, Sweden

Peter Almgren and Rashmi B. Prasad
Department of Clinical Sciences, Clinical Research Centre, Lund University, Malmö, Sweden

Leif Groop
Department of Clinical Sciences, Clinical Research Centre, Lund University, Malmö, Sweden
Finnish Institute of Molecular Medicine (FIMM), Helsinki University, Helsinki, Finland

Allan A. Vaag
Department of Clinical Sciences, Clinical Research Centre, Lund University, Malmö, Sweden
Department of Endocrinology (Diabetes and Metabolism), Rigshospitalet, Copenhagen, Denmark
Cardiovascular and Metabolic Disease (CVMD) Translational Medicine Unit, Early Clinical Development, IMED Biotech Unit, AstraZeneca, Gothenburg, Sweden

Charlotte Brøns
Department of Endocrinology (Diabetes and Metabolism), Rigshospitalet, Copenhagen, Denmark

Anne Brandes Aitken, Vishnu Prakas Nair, Gilberto da Gente and Molly Rae Gerdes
Department of Neurology, University of California, San Francisco, 675 Nelson Rising Lane, San Francisco, CA 9415, USA

Elysa Jill Marco
Department of Neurology, University of California, San Francisco, 675 Nelson Rising Lane, San Francisco, CA 9415, USA
Department of Psychiatry, University of California, San Francisco, 401 Parnassus Ave, San Francisco, CA 94143, USA
Department of Pediatrics, University of California, San Francisco, 550 16th Street, San Francisco, CA 94143, USA

Elliott H. Sherr
Department of Neurology, University of California, San Francisco, 675 Nelson Rising Lane, San Francisco, CA 9415, USA
Department of Pediatrics, University of California, San Francisco, 550 16th Street, San Francisco, CA 94143, USA
Institute of Human Genetics, University of California, San Francisco, 513 Parnassus Avenue, S965, San Francisco, CA 94143-0794, USA

Sean Thomas
Department of Biostatistics and Epidemiology, University of California, San Francisco, 550 16th Street, 2nd Floor, San Francisco, CA 94158-2549, USA

Leyla Bologlu
San Francisco, CA, USA

Pengfei Xu, Jian Yang, Junhui Liu, Xue Yang, Jianming Liao, Fanen Yuan, Yang Xu, Baohui Liu and Qianxue Chen
Department of Neurosurgery, Renmin Hospital of Wuhan University, 9 Zhangzhidong Road and 238 Jiefang Road, Wuchang, Wuhan, Hubei 430060, People's Republic of China

Alessandra Vidotto, Giovana M. Polachini and Tiago Henrique
Departamento de Biologia Molecular, Faculdade de Medicina (FAMERP), Av. Brigadeiro Faria Lima, 5416, Vila São Pedro, São José do Rio Preto, SP CEP 15090-000, Brazil

Eloiza H. Tajara
Departamento de Biologia Molecular, Faculdade de Medicina (FAMERP), Av. Brigadeiro Faria Lima, 5416, Vila São Pedro, São José do Rio Preto, SP CEP 15090-000, Brazil

Departamento de Genética e Biologia Evolutiva, Instituto de Biociências, Universidade de São Paulo, R. do Matão, 321, São Paulo, SP CEP 05508-090, Brazil

Marina de Paula-Silva and Sonia M. Oliani
Departamento de Biologia, Instituto de Biociências, Letras e Ciências Exatas (IBILCE), Universidade Estadual Paulista (UNESP), R. Cristóvão Colombo, 2265, São José do Rio Preto, SP CEP 15054-000, Brazil

Rossana V. M. López
Instituto do Câncer de São Paulo Octavio Frias de Oliveira – ICESP, Av. Dr. Arnaldo, 251 -Cerqueira César, São Paulo, SP CEP 01246-000, Brazil

Patrícia M. Cury
Faculdade Ceres (Faceres), Av. Anísio Haddad, 6751, São José do Rio Preto, SP CEP 15090-305, Brazil

Fabio D. Nunes
Departamento de Estomatologia, Faculdade de Odontologia, Universidade de São Paulo, Av. Prof. Lineu Prestes, 2227, São Paulo, SP CEP 05508-000, Brazil

José F. Góis-Filho
Instituto do Câncer Arnaldo Vieira de Carvalho, R. Dr Cesário Mota Jr, 112, São Paulo, SP CEP 01221-020, Brazil

Marcos B. de Carvalho
Departamento de Cirurgia de Cabeça e Pescoço, Hospital Heliópolis, R. Cônego Xavier, 276, São Paulo, SP CEP 04231-030, Brazil

Andréia M. Leopoldino
Departamento de Análises Clínicas, Toxicológicas e Bromatológicas, Faculdade de Ciências Farmacêuticas, Universidade de São Paulo, Avenida do Café, s/n, Ribeirão Preto, SP CEP 14040-903, Brazil

Yanjie Fan, Lili Wang, Yu Wang, Zhuwen Gong, Wenjuan Qiu, Huiwen Zhang, Xing Ji, Jun Ye, Lianshu Han, Bing Xiao, Lili Liang, Xia Zhang, Xiaomin Liu and Xuefan Gu
Department of Pediatric Endocrinology/Genetics, Xinhua Hospital affiliated to Shanghai Jiao Tong University School of Medicine, Shanghai Institute for Pediatric Research, 1665 Kongjiang Road, Shanghai 200092, China

Yanming Wu
Department of Pediatric Endocrinology/Genetics, Xinhua Hospital affiliated to Shanghai Jiao Tong University School of Medicine, Shanghai Institute for Pediatric Research, 1665 Kongjiang Road, Shanghai 200092, China
Department of Pediatrics, People's Hospital of Shanghai Pudong New District, 490 South Chuanhuan Road, Shanghai 201200, China

Yongguo Yu
Department of Pediatric Endocrinology/Genetics, Xinhua Hospital affiliated to Shanghai Jiao Tong University School of Medicine, Shanghai Institute for Pediatric Research, 1665 Kongjiang Road, Shanghai 200092, China
Department of Endocrinology, Shanghai Children's Medical Center, Shanghai Jiao Tong University School of Medicine, 1678 Dongfang Road, Shanghai 200127, China

Jingmin Wang
Department of Pediatrics, Peking University First Hospital, 8 Xishiku Dajie Xicheng District, Beijing 100034, China

Xingming Jin
Department of Developmental and Behavioral Pediatrics, Shanghai Children's Medical Center, Shanghai Jiao Tong University School of Medicine, 1678 Dongfang Road, Shanghai 200127, China

Fei Li
Department of Developmental and Behavioral Pediatrics, Shanghai Children's Medical Center, Shanghai Jiao Tong University School of Medicine, 1678 Dongfang Road, Shanghai 200127, China
MOE-Shanghai Key Laboratory of Children's Environmental Health, Xinhua Hospital affiliated to Shanghai Jiao Tong University School of Medicine, 1665 Kongjiang Rd, Shanghai 200092, China

Yongnian Shen
Department of Endocrinology, Shanghai Children's Medical Center, Shanghai Jiao Tong University School of Medicine, 1678 Dongfang Road, Shanghai 200127, China

So Yeon Kim, Tae Rim Kim and Kyung-Ah Sohn
Department of Computer Engineering, Ajou University, Suwon 16499, South Korea

Hyun-Hwan Jeong
Department of Molecular and Human Genetics, Baylor College of Medicine, Houston, TX 77030, USA
Jan and Dan Duncan Neurological Research Institute, Texas Children's Hospital, Houston, TX 77030, USA

Yan Gong, Caitrin W. McDonough, Mohamed H. Shahin and Taimour Y. Langaee
Center for Pharmacogenomics, Department of Pharmacotherapy and Translational Research, College of Pharmacy, University of Florida, Gainesville, FL 32610-0486, USA

Ana Caroline C. Sá
Center for Pharmacogenomics, Department of Pharmacotherapy and Translational Research, College of Pharmacy, University of Florida, Gainesville, FL 32610-0486, USA

Graduate Program in Genetics and Genomics, University of Florida, Gainesville, FL, USA

Rhonda M. Cooper-DeHoff
Center for Pharmacogenomics, Department of Pharmacotherapy and Translational Research, College of Pharmacy, University of Florida, Gainesville, FL 32610-0486, USA
Department of Medicine, Division of Cardiovascular Medicine, University of Florida, Gainesville, FL, USA

Julie A. Johnson
Center for Pharmacogenomics, Department of Pharmacotherapy and Translational Research, College of Pharmacy, University of Florida, Gainesville, FL 32610-0486, USA
Graduate Program in Genetics and Genomics, University of Florida, Gainesville, FL, USA
Department of Medicine, Division of Cardiovascular Medicine, University of Florida, Gainesville, FL, USA

Amy Webb
Department of Biomedical Informatics, College of Medicine, The Ohio State University, Columbus, OH, USA

Somnath Datta
Department of Biostatistics, University of Florida, Gainesville, FL, USA

Stephen T. Turner
Division of Nephrology and Hypertension, Mayo Clinic, Rochester, MN, USA

Amber L. Beitelshees
Division of Endocrinology, Diabetes and Nutrition, University of Maryland, Baltimore, MD, USA

Arlene B. Chapman
Department of Medicine, University of Chicago, Chicago, IL, USA

Eric Boerwinkle
Division of Epidemiology, University of Texas at Houston, Houston, TX, USA

John G. Gums
Department of Pharmacotherapy and Translational Research, College of Pharmacy, University of Florida, Gainesville, USA
Department of Community Health and Family Medicine, College of Medicine, University of Florida, Gainesville, FL, USA

Steven E. Scherer
Human Genome Sequencing Center, Baylor College of Medicine, Houston, TX, USA

Wolfgang Sadee
Department of Cancer Biology and Genetic, College of Medicine, Center for Pharmacogenomics, Ohio State University, Columbus, OH, USA

Bo Xu, Changlong Li, Hang Zhuang, Jiali Wang, Qingfeng Wang, Chao Wang and Xuehai Zhou
School of Computer Science and Technology, University of Science and Technology of China, Hefei 230027, China

Matthew Yen, John A. Cooper and Michael D. Onken
Department of Biochemistry and Molecular Biophysics, Washington University School of Medicine, 660 S. Euclid Ave., St. Louis, MO 63110, USA

Zongtai Qi, Xuhua Chen and Robi D. Mitra
Department of Genetics and Center for Genome Sciences and Systems Biology, Washington University School of Medicine, 660 S. Euclid Ave., St. Louis, MO 63110, USA

Huey Yi Chong
School of Pharmacy, Monash University Malaysia, Subang Jaya, Selangor, Malaysia

Nathorn Chaiyakunapruk
School of Pharmacy, Monash University Malaysia, Subang Jaya, Selangor, Malaysia

Center of Pharmaceutical Outcomes Research (CPOR), Department of Pharmacy Practice, Faculty of Pharmaceutical Sciences, Naresuan University, Phitsanulok, Thailand
School of Pharmacy, University of Wisconsin, Madison, USA
Asian Centre for Evidence Synthesis in Population, Implementation and Clinical Outcomes (PICO), Global Asia in the 21st Century (GA21) Platform, Monash University Malaysia, Subang Jaya, Malaysia

Pascale A. Allotey
United Nations University International Institute for Global Health, Kuala Lumpur, Malaysia

Qiong Xu, Chun-yang Li, Yi Wang, Hui-ping Li, Bing-bing Wu and Xiu Xu
Developmental and Behavioral Pediatric Department and Child Health Care Department, Children's Hospital of Fudan University, 399 Wanyuan Road, Shanghai 201102, China

Yong-hui Jiang
Department of Pediatrics, Duke University School of Medicine, Durham, NC 27710, USA
Department of Neurobiology, Duke University School of Medicine, Durham, NC 27710, USA
Program in Genetics and Genomics, Duke University School of Medicine, Durham, NC 27710, USA
Cellular Molecular Biology, Duke University School of Medicine, Durham, NC 27710, USA

Index